Psychological Processes of Childbearing

Joan Raphael-Leff
Psychoanalyst and Social Psychologist

D1323735

2009
NEW EDITION
with 125 page UPDATE SECTION

Introduction by **Professor Colwyn Trevarthen**
Foreword by **Professor Marshall Klaus**

The Anna Freud Centre

FOURTH EDITION 2005

First published by Chapman & Hall, 1991
Reprinted 1992, 1993, 1994,
Revised edition 1996, Taylor & Francis
Revised edition 2001 University of Essex

© 1991 Joan Raphael-Leff

ISBN 978-0-9549319-0-2

Printed and bound in Great Britain by
Biddles Ltd., King's Lynn, Norfolk

A catalogue record for this book is available from the British Library
Library of Congress Cataloguing-in-Publication Data available

Published by The Anna Freud Centre

Contents

Part Seven **Complications**

1006084152

Introduction

Childbearing is where the ambitions of human biology and the benefits and constraints of human society meet, where cultural belief about birth and maternity are tested against the facts of life. Science has, so far, made a poor job of understanding how a foetus and its brain, nourished within a mother's responsive body, connected directly to her visceral turbulence, can be born with the mind of a conscious infant, sensitive to the scent and touch of her woman's body, suckling skilfully while holding her hand and gazing at her eyes, knowing her voice, able to engage the expressions of her face, her talk and her gestures, sharing her joy and her depression intimately. Only in recent years has this unique attachment of two intending and aware beings, one ignorant of theories, reasons and language and dependent on the body of the other for support, protection, nourishment and responsive sympathy (<u>not</u> empathy!), the other transformed in her feelings, pride and physiology to give needed and attentions and to share the happiness of play, been given the respectful observation it deserves. The complexity of their innate impulses of intersubjectivity, of Dan Stern's 'attunement', on both sides has surprised medical and psychological researchers who had assumed the baby could feel no pain and had no self-awareness, or capacity for imitative and inviting engagement with a rational adult. Most surprising discoveries have come from brain science. The potent influence of emotions in the making of the neural systems of reason, perception and memory for significant experiences has been proven. Thanks to Jaak Panksepp, Alan Schore and others we see that the affective brain and its capacity for sympathetic attachment takes control in the wedding of mature adult and questing infant. We know the attentive infant's whole brain resonates with images not only of the mother's appearance and movements, but with the quality of motives that generate them. This gives natural sense to the rationalisations and verbalisations of psychoanalysis, vindicating Freud's early hope for a neuroscience of human impulses. And yet, the most important matters remain the real life benefits and hardships of a new mother's partnership with the father, her family, the community she lives in and the state that governs services that affect her.

Joan Raphael-Leff set herself the formidable task of reviewing the trials and tribulations of people bearing children, worldwide. Her book, full of information perceptively and sensitively interpreted against a background of clinical experience has been a success. This new edition swells the data impressively, tackling the dramatic changes of the past decade, of HIV-AIDS in South Africa, of single parenthood, of mothers who escape loneliness with drugs or alcohol, or who deal with a father's insecurity or violence, or enforced loss of homeland. This is a unique reservoir of factual information and psychodynamic wisdom. Professor Raphael-Leff has created original practical tools for observing the different ways parents meet the presence of a young child with companionship in joy, with distant incomprehension, or with fear and even anger. It offers advice to all those who wish to give therapeutic aid, or simply wish to understand better how being human comes about.

Colwyn Trevarthen, Edinburgh, 23 November, 2004

Selected Reading:

Corrigall, J. and H. Wilkinson, H. (2003). (Eds.) Revolutionary Connections: Psychotherapy and Neuroscience. London/New York: Karnak.

Gomes-Pedro, J., Nugent, K., Young, G. and Brazelton, B., (2002). (Eds.) The Infant and Family in the Twenty-First Century New York/Hove, UK: Brunner-Routledge.

Schore, A. N. (2003). Affect Dysregulation and Disorders of the Self. New York: Norton.

Stern, D. N. (2000) The Interpersonal World of the Infant: A View from Psychoanalysis and Development Psychology. (Second Edition) Basic Books, New York.

Trevarthen, C. (2005) Stepping away from the mirror: Pride and shame in adventures of companionship Reflections on the nature and emotional needs of infant intersubjectivity. In, C.S. Carter, L. Ahnert et al., eds. Attachment and Bonding: A New Synthesis. Dahlem Workshop Report 92. Cambridge, MA: The MIT Press.

Colwyn Trevarthen, 2004
Professor (Emeritus) of Child Psychology & Psychobiology
Department of Psychology, University of Edinburgh

Chapter 0:

Psychosocial Process of Childbearing Revisited

OVERVIEW:

Childbearing seems eternal, primordial and universal. Yet over the last decades human reproduction is in a state of flux. This book highlights changes that have occurred over the years. Updating it is a challenge, as there have been crucial developments in several relevant fields. These include:

On a global level, increased precariousness, with marked climate changes, widespread terrorism, massive migration, rapid urbanisation, economic instability, and the rapid spread of HIV infection now estimated at 56 million people worldwide. (The latter has crucial implications for maternity and neonatal care as many women, especially in sub-Saharan Africa, learn of their positive status when tested in pregnancy).

On a physiological level knowledge of the human body has changed dramatically with the 2003 completion of the Human Genome Programme which defines the boundaries of heritability, and the complex dialectic between genes and environment. Assisted Reproductive Technology has burgeoned, transforming modes of conception, evolutionary natural selection and patterns of family formation to include childbearing of genetically unrelated offspring. Evolution of the functional MRI has brought major leaps in brain research, revealing the <u>interpersonal</u> nature of brain growth, thereby affecting the ways we think about development in babies.

Finally, *on the psychosocial level,* 21st century life's increasing complexity and instability are accompanied by new challenges to mental health in child-bearing and rearing, with ramifications for maternity and child care policies. There is a growing recognition of the diversity of women's needs, which is the foundation of this book. I argue that each woman's expectations and desires are rooted in both her internal and her external realities, and vary with age, parity, interval between pregnancies, relationship to her own mother, degree of emotional support in her immediate environment, restrictions in her socioeconomic situation and cultural expectations and previous experience of parenting - all of which determine her current orientation towards pregnancy, motherhood and this baby.

The central theme of this book is *interconnectedness*. Even when alone others are embedded in our minds, and every aspect of our lives is interwoven. This updating section reflects such dynamic reciprocation by addressing four inter-related topics:

1. Maternity care services [see section O.2 below]:

Increasingly over the past years, the emphasis has returned to woman-led midwifery provisions - antenatally, during labour and birth, and in establishing lactation.   In the UK, beginning with the 1993 'changing childbirth' report, government policies are now in keeping with the foundational message of this book - *greater awareness of psychological issues and availability of choices* - to cater to personal preferences, special needs and diversity of expectations. Midwives and consumers concur on the importance of midwifery competence, but also stress building a relationship through communication, mutual respect and compassion throughout pregnancy and birthing. However, studies reveal failings in both *continuity* of maternity care and *quality*. Nursing shortages continue with lack of uniformity in antenatal provisions, closure of smaller maternity units and birth centres and a rising rate of caesarean sections. Few specialist mother and baby units exist for women suffering severe mental health problems after the birth and inequalities of access still affect women with disabilities or language problems. This is somewhat remedied by programmes such as Sure Start, encouraging families in disadvantaged areas to access ante-natal and baby clinics, and specialist services exist for children with Special Educational Needs. But lack of data on the socio-economic and ethnic status of pregnant women and mothers impedes maternity service planners and providers in assessing equity of services. A Mental Health National Service Frame-work [NSF September 15th 2004] advocates multidisciplinary collaboration to safeguard mental health through provisions geared to children, young people and maternity.

2. Perinatal disturbance [see section O.3 below]:

Almost half the population of western new mothers experience mild depression, with over one in ten suffering severe disturbance over the first postnatal year. Perinatal psychiatric disorder is the leading cause of parental morbidity, and suicide is the leading cause of maternal mortality in the UK, and probably northern Europe. Fathers are not exempt. Emotional distress during the childbearing period is associated with deteriorating family relationships and long-term adverse consequences for the baby. As evidence accumulates of the link between parental disturbance and emotional social and cognitive difficulties in the offspring, government policy makers hope to combat this damaging intergenerational transmission of distress.

However, while developmental psychology demonstrates the effects of parental mental states on their baby's cognitive and psychosocial development, this book draws attention to current social arrangements which exacerbate the emotional upheaval antenatally, and the little acknowledged postnatal impact of the infant on the parent. I suggest that intense arousal resonates with procedural 'autobiographical' memories relating to the parent's own infancy, which have not been processed due to changes in family structure. These emotional memories are reactivated both by disturbing exposure to the baby's inchoate feelings and through unmediated contact with evocative primary substances (urine, feces, milk…). Some new parents find the primal intimacy overwhelming, and unable to protect themselves from such *'contagious arousal'*, succumb to postnatal disturbance – a spectrum of depressive, persecutory, obsessional or anxious reactions. Mechanisms range from anxious overinvolvement and identificatory fusion/confusion with the idealised infant to projection and/or detachment (phobias, paranoia or extreme withdrawal) from denigrated or feared attributes of the infant associated with repudiated aspects of the carer's imagined baby-self).

Recognition of such processes necessitates *changes in training midwives and health visitors* to increase their understanding of perinatal psychological disturbances, and to promote supportive maternity care and prompt referral of troubled women for therapeutic help, ideally during pregnancy.

3. Infant mental health issues [see section O.4 below]:
1990-2000 was 'decade of the brain' and in recent years infant mental health issues have gained recognition due to dissemination of findings about the competence and sensitivity of babies, in the womb and after birth. *The hallmark of this decade is rediscovery of the interactive nature of our innermost beings – and the long-lasting reciprocal influences that make us who we are.* Neonatal research demonstrates how innate capacities for sociability, self-regulation, thought and language can only

be activated through intensely emotional interactions with others. The infant's range of arousal, his/her stress responses and biochemical patterns come to reflect parental handling. Neuroscience reveals influences of caregiver's behaviour not only on the patterns of growth but the very structure of the baby's brain. Geneticists illustrate ways in which genetic endowment is instigated, modified or inhibited by the specific emotional-social environment of the child's life. Similarly, within the family system, interactions between parent/s and child/ren are never isolated occurrences, but part of an intricate familial give-and-take, a constantly adapting and changing kaleidoscopic feedback loop.

These realisations have implications for safeguarding healthy family interaction and helping parents and their children when this is derailed. In the wake of the 1989 UK Children Act, changes in practice ensure primacy of child welfare and rights, with *guidelines to prevent, detect and treat emotional, sexual and physical abuse.* The 2004 Children's NSF is similarly committed to sustained improvement in children's mental health through integrated health and social care from gestation to adulthood, and early interventions.

4. Facilitator-Reciprocator-Regulator model [see section O.5 below]:
The framework of this book delineates three basic orientations towards parenting, revealed in different practices that reflect underpinning beliefs and unconscious representations.

- *Facilitators* who relish pregnancy and natural childbirth, and postnatally, adapt devotedly to the baby to gratify his/her perceived needs.
- *Regulators* who strive to control the discomforts of pregnancy, want a 'civilised' birth and aim to regulate the baby so s/he learns to be socialised.
- *Reciprocators*, who can tolerate ambiguity and uncertainty, and neither adapt nor promote adaptation but negotiate each incident as it arises, both in pregnancy and labour, and postnatally.
- Pathological reactions are found at the extremes and in a fourth *conflicted group*, whose internal confusion and inconsistency spills over into the family.

Over the past 15 years, independent researchers have replicated my model with interesting results from large scale and longitudinal research in England and elsewhere. The model is extended to elucidate some of the unconscious representations and anxieties underpinning attachment styles, and prospective research has validated my predictors of postnatal depression. Rather than treating 'women' as a single category, questionnaires enable differentiation between groups with diverse expectations, needs and symptomatic disturbance (depressive, persecutory, obsessional, anxious reactions).

Research papers in the first three areas run into scores of thousands – so this updating section cites only a fraction, but hopefully representative sample of recent studies, predominantly British but also around the world. As always, findings from other locations must be read in context, questioning whether and how these apply to our own increasingly multicultural and complex (and in some ways, 'de-developing') society. I have a dual motivation in providing this mixture of findings: with all the faults of the National Health Service, in the UK we may need reminding of our own highly privileged access to services still unavailable in many other developed, as well as developing, societies. Conversely, worrying trends and research findings from other places highlight gaps and offer a means to re-evaluate and hopefully improve our own provisions. I begin by sketching the background to these issues. [Numbers in brackets refer to references which, unlike the rest of the book, appear at the end of this chapter].

0.1. SOCIO-CULTURAL BACKDROP

0.1.1. New parameters of Childbearing:

Babies are the potential of any society. Their health status predicts the quality of the future. Paradoxically, their needs have changed very little over the millennia. *In societies in transition, this puts babies at risk of being at odds with their parents' rapidly changing lives.* Today half the world's population live in towns and in the more developed regions, Latin America and the Caribbean, this rural to urban shift involves 75% of the inhabitants and is projected to rise still further[1]. Rapid urbanisation has altered family patterns. Geographical mobility and trans-border migration dislocate communities, disconnecting generations and disrupting support networks. Adults tend to develop passionate (often, serial) sexual relations, and/or emotionally intense parent-child twosomes With dispersal of extended families the family unit becomes a small nuclear unit, often composed of a lone parent and child/ren.

The way western societies are age-stratified means that many adults have had little exposure to young children before becoming parents. This leaves them unprepared for the emotional impact of a baby on their lives, especially one for whom they are totally responsible. *I argue that growing up in smaller families reduces opportunities for us to emotionally work through infantile issues triggered by babies (siblings, cousins, etc) in the presence of containing adults, before becoming a parent oneself - thus raising the likelihood of perinatal disturbance* [2].

Ninety percent of infants are born in developing or low-income countries. Yet, as safer childbirth and lower child mortality diminish the need to have lots of children to ensure that some will survive, in many societies family size is decreasing. This is largely due to government policies and/or changing social attitudes, with safer abortion and efficient contraception. *Worldwide, women are having fewer babies than their mothers did.* Compared to the late 1980's, in societies where traditionally women had many offspring, now significantly more mothers of two children are saying they want no more − 60% of women in Bangladesh and Egypt; 38% in Guatemala, 33% of Kenyan women and 29% in Zimbabwe [3]. Similarly, in places as diverse as Brazil, Tunisia, Indonesia and Iran, women who had six or seven siblings now only have two children [4]. However, paradoxically, although the number of babies per woman has declined, millions are still added to the world's population annually as the number of women in their childbearing years has <u>increased</u> in most societies, due to high fertility in their mothers' and grandmothers' generations, and greater longevity of this generation. [UN predictions based on 'medium level' expectations state that fertility rates will decline significantly to two children per woman, even in developing nations, thereby stabilising at around 9 billion in three centuries].

However, one important effect of smaller families and scattering of extended families is to increase mutual-reliance within the isolated family and the intensity of interdependent relations in the small unit.

China, India and the United States are the three most populous countries and Africa has faster population growth, higher fertility and sadly, higher mortality than other parts of the world. Although there are still tracts of Africa and the Middle East where women will have three or more babies (and 6 or 7 in Somalia, Niger, Yemen and Uganda), in 2000-2005 in places as diverse as Hong Kong, Singapore, Korea (North and South) and Armenia to central Europe and even Catholic Spain and Italy *the average number of children per woman is just ONE* (or none)! [5]. Even in South Africa, there has been a dramatic fall from 5.75 live births per woman in 1970 to only 2.77 in 2004 − though this is not only due to socio-economic changes, but rural to urban migration and sadly, AIDS [6]. Overall, the patterns of westernised reproduction are shifting to concentrated, later or even negated reproduction. 12-20% of women are estimated to be childless-by-choice across Europe and birth rates have declined substantially, in some places to fewer than one baby per woman (Latvia has 7.8 births per 1,000 population; Bulgaria 8.6; Russia 9.02 and Greece 9.82). With the lowest birth rate of any region in world history Europe is now also the only region where the death rate exceeds the birth rate.

In western countries educational parity and career prospects delay childbearing, inevitably limiting reproduction. According to the Office for National Statistics in England and Wales birth rates have dropped to a record low of 1.64 births per woman of child-bearing age (this, despite a massive rise in the number of multiple births over the last ten years). Many women postpone starting a family until their thirties or later (the average UK age at maternity was 30.6 years in 2003, and this calculation includes teen age births!).   To counterbalance this, an industry of reproductive technology assists waning fertility in older women, and in turn produces new patterns of family formation – new kinship categories, such as surrogates, adopted embryos, lone-by-choice mothers, same-sexed parents, and post-menopausal parturients. With longer life expectancy, fertility treatments (and soon, egg-freezing) extend the upper range and versatility of prime adulthood, which is no longer dedicated to childbearing and rearing. However, despite technological solutions, infertility triggers emotional distress; increasingly bizarre treatments create painful tensions and raise false hopes (only about 15% of couples undergoing fertility treatment do achieve a 'take-home baby'), and despite the joy they sometimes bring, successful interventions are also accompanied by unprecedented anxieties, doubts and ethical dilemmas while the child is growing up. In addition, this trend towards postponed parenthood and decreasing fecundity increases the likelihood of only-children (or multiple births - twins, triplets or more), and newborns arriving during the turmoil of their parents' mid-life crises.

Conversely, the lower end of parenthood expands with ever younger mothers. In the UK one in ten babies is born to a teenage mother and infant mortality in this group is twice the average. Social circumstances, eating habits and access to services vary within subgroups and geographically. Low birth-weight, the primary cause of neonatal morbidity and mortality, is a common marker of maternal and child health. According to the WHO, Britain now has the highest western European rate of babies born below normal birth weight (5.5lb). Throughout the world, despite birth-control there are still many unwanted juvenile pregnancies attributed to earlier sexual activity, ignorance and/or casualness with contraception, and in impoverished communities also due to child-prostitution or child-rape associated with a range of emotional, health and socio-economic problems.

0.1.2 Teenage pregnancies:

Over the last few decades, the western age of menarche has dropped with improved nutrition. We demarcate adolescence as a prolonged transitional period of maturation and learning how to operate in our complex society. Yet, due to various factors including more relaxed social mores and disillusionment with contraception, in 1997 Britain was found to have the highest rate in western Europe for adolescent mothers - triple that of France and Sweden, quadruple that of Italy, six times that of the Netherlands and ten times that of Switzerland! [7]. Sex-education campaigns have been effective and between 1998 and 2001 teenage conceptions in England fell by 9%. Despite a slight rise in 2002 among 14, 15 and 16 year-olds, statistics were still lower than those for 1992, an improvement seemingly related to reaffirmed confidence in the pill (after the 1996 scare). Nonetheless, the number of babies conceived by teenagers in the UK is still very high (90,000 in 2003), and varies geographically - women in poor inner-city areas are six times more likely to become pregnant before age 20 than their counterparts in wealthier areas [8a]. Although half of adolescent pregnancies end in abortion, those who keep the pregnancy now choose to raise their babies (but are less likely to breastfeed). Many are excellent mothers but young parenthood is associated with particular emotional and economic hardships (see Chapter 27). The government aims to halve the teenage birth-rate by 2010 as part of a drive to reduce health inequalities, and to prevent child poverty and social exclusion. Among other proposals, a national media campaign to foster personal responsibility, offering advice and contraception for young people; Sex and Relationship Education (SRE) and Personal, Social and Health Education (PSHE) in schools, along with training teacher and involving parents in prevention of teenage pregnancies. In addition, support for young parents includes hostels and subsidised housing, providing job-training, benefits for co-habiting fathers, and healthcare and crèche facilities are being evaluated, especially for parents under 16 years old [8b]. The Independent Advisory Group for Sexual Health recommended free condoms, 90% of abortions funded by the NHS, and early detection and treatment of sexually transmitted infections [8c]. RESPECT, a recent campaign to end poverty and prejudice faced by young mums, has published a charter calling for extension of Sure Start, improvements in education, income and affordable, flexible childcare, and support services, including specialised midwives [8d].

In the USA, since teenage pregnancies peaked in 1991 these have fallen overall by 31% in the 15-19 group (and 42% among black women!), possibly related to campaigns for celibacy, delayed sexual activity and use of contraception. Nonetheless, with over 40% of adolescents becoming pregnant before age 20, *the US still has the highest rate of teen pregnancy and births in the western industrialised world*, twice as high as England, France and Canada. Eight of each ten of these US teen-pregnancies are unintended, and as only a third of these girls finish high school, many live in poverty and nearly 80% of them end up on welfare [9] thereby extending the cycle of deprivation, which is found to affect their sons and daughters in turn.

0.1.3. Gender inequality, parental grants and social 'revolution':

Despite our expectations for the improved quality of life depicted by the media depictions and feminist driven socio-political demands, women in the 21st century still suffer inequalities. This is reflected in basic education worldwide (even where it does accept girls, not only do pregnant ones drop out, but pre-teens are expected to miss school to do housework, help with child care or fetch water). Even in the privileged West, there are still disproportionately few female tertiary students. *Employment is still subject to sex discrimination. Earning differential and, segregated work conditions are commonplace, and downward post-maternal occupational mobility affects professionals too.* In the west, women earn 75% of what men do for comparable work, and gender interacts with other axes of social disadvantage such as race and class. In egalitarian Europe equity for parents remains a myth, with mothers striving to fulfil often conflicting domestic and work roles, both in traditional (largely Catholic) south-east European countries (where the fertility rate has now dropped below 1.7 births per woman), and in the more generously state-endowed north-western European countries. Despite growing appreciation of the importance of fathers, outside of Scandinavia paternity leave is meagre or non-existent. Similarly, despite awareness of the needs of young children, maternity leave is short, child-care remains problematic, and in Britain is the most expensive in Europe!

Clearly, the way welfare issues are addressed at governmental level determines the mode and quality of life for families. *The wealthiest 20% of the world's population consume 80% of resources.* Always in the vanguard, during the last decade of the century the Nordic countries decided to <u>decentralise</u> provisions to safeguard equity and welfare. The very human definition of 'welfare' is 'individual resources to direct the conditions of one's life' [10] - in other words, the means to maintain *a sense of agency or self-determination*. The Nordic changes were introduced as a response to the regional macro-economic crisis, with local recessions, deteriorating work and living condition for the lower income section of the population (usually single mothers and immigrants), and recognition that these increase poor health and raise anxiety, with special risks to babies and children. Sweden and Finland in particular, recognised that relative income poverty had spread with growing socio-economic inequalities despite strategies of even-handedness [11]. Denmark, too, addressed issues of social protection for weaker groups by extending the scope of services for children in the 1990's, improving full-time jobs for mothers and investing in equality-promoting policies of childcare and education [12].

0.1.3.1. Parental leave:

In Iceland, policies to combat the extensive rise in gender and economic inequality included income-tested child benefits and increased expenditure on healthcare. *Fathers' leave* increased from two weeks in 1997 to nine months parental leave [three months for each parent and the remaining three to be utilised by either, with fathers receiving 80% of their regular pay] [13]. Sweden entitled fathers to at least two months parental leave out of the 18 months allocated to both parents [14]. Over the 1990's Norway too, shifted from a policy of universalism aimed to diminish inequality to one of specifically improving welfare for the poorest. Relying on its oil economy to ensure generous benefits, Norway also extended its parental leave period from 28 to 42 weeks at 100% wage compensation, with fathers having a <u>minimum</u> of four weeks spread over the first year [15]. Compare this the recent (2004) British fathers' boost of two weeks to be taken within the first two months! And contrast the Nordic early parental leave policies with figures for maternity leave and pay in the rest of Europe: UK - 6 weeks at 90% of pay, then 20 weeks statutory maternity pay at £102.80 (with up to another 26 weeks unpaid leave); Austria - 16 weeks at 100%; Portugal – 13 weeks at 100%; France - 16-26 weeks at 84% pay; Ireland - 14 weeks at 70%; Switzerland - 8 weeks at 100% [16a]. A hidden drawback remains: as long as sex-based inequalities of pay persist with a payment ceiling for paternity leave, the choice of who takes leave is predetermined among higher earning men, as it makes economic sense for fathers to go back to work. (British fathers on average earn two-thirds of family incomes and work the longest hours in the European Union – 48 hours a week [16b]). *Furthermore, as the stay-home primary carer's total responsibility for the developing infant increases, with intimate knowledge of needs and wants, the working parent becomes further distanced as secondary and less familiar caregiver.* Nevertheless, in the UK 36% of fathers are the main carers while mothers are working, and many are involved in primary care on weekends.

However, it is not an all or nothing situation. Among working parents in Britain, a recent survey revealed a hidden social revolution taking place in public attitudes towards balancing work and parenting, with 61% saying that parents of young children spend too long at work. Since 2003 the younger workforce has been trying to change the balance of their responsibilities by taking advantage of the Government's 'family friendly' package which gives employees the right to request flexible working hours, to enable them to spend more 'prime' time at home. However, there is a need for further reform of early care, and 66% of all those polled expressed a desire to see families being given a Scandinavian style choice of mothers or fathers sharing parental leave, and 53% want more than the 'mean' current two-week paternity leave to enable fathers to have a chance to take a greater role in caring for babies and bringing up their young children [17a]. Once again, we may think in terms of the three basic orientations towards mothering, differing in behavioural practices that reflect underpinning beliefs and unconscious representations. The *'Facilitator'* mother who believes that pregnancy primes her for a unique and exclusive connection to her baby; the *'Regulator'* who sees mothering as one role among many and the *'Reciprocator'* who negotiates issues as these arise, rather than acting on set beliefs. Clearly, the pressure to return to work too soon affects Facilitators who wish to be sole provider for the baby. Craving adult company and application of their work skills, other mothers (namely Regulators) might be ready to go back well before the maternity leave is up. While Reciprocators may seek a combination. One neat (and cheap) solution that combats both social isolation and second-rate childcare is a PACT [Parent and Children Together] baby and toddler playgroup facility in which Facilitator mums stay with their own baby and in addition, take personal responsibility for the baby of a working Regulator.

However, sadly, for most mothers, decisions are determined not by desires but financial needs, as a family drops abruptly from two incomes to one at the very point of their biggest expenditure. In competitive professions, career women feel pressured to return to work for fear of losing out. Conversely, with high unemployment, some of those wishing to work may have no job to go back to. And for working mothers living in large cities, breastfeeding remains a problematic issue as long as work places do not provide on-site crèche facilities (see 0.2.9 below).

Once again, it is a matter of implementing policies which provide multiple choices to suit the needs of differing families. Yet far from providing such flexibility of choice, in Britain the current Government has veered from one extreme to another – providing financial incentives to encourage all mothers to go back to work, penalising stay-at-home Mums. Then, conversely, as awareness of the birth-rate falling below the critical replacement level created panic at the looming crisis of an ageing population. The projected soaring number of pensionless older citizens and shrinking work-force in 2050 induced the Trade & Industry Secretary to actually appeal in late 2004 to women's sense of 'national duty' to have more babies so 'crucial for the economic and social success of the country', pledging new family friendly policies [17b]. *This blurring of private and public zones, illustrates the dawning recognition that while reproduction is essential for species and state – for the individual woman, it is now an option.*

0.1.3.2 Mental Health of children and adolescents in Great Britain:

The one consistent precipitant of disturbance in children is parental disorder. As many people experiencing mental health problems go undetected or do not seek help, a series of nation wide surveys were undertaken to establish rates of psychiatric morbidity across Great Britain and England. These household surveys found that 1 in 6 (16%) of the population of adults have mental health problems and symptoms at any one point in time of which a higher proportion are women (in London 22.4% vs. 14%). Men have higher levels of generalised anxiety disorder and depressive episodes, personality disorders, drug and alcohol misuse and suicide, although women are at a higher risk for ongoing depression.

Rates of emotional disorders in children are directly associated with mental health problems in the parents, with a three-fold risk when mothers are disturbed, a two-fold risk in discordant or reconstituted families and in lone parent-families (whether single, widowed, divorced or separated). Apart from severe disorders, childhood disturbance manifests as 5% conduct disorders, 4% emotional disturbance (mainly anxiety and depression) and 1% hyperactivity, with a higher proportion of boys (11% vs.8%). Rates increase with stressful life events, poverty, geographical location (twice as many children have mental health problems in inner cities and 'striving' as opposed to 'expanding' or 'thriving' areas), linked to parental unemployment and low education [17c]. If this is so in the UK with its National Health Service and all its many resources, this is even more pertinent in le ss fortunate societies. As noted throughout this book, children are particularly vulnerable during *the early years of life* when the child's self is being constituted through interaction with caregivers [see section 0.4 below]. The detrimental effects of parental postnatal disturbance on the ir children's emotional, social and cognitive development often persist long after the carer's illness abates. It is crucial therefore to provide parents with resources to prevent disorder and opportunities to work through and resolve disturbance rather than inflicting this on their children.

0.1.4. Life Expectancy, infant mortality and relevant Epidemiological data:

0.1.4.1. Healthy life expectancy at birth has risen dramatically in the west over the past two decades but it varies between rich and poor, both within societies, and across the world - from just 25.9 years in Sierra Leone, and under 30 for many other sub-Saharan countries where it has dropped to medieval figures due to AIDS.

This new method of calculation developed by WHO [HALE or DALE] estimates the expected number of years a baby born today will live in full health, Years lost to disability are substantially higher in poorer countries (14% of life in blindness, paralysis or severe bouts of malaria) than the healthiest regions who lose some 9% to ill health. Healthy life expectancy in war devastated Afghanistan is a mere 33.8 years as opposed to 69.9 in the UK and 73.8 in low heart disease Japan (projected to fall as eating habits deteriorate). Preventable ill-health is still an issue - even Iceland and Norway (amongst the highest life expectancy in the world - 78.1 and 76.4 for men and 82.2 and 81.7 for women respectively) are still losing almost 6 and 9 years respectively on (largely alcohol related) conditions. In addition, an estimated 25% of preventable illnesses worldwide can be attributed to poor environmental quality!

The other top nations are France (73.1); Sweden (73.0); Spain (72.8); Italy (72.7); Greece and Swizerland (72.5). Australia is about to fall from 73.2 due to childhood obesity. USA came 24th, with 72.6 for females and 67.5 for males, largely due to poor minorities, homicides, HIV, obesity, drug and tobacco abuse. *As noted, within societies, health disparities can be marked, intrinsically related to income, education and access to health facilities.* The infant death rate among African Americans, American Indians and Alaska natives is twice that of whites – attributed to a complex interaction between environmental factors, genetic variations and specific health behaviours. Similarly, **gender disparities** exist within societies. In the early 1990s, the gap between female and male life expectancy was 2-3 years in richer countries, but by 1999, women live an average of 7-8 years longer (due to better diet and more exercise although recent increased smoking among women will soon translate into higher disability and earlier death). In the UK, the gender breakdown for current HALE figures is 69.1 for males and 7.2.1 for females with total life expectancy (LEX - uncorrected for years of illness and disability) at 75.8 for males and 80.5 for females born in 2004 (contrasted with 100 years ago when it was 45 and 49 respectively!). The greatest female/male discrepancy is Russia with 66.4 and 56.1 respectively due largely to male alcohol abuse with consequent accidents, violence and cardiovascular disease [18 a, b, c]. In general, differences in life expectancy have widened over the past decade between prosperous and deprived areas (counties and health districts) even within the same society.

0.1.4.2. Infant Mortality:
Medical care, especially targeted at weaker groups, with incentives to utilise antenatal care and early immunization initiatives are seen to pay off. In 1997, Sweden had the lowest recorded rate of infant mortality in history – 3.6 deaths per 1,000 live births. However, by the end of the millennium Iceland achieved an outstanding reduction in infant mortality to 1.2 per 1000 live births! (vs. 2.4-3.1 in the other Nordic countries). Deaths under a year result from extreme prematurity, birth defects and Sudden Infant Death Syndrome. The most recent UK figures put infant mortality rates at 5.5. But figures can be misleading as although similarly based on the number of deaths before the first birthday for every thousand live births, in Britain viability at birth is calculated from 24 weeks of gestation (and the USA at 20 weeks) – so figures may not be comparable to rates elsewhere which figure birth from 34 weeks gestation or later. Similarly, figures are biased as many societies do not register births of under 1,000 grams as opposed to highly industrialised societies with systems of intensive emergency intervention, who do register very low birth weight preterm babies, with an extremely high risk of dying.

A breakdown of UK infant mortality rates delineates: early neonatal deaths 2.7 (under one week); neonatal deaths 3.6 (per 1,000 babies under 4 weeks), post-neonatal deaths 1.8 (post 28 days but under a year) and 5.3 stillbirths per 1,000 births [19a]. Foetal and neonatal deaths are highly related to socioeconomic deprivation (whether measured by any of three population based indicators of material deprivation - Jarman index, Townsend score and percentage unemployed). One study showed that 30% of perinatal deaths were statistically attributable to social inequality [19b]. Similarly, regional differences in stillbirths and neonatal death rates can help to ascertain weak elements in quality of antenatal, delivery and neonatal clinical care, as studies in Wales and Sweden illustrate [19c,d].

Bearing these qualifications in mind, variations in infant mortality rates serve as a measure of *state health care policies and the socio-economic status of subgroups of a general population*. The USA, with 5% of the world's population consumes 40% of its natural resources. Nevertheless, this richest society in the world has a high infant mortality rate, and America's life expectancy at birth still ranks behind fifteen other nations, all of which spend proportionately far less on health care. In 2001 infant mortality rate reached an historic low of 6.8 deaths per 1,000 live births, but by 2002 it rose to 7.2, backsliding from 21st to 30th place in infant mortality, behind Cuba (at 6.45) with its socialist public health care system [20]. Infants die at a higher rate in America each year than in 29 other industrialized societies, including the Nordic countries, UK, Germany, Portugal, Israel, France, Singapore and Slovenia! The Center for Diseases Control and Prevention attributes the worsening US rate to very young or much older first-time mothers, inclusion of preterm very low birth-weight babies and multiple births rather than poor state health care provisions. However, examination of the figures reveals *large disparities among racial and ethnic groups*, with black infant mortality rates still almost three times greater than that of white infants which continue into the new millennium despite new initiatives of Medicaid and SCHIP (State Children's Health Insurance Program). And according to a 2004 study by the US Center for System Research (n=25,400 families), one in seven Americans – or 20 million families – are struggling to pay for food and shelter because of debt problems from medical care![21]

0.1.4.3. Cultural influences: Infant mortality is also compounded by *social mores*. In Asia, conservative estimates find that 90 million females are missing in societies which favour sons over daughters, practicing discriminatory abortion or female infanticide, especially in India, Japan, and China since the single-child policy. Laws prohibiting abuse of ultrasound for fetal sex-selection are finally becoming more effective but the social ramifications of the gender gap are enormous.

0.1.4.4. Crisis and conflict: Perinatal mortality also directly reflects *political realities.* The worst rates, like 165 babies of every thousand live births dying under one year in Afghanistan, reflect desperate poverty, poor sanitation and post-war difficulty implementing health programmes, such as immunization. In war-torn Iraq due to a collapse of the water and sewage systems, women are miscarrying and dying from a virulent form of hepatitis E infection particularly dangerous to pregnant women [22a]. Statistics from the Middle East demonstrate a similar story. Israeli figures indicate a steady decline in infant mortality since 1970. The most recent figures show a decrease from 5.5 per 1000 in 2002 to 4.94 in 2003. However, when broken down into ethnic groups, the figure for Jewish babies was 3.3 per 1000 (constituting a 10% drop) while in the Israeli Arab sector it was 8.36 per 1000, reflecting an 8% fall. The discrepancy is attributed to 'inbreeding [between first cousins] and poverty' [22b]. However, figures for Palestinians in the occupied territories (as opposed to Arab citizens of Israel) show a much higher figure despite a recorded fall from 32 in 1990 to 21 per thousand in 2001. Official figures are based on registered infant deaths, and some Palestinian professionals claim that infant mortality in the West Bank and Gaza far exceeds the low 20's (and UNICEF puts it at 23 for 2003). Quite apart from the chronic anxiety, food shortages nightly bombings and violence – curfews and travel restrictions affect antenatal screening and long delays at checkpoints when in labour greatly increase the chances of complications [23].

Throughout the world, in many places the devastating aftermath of wars creates large-scale population upheavals with displacement of refugees. In addition, internally displaced people (IDP), and voluntary or enforced rural to urban and/or trans-border migration have lead to a hundred million homeless worldwide (1,000 million if temporary or poor accommodation is included), with consequent problems of lowered self-confidence, disorientation, lost relatives and possessions, dependency and lack of protection. Starvation, illness, overcrowding and social isolation, mass unemployment, lack of access to medical care, drug addiction and sexually transmitted diseases all contribute to the medley of demographic and socio-economic reasons for a high prevalence of psychological distress, especially affecting parents, young children and vulnerable babies. Thus UNICEF cites 2004 infant mortality figures for Mozambique, a civil-war torn and climactically devastated country, at 197 deaths per 1,000 live births! As noted above, 165 under-one-year olds die in post-war Afghanistan with under-five mortality rising to 257 per 1,000 live births and over 400,000 displaced people. 129 infants per thousand live births die in the democratic republic of Congo where one of the bloodiest world conflicts rages, with disease, starvation and destruction of homes and hospitals. Conversely, with health and nutrition campaigns, Angola which had one of the world's worst infant mortality rates has now dropped to 154 deaths per thousand babies under one year, (and 260 for under-fives!) but hopes are high since the April 2002 peace accord, despite landmines, rising HIV/AIDS, lack of safe water and devastated health and education services.

0.1.5. Third World privations, AIDS and maternity:

In the relative luxury of our health services, we tend to forget that compared to Europe, the third world gap in life expectation continues to widen. Babies born now are doomed to an early death due to privation, famine, violence and disease, especially AIDS, in addition to poverty, dietary deficiencies and maternal mortality [see 0.2.9. below]. UNAIDS 2003 estimate the global total of HIV/AIDS-related deaths at 3 million, with 37 million adults and 2.5 million children living with HIV - 95% of those in the developing world [24] [This is a shocking 50% higher than the figures projected by WHO in 1991. However, UN predictions are that after an eventual peaking of AIDS deaths, rates of HIV transmission will start to decline from 2010 in the 53 countries most affected]. Antiretroviral treatments increase survivor numbers in high-income countries; however these have not been available in poorer societies, who are now negotiating the use of generic locally made cheaper drugs. As many African males find condoms objectionable, new preventive measures include protective microbicides, and diaphragms or condoms for use by females. Planning also includes a relatively cheap treatment for herpes infection as up to 70% of women in sub-Saharan Africa suffer from genital herpes which increases the risk of contracting AIDS by a factor of four or five [25]. Meanwhile, there are expanding geographical tracts in which the population is 'hour-glass' shaped and toddlers are cared for by grandparents as the mid-range generation of childbearing adults have died off. 14 million AIDS orphans live in slums around the world, joining other child-headed households and street-children who survive by prostitution or scavenging. Unlike women in other regions, African women are 1.2 times more likely than men to be infected [26a]. In many places, women are screened for HIV during pregnancy. This gives an indication of the rapid spread of the disease. In South Africa, HIV prevalence in antenatal clinics has risen from 0.7% in 1990 to 4.0% in 1993, to 17.0% in 1997 and 26.5% in 2002! [26b]. Throughout Africa between 5% and 40% of pregnant women are affected, with more than one child infected every minute of every day through mother-to-child transmission, occurring before, during or after delivery. A number of pilot projects started by UNICEF, USAID, UNFPA, UNAIDS, WHO, Medecins Sans Frontieres, the Therapeutic Solidarity Fund and other agencies aim to reduce the risk of transmission by lowering maternal viral load (using prophylactic anti-retroviral treatment, boosting the immune system, and reducing the baby's exposure).

My consultations to midwives, therapists and counsellors on different continents, show that wherever she lives, when an expectant mother discovers she is HIV+, the juxtaposition of a life threatening illness with a life-giving pregnancy is an impossible aporia. The diagnosis in the context of pregnancy is accompanied by stages akin to mourning – shock, confusion, denial, abandonment, anger and mixed feelings. Pleasure in the pregnancy mingles with anxiety about her own survival, guilt about bringing an orphan into the world, remorse at possibly infecting her baby, shame about having to break the news to her family (with the social stigma of AIDS still rife) and dread of the uncertain course ahead, including treatment (or its unavailability). In macho societies, many pregnant women are beaten or abandoned by their partners who refuse to be tested themselves. Some are ostracised by family and friends. In addition to being treated as potentially contaminating by maternity staff, a woman has her own fears about pregnancy exacerbating the illness, ambivalence about a C-section, crucial decisions about breastfeeding as fantasies merge with the reality of her body and milk being poisonous. (WHO stresses that forbidding breast-feeding where it is the norm marks the bottle-feeding mother as HIV-infected, and the risk of stigmatisation, possible violence and rejection [27]).

Every new physical twinge is treated with caution and confusion between symptoms due to pregnancy and others of unclear origin. These turbulent emotions often lead to inconsistent treatment of the baby who is both over-invested and envied, repudiated and/or blamed. Counselling is often restricted to only two visits and limited to the physical The need for ongoing psychological treatment and/or containment usually goes unrecognised, or is regarded as too expensive by perinatal service providers. However, work in Soweto and other HIV+ high-density areas, demonstrate the effectiveness of low maintenance leaderless pre and postnatal peer-support groups, and many women benefit from this self-help group. Nevertheless, some mothers choose to avoid these, feeling that being reminded of the diagnosis undermines their adaptive denial or need for secrecy.

Mother to child transmission is responsible for at least 50% of child cases. Breastfeeding by HIV+ mothers is usually counter-indicated [28]. However, often it is the only viable choice, as refraining from breastfeeding in areas of famine or polluted water increases the risk of infant mortality (and releases maternal fertility). Studies in Cote d'Ivoire and Burkina Faso of women who breastfed despite the risks, found that the initial benefits of prevention of vertical HIV infection are partly reversed through breastfeeding [29]. Another study in Durban, South Africa, shows that even in the absence of antiretroviral therapy to reduce mother-to-infant transmission, babies who were <u>exclusively</u> breastfed for three months or more by HIV-infected mothers had no excess risk of HIV infection over six months than those never breastfed [30]. Sadly though, exclusive breastfeeding can compound the risks as a cohort study of child survival in Uganda found. In many cases infant mortality associated with maternal death is not due to HIV infection but malnutrition or diarrhoeal disease because of sudden forced weaning [31]. Teasing out the complexities of these various findings is essential in view of the risks of NOT breastfeeding among disadvantaged populations in Sub-Saharan Africa and South Asia where clean water for formula feeding is not readily available. Finally, a new form of HIV infection has been disclosed in some hospital-born babies to parents not infected by the virus (thus unrelated to breastfeeding or sexual transmission). Fourteen such cases have been brought to light recently by parents suing the department of health in the Western Cape and elsewhere [32a]. The source of these infections may be blood transfusions, needle-stick, contaminated medical instruments or possibly, infection by another patient in the same hospital, indicating the need for greater HIV risk management and increased precautions.

Finally, there is no place for western complacency as the total number of people living with HIV continues to rise in high-income countries (now estimated at 1.6 million), largely due to widespread access to antiretroviral treatment, as well as the 80,000 new infections in 2003, due to risk-taking behaviours. Prevention activities are not keeping pace with the rapid and changing spread of HIV and AIDS continues to take its toll, claiming some 18, 000 lives in the past year. And the AIDS epidemic in Eastern Europe and Central Asia shows no signs of declining, especially in the Russian Federation, Ukraine and the Baltic states with some 230,000 newly infected in 2003 bringing the total number of people living there with the virus to 1.5 million (and 30,000 deaths last year). Similarly, over 1 million people acquired HIV in 2003 in Asia and the Pacific, bringing the estimated total there to 7.4 million. Infection also rose in North Africa and the Middle East. And more than 2 million people in Latin America and the Caribbean are now living with the illness [32b]. Since the 1996 introduction of anti-retroviral drugs, in some European countries, medical policy leans towards assisting HIV affected couples to conceiving safely through sperm washing and IVF, thereby treating it as a containable disease, like diabetes. However, worldwide, early and unprotected sex results in unintended pregnancy, in some cases with terrible repercussions. Over 90% of infected children in the world are babies born to HIV positive mothers who have not received protective drugs. Their care, education campaigns and prevention of HIV must concern us all. In these times of interdependent globalisation, none of us can ethically remain a protected isolate.

Changing parameters of childbearing, infant mortality and healthy life expectancy are indices of the complex interrelatedness of factors which determine any individual's quality of life, anywhere in the world. They indicate the necessity for a combined multidisciplinary effort towards health promotion, appropriate education, reduction in health disparities and improved emotional well-being, to which we can contribute, each in our own way, in our own corner.

KEY POINTS:

*The needs of babies have changed very little over the millennia. In societies in transition, this puts babies at risk of being at odds with their parents' rapidly changing lives.

*Scattering of extended families and eroded community networks increase mutual-reliance and the intensity of interdependent relations in the small nuclear unit.

*Gender inequalities of childcare within the family are fostered by governmental policies on parental leave.

*In western countries educational parity and women's career prospects delay childbearing, and work/home dislocation disrupts parental childcare.

*Conversely, western teenage births have increased, with attendant problems of low birth weight, poverty and parental immaturity.

* Urban stratification and reduced family size decrease access to babies and opportunities for us to emotionally work through infantile issues

before becoming a parent raising the likelihood of perinatal disturbance.
* The detrimental effects of parental disturbance on their children's
emotional, social and cognitive development often long after the carer's
illness abates. Preventive and therapeutic measures are a necessity.
* Both within and between societies, health disparities are intrinsically
related to income, education and access to health facilities, with higher
infant mortality and maternal morbidity.

0.2. MATERNITY CARE

0.2.1. Changes in maternity services in the UK:
Over the past few decades, advances have been led by both *provider
initiatives* (Health providers in the UK, Association of Radical Midwives
and ANACS – the Association of Nurse Advocates for Childbirth
Solutions in the USA) and *consumer pressures* (National Childbirth Trust,
Maternity Alliance, and AIMS – the Association for Improvement of
Maternity Services in the UK and the Maternity Care Coalition in the
USA) to improve maternity care. *The emphasis is on woman-led care -
antenatally, during labour and birth, and in establishing lactation.*
Concerted campaigns from courageous individuals to ensure women's
rights [33] have helped to change the climate of opinion. In recent years,
British Government policies indicate greater awareness of psychological
issues, and advocate availability of options to cater to personal
preferences, special needs and diverse cultural expectations. The 1993
'Changing Childbirth' report laid down guidelines for one-to-one
midwifery care and 'choice, control and continuity' for women and since
devolution, the Scottish Framework evolved 27 principles to improve
maternity services [34 a, b]. The Royal College of Midwives, the world's
oldest and largest midwifery organisation, published a report entitled
'Vision 2000' for future development of maternity services based on a UK-
wide consultation, conducted throughout 1999, of midwives and other key
stakeholders in maternity care. The vision called for maternity services to
provide high quality, evidence-based, cost-effective care which is
responsive to individual needs and preferences, and which promotes and
sustains public health according to twelve key principles:
- *User involvement.*
- *Public health (*including targeted support for women with special
  health and social needs, and measures to reduce inequalities).
- *Community focus*
- *Integration across acute and community sectors*

- *Normality (*an underpinning philosophy of pregnancy and birth as normal, with a commitment to positive reduction in unnecessary medicalisation)
- *Midwifery-led care*
- *Maximised and targeted continuity of carer*
- *One-to-one midwifery care in labour*
- *Family-centred care*
- *Clinical excellence*
- *Midwifery leadership*
- *Partnership* (between Midwives, obstetricians, paediatricians, GPs and health visitors)
- *Opportunities for change* (acknowledging variations in models of maternity care and geographical, demographic and staffing, pointing to the need for continuing flexibility and creativity in service planning and delivery) [35a,b].

Sadly this 'vision' is far from realisation. In fact a national survey investigating the experiences of 2,000 recent mothers (average age 29) published in March 2001revealed that most respondents were dissatisfied with the care they received during childbirth and less than half felt happy to return to the same hospital to give birth again. Three-quarters said they felt anxious during pregnancy and frightened during labour. Six in ten found the experience of giving birth more shocking than they expected. Four in ten said they were not allowed to move around during labour and take up positions they wanted, and 43% said they did not have the type of birth they sought. Only 8% of women had a completely natural birth, without the need for drugs or surgical interventions. A quarter had a caesarean section. Among those giving birth normally, 35% were induced, 45% had an epidural, 12% had a forceps delivery and 53% needed stitches. Half of all new mothers also said they had received poor postnatal care once they had taken their baby home and 79% said they were in pain after the birth for an average of two weeks. The women were also dissatisfied with their care during pregnancy. And only 4% had the same midwife for all antenatal appointments and delivery. Summed up as 'conveyor-belt birth experience to suit the hospital's agenda', these findings were partly attributed to 'overstretched maternity staff' and a 'lottery' of unevenly distributed resources and variations in standards in units across the country [36]. This situation lowers the morale of midwives who strive to provide good care as well as letting down the women who are entitled to it.

0.2.2. On the coal-front:

How has this situation come about? A National Service Framework (NSF) on maternity services enforced new national standards to ensure that every woman would have *'one-to-one' continuous care* by a midwife, dedicated to her throughout labour and the National Institute for Clinical Effectiveness [NICE] provided a review and guidance on Intrapartum Care [37a,b]. And to facilitate improvement the government promised £100 million to maternity services staff and agencies in May 2001. This 'cash injection' was to be supplemented by an extra 2,000 midwives on wards in England by 2005, 500 of whom were promised to be in place by the end of 2003. All 250 NHS maternity units in England were to receive 'extra funds 'to refurbish and modernise facilities in a bid to eliminate big variations in the standard of maternity care throughout the UK' [38]. This boost was intended for 'maternity services that give women and families more choice over the care they receive so that every child, regardless of background or circumstance, has the best possible start in life'. Nevertheless, a report by the Commons health committee a year later noted that maternity services were still lacking, with only 2% of babies being born at home (although 20% of mothers would prefer this type of delivery given a choice). Women were limited to bringing only a single birth partner and 'too many women were being given caesareans without having the opportunity to exercise informed choice'. In addition inequalities were still rife and maternal death rate in unemployed families in England was still 20 times higher (!) than among women in the two highest social classes, and a disproportionate number of women from traveller families died in childbirth or shortly afterwards. The Health Committee members concluded that 'the government should address concern that birth was no longer perceived as a normal physiological process'. These MPs also highlighted concerns about the closure of smaller maternity units and birth centres, midwife shortages and a lack of experienced obstetricians, lack of specialist mother and baby units for women suffering severe mental health problems after the birth, and little help for those affected by disabilities or language problems [39]. To date, the UK's midwifery shortfall shows no signs of improving, according to new figures unveiled by the Royal College of Midwives on March 18th 2004. Surveying 240 midwifery units across England, Northern Ireland, Scotland and Wales they found that more than three quarters of the maternity units who responded are still experiencing shortages, rising to 83% of those surveyed in England. In London a massive 18.3% of posts remain unfilled, whilst there has been a decrease in all categories of midwives joining the service, and no significant improvement on the previous year. In fact, in London and the South East the situation has deteriorated further. Bad conditions and low pay deterred trainee nurses from becoming midwives, and one sorry solution has been to poach qualified midwives from developing countries where they are sorely needed. Conversely, many nurses including midwives are seeking agency jobs or recruited to work in the USA, where flexible work hours and better conditions beckon. It is now estimated that the NHS lacks a further million nurses in 2005! Nevertheless it is not just a matter of numbers. In the debate that followed some adverse maternity incidents, one Director of Midwifery noted that simply increasing staffing levels may not resolve the problem as 'even on a well staffed labour ward there can be moments of crisis…because of the unpredictable nature of the service', especially f personnel are tied up in caesarean sections. She suggested deploying midwives to educate women antenatally to realise the 'cascade of interventions' that follow coming into hospital too early and to motivate doctors and midwives to reduce interventions [40].

0.2.3. Provisions for addressing anxiety - women:

Humans seem to be the only primates who seek assistance during labour. This is attributed to the discrepancy between the large-headed baby and the long axis of the birth canal since humans began to walk upright some five million years ago [41]. We are also the only species who can imagine our own death, and make connections between the aloneness of birthgiving and of dying. Ancient references to midwives and anthropological evidence indicate that provision of assistance was probably not merely physical but included emotional support at a time of pain and anxiety. These needs still exist. However, due to medicalisation, staff shortages and lack of psychological training, the anxieties of pregnant women tend to be overlooked antenatally. Like other research which asks about anxieties, a study of 481 women in western Finland found that 78% of respondents expressed fears relating to pregnancy, childbirth or both and that in some cases desire for a caesarean section was related to negative experiences in previous pregnancies, and a wish to avoid the birth [42]. Similarly, a Swedish study of 100 women with severe anxiety over childbirth found that intense psychological support reduced the rate of C-sections by half [43]. Antenatal classes are the ideal place for emotional support and exploration of anxieties. However, sadly, in the UK fears and fantasies are rarely addressed during pregnancy, and in the absence of continuous one-to-one midwifery care during labour, women are often left to their own anxieties, which increases the necessity for interventions. Within the NHS antenatal classes tend to focus on the physical aspects of labour and birth, and these lack uniformity, varying regionally, and even within the same hospital. In addition private classes (NCT, Active Birth, Yoga and others) focusing on breathing and relaxation strategies, may not prepare women for the unexpected and/or produce expectations which are at odds with hospital practices.

0.2.3. Provisions for addressing anxiety - midwives:

On the other hand, neither are the **anxieties experienced by midwives** addressed. Working within a cauldron of bubbling and highly disturbing emotions, a midwife is both absorbing the raw feelings of the labouring woman and dealing with life-giving and death-dealing issues in herself. In her daily job, a midwife is exposed to the naked physicality of a stranger, to the tidal contractions and unleashed eruptions of her innermost emotions and bodily fluids. A mid-wife inserts her hand into the stranger's vagina to sweep her membranes, she tidies tendrils of her damp hair, offer her water-sips, blows her nose, rubs her back and holds her hand. In helping the labouring woman, she accepts her leakages - bowel or bladder 'accidents'; vocalisations of pain - screams, curses and expletives; soothes her convulsions of fear and paroxysms of rage, coaches and wheedles the crowning and massages the parturient's trembling legs. Encouraging the birth, she slips her fingers beneath the bulging rim, and as the vernix-covered body slithers out, wipes away the filaments of sac, amnion, meconium and streaks of blood before handing over the glistening squirming bundle into the arms of the spent mother.

Reacting to rudimentary passion in the room through the filter of emotions stirred up inside her from her own unprocessed past experience, the midwife exudes her own anxieties while soaking up those of the woman whose perspiration she mops. She is both fulfilling her professional duty and unconsciously trying to live up to, or taken by surprise by, the labouring woman's unconscious projections of a harsh or protective archaic powerful maternal figure into her (which may or may not coincide with the midwife's own internal mother figure). She may have difficulties negotiating her (at times conflicting) dual identifications with, and envy of, both the mother and her baby during pregnancy, labour and birth. While indispensable she is secondary, a bystander and witness to bare emotional and erotic intimacies between the woman and her partner from which she is excluded, as she was from her parents' sexual relationship. In an emergency situation, providing psychological support for the labouring woman and her partner is difficult as the midwife confronts immediate dangers she alone can anticipate. Guiding and encouraging the birthing woman to 'pant' or 'push', her feelings wax and wane, aroused and yet resisting arousal by treating as ordinary the miraculous moment of birth. Confronted time and again, night after night, day in and day out by the mystery of origination - a new human being emerging from another (as she herself did, and each and every one of us who rarely have to think about it). And all this while also negotiating issues of control and its loss, authority and unequal power relations; containing the chronic stress and inevitable pain inherent in the job! These are but some of the complexity of feelings experienced by a midwife on the labour ward, but in addition, unlike therapists who are exposed to heightened emotions in their consulting room, she has not had the opportunity of exploring her own hidden feelings [see Chapter 16]

Not surprisingly, the midwife's anxieties and unconscious representations find their way into her practice. For instance, if the labouring woman's body is unconsciously deemed 'open', apprehension about her vulnerability may be formulated as fear that she is susceptible to entry or attack (by germs, bad thoughts, etc) or conversely, to seepages from within (amniotic fluid, loss of blood) leading to urgency about inducing, prepping, stitching, wadding, etc. Similarly, if the labouring woman is perceived as dangerous, a threat either to those around her or the baby, she may be avoided, kept away from others, and/or monitored to prevent her endangering the child. When socially unconscious representations take the form of cultural beliefs, practices become embedded in routine, ritual and unquestioned local customs (also see Chapter 18). These may be charted in **five childbearing configurations** :

	IMAGE of WOMAN:	CONDITION:	PRACTICE:
I	**Vulnerable**	*Open* ? in	closure, speed
		? out	protective devices
II	**Dangerous**	*'dark'* (supernatural)	seclusion
		'dirty' untouchable	avoidance
		'polluting'	purifications
		'damaging'	control
III	**Passive**	*inert container*	delivery/caesarean
		'resistant'	coaxing
IV	**Obstructive**	*'ignorant'*	coaching
		'difficult patient'	punishment
V	**Active agent**	*entitled participant*	informed choice

0.2.4.The five 'C's – choice, control and continuity, communication and compassion:

Birth is a highly private and cherished event which many women resent sharing with a stranger. Studies of thousands of women from places as far apart as Melbourne, Australia and Scotland [44a, b] provide evidence that not surprisingly, women desire care from a *known midwife*. However, few services outside of Scandinavia offer overall one-to-one antenatal, intrapartum and postnatal continuity. Nonetheless, although clearly important, there is a danger that focusing research on the issue of 'continuity' of care throughout pregnancy and labour may obscure the importance of *quality* of care, even by an unknown midwife [45].

To the Cumberlage '3C's' of a woman being granted *'choice, control and continuity'* during her labour, we may add two more – *'communication and compassion'*. The need for an empathic experience with the midwife is highlighted in studies around the world. For instance two centres in Sweden stress that women's experiences of childbirth are enhanced by creating a trusting relationship between the woman and her midwife, based on the latter's listening skills [46]. Good communication is an asset, but not the whole story as a large survey in Atlanta, Georgia stresses, adding the necessity for pain management and opportunities to discuss the birth postpartum to reduce the traumatic experience of childbirth (especially in women with a history of sexual trauma) [47]. Not only the vulnerable but everyone searches for meaning after a confusing or disturbing experience, especially if it has been traumatic. However, sadly, *'debriefing'* after birth is often separated from the event itself. A national audit of maternity care services in Scotland found that although 62% of women had talked to a professional about what happened during their delivery and labour, in more than half the cases this was not someone who had been present at her labour! [48a]. Feeling powerless and abused, damaged or betrayed, 'overwhelmed', 'mutilated', 'violated' or stigmatised are subjective descriptions of birth experiences. Women who do not have an opportunity to work through what they consider to be negative incidents, continue to mull these over for many years after the event, with all the characteristics of PTSD such as intrusive thoughts, flashbacks, hyper-vigilance, sleep disorders, preoccupation with minutiae of the labour and birth, somatic complaints, suicidal ideation, self-destructive behaviours, sexual dysfunction, marital difficulties, postnatal and ongoing depression [48b].

Researchers comparing maternity-care perceptions of child-bearing women and those of primary health care professionals stress that development of a *'consumer focused service'* means just that – understanding (rather than underestimating) the importance for women to have confidence in the providers. This includes a need to understand what is happening to them – to receive information about procedures and professionals' roles, and to be given a (personally and medically) appropriate degree of personal involvement in the process of decision making [49] about their own bodies and one of the most important experiences of their lives. Birth plans are a step in that direction, but in many cases these are overridden by hospital protocols. If stress and anxiety are provoked by feeling powerless in an unpredictable and depersonalised situation, *choice* (and realistic preparation) gives people a sense of personal control.

Anecdotal feedback from parturients in the USA and the UK indicate that the childbirth experience in the present context still reflects lack of control, choice, communication and compassion which are far from conducive to emotional well-being [50]. More importantly from the point of view of detecting anxiety and emotional problems during pregnancy, *discontinuous care* and multiple carers have an important side-effect. 'As a woman passes from family doctor to student midwife or to junior obstetricians for subsequent antenatal visits, then meets new faces in the delivery suite and subsequently in the postnatal ward where she must undergo checks from obstetricians and paediatricians before leaving hospital to go back into the care of the community midwives, health visitors and her family doctor, it is not surprising that changes in her mental state may be missed' says a psychiatrist-psychoanalyst [51]. This is compounded by the fact that even when vigorous attempts are made to detect women at risk of developing emotional disturbances, or those already suffering with psychiatric problems antenatally or after the birth, a significant proportion, nearly a third, fail to keep clinic appointments. It is possible that many such non-attenders are also the most needy or distressed; they may be overwhelmed by the problems of coping with other small children without a partner or too depressed or fearful to attend. Women suffering from phobias may find it hard to come to a hospital clinic. Others find the journey too difficult while feeling anxious, exhausted and run down, especially with an infant or toddler in tow. To address these issues, there clearly is a need for a *coordinated policy of care* based upon links between hospital and community primary health care services, Social Services and voluntary agencies. To be effective, such resources must also be capable of being delivered at home and the

contribution of child psychiatrists and parent-infant psychotherapists to
the development and shaping of these services seems indispensable.

0.2.5. Complementary and differing perspectives on birth:

In recent years a great deal of research has explored retrospective feelings
'service users' have about the care they receive during this momentous
event in their lives. Most findings indicate that labouring women wish to
be treated with respect and as individuals. The UK National Birthday
Trust Fund's semi-qualitative survey of over 15,000 women named <u>choice</u>
as the key factor. Women are satisfied with maternity care, whether at
home or in hospital, provided it meets their personal expectations [52].
Studies examining the inter-relationship between women's expectations
and their actual experiences of decision making, continuity, choice and
control in labour have implications for NHS maternity service policies.
Recent findings show a shift in parturients since 1987 towards greater
desire for involvement in both non-emergency and emergency decision
making (including caesarean section) and choices about pain relief.
*Overall, feeling in control during labour was associated with higher
satisfaction and better emotional well-being postnatally* [53]. However, as
I reiterate throughout this book, 'women' cannot be treated as a unified
group. They each differ in their needs and priorities, and hope to have
these respected. Thus, a small American study of women with high risk
pregnancies (hypertension or threatened preterm delivery) illustrated that
these women differed in the <u>degree</u> to which they wanted to be involved
in decision-making during this period, but both those wanting active
involvement and those who preferred a more passive role were satisfied if
health care professionals were congruent with their wishes [54].

In all these studies, the **method of data collection** is most
important. A large-scale nation-wide survey of *all* women giving birth in
23 consultant-led maternity units across Scotland over a ten-day period
emphasised *the need to compare user and provider views,* using this
complementary system of data collection to detect disparities and improve
the quality of care [55]. Similarly, the need for comparison was
emphasised by a review of all the UK literature relating to women's views
on community based care between 1970-1998 concluding that consumer
views must reflect <u>different</u> groups of women and their experiences of
different care processes [56]. It is also important to recognise that Britain
is now a pluralistic society with a diversity of cultural expectations, needs
and beliefs. Services must meet the wide variety of needs of the
populations they serve locally (see section 0.2.10 below). Evaluation of

the current success of projects within the 'ASQUAM' programme (Achieving Sustainable Quality in Maternity) claim that use of local guidelines, cyclical audit, monthly feedback meetings and training courses have led to significant improvements in clinical effectiveness in many of the 45 standards prioritised. However, they note there has <u>not</u> been the same success in achieving high standards in communication and informed choice [57]. Indeed, this is a recurrent theme, and a prospective study including in-depth interviews to assess women's views in north-east Scotland found that many consumers felt they were given insufficient information about the basics, such as available options of places of birth and pain relief [58].

Even women who try and glean as much knowledge as possible from external sources such as books and the internet, may find themselves caught up in a system where the rationale and implications of procedures are unknown. Clearly, information provision is a complex area, but in the absence of clear understanding, choices may be made by default.

Antenatal screening is a case in point. A review of 98 reports of 74 primary studies in 18 countries found that although ultrasound is attractive to women and their partners, they often lack information about its specific purpose and the technical limitations of the procedure and are therefore unprepared for adverse findings [59]. Indeed, a study of prenatal screening in two Finish towns raises the ethical issue of women being unaware that participation in screening procedures is not routine but a voluntary option [60]. Some tests (e.g. AFP and triple tests) with high false positive rates may cause unnecessary anxiety, followed by a cascade of diagnostic tests, some of which carry a risk of induced abortion and long waits for results. Counseling is rare and information-giving in itself is not always enough – ramifications of findings must be spelled out <u>before</u> a woman undertakes a test. Despite improvement on a previous multi-centre survey, a study in Glasgow similarly commented on women's compliance with antenatal serum-screening despite poor understanding of the nature of tests and their results [61]. Confronted with findings indicating that they have a high risk of a Down's baby, many women may not be aware that they will need further tests to confirm the veracity of the results, or are not even told of the small but real risk of miscarriage or infection amniocentesis holds. More importantly, they may not be informed about probabilities of false-positive maternal serum results, nor have contemplated the consequences of discovering their baby is imperfect, or the degree of abnormality they are willing to accept. A large scale trial in Helsinki reported on the need for written rather than just verbal information about serum-screening, and possibly a second leaflet for women receiving positive results [62]. Brief counselling would give a couple the chance to bring understanding and emotion together in exploring the options available to them.

Similarly, information, acknowledgement and humane care were the variables cited in a qualitative study of women's needs in response to discovering **a 'vanished twin'** through ultrasound [63]. These basic needs are also poignantly illustrated in in-depth case histories which reveal the often overlooked dual impact of technological screening - fostering parental faith in all-powerful medicine and yet also increasing the shattering experience if the familiar baby they have come to know through visualisations on the screen, dies in utero [64] or is born with a defect, despite screening.

Likewise, insufficient information about **the birth process** may lead to choices with unforeseen consequences, such as restricted mobility with drips and fetal monitors (and the latter's unreliability); the rapid acceleration of induced labour; catheterisation, raised uterine temperature, side–effects for the baby, maternal post-birth headache and backache associated with epidurals, and raised likelihood of caesarean, forceps or vacuum assisted deliveries, and possibility of severe perineal lacerations.

0.2.6. Caesarean sections:

In 1985 the WHO proclaimed that no region in the world was justified in having a caesarean rate of more than 10-15%. Despite this and the many medical risks involved for mothers and babies, in the past 20 years, rates in North America have nearly quintupled in the US (to 24%) and quadrupled in Canada - partly due to repeat C-sections, epidural analgesia, private medical insurance, and doctors' fear of litigation. In Britain too, figures have quadrupled over the past 30 years. One in five births in the UK are now by caesarean section - attributed to older primigravidae and a higher incidence of twins and triplets, conceived through IVF. However, caesarean rates also reflect the attitudes of the professionals involved. The doctor's age and gender, too, has been found to affect rates![65]. US studies of low risk cases also find that C-section rates vary between midwifery-led and physicians' wards even in the same hospital, and in free-standing midwives' birth centres rates are significantly lower. In the UK, disillusioned on the 5th anniversary of 'Changing Childbirth', in a 'Midwifery Matters' editorial the Association of Radical Midwives called for a midwife-led birth centre in every neighbourhood [66]. Caesarean section is also related to patient anxiety. A systematic Cochrane review of randomized controlled trials shows that continuous professional support during labour is associated with a reduced incidence of surgery and instrumental delivery [67]. If one-to-one support in labour reduces risks, yet labour ward midwives are no longer available to provide this (because of overseeing several labours at once), a trained 'doula' birth partner (or female friend) is effective in reducing duration and complications of labour [68].

There are **four primary reasons for 85% of C-sections** : repeat caesarean (29%), presumed foetal distress (22%), failure to progress (20%) and breech birth (16%). Collecting data on 99% of births in England, Wales and Northern Ireland over a three month period in 2000, a Department of Health audit in 2000 found that only 63% of all caesareans were emergency and 37%, elective [69]. [When my own study in 1985 showed a high proportion of elective caesareans among Regulators, the results were questioned as it seemed unthinkable that women could influence their doctors to conduct major surgery by request]. *The dramatic rise in caesarean rate is now ascribed to a combination of medical, organisational and socio-cultural factors with long-term impact of the mother's health, greater cost to the NHS and as yet unknown effects on babies.* **Depression** is now a recognised common post-surgical phenomenon. Caesareans are major operations, and not surprisingly, many women experience a deep sense of melancholy, partly related to the body's fallibility and the profound helplessness of having surrendered to being cut open while awake. Breastfeeding is more difficult to establish following a caesarean operation, it is difficult to lift the baby, cough or even laugh. Many women experience a sense of failure, shame and drop in self esteem at not having given birth 'naturally'/vaginally. Some feel embittered, alienated from the baby and or shocked by their scarred ('mutilated') body, and fearful that their fertility has been compromised.

Despite a fall in the mid-90's, worldwide the rate of Caesarean sections has climbed up again in recent years. In 2002 the US average rate rose to its highest ever at 26% (ranging from 31% in Mississippi (where midwifery is still illegal) to 19% in New Mexico where unusually, over 25% of babies are delivered by midwives) [70]. In Brazil it reached an unbelievable average rate of 40% (and over 80% in private hospitals). In the UK the NHS rate is around 20% of which the elective rate is 8.9% - usually attributed to women 'too posh to push'. However, a recent investigation into the rising rates in the UK found on the basis of NHS hospital data for 2001-2 that although women living in deprived areas are significantly less likely to have an elective caesarean, in the other areas this is <u>not</u> linked to increasing affluence. Nevertheless, this study excludes private hospitals which have very high rates [71]. The reasons for elective Caesars are complex, including a busy schedule and desire for control (by both private obstetricians and the women they serve); avoidance of pain; an intact 'honeymoon fresh' vagina; fear of labour... Financial gain and fear of litigation are among the reasons for compliance by private obstetricians. Accurate information about the postnatal incapacity involved, good birth preparation and timely counseling for women's anxieties may prevent some of these unnecessary operations.

0.2.7. Home births:

In Holland and Denmark, almost one in three children is born at home. In the UK, despite all women's entitlement to a home birth by law, in 1991 when this book was first published almost 98% of births occurred in hospital. However, by 1994, the 'changing childbirth' report indicated that women be referred to a midwife for a home birth on request. The National Birthday Trust conducted a prospective confidential survey of home births, following all women who booked a home birth in the UK in 1994. Results showed that planning a home birth <u>halved</u> the chances of assisted or caesarean births. The researchers concluded that home births would probably increase to 4-5% of all maternities in UK during the next decade, which is indeed the case.

I present these findings in some detail here as they strongly support the hypothesis that social and environmental factors can affect progress of labour and mode of delivery. This study included almost 6000 women at 37 weeks' gestation matched for age, parity and obstetric history by their midwives with a woman in their practice who was booked to deliver in hospital. The overall group profile was low-risk. 84% were expecting second or subsequent children. Mothers who had a previous Caesarean made up 1.4% of the home birth group, and 3% of the hospital group. It was found that despite matching the home-birth group had less incidence of high blood pressure between recruitment for the study, at 37 weeks, and the birth - possibly due to less stressful (midwife) antenatal care. (Alternatively, women who developed high blood pressure before 37 weeks had transferred their booking to the hospital).

	Planned home births *	**Planned hospital births**
Spontaneous vaginal delivery	94.7%	90.2%
Assisted (forceps, ventouse)	2.4%	5.4%
Caesarean	2.0%	4.1%

*(includes 16% transfers to hospital in late pregnancy or labour)

Home births, including those who transferred to hospital were less likely to involve post-partum haemorrhage. Home birth mothers had fewer episiotomies but more first-degree perineal tears. They were much less likely to use drugs for pain relief, despite availability of Entonox (nitrous oxide and oxygen, 'gas and air'), and Pethidine (called Demerol in the USA). And they were more likely than hospital births to use relaxation techniques, warm water, aromatherapy and homeopathy. At 1 minute, 5.2% of the planned home-birth babies had APGAR scores below 7, compared to 9.3% of the planned hospital babies. At 5 minutes, 0.7% of both groups had scores below 7. Babies planned for home birth were less likely to have bruising or 'resuscitation' interventions (both suctioning, oxygen with a bag and mask, or intubation). Exclusive breastfeeding rates 48 hours after birth were 80% in the home birth group and 58.1% in the planned hospital group; six weeks later, the figures were 65% and 44% respectively [72a]. [The relaxed nature of a home delivery, privacy, security, comfort and the absence of any separation of mother and baby clearly help to establish breastfeeding. However, since breastfeeding rates for the transferred home births were almost identical despite the difficult hospital delivery, perhaps figures reflect specific maternal orientations – Facilitators and Reciprocators – both of whom usually have high level of commitment to breastfeed whatever the circumstances (see Chapter 24, and 0.2.9 below)]. It must be noted that women planning home births have also been found to be highly motivated, better educated and more affluent and hence slightly lower-risk. However, despite the evidence of safety and advantages of home births, there is still a great deal of medical opposition, as a 2004 National Birth Alliance report attests, revealing a range of coercive measures and forcible hospitalisation of Irish would-be-home-birth mothers [72b].

0.2.8. Miscarriage, stillbirth and special care:

Finally, it is when things go wrong that the caregiving relationship is tested to its limits (see Chapter 30). New guidelines have been devised for management of women experiencing **pregnancy loss under 24 weeks**, with implications for provision of information, and improved choice and control by women themselves. Yet explanations are not always forthcoming, as the cause of the miscarriage may be obscure. Many women find the lack of feedback after a spontaneous abortion very distressing. More distressing still, is staff insensitivity. In one appalling incident, lack of foresight and storage facilities resulted in a 14 year old being given her aborted fetus in a jar and told to take it home and return with it at a later date when a specialist was available [73a]. Organisations like the Miscarriage Association publish guidelines for good practice following pregnancy loss, including study days for professionals to promote more awareness and sensitivity [73b]. Although midwives believe they are ideally placed to provide a holistic approach for women who have suffered a miscarriage [74] the many demands and restrictions of their job make this difficult. Similarly, while diagnostic techniques of antenatal screening are ever more sophisticated, the attention to psychological issues still lags behind. As noted above (section 0.2.5), women may not realise the implications of the seemingly harmless tests, and in the case of suspected abnormalities, they often face a brutal dilemma with little support or guidance. Disenchantment and guilt often follow spontaneous or induced pregnancy losses with a sense that 'the womb is not a safe place' and gestation cannot be taken for granted. A subsequent pregnancy may be filled with trepidation and concern.

0.2.7.1. In the UK, 1 baby in 100 is stillborn or dies within the first 4 weeks of life. Loss so late in the process is particularly poignant and parents are often traumatised and mull over minutiae of the events leading up to the death in years to come, wondering if it could have been forestalled. The institutional approach to **stillbirth or neonatal death** has changed in recent years. There is now greater recognition by maternity staff that perinatal loss is a serious bereavement and parents will experience grief for many months after the loss. The trauma of stillbirth can have long term effects with some 20% of women experiencing prolonged depression [75], and 20% post traumatic stress disorder (PTSD) in the subsequent pregnancy [76]. How it is handled by staff is crucial. Studies show that bereaved mothers report a sense of 'empowerment' from empathic and humane comfort rather than just competent physical care from their health care professionals [77]. Children who have eagerly (and uneasily) anticipated birth of a sibling are deeply affected by the loss (see pages 398-40) and an association has been found between anxiety disorder in adolescence and maternal experience of stillbirth [78]. Infants next-born after stillbirth show a significant increase in disorganisation of attachment behaviour to the mother, mediated not by maternal depression or anxiety, but by a measure of maternal unresolved mourning [79a,b] and the child's fear that s/he too may be doomed. Bereaved parents may not be emotionally available to talk over these painful feelings with the child and referrals for child psychotherapy or family therapy in later years may be necessary to address this unmetabolised family trauma.

Some decades ago, pioneering work in London [80] demonstrated the importance for crisis support to help parents feel less guilty, ashamed and stupified by the 'non-event' of stillbirth, and less likely to rush in with a replacement pregnancy before resolving their grief. However, the now usual practice of encouraging contact with the dead infant's body which they advocated to facilitate mourning and recovery, was not systematically evaluated. A new study now suggests that for some parents, close contact may be associated with adverse outcome [81]. Once again, this demonstrates differences such as those reflected in parenting orientations, and the need for individuals to follow their own emotional inclinations. Bereavement counselling now also stresses *diverse reactions and gender differences in mourning*. There is often a divergence in expression and duration of grief within the same couple. Most bereaved parents will feel somewhat better 6 to 9 months following a neonatal loss (and the anniversary of original due date, actual birth, burial are crucial events), but it is usually 2-3 years before they are close to full recovery. And even then, anniversaries or other reminders may trigger painful flash backs for years to come. Intense grief, self-blame and guilt have in the past been attributed to maternal ambivalence or unconscious aggression. However, these are now recognised as *a healthy adaptive reaction* to the traumatising helplessness posed by such a loss [82] especially when reproductive technology is accompanied by an illusion of control.

0.2.7.2. **Mourning:** A review of contemporary bereavement literature in nursing, medical and social science data indicates that a major change is occurring in the understanding of mourning in the United Kingdom and United States of America. This change particularly applies to bereaved parents in the West, where death of a child is seen to be against the natural order. Whereas traditional models of mourning (beginning with Freud) placed emphasis on bereaved people letting go of their emotional relationships with those who have died, *contemporary models accept the need for parents to hold on to their relationship with their dead children.* Therapeutic interventions of health professionals support parents in their grief and encourage them to talk about their loved one and incorporate him or her into their daily life [83a]. The difficulty with stillbirth and very early loss is the brevity of contact and absence of memories, combined with the long build up of now thwarted expectations and hopes invested in the baby. Acknowledged by professionals who knew the woman during her pregnancy is now recognised as a helpful bridge between past and present, as is the need for counseling or psychotherapeutic help with unmanageable feelings following a perinatal loss. Needless to say, subsequent pregnancies are fraught with misgivings and especially compassionate midwifery care is necessary [83b]. An innovative joint Australian-Canadian study advocates a midwife-managed Special Delivery Service programme and supportive health care services for women who have experienced loss of a baby in a previous pregnancy [84].

Similarly, following **Sudden Infant Death** the shock, confusion, guilt and self-questioning, sleep disturbance and distressing dreams, emotional withdrawal, and long-term grieving process may persist in parents, siblings and grandparents. In some cases, this is exacerbated by accusations and even imprisonment of parents. Despite much research over the past 15 years, the causes of SIDS remain controversial, and although recent guidelines reduce the risk of cot death, they have not prevented it. In this, as in all forms of sudden bereavement, counseling is a necessity.

0.2.7.3 The stresses of **premature births** are exacerbated by lack of preparation for the birth and feelings of shock, abandonment, self-blame and guilt. Uncertainty of outcome and the highly technological and frightening NICU (neonatal intensive care unit) and attendant worries about morbidity, separation and emotional and cognitive effects of incubation all take their toll on new parents. Observations show that staff, too, are challenged in this environment of chronic stress and fatalities, and many find defensive ways of reacting by becoming inappropriately over-involved or callously hardened to their painful tasks [85].
Although the percentage of low birth weight babies is increasing, the borders of viability (24-28 weeks) have hardly changed since 1980, with high mortality rates especially in the first 48hours, and risk of neurological damage in those who survive. Follow ups reveal that many children have multiple cognitive deficits in later life. Even among low-risk 27-34 week births the maximum survival rate is still 95% and has changed very little over the years [86]. However, a surprising innovation originates in third world countries lacking facilities for incubation. A recent randomised control trial in Southern Africa shows positive effects of immediately placing the baby between the mother's breasts in **skin-to-skin 'kangaroo' care**. This has been found to increase the survival rate even among very low birth-weight babies [87]. In fact the smaller the

baby the more important skin-to-skin care appears to be – as it stabilises the tiny baby more effectively than incubation. Through a fine-tuned process of thermo-synchrony, the mother's body temperature falls as baby's rises (while kangarooing father's tend to overheat the baby). Even six hours of such kangarooing following birth are effective in minimising hyper-arousal and the hyper-metabolic state of premature separation, and is advocated even when incubators are available. Intensive first week skin-to-skin kangaroo care also appears to have a positive effect on some mothers, too, increasing the duration of breastfeeding. For these mothers (namely Facilitators) keeping the baby between their bare breasts provides a continuity of the closeness disrupted by the birth, and possibly may help the grieving process if the baby dies. (This link will be studied in the near future). Regulator mothers find it difficult to have the tiny baby in such constant and intimate contact 24 hours a day, and counselling may be needed to sustain the prolonged skin-to-skin contact. Kangarooing is clearly very important in ill-equipped third world countries or rural districts without electricity, and has been used with good results in Columbia, Ecuador and Zimbabwe.

Finally, many **neonatal units** now encourage parental involvement in the care of premature babies as a means of increasing attachment and reducing parental anxiety. Not surprisingly given the scarcity of paternal leave, findings from a study of the degree of participation in caregiving activities show that mothers visit more frequently than fathers (85% vs. 45%) and for longer, although both parents engage in 'social' interactions such as talking, stroking and holding. A mother's greater involvement in cleaning and feeding activities is linked to the duration of her visits [88]. However, among mothers of incubated babies, too, Facilitator/Regulator orientations towards parenting operate differentially, with the former determined to visit her preemie as much as possible since she regards herself as primed by pregnancy to be the best interpreter of her baby's needs; while the latter (among the 15% who visit infrequently) relies on expert staff to care for the fragile baby until its needs are 'regulated' (see Chapters 6, 21 and 31).

0.2.9. Breastfeeding:

The benefits of breastfeeding are undeniable, and this past decade much effort has been devoted to the best way of encouraging and sustaining it. A Cochrane review of 20 separate controlled trials and observational studies in both developing and developed countries as diverse as Finland, Peru, the Philippines, Senegal and the USA provided evidence that babies who were exclusively breastfed for six months had less infectious diseases and grew as well as those given other foods [89]. This is particularly important in those many geographical areas where clean water may not be available for preparation of formula or gruel. It is therefore ironic that in many developing countries formula feeding is still being promoted at the very time when Western societies are raising women's awareness of the benefits of breast-feeding. Currently only 35% of babies world wide are exclusively breast fed during the first four months and malnutrition is highest in South Asia where despite the relatively low HIV infection, only 45% of 0-3 months old babies are exclusively breastfed, and in India, only 20% for 6 months [90]. Nonetheless, in some countries trends are being reversed, as in China, where after 20 years of sexual equality expressed in bottle feeding, breastfeeding was reintroduced by the WHO in 1992 and within one week, every parturient was suckling.

In the UK *the incidence of women breastfeeding at birth* rose from 64% in 1990 to 66% in 1995 to 69% in 2000 (most increases occurred in social class I, and in England and Wales), however by six months only 21% still feed and by nine months this drops to 13% [91]. Initial figures can be misleading - in Brisbane Australia, one 2002 study found that although 92% [!] of participants initiated breastfeeding by 4 months almost 40% had discontinued, and only 28% were breastfeeding exclusively, attributed to their sense of 'self-efficacy' [92]. In addition to class variations, there are considerable racial and ethnic disparities even in the same community. For instance, an American study based on data reported by parents in a national survey showed that the proportion of children ever-breastfed was 60% for whites, 26% among non-Hispanic blacks and 54% among Mexican Americans, decreasing by six months to 27%, 9% and 23% correspondingly [93].

Professionals have a great deal of influence for better or for worse. Seeming indifference of health carers and hospital staff is instrumental in influencing breastfeeding failure [94]. Various targeted programmes have been effective in actively encouraging ongoing breastfeeding, with hospital or community health interventions, the latter including home visits [95], and telephone support by peer counsellors or community health nurses, demonstrating that community health interventions induce longer breastfeeding duration, fewer sick visits, offsetting costs of health care and formula [96]. Similarly, a UK study showed that breastfed babies had 15% fewer GP consultations [97].

To successfully promote breastfeeding, health care professionals must understand the emotional intricacies of this intimate exchange. Some women feel revulsion or anxieties about the erotic experience of breastfeeding while others discover great pride in their capacity, and gain status by their power to make a baby grow. Exclusive breastfeeding can feel depleting – a vital demand on a woman's physical resources, requiring her bodily availability, and drawing on her internal resources. It may interfere with her sexual partnership, her work patterns and relationship with her other children. Some mothers feel endangered by the needy, seemingly insatiable or even 'devouring' baby; indeed, some see breastfeeding as 'cannibalistic'[98]. Conversely, due to her own low self-esteem, a woman may regard her milk as lacking – too 'thin', inferior or even poisonous. The bottle may seem to offer protection and a means of monitoring the baby's intake which feels reassuring to an anxious mother. The fact the amount of milk consumed is <u>measurable</u> is of considerable importance to women who have doubts about adequacy of their own resources or concerns about nourishing the infant - neither starving nor over-stuffing. Indeed, for a mother with eating disorder, or one who dreads her own pathogenic tendencies (reflected in anxieties about the quality of milk), bottle rather than breast feels 'best'. Feeding becomes a rational, shareable, measurable activity. If therapy is not available to the mother, the emotional advantages of bottle feeding outweigh other considerations.

0.2.10. Ethnic minorities, inequalities and disadvantage:

The population of Britain has changed over the past decades. Estimates based on the Labour Force Survey suggest a steep rise in ethnic minorities within the population from 3.9% in 1981, to 5.7% in 1994 to 6.4% in 1997. Since 1991 the Census has included a question of ethnic origins and the latest Census publication 2003 charts the composition of origins of the British ethnic minority population as follows:

28.1% Indian; 16.9% Black Caribbean; 15.4% Pakistani; 7.1% Black African; 6.0% Black other; 5.0% Chinese; 5.5% Bangladeshi; Other Asian 6.5%; Other 9.0%. [99]. Absolute figures have changed, but the geographical distribution of ethnic groups across the country is still as reported previously (pages 22-26).

Circumstances, nutrition and access to services vary within subgroups in each population. For instance, Birmingham Health Authority's 1999 Report cites the babies of women of Pakistani and African Caribbean origin having twice the chance of infant mortality than white European (with poorer material circumstances of income, employment, housing, education and nutrition), and USA figures show similar discrepancies (see section 0.1.4. above on infant mortality). Recent NICE guidelines aim to reduce NHS variation across the country. However, contact with services does not accurately reflect prevalence, as people may opt out of formal health care, and cultural expectations and concepts of illness vary.

Indeed, a recent parliamentary enquiry found that unfortunately the statistics that are routinely available for maternal and perinatal health care in England are inadequate for measuring the level of access to maternity and neonatal services for groups within the population, including minority ethnic groups and socially disadvantaged groups. Maternity service planners and providers are 'impeded in their work' by lack of data on the socio-economic and ethnic status of pregnant women and mothers, making any comparisons of inequalities in health outcomes along with any assessment of equity of access for vulnerable groups, impossible [100]. Similarly, an important gap in knowledge about inequalities in access to maternity care has been created by the lack of information on women who give birth to their babies without having booked any maternity care at all. A survey showed that at least 4% of women receive no antenatal care whatsoever. One study undertaken in the mid-1990s suggested that on average, women from South Asian backgrounds started maternity care later and made fewer visits than white women. The NPEU also found evidence that South Asian women might be up to 70% less likely to be offered/receive prenatal testing for haemoglobin disorders and Down's Syndrome. Information about differences in access to postnatal and infant care was even more limited although evaluations of new initiatives may increase that [101].

Like Healthy Start in the US, the Sure Start programme was introduced in the UK to ensure families in disadvantaged areas had equal access to services and practical help which enable young children to 'flourish from birth'. This includes help from the first antenatal visit, advice on health in pregnancy and preparation for parenthood.

Sure Start programmes are led by local partnerships with strong parental and community involvement to promote the physical, intellectual, social and emotional development of young children through a range of childcare, preschool education and parent support. The programme offers enhanced childcare, play and early learning opportunities and better access to health services - from ante-natal and baby clinics to specialist services for children with special educational needs. Services are delivered in new 'seamless' ways, by staff working together across health, care and education. It is still too early to assess its effectiveness but underpinning this programme is a recognition that children's experiences in the earliest years of their life are critical to their subsequent development (see, section 0.4 below) and that psychosocial adversity is damaging. In keeping with this, the Government has also begun a drive to halve child poverty in 10 years and to eradicate it in 20.

0.2.11. Maternal mortality, reproductive rights and safer childbirth:

Finally, a reminder of our own privileged experience in the West. *Every minute a woman dies from complications related to pregnancy and childbirth and 99% of these deaths occur in the developing world.* Globally, only 62% of births are attended by a skilled attendant [102].

A decade has now passed since the UN 4th Conference of Women, in Beijing and the UN International Conference on Population & Development ICPD in Cairo. The latter concluded with a plan of action adopted by 179 countries – a programme for the empowerment of women, which committed nations to work towards guaranteeing access to reproductive health services for all by 2015. This goal included not only improving provisions but educating women about their rights and choices regarding contraception, pregnancy care and postnatal help. Today, there are still many societies where socio-economic conditions, religious injunctions, male dominance and female ignorance of reproductive rights means that women have no access to contraception. Such 'unsafe motherhood' is a function of both poor health systems and societal causes, including women's powerlessness over their reproductive lives, and dependent status. It is ironic that leaders such as George Bush contribute to this powerlessness by stipulating in 2003 that legal abortion clinics be excluded from multimillion dollar grants to combat HIV/AIDS in developing countries. Abortion is often the last desperate resort for women whose lives cannot stretch to accommodate a(nother) baby.

For example, in Kenya, 700 women daily resort to illegal back street abortions, with 5000 dying annually of complications. In addition to unsafe abortion, haemorrhage, infection, eclampsia and obstructed labour account for 70% of maternal deaths, while over 20% of women die as a result of diseases aggravated by pregnancy, such as malaria, anaemia, TB and increasingly, HIV/AIDS. The rate of maternal morbidity in childbirth is still very high in many parts of the third world, particularly sub-Saharan Africa [103]. In Nigeria, for instance, where it is estimated about 8-10 women die per 1,000 live births, a recent National Health Survey showed that only 31% of deliveries are attended by trained personnel. Many Nigerian women forgo hospital births, preferring to have traditional birth attendants at home, or in a church. Thus, though facilities for obstetric care exist, utilisation of these services during labour is poor. It seems women are deterred by pubic shaving, enema, lithotomy and other restrictive practices. Indeed, systematic reviews highlight potentially harmful hospital birth practices, such as routine episiotomy or ruptured membranes, which possibly increase the risk of HIV transmission to the baby [104]. In societies where women are relatively powerless, hospital nurses may express their own limited autonomy and frustration in punitive behaviour towards their clients. In many places in Africa, *'Better Birth Initiative'* (BBI), a collaborative project is now in place as a strategy to improve care, to reduce maternal morbidity and to encourage utilisation of health facilities [105].

The safest countries for delivering babies include Sweden, Iceland, Slovakia and Austria. High maternal mortality countries, in rank order, include Malawi, Angola, Niger, the United Republic of Tanzania, Rwanda, Mali and Somalia. Due to their physical immaturity, very young women are especially vulnerable to maternity complications, some of which are also related to female circumcision and infibulation which is still widely practiced. Recent findings by WHO, UNICEF and the United Nations Population Fund (UNFPA) show that over her lifetime a woman living in sub-Saharan Africa has a 1 in 16 chance of dying in pregnancy or childbirth. This compares with a 1 in 2,800 risk for a woman from a developed region. The next highest maternal mortality rates globally are in south-central Asia. According to the World Health Organisation, the greatest risk for Asian women in childbirth occurs in Sierra Leone and Afghanistan, where one out of every six childbearing women will die from complications related to pregnancy and childbirth. In India alone, 136,000 women die in pregnancy and childbirth every year [106].

Sadly, women need not die in childbearing. The vast majority of maternal deaths could be prevented if women had better nutrition before conceiving, access to, and use of, skilled care during pregnancy, childbirth and the first month after delivery. Newborns, too, die or are disabled because of poor maternal health or lack of perinatal care, and some <u>one million</u> children are left motherless each year as a result of maternal deaths. These children are three to 10 times more likely to die within two years than children who live with both parents.

In conclusion, maternal mortality is a Human Rights and Equity issue. The Millennium Declaration aimed to reduce maternal mortality by ¾ by 2015, by training skilled birth attendants, improving family planning services and strengthening health systems to provide a 'continuum' of care, including maternity services, abortion and post-abortion care. This will be complemented by educational programmes encouraging self-care by individuals, families and communities and fostering collaborative links with other key primary health care programmes. Babies are the future citizens of any nation. In developed as well as developing societies, providing optimal conditions from the start increases long term physical and mental health and quality of life of the nation.

KEY POINTS:

* Woman-led midwifery provisions - antenatally, during labour and birth, and in establishing lactation involve greater awareness of psychological issues and provision of choice to cater to personal preferences, special needs and diversity of expectations.
*'Consumers' emphasise the importance of choice and control, midwifery competence, communication and compassion throughout pregnancy and birthing in addition to continuity in maternity care.
* Anxieties contribute to increased interventions. Antenatal classes are the ideal place for emotional support and exploration of labour fears and fantasies in expectant parents.
* Midwives work in situations of chronic anxiety and emotional arousal, including evocation of primal material. Peer supervision and experiential group support can mitigate these.
* When socially unconscious representations take the form of cultural beliefs, practices become embedded in routine, ritual and unquestioned local customs.
* The dramatic rise in caesarean rate is ascribed to a combination of organisational defences and socio-cultural pressures with long-term impact of the mother's health, greater cost to the NHS and as yet unknown effects on babie s.
* Social and environmental factors can affect progress of labour, mode of delivery, bonding, and breastfeeding duration yet home births still constitute only 2% of deliveries although desired by 20% of women.

0.3. PERINATAL EMOTIONAL DISTURBANCES:
0.3.1. Partners becoming parents:

Becoming a parent is not easy and rates of perinatal disturbance are high. As this book demonstrates throughout, conception alters the balance in even the most egalitarian couple's relationship, as she grows <u>their</u> baby in her own body. Pregnancy sets in motion a mass of arousing, often contradictory physical and emotional experiences to which each expectant parent responds differently. These interact with trans-generational narratives of childbearing that each partner brings from their own families, informing their current expectations of parenthood and representations of the unborn baby. Labour and birth then bring about further extraordinary experiences which each parturient (and her partner) interprets in her own way. Some women suffer excruciating contractions and humiliating loss of control while others think in terms of surrender and exaltation. Witnessing her pain, her mate's response may accord with or contradict her own. Then with arrival of the baby, a further avalanche of unexpectedly intense emotions erupt - profusions of sadness and rapture, deep troughs of exhaustion, confusion, rage at the heaviness of responsibility and realization that life has changed irreversibly which affects each partner differently. In addition to sleep deprivation, stress, hormonal fluctuations, and after effects of birth, the breastfeeding mother has specific anxieties about her suckling (see 0.2.9.). She may feel accused by the baby's inconsolability, blaming herself irrationally for any unhappiness, attributing it to the quality of her milk as she deems herself unconditionally accountable to the baby who, having grown inside her, knows her innermost secret ambivalence and shortcomings.

The transition to parenthood transforms the interaction between partners [107]. Childbearing is a particularly stressful period for women, with a threefold increased rate of depression within five weeks of delivery [108]. In the 'first world' <u>half the population</u> of new mothers experience milder forms of perinatal disturbance, and at least one in ten mothers suffer severe depression over the first postnatal year. *Like happiness, disturbance, too, is interactive.* While mood fluctuations are associated with hormonal changes in the early postpartum weeks (especially the sudden drop in prolactin, cortisol and HGG), depression over the next year or two is clearly related to psychosocial factors.

In **traditional societies** new mothers are cosseted for the first month or 40 days, mothered and offered special attention and nourishing foods, while experienced helpers assist with baby care (see Chapter 23 section 23.8). Then again, although formal postpartum support (such as the Chinese *peiyue)* protects the mother from exhaustion and ensures transmission of baby-care lore, the close contact with significant others at this vulnerable time, and particularly conflicts with the mother-in-law, may increase rather than reduce postnatal distress [109a]. A poor relationship with in-laws is associated with depression in societies where the woman leaves her own parents to live with her husband's family, or comes under their subjugation. In Turkey, for instance, her dependent position increases the likelihood of postnatal disturbance [109b]. (Also see the case of a Zulu woman 0.3.11). Conversely, western mothers who are sent home from hospital after a few days (or even hours) with an expectation that they, and they alone, will take full exclusive care of the newborn, with no-one to care for them, justly feel unsupported, and many receive little practical help from either parents or in-laws. A woman's archaic relationship with her own (generous and supportive or forbidding) 'internal' mother may take on prime importance even (as perhaps, especially) in the absence of her real, live mother.

Thus, a crucial factor in mental ill-health in westernised societies, relates to the *changing patterns of family relationships with few support networks, and high reliance on the sexual partner.* Intimate relationships often take the form of serial cohabitations (or perhaps, serial disillusionments), and separation is common. In Britain, more than one in three children are born to unmarried parents, and over half these births are registered by the mother alone. Social mobility which erodes extended-family and community networks, also produces increased strain on nuclear households. In the absence of other support-systems a couple's relationship is highly interdependent and partners must often be 'best friends' and mutual carers, as well as lovers. However, birth of a baby skews the once equal relationship, as the bulk of intensely demanding baby-care falls on the mother, whose breasts dispense milk and whose salary is usually more dispensable than the father's. Furthermore, it is a circular process. Day-to-day care affords the mother intimate understanding of the baby's needs who then becomes treated as her responsibility even in the presence of a 'hands on' father who is eager to 'help out', yet lacks exact know-how of the minutiae of the baby's experience. Unlike any other job, a primary carer is 'on call' 24 hours a day. The concentrated parent-baby bond, lonely, and unmitigated by other adults, may be both a burden and provide solace to the mother in the absence of her partner (whose 'working for two' now often involves longer hours on the job). Both parents tend to feel overworked and exploited. He often feels ousted from his previous special place in their relationship. She has lost her position as equal partner. Her loss of earnings often subtly affects the balance of her spending power, as their mutual financial assets now become 'his'. And if she wishes to return to work she must justify doing so by covering costs of child-care, although in the absence of good, reasonably priced day-care, these may swallow up her entire salary. Furthermore, when she does return to work, domestic chores usually remain her domain, as traditional family patterns reassert themselves.

A *Regulator* who resents being demoted from equal 'career woman' to taken-for-granted mother in 'solitary confinement' with her baby, or a *Facilitator* who chooses to stay home, may exercise the only authority remaining to her, by controlling her partner's interaction with the child, allocating tasks or cutting him out - which may suit a *Renouncing* father, but not a *Participator* who wants to be an equal partner in nurturing. Clearly, interactive dynamics vary according the permutations of partners' combined orientation [see Chapters 24 and 25). The couple relationship is irrevocably changed and where intimate communication ceases, many couples split up in the course of the first two postnatal years as their relations deteriorate [110a,b].

In addition, as noted, few parents have had experience with young children, and many feel unprepared for this most important task. **'Parenting programmes'** have flourished in the UK as in the USA, some with an emphasis on parenting skills or education, while others focus on providing support or help towards some in-depth change. A survey of 38 group-based parenting programmes in the UK found three groups of participants according to types of motivation – those who want to 'do the best for their children'; parents of children with behaviour problems of varying severity; and parents with multiple problems, including depression and extremely low self-esteem(some of the latter projects are described in 0.3.7 below). Some, like PIPPINS, offer a structured preventative educational programme beginning in the fourth month of pregnancy (complementing antenatal classes) and providing 17 sessions and a home visit. Most others are community based and operate only postnatally. Some, like Parent Network, operate informal support groups with periodical follow-up modules. Sadly, few programmes involve fathers or focus on the couple relationship as they become parents. A number of programmes operating in the UK were developed in the United States – Family Nurturing Network, Parent Efectiveness Training (PET), Systematic Training for Effective Parenting (STEP), Webster-Stratton Parents & Children Series. The main difference in approach is that unlike the USA where parent education has developed into a separate profession, in Britain facilitators come from a large number of professional backgrounds ranging from psychologists, health visitors, midwives, social workers, teachers, counselors and community workers [111]. In general, aims differ from psychodynamic psychotherapeutic groups in focusing on current conflict resolution, problem solving and behaviour changes geared to improving social and relational functioning rather than seeking to address the residue of past experience in unconscious defences and communications.

0.3.2. Antenatal and postnatal disturbances:

New parents are particularly susceptible in societies in transition, A transcultural study in 15 centres found that postnatal depression or commensurate morbid unhappiness after childbirth are consistently attributed to *loneliness, lack of emotional and practical support, poor relationship with one's partner, family conflict, tiredness and problems with the baby* [112]. The 'spiral of demoralization' is further exacerbated by fragmentation of health care, critical attitudes and conflicting advice from midwives in hospital, and health visitor, GP and relatives at home [113], bereavement and loss in people who are prone to develop depression.

Postnatal depression occurs in fathers too [114a], albeit manifesting differently. One study found that new fathers were more troubled by unresolved past events and difficulties in the relationship and its change after the birth of a child; while new mothers primarily felt distressed by perinatal and infant influenced factors [114b]. The important point is that ***perinatal disturbance is interactive***. A review of twenty recent studies found that commonly depression in one partner is significantly correlated with depression in the other [115]. *As with antenatal depression, vulnerability to postnatal disturbance is increased under conditions of stress and psychosocial adversity, and is significantly related to couple discord.* There is a substantial overlap between depression and anxiety in the prepartum and postpartum periods [116]. Antenatally, the higher incidence of depressive symptoms in inner cities is also associated with poor emotional support, no partner in second or subsequent pregnancy as well as socio-economic disadvantage – unemployment and lack of educational qualifications [117]. In addition to the distress experienced by the woman and her family, maternal antenatal depression has implications for the unborn child, as it is also associated with poor antenatal clinic attendance, low birth weight and preterm delivery [118] and risk-taking behaviours such as smoking and unhealthy eating, which may also signify disregard for, or rejection of an unwanted baby.

Yet antenatal depression often goes unrecognised by professionals. Some suggest it may have a higher prevalence than postnatal depression, which it frequently precedes [119]. Its effects may be crucial for the baby. Although as yet no causal connection can be sustained by available evidence [120], there is a growing body of work linking maternal emotional distress in pregnancy and later behavioural problems in the offspring. In addition to direct effects on the gestating fetus of toxins such as alcohol, nicotine and opiates imbibed by the mother, **antenatal maternal stress** and its concomitant high cortisol levels may be transmitted to the fetus, possibly producing a hyper-reactive baby. A longitudinal study of over 10,000 women examined antenatal disturbance separately from postnatal depression, finding that anxiety in late pregnancy posed an independent risk associated with behavioural/emotional problems in the child at 4 years of age [121]. Similarly, maternal antenatal and postpartum stressors are correlated with the temperament of their three year olds [122]. *Clearly, it is essential to identify antenatal stress and distress and to offer counselling or psychotherapy before the baby is born.*

At this time of intensely demanding responsibility yet greater dependency, the drop in a western woman's self confidence is related to lack of preparation for the most challenging job of all, coupled with her isolation, and sudden demotion from a position of seeming equality. Unlike new fathers, there is still an expectation that 'good' mothers stay home with their infants. Yet contradictions abound and sentimentalisation of the mother-infant bond is often accompanied by societal denigration of her role ['Do you work?' new mothers are asked, as if what they do is not] or an assumption that she will drop her emotional concern for the baby when she rejoins the work force.

In addition, throughout this book I suggest that this is *a hypersensitive period.* The enforced intimacy of sharing her body in pregnancy reactivates unresolved emotional issues which continue to reverberate postnatally, and close contact with a young baby is a highly evocative experience, which re-opens old wounds in vulnerable people. Although many depressed women make very good mothers, micro-analysis of videos reveal disrupted patterns of interaction with their infants, featuring maternal withdrawal and reduced emotional availability, or bouts of intrusion and hostility [123]. In other words, depressed mothers may find i necessary to protect themselves (and/or their babies) from contact that feels too close and endangering.   Risks are elevated with personal predisposition - about one third of all women with postpartum depression have a history of previous depression. Continuous responsibility without opportunities for self-replenishment and economic insecurities also contribute to her distress. A depressed mother may be preoccupied with her own sad childhood experiences. If these resonate with the crying baby's misery she may feel too overwhelmed to respond. The unhappy baby provides an ongoing emotional reminder of her own early suffering, and in addition provokes guilt at the suffering she herself inflicts. Feeling that she has been irrevocably failed as a child and is now constantly failing her own child a depressed mother may become suicidal. Only death seems to offer a resolution to her double anguish.

Other mothers manage to maintain their defences yet are threatened by the risk of baby's raw emotions triggering their own. Feeling persecuted rather than depressed, such a mother may resent mothering as exploitative.   Regarding her baby as intentionally malevolent, she may retaliate in kind. In extreme cases, punitive interaction towards a 'demanding' baby may escalate into verbal abuse, hitting or even infanticide, with the unconscious aim of ridding herself of the needy, greedy or bad reminder of her own repudiated 'baby-self'. Yet other parents may become self-critical and so anxious about possible loss of control in public, that they become agoraphobic and housebound to avoid exposing themselves to a disapproving world. Another form projection takes is the parent who invests all the badness in others and treats the world as unsafe, reluctant to expose the baby (and the baby-part of themselves) to its dangers.

As noted, in nuclear families, the baby is often alone and totally dependent on the primary carer, who constitutes the medium of emotional and physical growth for better or worse. It is in cases such as all these, that the British tradition of home-visits from health visitors is invaluable.

0.3.3. Generative Identity:

To understand the nature of the emotional 'predisposition' to perinatal disturbances, it is necessary to explore subjective meanings attributed to becoming a parent – and their rootedness in generative identity. Each of us is gendered – a sexed psychic structuring we acquire that is partly defined by the society in which we live, and partly inscribed with our own personal formulations filtered through our caregivers and peers. Gender is thus a complex identity and I have proposed the concept of 'generative identity' as one of the components of gender formation:

1. *core gender identity* - the mental representation of oneself as anatomically <u>male or female.</u>
2. *gender role* - relating to <u>feminine or masculine</u> cultural roles and psychosocial ideas of the self
3. *sexual partner orientation* which focuses on articulation of <u>hetero /homosexual desires</u>
4. *generative identity* - the psychic construction of oneself as <u>a potential progenitor</u> [124].

Generative identity means recognising one's own reproductive capacities in the context of basic facts of life. I suggest it is consolidated some time between 18-36 months when the child who previously imagined s/he could be 'everything' now has to accommodate four basic restrictions:

- of *sex* (I am only female or male, not the other sex, neither or both)
- of *genesis* (I am not self-made)
- of *generation* (adults have babies; children cannot)
- of *generativity* (females carry/suckle babies, males impregnate).

For a toddler, these restrictions mean facing painful loss of omnipotence. Relinquishing a belief in bi-sexual over-inclusiveness results in acute feelings of jealousy towards adults and 'penis envy' or 'womb envy' of the other sex. In other words, childhood acquisition of generative identity is a struggle. It entails recognising one's limitations - being only <u>one</u> sex (rather than both and unlimited); being <u>pre</u>-potent (rather than omnipotent) and interdependent (<u>half</u> of future procreative coupling rather than autonomous). *In heterosexual two parent families, it also means accepting that they have a sexual and potentially reproductive union from which the child is excluded.* Depending on emotional circumstances at this crucial time, the growing child may come to accept these facts of life creatively, or overreact by stereotypical adherence to, or rebellious refusal of the reality. Some children feel inhibited by the pressure to comply, or depressed by their losses. While others rebel, becoming engrossed in compulsive re-enactments of omnipotence. Clinical experience suggests that disturbances in acquisition of generative identity are more likely to occur when traumatic external events, especially reproductive disasters in the family, severe bodily trauma or sexual abuse coincide with this critical period of demarcation of the child's own generative potentialities. In adulthood, gender disorders and sexual aberrations (such as sex-change or paedophilia) exemplify denial of, or unresolved issues with one or more of the four fundamental restrictions above.

By contrast, when a child does achieve generative identity several momentous conceptual shifts become possible:

- a shift from being someone else's creature or creation to becoming a potential creator in one's own right
- some children make an imaginative leap, freeing themselves from the biological determinism of sex by utilising <u>psychic</u> cross-gender potentialities. Others adopt formulaic gender identities.
- some children manage a shift from emphasis on physical procreativity of a baby to a more abstract and general notion of creativity. Others persist in treating future reproduction as the height of creativity.

The outcome is that some children grow up with a sense of <u>agency</u>, feeling that irrespective of whether they are male or female, through identification with significant others they can encompass mental characteristics socially attributed to the other sex without having to restrict themselves to being conventionally 'feminine' or 'masculine'. They express their generativity in various non-reproductive ways, rather than having to wait for a baby to fulfil it. In adulthood, comprehensive gratification from their wide-ranging potentialities is such that some people feel no need to embark on parenthood at all. Others do go on to reproduce, with a sense of emotional wellbeing rather than compulsion, but may feel denigrated if confined to a maternal role.

Conversely, when the sense of generative identity remains embedded in procreation, having a child may come to seem to be-all and end-all of adult self-expression. To such a person, diagnosis of infertility can be devastating. Pregnancy when it occurs represents culmination of the precious childhood promise and parenthood is invested with idealised dreams that reality cannot possibly match. Depression commonly follows disappointment with birth of an ordinary (rather than wondrous) baby; or discovery that caregiving is a difficult and demanding occupation (rather than a magical transformative vocation) or when conditions exist that prevent optimal parenting according to their own ideal standards.

To others, having a baby may seem fraught with anxieties relating to fears of usurping their own parents. These may be expressed in an inability to nurture unreservedly, or a strict adherence to the 'rules'. For yet others, parenting may seem antithetical to fulfilment of their own sense of agency and autonomy. Pregnancy is resented, the interdependency of parenthood may feel restrictive. In all these cases, ante or postnatal depression or persecution follow *disillusionment of unrealistic expectations*, rooted in their long-held unconscious sense of generative identity, within their own particular wider psychosocial context.

0.3.4. Different patterns of perinatal disorders:

Perinatal disorders affect women in many cultures. They manifest both ante- and postnatally. Using standardised diagnostic assessment procedures a multi-centre pilot study across Europe and in the USA found that *antenatal 'caseness'* (including depression and anxiety disorders) averaged at 11.8% across cultures, with diverse rates in different places, ranging from 0% in Vienna to 23.3% in Bordeaux [125]. [Significant differences among the various centres are attributed to between sample differences in terms of demographic characteristics, health care delivery systems and local variables such as attachment types, life events and chronic stresses]. The number of people found to have *major postnatal depression* was 12.3% in this study (overall 6 month period prevalence rate). This is almost identical to the 13% mean prevalence calculated in a meta-analysis of 59 postpartum depression studies conducted in European western and non-western countries over the past 20 years [126].

Puerperal Psychoses are much rarer – about 0.2% of the population. Mothers have a 16-fold risk of developing psychotic illness within three months of the birth as opposed to the rest of their lives with highly disturbing hallucinations, delusions and incongruous feelings. This cannot be merely 'hormonal' as fathers also suffer psychiatric morbidity, including 40% of those whose wives are among the two in a thousand women suffering from puerperal psychoses! [127]. The high rate among partners may be caused by 'assortative mating' (vulnerable people choosing each other), or by the emotional effect of one or each of the partners' illness on the other.

In northern Europe perinatal psychiatric disorder is the leading cause of maternal morbidity, and suicide is the leading cause of maternal mortality in the UK [128]. At risk are not only deluded and acutely depressed women but perfectionistic mothers with good social skills, who often go undetected as they hide their severe disturbance under a façade of bright coping mechanisms. Reluctant to admit defeat or to ask for help, there is a high risk of suicide without warning when their defences fail them.

Perinatal disturbance is characterised by emotional upheavals. The predominant symptom for most new parents is exhaustion caused by sleep deprivation and the psychologically demanding experience of fathoming and then meeting a (non-verbal) baby's needs. Disturbance may feature extreme concern for or difficulty in expressing love of the baby, depression and excessive crying with low self-esteem, reduced creativity and impaired concentration. For some this is coupled with distressing fluctuations of mood such as bouts of intense anxiety or guilt and panic states. In others, obsessional-compulsive or persecutory syndromes and paranoia predominate, coupled with doubts, irritability, anger, suspicion, thoughts of harming the baby, difficulty concentrating, or a sense of deprivation or exploitation. In a few, delusions, hallucinations or manic states prevail.

As noted, perinatal disturbance is often associated with a relational problem and in many studies, including cross-cultural ones, poor rapport with the partner (along with adversity and negative feelings about the pregnancy) actually predicts perinatal depression [129]. Again, it is unclear to what degree depression aggravates a poor relationship or is aggravated by it, but numerous studies have found that *lack of a confidante* (whether partner or friend) is associated with depression. At a time when there are so many new experiences and turbulent feelings to process, caregivers need a supportive and trustworthy companion in whom they can confide and from whom they can expect some care, while they give out so much of themselves in nurturing the baby. In the absence of such, a professional counsellor or psychotherapist is a necessity.

Following depression, the most frequent adult diagnoses these days is **post-traumatic stress disorder** (PSTD) manifesting in hopelessness, dissociation and/or excessive vigilance, or anxiety disorders, lasting for months and often years following a traumatic event. These symptoms are heightened during the period of expectant and early parenthood, particularly when vulnerability is rooted in childhood privations and deprivations which are then reactivated by taking on responsibility for a child of one's own. Preoccupation with his/her own early suffering makes a troubled parent unlikely to be emotionally available to the baby. Prolonged pain, loss of self-control and harsh treatment by staff during delivery often constitute retraumatising experiences in their own right. Repressed incidents of sexual abuse or rape may be reactivated during labour, triggering flashbacks of unprocessed trauma in either spouse. Sex may become a nightmare experience for the parturient for months after the birth due to internal bruising, painful episiotomy or a caesarean, in addition to changes in body image changes.

Her partner too, may be inhibited by her leaking breasts (no longer erotic but matronly and belonging to the baby) or the memory of having watched her go through the agonies of birth. Traumatised people often feel the need to avoid mental pain by discharging rather than experiencing it. Traumatised parents thereby often inflict similar experiences of emotional, sexual or physical abuse on their offspring as a means of momentarily relieving themselves of internal distress.

A further common disturbance is use of vulnerable body-systems to express psychic complaints through **stress related symptoms/illness** such as headaches, digestive problems, allergies and exhaustion, all of which affect the capacity to fully engage in work, love or play. Pregnancy, with its altered physiological state lends itself to psychosomatic expressions of distress thereby bypassing psychological understanding of painful issues. Increasingly, studies of expectant fathers reveal they too may express distress psychosomatically, often presenting to their GP with pregnancy-like symptoms of nausea or backache.

It is noteworthy that the distribution of emotional disturbance is sex-related. Traditionally depression has been cited as twice as common in women than men. This difference has been accounted for by women worldwide experiencing greater poverty, inferior social roles and sex discrimination, which lead to more negative life events, including violence and abuse [130a] Put differently, the tendency to depression in women has been linked to their greater experiences of loss, humiliation and family entrapment [130b]. However, based on evidence from studies, the Royal College of Psychiatrists suggests that depression is just as common in men but women are twice as likely to be diagnosed and hence treated [131]. Other disturbances in men tend to take the form of substance abuse, alcoholism, suicide (especially between 15-34) and violent enactments which affect both wives and children. Women are said to experience a higher incidence of anxiety and panic attacks, PTSD and eating disorders. However, women also tend to be better at requesting therapy, and do so for relational issues, low self-esteem, bodily vulnerability and/or unexpressed anger.

0.3.5. Antenatal distress and the 'Placental paradigm':

During pregnancy, the expectant mother provides nutrients and excretes the baby's waste products through the placental connection. I have suggested that for many pregnant women this informs a mental image of the emotional connection between herself and her tethered baby. Depending on her self-esteem and experience, she may regard herself as an abundant or inadequate nurturer linked to a benign baby or to a parasitic invader. Her self-regard inevitably contains some residues of her own experiences of being mothered, while the image of her unborn baby represents not only a fantasy child, but one unconsciously imbued with aspects of her own (imagined) baby-self.

While most pregnant women experience a variety of mixed feelings fluctuating over the course of a day if not an hour, some take a fixed and intense stance to this continuous placental connection with the baby. A fixed attitude may be composed of one of the perinatal syndromes (section 0.2.6), an exacerbation of her customary tendencies. For instance, a woman who is quite fastidious may intensify her *obsessional type defences* at this point, when her usual means of regulating closeness become threatened by the ultra-intimacy of having two people in one body. *Compulsive actions* fail to ward off the dangers of invasion, and the perfectionist struggle to keep internal good and bad aspects apart is imperilled by the uncontrollable intruder. In addition there is the uncertainty (s/he may be less than perfect), and the threat of revelation, as the baby 'knows' her inside out and when born, will reveal her own hidden faults. *Intrusive thoughts* about controlling or punishing the baby now break through her defences, posing the risk of enacting these antenatally in physical attacks on the fetus, or in postnatal violence or sexual abuse (for clinical examples see 'placental paradigm', [132]). These are not rare conditions as between 20-40% of depressed mothers also report obsessional thoughts about harming the child [133]. For teaching purposes the various positive and negative permutations of these 'fixed' representations on the '**Placental Paradigm**' may be charted as follows:

Self-as-mother	Baby	
+	+	*idealisation*
-	+	*depression*
+	-	*persecution*
-	-	*anxiety*
+¦-	+¦-	*obsession*
+/-	0	*detachment*

0.3.6. A spectrum of perinatal syndromes:

For some pregnant women, having another (possibly male) growing inside her body blurs or intensifies distinctions between self and other, female and male, outer and inner, past and future with attendant anxieties and emotional disturbance. Motherhood, too, causes a crisis of identity as a woman finds herself in a state of internal contradictions and external unpredictability, neither able to return to her previous life nor yet to foresee the future priorities. Distress takes many forms. Although development of the popular Edinburgh Postnatal Depression Scale (EPDS) has focused research on postnatal depression, let us not overlook the full spectrum of perinatal disturbance, which occurs with some overlaps between categories. These are based on my own clinical experience or supervision of therapists working with women, both self-referred or sent by clinics:

Depressive disorders
- a range of symptoms, including feelings of despair, emptiness, guilt, inferiority and self-criticism, mainly about being insufficiently nurturing in pregnancy or a 'bad' mother;
- inhibition of thinking; libido and sleep disturbances, eating disorders and psychomotor retardation which may exacerbate the progress of pregnancy or process of caring for a baby.

Persecutory syndromes
- social and other phobias [contamination anxiety; tokophobia (fears about labour and birth);
- feared depletion/exploitation by the fetus or baby; claustrophobia, agoraphobia];
- generalised anxiety disorders and panic states (usually 'free floating anxieties which attach themselves to any 'hook';
- paranoia (irrational fears and projections making others or external events a source of danger).

Schizoid withdrawal
- defensive detachment (avoidance of feelings);
- dread of intimacy (desire for but fear of closeness);
- intellectualisation (replacement of emotion with rationality).

Obsessive-compulsive syndromes
- ruminations (mentally going round in circles);
- ritualistic activities (magical thinking and repetitive deeds to avoid danger);
- intrusive thoughts ('out of the blue' pictures, ideas or instructions).

Psychosomatic and behavioural manifestations

- hyperemesis (extreme nausea/vomiting), compulsive, anorexic and bulimic eating disorders;
- alcohol, nicotine and substance abuse (escape from, or avoidance of, mental pain);
- violence, self-harm and direct attacks on the fetus by the woman or her partner (action as a means of ridding oneself of internal stress).

Manic mood disorders
- idealisation (of pregnancy, motherhood and/or baby);
- grandiosity (a sense of omnipotent capacities or excessive generosity);
- psychomotor excitation (rapid thought, speech, actions).

0.3.7. Specific programmes for mothers at risk:

Not surprisingly, women who are worn down by persistent socio-economic deprivation and chronic oppression are often apathetic, demoralised and powerless, displaying emotional numbness, low self-confidence, depression and insensitivity to, and/or over-reliance on, their children for support. *Increased life stresses and lack of social support raise the incidence of depression.* For instance, the prevalence of postnatal depression in Khayelitsha, a township near Cape Town, is 34.7% [134], almost triple that among the white middle class population. Similarly, in Chile, the rate rose to 36.7% in the lower socioeconomic strata of Santiago [135]. Studies from south Asia demonstrate how severe poverty, social stressors and societal sex-preference act as predisposing causes of perinatal disturbance. A depressed woman's poor nutritional intake affects her baby's development during pregnancy. Postnatally, baby girls are found to be especially at risk of under-nourishment in cultures which favour males, suggesting the need for intervention programmes that focus on improving maternal mental health alongside those targeting infant nutrition [136]. And political stressors and chronic anxiety also contribute to high levels of postnatal distress – for instance, an Israeli study found a prevalence rate of 22.6% [137]. In addition, hidden urban stressors relate to spatial and practical drawbacks and dangers in domestic, community and public spaces - usually planned, designed and implemented by men with little regard for safety, ease of transport, shopping, surveillance of children at play, female cameraderie, use of pushchairs, etc.

In common, all intervention programmes for high risk mothers and traumatised or overburdened families aim to enhance quality of life and reciprocal interaction. Most recognise the intergenerational repetition of unintegrated experiences. Depending on the nature of the problem, treatments may take the form of **brief crisis intervention** or ongoing **case management** of individual families. Some therapeutic projects focus on the immediate interaction between parent and infant, making links with the past and increasing parental awareness of the baby as a sensitive person with feelings and a mind (also see 0.3.11.2 below). This may be achieved by the therapist modelling appropriate receptiveness. In some cases video feedback is used to show-up mismatched sequences of parent-child interaction, and to encourage intrusive carers to tone down their pursuit, or inactive parents to increase their engagement. Similarly **psycho-education** fostering age-appropriate expectations may help carers to relate more realistically. **Psychodynamic approaches** offer the parent an opportunity to have someone listen intently while s/he reflects upon feelings, which is restorative in itself, and, when internalised, enables the parent to similarly listen to their child (see 0.3.2.10-11 below). **Community programmes** such as Sure Start in the UK and CBFRS (Community-based Family Resource Service Programs) in the USA offer a range of collaborative and interdisciplinary community services, some of which are targeted towards families at risk. [Fathers complain that in their hours of operation and activities, these tend to exclude them]. Most **home-based therapeutic interventions** originate in Selma Fraiberg's combination of social-work methods and psychoanalytic understanding [see Chapter 27.3]. Randomised trials of supportive home-based counseling by health visitors or paraprofessionals health care workers show twice as much recovery in the treatment group compared to the control group [138a]. Similarly a Swedish study found that brief training for healthcare workers in non-directive counseling produced excellent results when visiting mothers at home, even for as little as ½ hour over a period of eight weeks [138b]. Some programmes involving home visits may use eclectic practices. For instance the Solihull approach in the Midlands, offers an innovative combination of psychoanalytic and behavioural theories in interventions with disadvantaged families at points of developmental challenges or 'derailments' [138c]. Another 'mixed' example is a UCLA project for high risk mothers offering home visits plus a 'relation-based' therapeutic group which made a significant positive impact on maternal responsiveness and encouragement of autonomy in the child, and after two years of therapy verbally persuasive control replaced physically coercive methods [138d]. **Family programmes** attempt to 'optimalise' the relationship by helping parents recognise the child's developmental milestones, emotional, linguistic and social needs, either through health visitors in the UK or home visits by child development specialists in the USA [139]. Recent interventions involve training health visitors in running parenting groups using a Webster Stratton programme for 10 weeks. When resources are scarce, home-outreach or individual sessions are often too costly or time consuming, and isolated mothers benefit from community support. **Mother-infant group work** is effective in establishing a support network. These may target hard-to-reach or deprived mothers, or those with personality disorders. Help is usually offered in the context of community based mother-child play groups. Or toddler's stimulation groups while mothers receive community-liason supervised work-rehabilitation. A British project 'Mellow Mothering' set up a community base on a troubled impoverished estate, delivered the programme within the immediate territory, teaching the principles of good interactive childcare and facilitating play (an activity which many mothers had not experienced in childhood). Disturbed women were taught dietary standards, cooked communal meals, and were lent a video camera to film a neighbour at home feeding and hair-washing her baby, and then discussed each others' observed interaction in a small therapeutic group. Evaluation proved positive and all these personality disordered mothers (many of whom had previously had children removed while on the 'at risk' register) kept their babies [140a]. Similarly the Charles St. parent and baby unit and various NEWPIN **drop in centres** are examples of British projects specifically designed for women with postnatal depression offering befrienders, peer group support and 24 hour telephone contact, as well as play facilitation for the babies and a therapeutic support group and personal development programme for the mothers encouraging exploration of underlying problems [140b]. A Swedish **therapeutic centre** 'Maskan' (meaning a 'dropped' stitch in knitting) has also been in existence for over 15 years, utilising a combination of twice weekly three hour groups and individual psycho-educational and psychotherapeutic methods to treat relationship disturbances between mothers and their babies during the first year [140c]. Other examples are of **centres for child development,** such as one in New York, which sees self-referred mothers and their children in small groups, holds psychoanalytically informed discussion groups and provides interventions for self-referred mothers re-experiencing conflicts, deficits or impairments which impinge on the child [141a]. Or another in Cleveland, Ohio which provides a nursery group and Mother-infant intervention consists of support, education, interpretation and developmental help [141b], and a similar set up at the Anna Freud Centre in London [141c] . The Cassell Hospital in London offers a live-in **Psychotherapeutic Community for the whole family** to deal with issues such as child abuse [142a], while the Marlborough Family Service in London offers evaluation and therapeutic intervention for multiple disturbed families seen simultaneously [142b]. [Psychodynamic forms of psychotherapy will be dealt with below (section 0.3.11)].

It is estimated that 11% of women are substance abusers. **Drug misuse** in pregnancy and early motherhood is a complex problem and care management cannot be constructed in isolation from the social and psychological factors contributing to that lifestyle. Realistically treatment goals hope to focus on harm reduction rather than 'cure' [143]. However, antenatal work can be beneficial. A recent study showed that drug addicted pregnant women who attended even four brief motivational therapy sessions of behavioural reinforcement of drug abstinence gave birth to higher birth-weight babies compared to mothers who did not comply with the full therapy course (attending none to three sessions) [144]. A review of 55 similar multi-component programs for expectant mothers concluded that discriminatingly targeting women with specific risk factors is effective in reducing prevalence of drug abuse, alcohol and tobacco use, with raised birth weight [145]. However, as the early weeks of gestation are the most crucial ones, prevention programmes must find ways of reaching women <u>before</u> they conceive, by using schools and media to address issues of growth deficiencies, and publicising the effects of smoking in pregnancy, or alcohol related neuro-developmental defects and Fetal Alcohol Syndrome (FAS).

Various intervention programmes focus on **psychotic mothers.** For instance, CHILD, an American project includes home visits, stimulation groups for toddlers and preschoolers, community liaison and three times a week 'mother-baby school', in which the focus is on modelling and helping mothers in the group identify their babies' needs and reinforcing effective age appropriate interactions [146]. Other projects like the 'Threshold nurseries' in the US for psychiatrically disturbed mothers living in 'socially disorganised families and chaotic communities', promotes a supervised work-rehabilitation course and quality day-care for their children, aiming to reduce their high (35%) rate of rehospitalisation.

0.3.8. Fathers:

Although her swelling body galvanises interest in the childbearing woman's experience, fathers too are deeply moved by their partner's pregnancy and birth. Nine out of ten fathers in the UK attend the delivery indirectly of their babies and whether resident in the home or absent, have a crucial influence on infant mental health. In non-traditional societies such as our own, fathering, like contemporary mothering, follows subjective choices, with each man's parenting orientation dictated by his own conscious beliefs and unconscious identifications. We may distinguish some approaches to fathering as follows (also see Chapters 11 and 24): drawing on primary identification with his archaic mother a *Participator* father wishes to be fully involved with early child care. The *Renouncer* father would rather wait until the child is older. (This paternal orientation is based on a traditional male/female divide that renounces femininity and regards pregnancy and early nurturing as the province of women). A *Reciprocator* father appears to be a mixture of the other two but unlike them, bases fathering neither on identification with mother or baby, nor emulation of a powerful father and dis-identification with femininity, but on personal assimilation of qualities of all his significant relationships, including both mother and father, siblings, teachers and other caring figures (see Generative Identity, 0.3.3.). His capacity for nurturing draws on sympathy which enables him to switch perspective and reflect on the emotional effect he is having on his loved ones, and they on him. Research findings show that fathers prefer play to caretaking and have a distinctive interactive style of play ('roughhousing' type stimulation vs. maternal containment). However, other findings point to similar styles and degree of attunement. Once again, these conflictual reports do not take account of different parental orientations.

In addition to personal orientations, there are mutual influences and forces within a couple's relationship that shape their respective parental interactions, along with societal demands (see Chapter 24.3). During pregnancy, unlike his pregnant woman for a man taking on the role of Father leaves no physiological traces but entails psychologically assuming his virile manhood within himself. For men who have resolved their basic early conflicts and relinquished untenable desires, parenthood offers a rich opportunity to further their relational capacities. For others, paternity may continue to feel fraught – feeling they are being put to the test or accompanied by guilt and a sense of danger at usurping the archaic father of their own childhood. An expectant father may also experience a poignant sense of exclusion. Feeling displaced by the twosome inside his partner's body he may try to appropriate the pregnancy. This may reflect his unconscious pervasive longing for the blissful state of 'oneness' that he enviously feels the fetus has achieved. For men who have not satisfactorily consolidated their generative identity, fatherhood may retrigger unresolved envy of the female capacity for childbearing, and in extreme Participators, anger and frustration at being dependent on the pregnant partner to produce (and then breastfeed) the baby, rather than being able to omnipotently do it all himself. Conversely, an extreme Renouncer may feel threatened by the painful or needy feelings the baby arouses in him, and resents the care his partner gives the baby, experiencing it as a risk to his special position (as he may have felt usurped by a younger sibling in childhood). Some fathers may even prohibit the mother from breastfeeding. Fathers who are unable to address these disturbing feelings in themselves may find them reverberating uncontrollably in their ongoing relationships with both mother and child, in some, escalating in envious and violent attacks (see section 0.3.8 below).

At this critical point in their lives, most new fathers experience some confusion, concern for their partner, frustration and helplessness in the face of multiple responsibilities, uncertainty about the future, anger at the many sacrifices and disrupted family, social and leisure activities, not to mention worry about financial problems. Whereas in the early months of fathering a man's relationship to his own parents is vital, later in the first postpartum year the dynamics and functioning of the parental couple are a more significant predictor of depression [147]. In addition, confidence in the reciprocal partnership is important. Men in stepfamilies and partners of single mothers have been found to have higher levels of depressive symptoms than those in traditional families [148], and unskilled occupations and prior poor social functioning have been identified as significant risk factors for depression in new fathers [149].

As noted many men go on to develop postnatal disturbances - a quarter of men with depressed partners develop depression themselves, and this incidence increases significantly when the woman is severely depressed. Up to 50% of the partners of women admitted to psychiatric mother-and-baby units meet diagnostic criteria for psychiatric morbidity, compared with only 4% of men whose partners are not depressed [150]. *Most of these fathers suffer major depressive disorder and generalized anxiety disorders.* Paternal depression is not short lived. Of the 10% of fathers who are depressed when the baby is 6 weeks old, more than half remain depressed at 6 months [151] and 60% of fathers diagnosed with psychiatric disorder at 2 months postpartum are still symptomatic at 6 month follow-up [152a]. Paternal depression is related to both internalising and externalising psychopathology in adolescents, and maladaptive father-child relationships [152b].

In sum, a new father's postnatal emotional reappraisals, conscious goals, nurturing capacities and immediate priorities are rooted within the context of his own internal world. How he has processed his past will determine how he faces the changing configurations of his intimate relationships, with his parents, the woman and child(ren) in his life. And the external pressures of new social, work and domestic demands, and loss of (usually female) earnings at time of the family's greatest material expenses. Most research focuses on mothers and knowledge of the emotional influence of fathers on their children's development is minimal. However the evidence from two-parent families suggests they do play an important role, especially through play, and interestingly, are better predictors of offspring's adult adjustment than mothers. Further investigations are needed using specifically devised paternal measures rather than those borrowed from exploration of motherhood [152c]. In my view, to increase understanding, research must also differentiate between diverse orientations to fatherhood.

0.3.9. Disturbance and violence in the relationship:

The transition to parenthood involves changes, pressures and role adjustments which crucially affect the couple relationship (see Chapters 13, 14, 15, and 24, 25 and 27). Their lives are irrevocably transformed with the birth but demands escalate and continue to build as the baby grows. *Many studies find that the increase in couple morbidity peaks for both partners at one year, when over half of all new parents are depressed!* As noted, a non-supportive partner increases the likelihood of depression in new mothers (see 0.3.2.-4.). Not surprisingly, the same is true of new fathers. A literature review of twenty research studies found that during the first postpartum year, the incidence of paternal depression ranged from 1.2% to 25.5% in community samples, and from 24% to 50% among men whose partners were themselves experiencing postnatal depression [153]. [This rises to almost 60% when antenatal depression is included]. In other words, a man whose partner is depressed, is unlikely to find her supportive at this time of his own vulnerability, and he in turn may be unable to provide the support she needs in stressful early motherhood.

Main predictors of **postnatal depression** in both men and women:

- a personal history of depression
- depression in partner, either antenatally or during the early postpartum period
- a dysfunctional couple relationship.

The high prevalence of parental postpartum depression clearly has implications for the well-being of the child. Research has focused on ways in which maternal depression negatively affects mother–infant interaction and child development [154a] (and see 0.4.7 below). A healthy parent can buffer the effects of a depressed one, and infants of depressed mothers are known to have more positive interactions with their non-depressed fathers [154b]. However when <u>both</u> parents experience depressive symptoms during the postpartum period, the interaction between the mother's and father's respective depressions may further the risk to their child's development.

As noted above, women tend to experience more depression, anxiety and panic attacks while in men disturbance tends to take the form of substance abuse, alcoholism, verbal and violent enactments. Recently, in addition to acknowledging ante and postnatal distress in fathers, there is growing recognition of **violence during pregnancy** – 30% of domestic violence either begins or intensifies during pregnancy and is associated with increased rates of miscarriage, low birth weight, premature birth, fetal injury and death. In the UK, a statement by the Public Health Minister in October 2004 promised to introduce routine antenatal clinic enquiry into domestic abuse, and referral for help.

Violence unleashed during pregnancy may be embedded in a culture of male control over women and their bodies. It may be a continuation of a more generalised domestic abuse cycle (*battering? contrition? 'honeymoon'? re-escalation of violence*) or a new phenomenon, in which the man specifically directs his aggression at his pregnant partner's belly. In these latter cases, an expectant father experiences bouts of uncontrollable anger, stemming either from envy of her creative capacity or jealousy of the intimacy of mother and fetus. While etiological pathways vary, the relationship to his own father may have been marked by a real absence or an emotional withdrawal by a man who failed in his paternal role. In such a case, the growing boy's closeness with an over-involved mother may have been aided and abetted by her belittling the father's authority and competence. The expectant father now rages against feeling placed in that 'excluded' position during his partner's pregnancy, and his violence is a demonstration of both his childish fury and a cruel parody of 'manly' domination. In others, violence directly imitates paternal violence in their own childhood, in identification with the brutality of their own sadistic father. Without therapy the underlying deep-seated problems and lack of empathy will remain unresolved.   Group sessions for *'anger management'* offer a platform for exchange, and teach 'conflict resolution' strategies for abusive men, some of whom have suspended sentences. These courses foster welcome self-restraints for people who as children lacked guidance about containing their aggressive impulses. However the courses fail to engage with unconscious issues that resolved, could enable such a man to become a reasonable father to his own child. Individual psychotherapeutic sessions or group therapy can allow space for exploration of the issues underpinning violence. *Couple therapy* may provide the necessary help to find a different balance between the partners. This is crucial, as at this time of increased dependency and vulnerability many a pregnant woman chooses to stay with her abuser for the sake of the child, believing his promises of change, or worse, accepting his excuse ['You drive me to violence but I still love you'] and abjectly agreeing that it is her own fault.

However, many opt for lone motherhood. The National Survey of Mental Health conducted by the Australian Bureau of Statistics in 1997 found that lone mothers were more likely than partnered women to have experienced domestic physical and sexual violence, and childhood sexual abuse, which accounted for a greater prevalence of depressive and anxiety disorders in this group [155] (and probably explains their lone status as a distrust of or abandonment by men). Because of the private nature of the true scale of domestic violence is unknown. In the USA, it is estimated that at least 20% of pregnant women are subjected to violence, and their children under-five are emotionally affected by exposure to this aggression, which undermines trust in attachment figures [155b]. However, the damage is already done antenatally. Women who experience violence during pregnancy reveal more negative prenatal representations of the baby, characterised by less flexibility and caregiving sensitivity, greater anxiety, and a lower sense of self-efficacy. These expectant mothers also tend to interpret fetal movements as abusive, or view the baby as aggressive 'like his father' [156], which sets the scene for a distorted relationship. *Once again, to be effective, preventive intervention work must begin antenatally, either to help the mother leave the abusive relationship, or, in less pathological relationships, couple counselling with both parents (and complementary therapy for the male partner) offers motivated expectant parents a chance to work through some of the pernicious interactive tensions before the birth of their child.*

0.3.10 Reproductive trauma and unsymbolised/unresolved losses:

Finally, in all these emotional disturbances, we must bear in mind that human behaviour is very complex, reflecting a variety of over-determined meanings, stemming from multiple past and present conscious and unconscious sources. While there is no one-to-one correspondence, *because of the fundamental nature of reproduction, becoming a parent serves as an acute catalyst, reactivating unintegrated denied, disavowed and/or unprocessed memories of being parented in one's own childhood, some of which can never be retrieved.*

Where there is a history of reproductive trauma in the family of origin, including unsymbolised ordeals or ungrieved losses (such as early death of a sibling, secrecy around maternal abortions or miscarriage, infertility and inexplicable absences and loss) these may be re-enacted by the next generation in physical symptoms or actions, bypassing conscious reflection. As case histories illustrate, the ungrieved 'presence of absence' is a potent factor that can operate after many years. Reactions to an unmourned stillbirth can erupt decades later. Similarly, unprocessed grief may materialise in birth of a replacement child. Unconsciously absorbed maternal secrets may motivate a daughter to give up her baby for adoption. And guilt-ridden non-representation of an abortion may result in a couple's psychogenic infertility - all reflecting the internalised presence of an unresolved absence or loss [157]. The subtlety of multigenerational transmission of trauma is revealed in a detailed clinical case showing the devastating effect of a mother's termination of a (female) Down's fetus. Following this abortion she unwittingly began to repeat with her small son the painful experience she herself had experienced in early childhood, of being emotionally abandoned by her own depressed mother after the death of a female child. Unconsciously appropriated and annihilated by his mother, the traumatised little boy felt unwillingly transformed into a girl, with attendant confusion of gender [158].

Therapy is essential when pregnancy, early parenting and reproductive events revitalise people's unresolved traumatic experiences with their own carers. These may include incestuous abuse, cruelty and violence, neglect, abandonment or invalidation, or more subtle forms of dehumanisation in which the child's only solution is dissociation, fragmentation or taking the guilt upon his/her self. The sudden release of unconscious forces in early parenthood may flood the person with traumatic flashbacks, overwhelming rage or self-hatred and/or terrifying helplessness which inhibits their adult capacities, and may trigger re-enactments, inflicting their own fears and sense of rejection on the infant in their care with detrimental and long lasting effects.

0.3.11. Talking therapies:

People experiencing perinatal distress, whether expressed emotionally or in physical or interactional enactments, benefit from therapeutic support. Acceptability of psychological therapies varies cross-culturally, and alternative or complementary treatments are often sought in preference to, or in conjunction with, established treatments. *Therapies are divided between psychotherapeutic, biomedical and traditional health care systems according to local explanatory models of mental disorder.* We see this clearly in a case study of Nonhahle, a 19-year-old Zulu girl whose family became concerned because she ignored her 5 week old baby, saying she heard a female voice telling her to leave her partner. First she was taken to the hospital to cure her insomnia and headache, but then to the diviner as her strange behaviour was attributed to bewitchment by her man's new girlfriend. In hospital she was diagnosed with puerperal depression and given antipsychotic medication, while the Insangoma referred her to an herbalist who also met with the partner and insisted that he have no further contact with the new girlfriend. At follow up two weeks later, she had completely recovered but continued taking a small daily dose of chlorpromazine [159]. However, this is not restricted to other cultures. In addition to ethnic minority groups in western cultures who continue to visit traditional healers sharing their value systems, there are currently 18,000 spiritual healers in Britain, and many are consulted alongside conventional medicine. Similarly, many alternative treatments, such as hypnotherapy, acupuncture, aromatherapy, yoga, reflexology, reiki, cranial osteopathy are utilised alongside mainstream services during pregnancy and labour. And bright light therapy, massage, relaxation to produce improvements in postnatal mood. Although symptoms may be somatised by some, where emotional disturbance is recognised and professional help is sought by westernised cohorts, 'talking' therapies are the preferred option [160].

Women with major mental illnesses such as schizophrenia, schizoaffective or bipolar disorders are particularly at risk for decompensations during pregnancy, and the illness is often complicated by substance abuse, resulting in poor prenatal care. Although some do require hospitalisation and psychotropic medication 'talking cures' such as supportive counseling or psychotherapy are also regarded as a preferential treatment option for perinatal <u>psychiatric</u> disorders since most antipsychotic medications cross the placental barrier in pregnancy and prevent breastfeeding postnatally [161a,b]. But when maternity is hyped up as a joyous process, shame and fear of stigma prevents many depressed mothers from seeking help [162] and take-up rates for treatment vary geographically, as do mental health care and perinatal psychiatric provisions [163]. Furthermore, referrals may not be forthcoming as maternal emotional disturbance is often under-diagnosed by paediatricians [164], and overlooked by GPs and health visitors [165]. Some clinicians question the usefulness of postnatal depression as a separate diagnostic category [166]. But whatever the similarities across depressions, in other periods, the juxtaposition of parenting a young baby and depression is a toxic combination for all concerned, and it is important that professionals learn to detect postnatal disturbance.

0.3.11.1.   Psychoanalytic Perinatal Therapy -
individual, couple, group or family:

Throughout this book it is emphasised that to alleviate mental distress and disorders, ideally psychotherapy should begin antenatally and continue for some time after the baby arrives. Such *perinatal psychotherapy* can reduce postnatal disturbance in expectant mothers experiencing emotional overload. It can modify negative representations of the baby, pregnancy or motherhood; and disentangle reactivated troubling experiences of trauma or previous loss from the current situation. Treatment may vary from **individual sessions** of brief psychodynamic psychotherapy before the birth, usually continuing after the birth with the baby, and/or longer term psychoanalytic treatment. Other options are preventive **antenatal group interventions** in pregnancy for women at risk which may or may not continue postnatally.

Principles of Perinatal Psychotherapy:
- utilising the perinatal permeability of internal boundaries in pregnancy
- making the most of the high motivation to become a better parent by reworking unresolved issues before the birth

- processing 'contagious arousal' and the parent's own reactivated infantile 'procedural' memories, thereby integrating these to prevent repetitious enactments and attachment problems
- modifying negative unconscious representations during pregnancy

before these are imposed on the baby

Couple therapy during pregnancy may tackle seemingly irresolvable antagonisms between the partners, relating to unequal division of emotional responsibilities, or mismatched unconscious fantasy baby or discrepant concepts of childrearing.

Every couple acquires an identity of its own. Sexual partners are often unconsciously selected for their resemblance to early 'objects' of desire and each partner brings to the intimate relationship their cumulative past including emotional relationships, unresolved conflicts and unfulfilled cravings that they wish to satisfy alongside hopes of adult development (see Chapter 15). *Healthy unions which respect difference and allow each partner to flourish, facilitate further growth and self-individuation within the partnership despite the counter-pull to repeat and gratify unprocessed archaic desires.* In others, enmeshment of the couple's unconscious contracts is thrown into turmoil by pregnancy, and if untreated, the pathological nature of their interaction may try to enlist the new baby in fantasy enactments.

This may continue postnatally in **parent-infant therapy** (see 0.3.11.2 below) to prevent parenting dysfunction consolidating into an intractable interactional pattern. Psychodynamically orientated **family therapy** similarly focuses on unconscious patterns within the interactive 'system', not only between the partners but with each of their offspring [167]. [This differs from cognitive-behavioural family intervention programmes which aim to improve parental capacities (see 0.3.7. above)]. Finally, disturbed parents with particular parenting difficulties may benefit from specialised **group therapy** for parents [168] or group therapy for depressive mothers.

3.11.2. Parent-Infant psychotherapy:

The 15 year old message of this book advocating prevention, identification of high risk groups and early treatment is finally being heeded. In recent years therapies which directly engage parent/s and infant together, have arisen out of the growing recognition both of the crucial importance of the relationship, the family as a 'system' in which the representational world of the parents is constitutive of the baby's mind. Sadly, as yet there is very little prophylactic antenatal therapeutic work. However, over the past decade in Britain, psychoanalytically informed Parent-Infant treatments have been developed by the Under-5 section of the Tavistock Clinic, the Anna Freud Centre Parent-Infant-Project and the Infant-Parent-Clinic in London. Babies are referred with a variety of compla ints that are seen to indicate family disturbance. In the first year of life these may take the form of *'behaviour disorders'*: sleep problems [169], incessant rocking, breath-holding, persistent masturbation, head-banging and other forms of self-harm. Symptoms may manifest in *'disorders of mood'*: persistent crying and screaming [170], whining and misery, apathy and withdrawal or even autistic features. Or a range of *feeding disorders* [171] such as failure to thrive, food refusal, pica (eating non-food substances) and rumination (chewing regurgitated food) or illnesses traditionally termed *'psycho-somatic disorders'*: vomiting, diarrhoea, constipation, asthma, eczema, some allergies and unusual susceptibility to infectious illness.

Psychoanalytically oriented parent-infant therapies all share an assumption that the internal world of the child is constituted in interaction with primary others, that his/her ability to appraise the emotions of others means that emotional disturbances in the parent/s, their negative representations of the baby and unconscious psychic defences all affect the developmental process, in some cases, causing its 'derailment'. In the sessions, the therapist observes the moment to moment give and take with the infant, and makes connections between this exchange and the emotional climate of the parent's childhood as remembered and reported. However, it is difficult to reach the deeper, unknown 'procedural' memories reactivated in the parent through 'contagious arousal' (see 0.4.6). Some emotional understanding of inter-generational transmissions of which the family members may be unaware comes about through the therapist's own counter-transference feelings during the sessions. For instance, one therapist describes how while listening to the parents' story, and trying both to engage them and to establish the baby as partner in the therapeutic process, she finds her identifications oscillating from parent to baby to grandparent during their interaction [172]. Whatever the specific techniques employed, in general, early sessions are utilised for observing the interaction, assessing risks to the baby's development, evaluating parental defensive functioning and their capacity for change. Gradually, the therapist explores links with the adults' own childhoods, and by stressing their strengths provides a generous model and an incentive for them to become more aware and self-reflective of their own negative as well as positive contributions to the relationship with the baby.

There are many commonalities and some variations in the techniques of parent-infant treatment across the world – as practiced in countries as far apart as Sweden [173], Australia [174], Japan [175] and South Africa [176]. Clinical practice may also vary locally. For instance, a Canadian study compared two different parent-infant interventions (infant led 'Watch, Wait and Wonder' and traditional Psychodynamic Psychotherapy) conducted weekly for five months in Toronto. Both had positive effects in reducing infants' symptoms and parental stress, which were maintained at 6 month follow-up. However the WWW group was found to <u>immediately</u> decrease maternal depression and improve the baby's attachment security (see 0.4.6.) which the other group only achieved during the post-treatment period. This difference is attributed to teaching the parent to appreciate the infant's status as 'initiator' as the name 'Watch, Wait and Wonder' suggests [177a]. This deceptively simple but highly effective intervention is also used in Australia [177b].

Sadly, most forms of parent-infant therapy still tend to focus on mothers. However, an unusual method of brief treatment of relational disturbances has been developed in Israel, which sees family members in weekly alternating couples – of mother-child; father-child and mother-father in addition to individual sessions if necessary [178a]. A manual for this form of treatment and several other handbooks now exist, documenting treatment process and techniques [178 b, c]. Several measurements exist to evaluate parental psychopathology around birth and early childhood to provide a base for therapeutic interventions. For instance scales developed in Munich, are used to assess the quality of intuitive parenting and degree of co-regulative behaviour in mother-child interaction [179a]. Another, Swiss method of structured therapeutic assessment of triadic family relationships is also used for training professionals in early childhood psychiatry programmes [179b].

Finally, Parent-Infant therapy capitalises on rapidity of change due to the plasticity of development of the baby within the primary relationship, which may serve as an incentive for growth even in unlikely parents. Given some motivation for change therapy may be utilized even in extreme conditions (antenatally as well as postnatally), such as with women with a criminal life-style or drug addiction. A San Francisco project suggested a modification of Parent-Infant therapy for use in such cases, where in addition to assessing child protection issues and risk to the baby, therapeutic intervention is comprised of three main components, the last of which differs in degree from other situations:

- Linking the past with the present to increase the mother's awareness of her own conflicts;
- Developmental guidance about the uniqueness, needs and capacities of the baby and his/her dynamics with the parent/s;
- The therapist taking action in the 'real' world if necessary to change a potentially destructive situation [180].

In sum, early intervention, even when it occurs postnatally, is a crucial preventive measure. As we shall see (0.4. below), not only is a baby's future mental health determined by the level of parental attunement but dysfunctional interaction can affect the actual structure of his brain. Perinatal therapy enables primary relationships to run a healthier course, by combating negative representations during pregnancy; and postnatally, by fostering a capacity for parental reflectiveness and interactive repair, based on their own strengths and the baby's resilience.

KEY POINTS:

*A crucial factor in mental ill-health in westernised societies relates to changing patterns of family relationships with few support networks and high emotional reliance on the sexual partner.

* The transition to parenthood transforms the interaction between partners as gender differences peak during pregnancy, with arousing physical and emotional experiences to which each expectant parent responds differently, thereby destabilising the couple's relationship.

* Ante and postnatal disturbance are attributed to loneliness, lack of emotional and practical support, poor relationship with one's partner, family conflict, tiredness, complications and disillusionment of unrealistic expectations.

* Most pregnant women experience a variety of mixed feelings about their 'placental connection'. Those who take a fixed and intense stance towards pregnancy, the fetus and/or motherhood (whether idealised, depressed, persecuted, anxious, obsessional or detached) may benefit from therapeutic help before the birth ['placental paradigm'].

*Exposure to a baby is a catalyst, reactivating unintegrated denied, disavowed and/or unprocessed memories of being parented in one's own childhood. The sudden release of unconscious forces in early parenthood may flood the person with traumatic flashbacks, overwhelming rage or self-hatred and/or terrifying helplessness which inhibits their adult capacities, and may trigger re-enactments with detrimental and long lasting effects.

*The increase in couple morbidity peaks for both partners at one year, when over half of all new parents are depressed. At least one in ten mothers suffer severe depression over the first postnatal year and the incidence of paternal depression ranges from 1.2% to 25.5% in community samples, and from 24% to 50% among men whose partners were themselves experiencing postnatal depression . [This rises to almost 60% when antenatal depression is included].

*Intervention programmes for high risk mothers and traumatised or overburdened families aim to enhance quality of life and foster reciprocal interaction (by recognising intergenerational repetition of unintegrated experiences).

*Perinatal therapy is essential when pregnancy, early parenting and reproductive events revitalise people's unresolved traumatic experiences with their own carers, including incestuous abuse, cruelty and violence, neglect, abandonment or invalidation. Ideally this should begin before the baby's birth increases the potential for crossgenerational transmission.

*Psychodynamic 'talking cures' include individual, couple, family, group or parent-infant therapy, in which observing the moment to moment give and take within the consulting room, the therapist can make connections with the emotional climate of childhood as remembered and unknown 'procedural' memories reactivated in the present through 'contagious arousal'.

* Parent-infant therapy is specially efficient because of rapidity of change.

0.4. INFANT MENTAL HEALTH

0.4.1. Human inter-relatedness:

Into this complex world babies are born. The years 1990-2000 were declared the 'decade of the brain' imaging techniques there has been a rapid expansion of **neuro-scientific information** concerning links between brain growth occurring in the early stages of human life and the psycho-social environment in which babies develop. In the current biologically-oriented climate of opinion, this concrete evidence seems to have impressed the government, leading to provisions for enhancement of early childhood experience (such as Sure Start). And with growing awareness of the *interconnectedness of infant and parents* – services offer greater family support.

However, **neonatal developmental research** had long established that even newborns are far more capable and discriminating than previously suggested, endowed with exquisitely sensitive feelings and an innate ability for reading the emotions of others, and sustaining proximity to carers. That relational capacities exist from the start was demonstrated decades ago in a landmark article showing turn-taking proto-speech in 'conversations with a two-month old' [181]. Since then we are more aware of this innate desire for dialogue and researchers have filmed non-verbal turn-taking 'conversations' between ever younger babies and their caregivers. Further evidence accumulates about ways in which babies seek out the mother's smell and voice and can imitate adult expressions within hours of birth. As anyone who has been wooed by a baby knows, from the start an infant wants to share and when others respond sensitively, this repeated 'interactional synchrony' fosters their growing self-awareness and understanding of their world and people in it.

What happens is not a pre-programmed unfolding of cognition but *a gradual evolution of innate capacities for sociability, thought and language through intensely emotional interactions with others* (not just mothers). Babies learn to think, play imaginatively and recognise themselves and others as having feelings, minds and subjective selves, through rich social engagement with their mothers, fathers, siblings, relatives, other babies and even strangers. Optimally this consists of finely coordinated 'joyful' attuned exchanges of mutual delight, in which the infant's communicative expressions and excited or subdued feelings are sensitively recognised and closely matched by an attentive companion [182]. We adults tend to devalue play but it is the prime medium of learning – for us all. *Play helps the child express and explore feelings and make sense of the world s/he inhabits.* Through play s/he masters difficult situations, communicates anxieties and extends the self by imaginatively testing out and practicing potential aspects of objects and relationships.

Every relationship is different. Through back and forth bi-directional influences between baby and carer, each specific pair co-contructs a particular interactional *'emotional climate'* as we may call it, developing their own mutually generated patterns of expressive exchanges and interweaving rhythms of activity. What is permitted or forbidden in this specific ambiance depends on the degree to which the older companion allows him/herself to enjoy the interaction and feels unthreatened enough to be attuned to the full range of the baby's affects.

The key to sensitivity lies in the carer's accessibility of his/her <u>own</u> emotions.   Recognition and acceptance of these enables him/her to acknowledge the baby's feelings, including negative ones. In turn, his/her verbal commentary, mirroring facial expressions and unconscious communications provide an emotional commentary about the baby's feelings which helps him make meaning of his interrelationships. This <u>profoundly social interchange</u> also embeds the baby in the local language, customs and sociocultural expectations.   The parent's elaboration of the infant's responses and modulation of his emotional state of arousal help him to gradually become aware of the nature of his own feelings and how to manage them. The child develops the capacity to differentiate feelings, modulate and eventually express them in words, as well as recognising the existence of inner states and feelings in others. Thus, in time, a child comes to appreciate herself as a thinking/feeling and embodied person among others, a member of a particular family within a wider societal context.

0.4.2. Development and Intersubjectivity:

Inherently distinct ways of relating to humans and objects change towards the end of the first year as the infant's enjoyment of sharing an object or experience with other people comes to include awareness of their differing responses to it. If initially *'primary intersubjectivity'* involved sharing emotional experiences, this *'secondary intersubjectivity'* now involves communicating experiences about objects in their shared world [183] from which symbolic functioning gradually emerges. The baby begins to recognise himself and his carers as subjects in their own rights (rather than a merged twosome or the one as 'object' of the other's needs or desires). (How exactly this happens and what i means has given rise to diverse theoretical considerations of Intersubjectivity [184]).

Most carers of young babies intuitively speak a form of 'motherese' – a high pitched, repetitive, rhythmic babytalk. They spontaneously match the baby's prevailing emotional 'mood', and then tend to 'mirror' it back. What is interesting is that they do so in an exaggerated way, thereby providing 'social biofeedback' which gradually enables the baby to recognise his or her own emotions, and to differentiate these from the carer's own feelings (which are not overstated) [185]. In healthy development, the caregiver's capacity to extend a view of the child as feeling and thinking (having a mind), helps him to think about his own and others' mental experiences.   Through 'pretend' play the child practices and explores and gradually integrates earlier modes of understanding into a 'reflective mode' of experiencing and recognising psychic reality [186].

Empathy, or sympathetic consideration of the feelings of others similarly arises through the baby's emotional responsiveness to, and identification with, the 'stance' of the other, by a developing capacity to temporarily shift his/her own perspective [187]. And, once again, the corollary of the baby's growing sensitivity to other people's differing views of the same reality, and to the meaning they ascribe to objects, events and to oneself, is enhanced self-awareness – the infant's dawning self-consciousness of being seen through the eyes of the other. This in turn allows for an altered form of psychic and reflective (rather than emotional) intimacy.

Greater complexity of symbolic thinking and use of language also evolve through ongoing interpersonal engagement. This promotes a growing understanding of *meanings* - the meaning of having different points of view, and understanding of differences between appearances and reality, between false and true beliefs, presence and representation, pretence and truth. Thus, over the first year of life the deepening social exchange with sensitive carers refines the infant's understanding of reality while serving as 'a fountain of pleasure, a reservoir of reassurance, and a well-spring of mischief' [188].

0.4.3. Proto-conversational exchanges:

Infant mental health is thus a function of shared emotions and intentions within the family system as a whole. Communication is a matter of a complex exchange of 'infectious' alternating or complementing emotions, rooted in psychobiological attunement. Even very early on *turn-taking* is apparent in 'proto-conversation' in which the infant responds in kind, or terminates the exchange, by turning away or withdrawing his/her gaze alternating periods of engagement and disengagement. The exchange is thus both a function of the communicative baby's mood, temperament and psychosocial needs, and of the sensitive carer/companion's receptivity, lively recognition and reciprocity [189]. What is more, in this intensely intimate exchange, each partner comes to incorporate 'meaning assemblages' of the other into his/her own state of consciousness [190].

It is important to note that in these exchanges, the emotional balance is affected not only by the baby/carer's mutual delight, but its absence. Their respective anxieties and pain impact also on each other. This explains the skewing effect on the relationship of parental postnatal depression – the carer's over-involvement, withdrawal or heightened anxiety and corresponding over-sensitivity and defences in the infant. In turn the baby's agitation and reluctance to be soothed aggravates the adult's state of mind. Experiences with primary caregivers shape the vulnerable baby's emerging self. *Carers who are unable to monitor and modify their own negative feelings also have difficulty modulating the infant's levels of affect when these are too high.* In fact, the interaction with a stressed adult actually <u>creates</u> stress in the infant, leaving him/her with an intrusion of chaotic feelings, undifferentiated embedded in his primitive states of mind. Thus parental stresses come to manifest as behavioural and personality disorders in their children. When misattunement is a chronic situation, the baby cannot learn to develop a smooth transition between emotional states, living in a state of hyper-arousal with deficits in self-regulation. Defences, such as hyper-vigilance or dissociation are brought in as strategies to avoid unmanageable affects and ward off unpredictable intrusions. Insensitively raised babies have difficulty in organising and modulating their emotional states although by digesting their trauma, many grow up to develop empathy or fine-tuned social understanding.

Given our individual differences, each primary relationship is unique. However, all relationships are built of exertion and none are perfect. Even mother-infant communication is not the lovely synchronised 'dance' once depicted. Inevitably misunderstandings and interactive mismatches occur. Ideally, even with very young babies, these 'errors' are followed by energetic attempts to understand the 'sloppiness', and to repair miscommunications through reciprocal feedback [191]. *Interactive repair and repeated misattunements followed by re-attunements contribute to the infant's growing capacity for self-organisation.* Gradually, this expands the complexity and coherence of the *'dyadic consciousness'* - the interweaving of co-created processes between the baby and the carer that is unique to that particular relationship [192] and will be different with other carers.

In addition to formal neonatal research in laboratories, numerous 'infant observations' have been conducted by psychotherapy students, psychoanalytic candidates and other professionals in training all over the world. This usually consists of longitudinal observation of infants and their carer/s in the home, in toddler groups, nurseries or elsewhere, starting as early as immediately after the birth [193]. These weekly hour-long observations following the development of patterns of interaction over time reveal that *resilient babies of sensitive caregivers can afford to maintain an open receptivity that fosters flexibility and variety of interchange, rather than fixity of emotional experiences.* Conversely, it is apparent that persistent exposure to unresponsive, chronically misattuned or intrusive carers forces a baby to withdraw defensively, to comply and create a 'false self' or to rely prematurely on self-regulation. (The rapidity of this effect has been demonstrated effectively in video filming of laboratory interactions in which the mother is asked to keep a 'still face' and not respond to her infant who then wilts and withdraws).

0.4.3.1. Seen in the context of the **Facilitator/Reciprocator/Regulator model** of this book, observation reveals that normal parental styles of interaction differ according to orientation and the underpinning representations of each. [These subtle differences are obscured or conflated in research that treats all 'normal' mothers as one homogeneous group].

- *A Facilitator* mother who believes in adapting, closely follows the baby's emotional initiative in 'communing'. She keeps the baby close at all times cuddles, chats and croons, her high pitched tonal expressions interspersed with kisses and rhythmic rocking. An observer would note that the unself-conscious content of her vocalisation emphasises <u>similarity</u> between the baby and herself, with sympathetic arousal and exaggerated affect. (Over-involved Facilitating mothers who are hypersensitive to the baby's disengagement, may meet his/her temporary withdrawal or focus of interest elsewhere with intense attempts at persuasion towards emotional acknowledgement. Similarly, <u>over</u>-attunement may prevent differentiation and the infant's ownership of his/her own feelings).

- *A Regulator* mother who expects the baby to adapt, tends towards a didactic stance to encourage independence. She often utilises nursery rhymes, action games and books in the exchange between them with the intention of 'socialising' the infant. This 'readymade' form of interaction also reduces the need for her own spontaneity, preserving her adult dignity (although sometimes interspersed with maternal 'swooping'). Somewhat wary of being drawn in emotionally, her verbal content tends towards an intellectual (correctional) running commentary and/or emphasizes <u>difference</u>, encouraging and applauding physical advances, and dismissing 'clinging'.

- *A Reciprocator* mother both follows the baby's lead but initiates her own interaction of playful sometimes teasing communication initiatives, imaginatively co-extending spontaneous play, improvised games, sing-song and chat to include physical 'banter' and lively romping. Verbal content tends to be both emotionally empathic and matter-of-fact informative, relating to the baby's state of mind and fostering self-regulation. While 'similarity' is emphasised in attuned empathic mirroring, 'difference' comes into play in inventive variations.

As noted in my early work [194] different mothers are good at meeting the baby's needs at particular time periods, and find other phases more difficult according to their orientation (and their own weakest developmental stages).

What is also evident are *mismatched baby and mother pairs*. This does not refer to momentary mismatches in affect states, or pathologically preoccupied or disordered mothers, but to rhythms of personal 'dynamism'. A habitual qualitative disparity of intensity, timing and rhythmicity – when a sparky woman is mother to a languorous baby, or a 'slow' mother to a speedy, vivacious one. Not only is conversational turn-taking disrupted by their different tempos, but unless they can attune to each other's pace, the whole interaction may be out of synch as observed in <u>duration</u> of temporal sequences – a baby being fed, changed, tickled or responded to too rapidly for his slower tempo; another having to wait too long for the carer's responsive gaze to acknowledge his, or the feeding spoon to meet his mouth. Occasionally there are also temperamental mismatches of orientation such as a regulated baby who prefers to be facilitated or vice versa. In some of these cases, where the carer is sufficiently receptive and mature, the baby can teach the parent to shift orientation. In others, it is the baby who has to comply, or the mismatch is uncomfortably played out in battles of will between adult and child.

0.4.4. Interpersonal Neuro-psychology:

Clearly a baby's psychosocial development is rooted in interaction. However, in recent years there have been exciting developments which have shown that neurobiology too, is 'interpersonal'! In early infancy, the overabundant production of synaptic connections in the baby's brain are constantly being flexed, fine-tuned and pruned not only by nutrition and background environmental events - but mainly by the responses and stimulation of caregivers. The primary carer is not only modulating the baby's emotions but regulating the infant's production of hormones that influence structural growth of the brain. Ongoing interpersonal experience both strengthens existing neural connections and also fosters <u>new</u> ones, laying down much used pathways and eliminating others - thereby altering the configuration of the brain itself. Pleasurable experiences with others trigger biochemical reactions, releasing opioids which promote neuronal growth by regulating glucose and insulin.   Impingements, traumatic events and negative emotional experiences trigger stress hormones and a high state of arousal which may prune vital connections [195a,b,c]. *In their emotional interaction with the infant, carers thus enable or constrain not only function but the actual structure of the developing brain!* MRI evidence has established that accelerated brain growth from the third trimester before birth until about two years postnatally, renders this a crucial period of great change during which brain circuits are formed, shaped by interpersonal exchanges during these early years.   This plasticity allows for adaptation of each baby to his particular family and its emotional climate, especially in the second half of the first year.

Although flexibility slows with age and early experiences leave an indelible permanent trace, the brain remains remarkably pliable. [As Russian neuro-psychologist Luria documented half a century ago, even split brains, where the hemispheres have been surgically or accidentally severed, have the plasticity to create new pathways]. Hence the ability of long term psychotherapy to alter pathological set patterns by gradually fostering alternative ways of managing emotional experiences.   This new evidence of responsive growth resolves the old nature/nurture debate by showing that developmental processes are a product of the interaction between both genetic disposition and childrearing. *Endowment is activated, modified or inhibited by the specific emotional-social environment.* The innate core-brain is the seat of automatic responses of survival, but the 'social' brain is the seedbed of the ever-evolving mind, and this is constituted interpersonally, between carer and baby. One psycho-neurologist described this process: 'human connections create the neural connections from which the mind emerges' [196].

Our 'self' is a product of others. As noted, infants feel intensely and utilise emotions to understand the world - projecting them out into the world and taking them in by responding acutely to nonverbal rhythms, tonal expressions and emotional facial expressions and gestures [197]. Parents too, tend to experience a state of heightened sensitivity in the early months following the birth. The more differentiated the 'vocabulary' of emotions each carer applies to the infant, the greater the versatility and range of subtle internal distinctions the baby can develop. Depending on parental attentiveness and capacity for responsive mirroring and sensitive emotional feedback, the infant gradually converts feelings created by events into mental representations and memories. These allow for elaboration of thinking, planning and learning from experience. (That these representations are both very real and yet not real also provides an ambiguity which permits the growing child to find a flexible perspective, a means of symbolising, exploring and <u>playing</u> with reality in his search for a more comfortable and personal way of living with/in it [198] and see 0.4.2. above).

Interestingly, early emotional communication between infant and carer is found to involve the *right* hemispheres of both their brains. Long before language develops, the maturing brain evolves through these spontaneous emotional exchanges. Modulated by reciprocal influences, organisation increases with the baby's non-conscious appraisal of positive and negative emotional significance of social stimuli. Gradually these take the form of *'somato-sensory' representations*, enabling the baby to recognise his own internal bodily states which in turn, induces a gradual transformation of the baby's external dependence on others as interpreters of his/her emotions, into capacity for <u>internal</u> self-regulation [199a] and cognitive elaboration [199b]. Clearly then, the particular patterns of early attachment, and the flow of 'energy and information' between infant and significant others powerfully affect *self-other internal representations* (see 0.4.2 and 0.4.3 above). And these intense early experiences create expectations, in anticipation of patterns of future emotional engagement.

0.4.5. Procedural caregiving and autobiographical memory and transgenerational transmission:

Initially infants assimilate cognitive structures in deeply affective ways – mediated through feelings such as curiosity, rage, lust, fear and play [200] from which representational processes of the 'core self' can begin to emerge [201]. This makes babies highly vulnerable to stimuli overload as Freud anticipated almost a century ago [202]. Recent research suggests that where parents allow experience to exceed the baby's threshold barrier, or when chronic deprivation and unpredictable, disrupted care predominate, these necessitate continual over-activity of the infant's own emotional systems. Findings show that a child may then become habituated to stress overload. When carers do not help the stressed baby to recover, this may lead to chronic states of intense arousal, a distorted biochemical baseline (high levels of cortisol), and may possibly provoke neuronal loss. Chronic high levels of arousal in infancy have been linked to ADHD, over-vigilance, anxiety and panic disorders, depression, eating disorders, addictions and borderline personalities in later life. Conversely, under perpetual bombardment, innate 'alarm systems' that usually activate appropriate responses to danger may defensively shut down, or be managed by obsessional-compulsive defences, including harm-avoidant preoccupations and rituals intended to control all unpredictable eventualities.

Interestingly, even non-psychodynamic theoreticians now agree that high levels of early stress may be accompanied by chronic feelings (such as sadness and alienation), possibly leading to persistent traits of shyness, guilt, shame or depression [203]. No surprise there - virtually thousands of psychoanalytic case histories link anxiety, panic disorders and depression in later life to toxic experiences of early neglect or abrupt separation, insensitive, intrusive or abusive events. These are often retained as self-other representations and procedural memories which organise expectation of relationships. Persisting into adulthood, these affect all intimate relationships. For example, a clinical case illustrates the confusing persistence of multiple inconsistent and contradictory implicit relational models stemming from serial mothering and traumatic early losses, and the way these perpetuate reliance on non-verbal cues in adulthood [204].

Maturation both regulates, and is regulated by reciprocal influences in spontaneous emotional communication between infant and carer. Seen neurologically – development (conceptualised as increasing organisation and gradual transformation of external dependence into internal regulation) – occurs with the growing complexity of maturing brain systems. *As language develops, a shift occurs from right to left hemisphere dominance.* However, it is the right hemisphere rather than the verbal-linguistic left one, which implicitly continues to perform a role in non-conscious appraisal of the emotional significance of social stimuli through 'somato-sensory' representations [205]. Many aspects of our interactions with others are implicit – non-verbally transmitting, registering and processing facial and bodily cues, and our own reactive sensory bodily information, outside awareness of either participant.

As we have seen, synchrony and responsivity are crucial factors in the early interaction. Babies are acutely aware of unconscious transmissions, and in turn react to the emotional climate of the relationship. They gradually evolve a pre-symbolic network of sensory representations of each primary attachment relationship – what Bowlby called an 'internal working model' – redolent with unprocessed emotion. (It is hypothesised that this is 'stored' in the right hemisphere in the form of implicit-procedural 'autobiographical' memory [206]). It is these unsymbolised anticipatory images and intense feelings which are reflected in the primitive form of automatic primal re-awakenings (which I've termed 'contagious arousal' in new parents), differing from the more developed reflective capacity to compare situations, think about differences and process feelings rather than acting blindly. I suggest that it is this rich and emotionally saturated (but un-narrated) procedural earliest 'autobiographical' memory that is reactivated when people fall in love, and stirred up in early parenthood. In the latter case, *'contagious arousal* is triggered by disturbing contact with evocative sensory experiences as well as direct exposure to the baby's inchoate pre-verbal emotions.

0.4.6. Impact of the baby on the carer –
unconscious identifications and 'contagious arousal':

Contagious arousal explains why the first few weeks of caring for a newborn are so intensely disturbing for most caregivers. Thrust into close contact with raw feelings of the pre-symbolic baby, and the redolent smell of primary substances (amniotic fluid, lochia, breast-milk, urine, feces, 'cradle cap', posset, etc), the new parent experiences a reawakening of procedural memories. *The ongoing intimate, emotional exchange with a newborn's right brain, reactivates the parent's own early* unprocessed *feelings* – infantile somato-sensory representations (of her/his own baby-self seen through the eyes of archaic caregivers) and implicit memories of being parented, for better and for worse. The nature of these unconscious representations reflect repeated experience of a myriad subjective schemas of sensations, affects, actions, arousal and motivation which form a network system of 'being-with-another-in-a-certain-way' [209].

People whose infantile experience has been largely positive, can relish this reactivation, delighting in the baby's dependence as reminder of their own baby-self in relation to an archaic carer. (They temporarily become totally engrossed in the baby, reflecting what Winnicott called 'primary maternal preoccupation' – see pp.315-6). From my clinical observation of new mothers, those who are resilient actively utilise the process of mothering to vicariously rework their own less than optimal early experiences. For others, this is a risky encounter, a powerful state of heightened arousal that threatens to evoke negative or traumatic experiences. They then try and control the risk by maintaining an emotional distance from the infant, through co-carers, routines and regulation (see Chapter 21). Some parents cannot withstand the negative aspects of this arousal. Finding this state overwhelming their experience is of 'primary parental persecution' [207]. Some new parents retreat into splitting of 'good' and 'bad', controlling the latter through compulsive rituals and avoidances or locating the 'bad' in external dangers and developing phobias or paranoid anxieties. Those who are unable to protect themselves, find this primitive state overwhelming and succumb to a spectrum of depressive, obsessional or persecutory disturbances which range from identificatory fusion/confusion with the idealised infant, to extreme withdrawal, disassociation or detachment from the denigrated or feared infant, representing repudiated aspects of the carer's own baby-self. (These disorders are elaborated in Chapter 33 and in section 0.3 above).

Once again, relating the effect of unconscious identifications on mothering to the **Facilitator/Regulator/Reciprocator model** presented in this book:

- A Facilitator mother regards the baby as similar (unconsciously associated with her own baby-self), inviting connectedness and resenting separateness. Over the early months she is preoccupied with her infant and resists any diversions. Failure to resurrect the ideal narcissistic state she imagines her baby experienced during gestation and loss of the close intimacy she experienced in pregnancy may result in guilt and depression. As the growing infant begins to separate, her own separation anxieties and fear of loss may lead to over-involvement with the infant. And similarly, denial of the negative axis of her own postnatal ambivalence increases anxieties about the baby's vulnerability to being harmed, and hence may result in over-protectiveness.

- A Regulator mother experiences different anxieties about being invaded in pregnancy, and swamped postnatally by repudiated needy or greedy aspects of her baby-self. Her own postnatal disturbance arises from the threat of contagious arousal of her own early feelings. This experience is one of primary persecution from which she tries to distance herself, by treating the baby as different and separate from herself. Similarly, denial of the empathic/positive axis of her ambivalent feelings renders her unable to enter full-bloodedly into the exchange.

- Finally, the Reciprocator manages to simultaneously hold both sides of the equation in mind – the baby as both similar in having (mixed) human emotions, yet different in being a baby. Similarly, she sees herself as both adult and rational/verbal yet motivated by emotional and partly irrational forces, both negative and positive,. She channels her own primary parental arousal into empathising (rather than identifying) with the infant.

0.4.6. Attachment issues:

Over the past 15 years attachment theory which offers a means of assessing the quality of *security* of a primary relationship, has burgeoned. Hundreds of research projects confirm and further John Bowlby's work of the late 1960's. The basic assumption is that like all helpless young primates, human babies seek proximity to their carers as a means of protection against danger. In Bowlby's view the primary function of this 'archaic heritage' is to ensure survival of the species by safeguarding the young [210 a,b,c]. An inborn, biologically adaptive, motivational system drives the newborn to form a close bond with a few selective meaningful figures. A 'secure base' of emotional stability is formed through the child's confidence in the availability and attunement of the attachment figure/s. Attachment also fulfils an important social function, and offers a sense of recognition by others. While attachment opportunities are multiple in traditional extended families and innovative co-parenting systems, in the small nuclear family there often is only one prime attachment figure, and erroneously the tie to the mother was regarded as 'monotropic' with all anxiety related to separation from this single carer. However, further research has confirmed that several primary attachments can coexist, and that *security is not a trait, but a connection* – which varies in degree of security from one primary carer to another. A child may be securely attached to the father or aunt but feels insecure with the mother, grandmother or babysitter, or vice versa. On the basis of the specific pattern of each primary relationship the infant establishes mental modes of relating and forms *'internal working models' of expectations* which, unless consciously processed and revised through later experience, are applied unmodified to other intimate relationships. Although they may not be apt in the present, these mental representations of carer, self and environment form expectations which are regarded as accurate reflections of 'implicit' memories of actual past experiences (as opposed to mere internal 'fantasies').

In small isolated families, if the core primary relationships cannot provide a sense of security this results in the toddler feeling unloved or rejected (and carries an internal model of the other as unloving or rejecting). When primary carers are unpredictable and inconsistent, a one-year old's *anxious-ambivalent insecure attachment* is manifested in clingy or agitated behaviour following separations. In other cases, where the carer is 'dismissive' (rejecting or neglectful) and/or controlling, the child defensively 'deactivates' the need for attachment resulting in *avoidant attachment behaviour*, cultivating pseudo-independence or seeming indifferent to the carer's whereabouts and responses (although physically aroused after separations). Recently, a further category has been delineated [211] - when a carer has not resolved his or her own early traumatic experiences, the infant manifests a form of *disorganised insecure attachment* with bizarre and dissociative reactions to separation (freezing or headbanging for instance) and disorientation in response to the carer's frightening and often abusive responses. A procedure called the 'Strange Situation' is used as a standard measure of one-year-old's responses to a brief separation and reunion with mother or father and interaction with a stranger under replicable laboratory conditions.

Once again what is apparent is *the intra-psychic/inter-personal exchange between carer and baby.* Security lies in learning to manage one's own sadness, anger and anxieties in a safe context with a sensitive carer who responds accordingly, rather than collapsing, retaliating or attacking. In later life, this secure inner core offers protection during periods of high stress. Interestingly, the unborn baby's attachment patterns at one year can already be predicted during gestation from interviews with the expectant mother about her own early attachments [212a]. Similarly, the way fathers recall their own childhood attachments is predictive of their infant's attachment at age one [212b]. The Adult Attachment Interview enables researchers to gauge not only how an expectant mother views her own childhood but whether this has been processed and how in turn it informs her relationship with her unborn baby, shaping the quality of that future attachment. This accords with studies in which **Facilitator/ Regulator/ Reciprocator parenting orientations** are already apparent and may be studied during pregnancy, long before their activation with the birth.

These orientations are based on unconscious representations of self and baby reflecting the degree to which past experiences are metabolised (rather than still 'raw') and how present ambivalence is tolerated or denied. Both idealising mothers and persecuted mothers are unable to accept the coexistence of good/bad ambivalent emotions – and hence, are cut off from one or other hidden aspect of their own mixed feelings about their mothers, self and baby. Regulators find it hard to tolerate the baby's neediness which reminds them of cravings they themselves feel but have dismissed. While Facilitators who vicariously indulge their own baby-selves through unlimited gratification (and adult desire to be needed), find it difficult to tolerate the infant's mixed feelings and growing independence. Under stressful conditions, Regulators may become controlling and/or dismissive of dependency and emotional outpourings, while the Facilitators become anxious about the baby's unhappiness or any hint of criticism. *Research linking these orientations to attachment theory shows that maternal orientation measured as early as 6 months postnatally discriminates among Secure & Insecure infants (as measured later by the Strange Situation at one year). Extreme (enmeshed) Facilitators breed ambivalent babies. Extreme (dismissive) Regulators have avoidant babies. Moderate Facilitators and Regulators, and Reciprocators raise secure toddlers [213].*

Longitudinal research rates children with a history of secure attachment as more socially oriented, resilient and empathic. Insecure attachments are related to less self-control, poor social relations and an unstable sense of self. In later life early insecurity (anxious-ambivalent; avoidant or disorganised) manifests in severe depression, compulsive self-reliance or antisocial behaviour; and borderline personality disorders respectively. Research from all over the world has consistently found around 35% of children are insecurely attached. (see [214 a,b,c] for more detail explications of Attachment theory). *Attachment theory confirms the message of this book – the necessity to help expectant parents to work through their own unresolved or traumatic early issues before these unprocessed early experiences come to be reenacted in interaction with the baby.*

0.4.7. Transgenerational impact of
parental disturbances on the infant:

Disturbances in early parenthood are dealt with in depth in section 0.3 above and in Chapter 33. The effects of the most common of these, postnatal depression, manifests in emotional unavailability - pervasive low mood, diminished pleasure, energy loss, guilt and sense of worthlessness and difficulty concentrating – all of which affect the nature of the relationship with the sensitive infant. PND also has high co-morbidity with anxiety disorders, substance abuse and eating disorders, all of which also impact on the baby. Above all, in their own ruminations over conflictual feelings, or emotional involvement with the past, these parents often lack awareness of the infant's needs. The disconsolate carer may feel compelled to re-enact with his/her own child the traumatising experiences encountered in childhood, leading to a sense of failure, abandonment and low self-worth in the child (and estrangement from their own needs and feelings) which in turn, may manifest as depression when s/he too becomes a parent. Transgenerational transmission of depression, low self-esteem and learned helplessness are common.

Serious mental illness in primary caregivers has long-term repercussions. But video studies show that even mildly disturbed parents are less responsive, less attuned, at times rejecting or hostile, inconsistent or ineffectual, and that when this is a chronic situation it can lead to developmental impairments in the child. Detrimental effects of early maternal depression have been found to result in cognitive, emotional and social developmental deficits [215] which persist in the child long after resolution of the maternal illness [216]. Faced with disturbance in a caregiver babies tend to develop one of three typical defences – *'fight', 'flight'* or *'freeze'*. When the danger is a chronic one, protective aggressiveness, defensive avoidance of emotion or disassociation may become ingrained.

If the children of a violent parent who cannot manage his anger have no access to someone who can teach them to trust in the possibility of discussing or repairing disagreements, they will find it hard to empathise or manage aggressive feelings, in themselves or in their dependents when they have children of their own. A child whose parent's depression or preoccupation with the past prevents him/her from holding the child in mind will have to flee elsewhere to resolve his worries, or may go to great lengths to avoid them, since he can't contain them within his own mind. Parental inconsistency, rejection coupled with over-intrusiveness, may produce both states of hyper-vigilance and anxiety disorders, and escapist addictions in borderline personalities in later life. A fine tuned match arises between parental disorder and the necessary coping strategies which may be reactivated in later life by similar situations to the original stressor.

Psychodynamic therapy offers an opportunity to break the cycle of cross-generational transmissions. In the therapeutic space, a person can verbalise, process and integrate implicit emotional forces, memories and attachment experiences, however traumatic. This working through takes place in the context of a caring attuned relationship with the empathic therapist who helps them voice and understand their feelings (an experience these people may not have had in their own infancies), which in time can be internalised as a basis for sensitive parenting. The capacity for healthy nurturing is associated with the carer's realistic self-esteem, enabling appropriate management of sadness, anger and anxiety. As an expectant parent's self-confidence is enhanced through therapy, and negative forces subside as the past becomes more understandable, obsolete defences may be shed. When this happens during pregnancy, modification of unconscious 'baby-carer representations' from their own childhoods alters expectations of the unborn baby (see 0.3.11.1 above). *To be effective, postnatal therapy must deal with the two interleaving parent-baby systems – the parent's internal representations of the past and their own current interaction with the real baby.* As they recognise their own difficulties, they can become more forgiving of the conflicts, shortcomings and fallibility of their own parents.

Needless to say, deep-seated changes such as these cannot be expected to occur through brief intervention. A recent controlled trial comparing the effect of three different psychological treatments for post-partum depression delivered at home (in 10 sessions) found that although CBT (Cognitive Behavioural Therapy) and non-directive counselling produced short-term mood changes and relief in early relationship difficulties, only psychodynamic psychotherapy produced a significant rate of reduction in depression, but these benefits did not persist beyond 9 months postpartum [217]. Another study found that 12 weeks of interpersonal psychotherapy was effective in relieving major postpartum depression (DSM-IVcriteria) compared to the waiting list group [218]. (However, there was no follow up). The need for more prolonged intervention and time to consolidate changes is one reason I advocate beginning therapy with people at risk early on, preferably during pregnancy. In the case of antenatal depression/persecution, a further reason is the hope of changing negative representations before these materialise in actual interactions with the new baby.

Borderline and psychotic parents are usually identified by midwives, health visitors or GP's as bringing their own intense and often chaotic uncontained emotions into the relationship in ways which are bizarre, confusing and terrifying for the infant. Therapeutic treatment may have to take place in a hospital setting or mother-baby unit, and must involve a team of professionals to ensure the baby's safety. However, it is crucial to note that many disturbed carers go unidentified and do not seek help. Community wide studies indicate that about half of all new mothers who meet operational clinical criteria for psychiatric 'caseness' go undetected by family doctors and other professionals [219]. As noted, there are also high rates of couple disharmony, conflict and separation, and cotemporaneous psychiatric morbidity in partners [220], seemingly associated with the unconscious choice of an equally vulnerable spouse ('assortative mating'), all of which lead to high levels of stress which are pathogenic to the vulnerable, immature brain [221] and emotionally detrimental to the growing infant.

Clearly, the child's physical and mental safety is paramount and assessment of parenting capacity must focus on the level of disturbance, instability, paranoia and impulse control, responsibility and the degree to which a child is involved in the parental psychopathological system [222], or deprived by the quality of their emotional functioning. Mother and baby units, residential and day placements for disturbed families may be an option, in addition to a variety of individual, couple, family or group therapeutic interventions (see 0.3 above).

0.4.8. Extreme Facilitator, Regulator
and conflicted postpartum adjustments:

Clinical experience reveals that perinatal emotional disturbances are most acute in parents who have not previously worked through and integrated their own infantile feelings and so remain under the powerful influence of unmitigated unconscious experiences. I suggest that the high incidence (12-22%) of severe depression and widespread prevalence (50%-60%) of milder forms of postnatal distress in western societies, are attributable both to inexperience and to *discrepancies between expectations and parental reality* (the latter particularly for Regulator mothers - for statistical confirmation see [223] and 0.5.1 below). Moreover, as I suggested above these disorders now occur in a generation of new parents who, having grown up in small and isolated nuclear families, have had limited opportunities to re-experience infantile feelings and work them through in childhood. Our culture demands that from a young age we control and suppress intense emotional experiences. Acute anxiety, passionate love and hatred, jealousy and rivalry, deep confusion, humiliating helplessness, excruciating dependence and sweet surrender have all been kept at bay rather than experienced repeatedly in relative safety, with the birth of siblings or cousins, and the help of an accepting adult.

In these cases a person finds it difficult to be in touch with the full range of their feelings – as noted, **Facilitators** are prone to suppress their own mixed and negative feelings (and those of the baby), while **Regulators** dismiss 'sentimentality' or 'soppy' feelings of dependence in themselves and the infant. Taking on full responsibility for one's own child unexpectedly unleashes a host of these intense and unprocessed infantile emotions. In addition, when this is combined with the trials of social adversity the risk of breakthrough emotions is exacerbated. **Conflicted parents** and those at the extremes of facilitation or regulation often experience disillusionments, disappointments, clashes and internal collapse of self-esteem during the early weeks and months. These are intensified for parents who have suffered early experiences of neglect, emotional, violent or childhood sexual abuse and their own past experience may be abusively re-enacted with the baby (see 0.4.9 below).

In most forms of postnatal disturbance, either the parent's emotional preoccupation with unresolved past issues or conversely, their disassociation from, and avid avoidance of the past interferes with empathic receptivity – with the ability to recognise, understand and respond sensitively to the emotional experience of the infant in their care.

The nature of parental early disturbance is reflected in their patterns of interaction with the infant – depending on their own internal realities, some mothers or fathers become distressed and overanxious while others withdraw, becoming avoidant and less emotionally available while yet others become inconsistent, or intrusive, or abusive and intimidating. How parents react is determined by their unconscious representations of the baby or of themselves. As disturbance occurs, an extreme Regulator may come to feel so persecuted that she is unable to distinguish between assertiveness and aggression in the baby, while an extremely idealising Facilitator may become anxiously overprotective towards her infant to ward off her own negative feelings. Unless a parent can tolerate the mixture of ambivalence within themselves, 'badness' is either projected into others, the parent thus becoming paranoid or phobic and isolated. If the baby becomes incorporated in the persecutory system, there is a risk of infanticide. Or, if invested in him/herself, the parent in whom internal strengths become eclipsed becomes depressed, guilt ridden, hopeless and suicidal.

This accords with the distinction between depression on the one hand, and persecutory disorders (phobias, paranoia, anxious avoidance of intimacy, obsessive-compulsive syndromes, contamination fears and hostility related to the baby, etc), or the latter with a possible overlay of depressive or PTSD features, especially in conflicted and borderline parents. Clinical material reveals in some disturbed parents an underpinning compensatory fantasy of merger, an unconscious desire for a 'saviour', an all-providing mother or unconditionally loving carer who will transform one's internal state. (Eating disorders, alcoholism, substance abuse and gambling may reflect a similar need for magical recompense or reduction of mental pain without having to recognise and process it).

When this wish for a 'transformer' is displaced on the infant, it creates a role-reversal. Inevitably, a young baby struggling to regulate his/her own feelings is unable to meet the parent's psychological needs which leads to an overburdened infant and a dissatisfied adult, whose frustration manifests in postnatal depression, emotional avoidance, or inconsistent closeness with hostility, impulsive rage or shut down. A parent who is unable to reflect psychologically about their own dismissed suffering and dependency needs, or one who is preoccupied with the past, is unable to help the baby to learn about his/her own feelings and to internalise sensitive awareness as a model for self-care. Some parents resent or envy the care the other lavishes on the baby and may retaliate by having an affair or resolves the feeling of being left out by separating.

0.4.9. Impact of emotional and sexual abuse or violence:

Research has proved that physical and sexual abuse are significant risk factors for many mental health disorders and abused children develop serious emotional and behavioural difficulties. Parents who have experienced early trauma may find themselves compelled to enact this. The dissociative detachment ['freeze'] or repression that often accompany unresolved and/or unnamed/unnameable scenarios is conducive to replacing these with a real life drama, in order to temporarily relieve some of the internal tensions and confusion. This has important implications for the understanding of the trans-generational nature of early abuse. Part of the devastating long-lasting effect is attributable to the dependent child having to rely upon an abuser. Violation of trust and deep confusion arise when the abusing person is one of the child's primary attachment figures and should be a source of protection rather than danger. Appropriation of the child for the abuser's own needs, coupled with invalidation and denial of the child's experience, presents the gravest obstacle to the kind of symbolic repair and transformation that must done on the attachment relationship if the child is to restore a viable sense of self [224]. When this confusion threatens to break-through in parenthood to be re-enacted with the next generation, ongoing perinatal psychotherapy can offer a safe place to explore these feelings and to break the cycle of mindless repetition that operates to alleviate the internal tension. Through recall and verbal processing in psychotherapy, implicit emotional trauma is transformed into explicit memory which can then be thought about. However, the intensity of raw emotions and newly recovered memories may feel overwhelming to the sufferer and therapist alike, especially when these are re-experienced in the sessions.

Intra-familial child abuse has long lasting effects. There are extra horrific residues when perpetrated by perverse adults who are members of cults, and sacrifice the child to others. Ritualised cruelty and organised sexual abuse of children are particularly pernicious in inflicting upon the victims unthinkable acts which mingle with terrifying elements of infantile fantasy [225].

Effects of abuse depend on the age of the child, the duration and nature of the abuse, whether it included violence; whether the child had loving figures around, and if s/he told, was supported or ridiculed and blamed. Above all, the *identity of the abuser* is crucial and worse effects are found with a close or known than unknown abuser. Child abuse is 15 times more likely to occur in families where spousal abuse occurs. Children are three times more likely to be abused by fathers than mothers, and societal factors, such as lack of social support, poverty, and a history of childhood abuse or depression (and substance abuse) feature, as well as the emotional immaturity of parents and their poor self-esteem. **Post traumatic symptoms** include difficulty with close relationships, mistrust, anxiety, fear, depression, low self-esteem, sexual difficulties, disruptive behaviour, aggression and stigmatisation. **Treatments** usually involve either dynamic play therapy with very young children, child psycho-therapy or intensive psychoanalysis, or family therapy, or briefer cognitive-behavioural approaches for older children and their non-offending caregivers. All these treatments strive to acknowledge the child's painful experiences and characterise these as wrong, unlawful and harmful [226].

Incidence: because of its hidden and unreported nature the incidence of abuse is difficult to estimate and statistics are controversial. US Department of Health and Human Services indicate that in 2000, substantiated victimisation rates of children up to three years old were 15.7 per 1,000 which included 63% neglect; 19% physical abuse; 10% sexual abuse and 8% psychological (although clearly, all these have deep psychological effects). However, adult retrospective studies indicate a much higher rate with 27% of women, and 16% of men reporting childhood victimisation. The single most comprehensive source of information about the current incidence of child abuse and neglect in the United States, the congressionally mandated Third National Incidence Study of Child Abuse and Neglect (NIS-3), reports *substantial and significant increases in the incidence of child abuse and neglect.* According to calculations based on a nationally representative sample of over 5,600 professionals in 842 agencies serving 42 counties, a child's risk of experiencing harm-causing abuse or neglect in 1993 was one and one-half times the child's risk in 1986. Two sets of standardized definitions of abuse and neglect - the *Harm Standard*, identified children who had already experienced harm from abuse or neglect, and *the Endangerment Standard*, of at-risk children. Physical abuse nearly doubled, sexual abuse more than doubled, and emotional abuse, physical neglect, and emotional neglect were all more than two and one-half times their NIS-2 levels. *The total number of children seriously injured and the total number endangered both quadrupled during this time* [227].

In addition to actual increase, figures indicate greater awareness of the problem, and a higher incidence of reporting. In the UK, the Children Act 1989 defined *'abuse'* as actions which 'cause a child to suffer significant harm to their health or development through excessive punishing, by hitting or shaking a child, by constant criticism, threats or rejection, sexual interference or assault. And *'neglect'* as not looking after a child – not providing enough to eat, ignoring them, not playing or talking with them, or neglecting their safety. In 2002 the Royal College of Psychiatrists brought out fact sheets for parents and teachers to help prevent child abuse and neglect, and recognise the emotional effects of it. *This is a reminder that children are usually abused by someone familiar or in the immediate family circle and that the child will suffer severe long-term consequences of repeated violent attacks, sexual abuse or severe neglect.*

- After-effects of traumatic experiences - distressing fears, flashbacks, poor sleep and difficulty in concentrating, are intensified if the child is also being emotionally abused or neglected.
- Identifying symptoms of physical abuse are the child's watchful, cautious, wariness of adults; inability to play, make friends and be spontaneous. Aggressive or abusive behaviour, bullying other children, or being bullied. Underachievement, temper tantrums, lying, stealing.
- Sexually abused children may suddenly behave differently when the abuse starts - withdraw into themselves or be secretive, regress and start wetting or soiling themselves. Be unable to sleep, behave in an inappropriately seductive or flirtatious way, be fearful, frightened of physical contact.
- Emotionally abused or neglected children may have delays in learning to walk and talk, be very passive, have feeding problems and grow slowly; find it hard to develop close relationships, yet

be over-friendly with strangers, get on badly with other children of the same age, be unable to play imaginatively and think badly of themselves [228].

Clearly, in the case of suspected abuse, Social Services will ascertain what has happened and the likelihood of it recurring. The child's name may be placed on the child protection register – and occasionally a child may have to be removed from the family because the risks of physical and emotional harm are too great. Safety is the prime issue. Their emotional and physical safety is assessed and reassessed at intervals. Many young children need specialist treatment from child psychotherapists or psychiatrists, and the abuser or entire family may require therapeutic treatment. In the USA too, guidelines and protocols for treatment are constantly evaluated.

In conclusion, preserving and fostering the mental health of children is a necessity for any nation. There can be 1,2,3 different levels of operation – *Primary* - **prevention** through anticipatory information and education about the capacities and needs of infants or programmes to increase awareness of healthy parenting practices. *Secondary* - **screening,** and early detection or preventative measures in high risk groups (including home-visitation programmes to prevent abuse, toddler groups and programmes to strengthen family and community connections and interventions enhance coordination of services). *Tertiary* - **treatments**, such as Parent-Infant Therapy or child psychotherapy aiming to minimise the impact of established conditions. In the case of emotional disturbances or potential abusive behaviours, it is clearly more effective to provide therapy before people conceive, or for expectant parent/s before their own problems are inflicted on offspring. It is therefore most important to define precipitants, evaluate risk factors and detect early indicators of vulnerability to disturbance, and to provide services on all three levels.

0.4.8. Summary - Developmental overview:
How better to conclude this section on infant mental health, than to cite the core concepts of development as defined by a large group of experts?
1. Human development is shaped by a dynamic and continuous interaction between biology and experience

2. Culture influences every aspect of human development and is reflected in childbearing beliefs and practices designed to promote healthy adaptation.

3. The growth of self-regulation is a cornerstone of early childhood development across all domains of culture.

4. Children are active participants in their own development, reflecting the intrinsic human drive to explore and master one's environment.

5. Human relationships, and the effect of relations on relations, are the building blocks of health development.

6. The broad range of individual experiences among young children often makes it difficult to distinguish normal variations and maturational delays from transient disorders and persistent variations.

7. The development of children unfolds along individual pathways whose trajectories are characterized by continuities and discontinuities, as well as by a series of significant transitions

8. Human development is shaped by the ongoing interplay among sources of vulnerability and sources of resilience

9. The timing of early experiences can matter, but, more often than not, the developing child remains vulnerable to risks and open to protective influences throughout the early years of life into adulthood.

10. The course of development can be altered in early childhood by effective interventions that change the balance between risk and protection, thereby shifting the odds in favour of more adaptive outcomes [229].

KEY POINTS:

* Endowment is activated, modified or inhibited by the specific emotional-social environment into which a child is born.

* Young babies learn to think, play imaginatively and recognise themselves and others as having feelings, minds and subjective selves, through rich social engagement with their mothers, fathers, siblings, relatives, other babies and even strangers.

* Every relationship is different. Each specific pair co-contructs a particular *'interactional climate'* developing their own mutually generated patterns of expressive exchanges and interweaving rhythms of activity

* Most sensitive carers of young babies intuitively speak a form of 'motherese' – a high pitched, repetitive, rhythmic baby-talk, spontaneously matching the baby's prevailing emotional 'mood' and 'mirroring' it back.

* The key to sensitivity lies in the carer's accessibility to and self-regulation of his/her <u>own</u> emotions. Recognition and acceptance of these enables him/her to accept and acknowledge the baby's feelings.

* Communication is never perfect and repeated misattunements followed by repair and re-attunements contribute to the infant's growing capacity for seeking meaning, thinking and self-organisation.

* Primary carers not only modulate the baby's emotions but by regulating the infant's production of hormones that influence structural growth of the brain. Ongoing interpersonal experience also both strengthens existing neural connections and fosters <u>new</u> ones, thereby altering the configuration of the brain itself. This plasticity allows for adaptation of each baby to his particular family and its emotional climate, especially in the second half of the first year.

* A pre-symbolic network of sensory representations of each primary attachment relationship forms an 'internal working model' reactivated in adult intimate relationships.

* In early parenthood *'contagious arousal'* triggered by disturbing contact with evocative primary substances and direct exposure to the baby's inchoate pre-verbal emotions, revives childhood experiences which preoccupy the withdrawn parent or are re-enacted in the relationship with the child.

* Experiences with primary caregivers thus shape the vulnerable baby's emerging self. Carers who are unable to monitor and modify their own negative feelings also have difficulty modulating the infant's levels of affect when these are too high. The interaction with a stressed adult actually <u>causes</u> stress and inconsistent, controlling or disturbed parents foster defensive, insecure ambivalent-anxious, avoidant or disorganised babies.

* Unless processed or resolved through psychotherapy, patterns of familial disturbance are transmitted cross-generationally as troubled and traumatised children grow up to become parents themselves.

0.5 FACILITATOR-RECIPROCATOR-REGULATOR MODEL:

Over the past 15 years since this book first appeared several independent researchers have replicated my model in large scale studies and longitudinal research, thus empirically substantiating clinical findings and observations. Studies have been conducted in the UK, Australia, Austria, Belgium, Canada, Israel, Italy, Peru, Sweden, South Africa, The Netherlands, USA and elsewhere. Some were BA projects or MA dissertations. Others at PhD or postgraduate level. In common, these projects confirm that by delineating these subgroups, the model allows for differentiation of variables that otherwise cancel each other out. The model has also been found to elucidate anxieties underpinning attachment styles, and prospective research has validated my predictors of postnatal depression. I will not attempt to bring all the many findings or data but will summarise a few of these research projects here:

Main Findings:

- The three orientations are found to cluster significantly, manifesting as conscious cognitive and behavioural expressions of underlying intrapsychic processes.

- Postnatal practices are predictable from pregnancy, and behaviour is underpinned by beliefs and unconscious representations which can be tapped by questionnaires [attitudes to pregnancy; expectations of labour/birth; representations of the fetus/baby and postnatal childcare practices as described here in Chapters 6, 13, 17, 19, 24 and 33]

- The discrepancy between a woman's expectations and subsequent experience of events is significantly predictive of multiple indices of postpartum depression

- Postnatal depression is triggered by different precipitators in Facilitators and Regulators, and attributable to discrepancies between antenatal subjective expectations and postnatal experience

- Women reporting a Regulator mothering orientation are at increased independent risk for above-threshold postnatal depression symptom levels

- Night waking is more frequent among first-born Facilitator babies compared to Regulators'. Both Facilitators and Regulators reported high levels of maternal separation anxiety as opposed to a low level of anxiety among the Reciprocators

- Links to attachment theory: maternal orientation at 6 months discriminated among Secure & Insecure infants (as measured by Strange Situation at one year). Extreme Facilitators: enmeshed (babies ambivalent); Extreme Regulators: dismissive (babies avoidant); Reciprocators: secure

- A correlation between discrepant expectations and perception of labour and delivery, and antenatal depression. Induction, episiotomy, Caesarean, ventouse, forceps and analgesia influence Facilitators' perception of labour but not Reciprocators'

- This model has also been applied to <u>caregivers</u> (other than parents), such as attitudes of breastfeeding counsellors, midwives, etc [230]

- Several questionnaires based on this model (drawing items from my original questionnaires) have now been developed and standardised including AMOM – delineating orientations antenatally and PPQ, tapping into antenatal representations (see Appendices C,D).

RESEARCH DETAILS:

0.5.1   THE LEICESTER STUDIES:
HELEN SHARP (1995) [231]

At the time this study was conducted in the early 90's, there was very little prospective research examining women's prior expectations in relation to outcome of events and development of postpartum depression. My own studies had been conducted on samples of highly privileged professional women, as I wanted to examine the choices of people who had few external restrictions. The prospective study reported here drew on a large socio-demographically representative sample of 205 primiparous women in Leicester, interviewed in the third trimester of pregnancy. Data collected included psychiatric history, life events, perceived quality of intimate bond, antenatal psychiatric symptomatology and cognitive style. Objective obstetric outcome information was collected from medical records and women completed an EPDS, and GHQ at 3 months postpartum, as well as being interviewed about their subjective experiences of labour, birth, the baby and early motherhood. High scorers on the two measures were given a Present State Examination [PSE].

Results:

The findings showed fundamental Facilitator/Regulator differences in individual expectations, antenatal preferences and postnatal subjective experiential reports of labour, birth, the new baby and motherhood. [At this point the Reciprocators were still regarded as an intermediary group].

Brief distillation shows that findings were in line with orientations elaborated in various chapters of this book:

1. Expectations differed according to orientations and respondents' postnatal experiential reports of labour and birth reflected these subjective expectations, and discrepancies between expectations and experience.

- **Facilitators**: looking forward to the birth, regarding it as exciting, and wanting a 'natural' birth;

- **Regulators**: dreading birth, hoping for a 'civilised' experience.

- **Regulators** had higher ratings on external locus of control (towards labour) vs. **Facilitators** whose locus was internal.

2. Approaches to the new baby and motherhood differed:
- **Facilitators**: experience the baby as familiar
- **Regulators:** as a stranger.
- Only 37% of Regulators reported enjoying mothering newborns vs. 60% later
- more Facilitators breastfed and differed significantly from Regulators in their ideal duration of breastfeeding.

3. The nature of external stressors and internal vulnerability factors differed as a function of mothering orientation and were found to be significant predictors of poor outcomes.

4. High EPDS score at six weeks postpartum:

- Among **Facilitators:** associated with higher neuroticism scores and medical complications.

- Among **Regulators:** associated with antenatal hospital admissions (disrupting her life-style), and a shorter hospital stay.

5. The discrepancy between a woman's expectations and subsequent experience of events was significantly predictive of multiple indices of postpartum depression

6. Postpartum depression

- **Regulators:** Lower socio-economic status (precluding paid child-care?) was significantly predictive

- **Facilitators:** Being single, viewing the partner as less caring; or one's mother as highly controlling were significant predictors of caseness in Facilitators at 6 weeks postpartum.

0.5.2. SHARP & BRAMWELL, 2004 [232].

Reciprocators were delineated in a subsequent study by the same researcher and a colleague using the same sample. This study explored maternal orientations and relative risk for early postnatal depression. It was designed to determine whether women's antenatal expectations of childbirth, of their future baby and of early motherhood accord with the Facilitator–Reciprocator–Regulator model of mothering orientation, I proposed in the 2001 revised edition of this book on the basis of my own studies.

A second question was whether a Regulator orientation confers greater relative risk for early postnatal depression. A socio-demographically representative sample of 205 primiparous women in Leicester completed a maternal orientation measure and the General Health Questionnaire (GHQ) in late pregnancy and the Edinburgh Postnatal Depression Scale (EPDS) at 6-8 weeks postpartum.

- Hierarchical cluster analysis was employed to cluster cases on the basis of antenatal expectations of their future baby and early motherhood and yielded a clear three cluster solution.
- Between-cluster comparisons of women's ratings on these variables, and of childbirth and feeding expectations did correspond with Facilitator, Regulator and Reciprocator mothering orientations.
- In line with the theory, *women reporting a Regulator mothering orientation were at increased independent risk* (OR 3.28, 95% CI 1.23 – 9.25) for above-threshold postnatal depression symptom levels (EPDS > 10.5).
- Regulator orientation confers greater relative risk for early postnatal depression. (GHQ; EPDS; Beck)
- Furthermore, in a hierarchical regression analysis, Regulator mothering orientation accounted for a significant proportion of variance in postnatal symptom level even after controlling for antenatal depression symptom level[232].

Two of my questionnaires were standardised and validated – AMOM and PMOM [see Appendix C]. Further studies are being conducted in Liverpool.

0.5.3. THE ISRAELI STUDIES:

1. SCHER & BLUMBERG, 1992 [233]:
cross-cultural and Methodological considerations.
An early study by the Department of Education at the University of Haifa, Israel delineated the orientations, and found significant differences

among Facilitator, Regulator, Intermediate (Reciprocator) and what they termed 'Bi-polar' (meaning conflicted) subgroups.

2. SCHER & BLUMBERG, 2000 [234]
Orientations and sleep patterns:
A later study by these researchers in the Department of Education at the University of Haifa found:
34% Facilitators; 34% Regulators; 15% Reciprocators and 17% Ambivalent-inconsistent 'bi-polars'. (1st born babies more common among Regulators).

The study looked at sleep patterns in infancy, on the assumption that these reflect negotiation about separation and reunion in both mothers and babies. Consistent with attachment theory and object relations theories, it was suggested that difficulties with separation are further reflected in problems of differentiation, distancing and boundary-formation for both mother and child. And that these were consistent with the Facilitator orientation and attitudes towards separation – her idea of maternal exclusivity of care, need for proximity and anxiety about separation.

Examining night waking among one year olds, they found that *mothers with high separation anxiety had babies who were frequent wakers and required/received parental intervention to regain sleep.*

Contrary to their predictions, both Facilitators and Regulators reported high levels of maternal separation anxiety (3.23 and 3.03 respectively) as opposed to a *low level of anxiety among the Reciprocators* (2.28). This is consistent with my own reasoning that suppressing one 'arm' of ambivalent feelings creates anxiety, arguing for a multifactorial model of separation anxiety in which maternal characteristics as well as child attributes co-vary with mother-child relationships (see [235]

Findings:
- high maternal separation anxiety is related to infant night waking
- these babies require/receive parental intervention to regain sleep
- night-waking is more frequent among first born Facilitators compared to Regulators.
- Maternal separation anxiety is significantly associated with both Facilitator and Regulator mothers vs. low level in Reciprocators.
- Infants of 'Bi-polar' conflicted mothers take significantly longer to fall asleep (25 vs.11 minutes) and wake later.
- First born babies of Reciprocators and Bi-polars woke more frequently (1.67 & 1.17) than Regulators (.45) and less frequently than Facilitators (2.00). [As predicted by the model, Regulators establish a set routine, including sleeping patterns while

Facilitators more frequently attend to their babies at night. In my own 1984 study with mothers of two year olds, Facilitator mothers reported still having interrupted nights while many Regulator mothers reported having slept through the night from around five weeks postnatally].

- Settling routines – 51% of low anxiety mothers used pacifiers vs. 79% mothers with high maternal separation concerns;
- Self-soothing: 36% infants of low-anxiety mothers sucked their thumb/fingers vs.4% of babies of the high-anxiety mothers [who presumably relied on their mothers for relief]

3. SCHER (2001) [236]:

Attachment:
This study was designed to go beyond the idea of parental attachment working models as a predictor of child's future attachment pattern, by exploring a mother's approach to her parenting role as a means of tapping into how representations, beliefs and attitudes affect baby-care strategies and serve as predictors of mother-child attachment relationships. It was assumed that distinct conceptualisations of the infant's nature and needs would be reflected in the meaning the mother assigned to gestures and messages of the child, and be expressed in the childcare strategies.

The aim of the study was to examine whether orientation could predict attachment.

The main finding was that *maternal orientation at 6 months discriminated among Secure & Insecure infants (as measured by Strange Situation at one year).*

This Israeli study delineated the parental orientation, and found significant differences among Facilitator, Regulator: using a postal FRQ at 6 months supplemented by home visit at 9months and at 12 months a Strange Situation:
Findings:
- SECURE infants more likely to be Facilitators
- PREDICTIVE VALUE of developmental outcomes

77% secure; 23% ambivalent (no avoidant responses in this study as in all Israeli studies to date)
34% Facilitators; 34% Regulators; 15% - Intermediate; 17% ambivalent-'bi-polar'

4. LULAV-GREENWALD D (1994) [237]

A further Israeli study associated Orientations and attachment patterns in Kibbutz mothers – their attitudes to raising children and the adjustment of the children to different sleeping arrangements.   Findings were in according with the hypotheses.

0.5.3. THE LEUVEN STUDIES, Belgium:

JOHAN BUSSEL (2001)[238]:

A study of 264 women (mean age 29.7) in Leuven, Belgium focused on antenatal maternal orientations, expectations and retrospective perception of labour and birth (47% primiparae). Findings mainly related to two groups, reflecting local cultural differences.

- Facilitators had higher 'social desirability' scores (MC_SDS) compared to Reciprocators (in the hospital clinical setting), ranging towards an 'archetype of good mother'.
- a correlation between the maternal orientation (Facilitator and Reciprocator) and expectations of labour and delivery
- a relation between maternal orientation and the perception of labour and delivery
- an influence of induction, mode of delivery, analgesia, Apgar-score after 1 minute and the transfer of the baby to the neonatal ward on the perception of labour and delivery
- Instrumental deliveries - induction, episiotomy, section, ventouse, forceps and analgesia negatively influenced the perception of Facilitators but not that of the Reciprocators.
- Both Faciltators and Reciprocators were influenced by the Apgar-score (lower then 7) after 1minute, but only the Facilitators remained negatively influenced after 5 minutes – experiencing 'less fulfilment and delight'.
- C strong significant (p=.001) correlation (r=.566) between antenatal and postnatal depressive symptoms. Women with BDI-score>13 expect less fulfilment (p=.007); less delight (p=.44), more distress (p<.001) and more difficulties (p=.024).
- a correlation between discrepant expectations and perception of labour and delivery and antenatal depression
- significantly (p=.003) more Facilitators than Reciprocators breastfeed before leaving hospital

This work is now being extended to include all orientations, and using the newer questionnaires.

0.5.4. 1. LINDA CHARLES – development of the PPP (2001) [239]:

In another independent study, for a Clinical Doctorate a questionnaire based on my **'Placental Paradigm'** was developed and piloted, with a focus selecting items. The purpose of the research was to develop a psychometrically-sound, self-completion scale for use during pregnancy to identify women who may be experiencing, or at risk of future, psychological distress. Analysis of data focused on the development and the refinement of the PPP as a measure of pregnant women's fantasies, conceptualisations and feelings towards themselves, their babies and their pregnancies in positive and negative terms. Out of a pool of initial items developed from the 'Placental Paradigm' model (Raphael-Leff, 1989, 1993, 1996), with slight modifications to some items, 40 were judged to be content valid by 3 experts, and face validity was confirmed in a pilot study. Items were initially selected according to their facility index, discrimination and range of responses produced. Their provisional exclusion was subsequently confirmed by reliability analyses of each subset. There was evidence of good internal consistency for 5 out of 6 of the subsets of the PPP (varying between .72 and .8) and good split-half reliability for all 6 subsets (varying between .72 and .86). Thus all but the 'Negative Self' subset (alpha = .67) were found to be internally consistent and reliable according to the recommended minimum correlation coefficient of .7 for person-based questionnaires (see Table 2). [Results of the 'Negative Self' subset were retained for further analysis at this stage, despite the slightly lower than recommended alpha since tests of fewer than 10 items are unlikely to be highly reliable]

As expected, the total scores of the refined positive subsets were negatively correlated, and the total scores of the refined negative subsets were positively correlated, with the total scores of the GHQ-12. All correlations, except that with the 'Positive Baby' subset, were significant. The strongest positive correlation was found with the 'Negative Baby' subset scores and the strongest negative correlation with the 'Positive Pregnancy' subset scores, suggesting that those women who experience the baby they are carrying in negative terms are the most susceptible to psychological distress during pregnancy. It was concluded that additional items needed to be generated and piloted to improve the internal consistencies of each of the subsets (although noted that there is some disagreement among psychometric experts that high internal consistency is desirable as it requires tests to be narrow and specific and may therefore be antithetical to validity). 20 items were selected as discriminating.

The PPP nevertheless provides more information than the GHQ-12 for pregnant women, in that while it correlates with the distress detected by the GHQ-12 it also has the potential to identify *where* the problem may lie in terms of self, baby or pregnancy.

0.5.4.2. JOAN RAPHAEL-LEFF – PPQ (2004)

A second questionnaire was developed having generated additional items (while retaining some of the original items selected for the PPP), and applying them in a different format [see Appendix C] clearly delineating not only the positive or negative quality and focus of representations (self, baby, pregnancy) but also the nature of disturbance.

This questionnaire is intended as **a screening device for specific antenatal emotional disturbance.** It detects depression and anxiety and in addition, delineates the predominant defences – idealisation, persecution, obsession and detachment. It may also be used to determine Orientation. The questionnaire is being administered on large samples in studies at Yale University, USA, Liverpool University, UK, Leuven University, Belgium and possibly Rimini in Italy and Cape Town, South Africa. This will provide standardisation and address test-retest reliability during pregnancy. Predictive validity across the antenatal and postnatal periods will be assessed by comparison of orientation and risk, as determined by the PPQ, complemented by existing measures (for example, Adult Attachment Interview, Main *et al.*, 1985; Dyadic Adjustment Scale, Spanier, 1976; Edinburgh Postnatal Depression Scale, Cox *et al.*, 1987; Strange Situation, Ainsworth *et al.*, 1978; Working Model of the Child Interview, Zeanah *et al.*, 1994).

SUBJECT INDEX FOR UPDATE SECTION

[All page numbers refer to this update section only (even when no'U' is shown); see end of book for larger Subject Index]

References:
[1]   Trends in urbanization by region, UN, *World Urbanization Prospects*, 2004.
[2]   Raphael-Leff, J (2005) 'Psychotherapy in the Reproductive Years', Chapter in *The Concise Oxford Textbook of Psychotherapy*, G Gabbard, J Beck & J Holmes (eds), Oxford: Oxford University Press
[3]   Desire for smaller families ORC Macro, Demographic and Health Surveys, 1988-2000, UN 2003 *Population Reference Bureau.*
[4]   UN, Diverging Trends in Fertility Reduction, United Nations, World Population Prospects: the 2002 revision, 2003 *Population Reference Bureau*
[5]   *United* Nations, World Population Prospects: the 2002 revision, 2003 *Population Reference Bureau.*
[6]   *South African News* 24, August 19th 2004
[7]   Kiernan K (1997) Becoming a young parent: a longitudinal study of associated factors *British Journal of Sociology,* **48**
[8]   a. www.teenagepregnancyunit.gov.uk
        b. 28241/Government response to the first Annual Report of the Independent Advisory Group on Teenage pregnancy. 27.06.2002
        http://www.dh.gov.uk/PolicyAndGuidance/HealthAndSocialCareTopics/ChildrenS ervices/fs/en
        c. First annual report from the Independent Advisory Group for Sexual Health *Department of Health press release* 5.10.2004
        d. RESPECT campaign challenging attitude to young mums, *YWCA press release* 5.10.2004
[9]   www.pregnancy-info.net/teen_pregnancy_statistics.html 2004
[10]   Lundberg O & Palme J (2002) A balance sheet for welfare: Sweden in the 1990's. Editorial, *Scandinavian Journal of Public Health,* **30**:241-243
[11]   Kautto M (2003) Welfare in Finland in the 1990's *Scandinavian Journal of Public Health,* **31**:1-4
[12]   Kvist J(2003) A Danish welfare miracle? Policies and outcomes in the 1990's. Editorial, *Scandinavian Journal of Public Health,* **31**:241-5
[13]   Ólafsson S (2003) Welfare trends of the 1990's in Iceland, Editorial, *Scandinavian Journal of Public Health,* **31**:401-4
[14]   Columbia University Clearinghouse on International Developments in Child, Youth and Family Policies – Sweden, 2004, www.childpolicyintl.org/countries]
[15]   Botten G, Elvbakken KT & Kildal N (2003) The Norwegian welfare state on the threshold of a new century. Editorial, *Scandinavian Journal of Public Health,* **31**:81-4
[16]   a. Maternity protection ILO, www.icftu.org, Sept. 2002
        b. for a review see Burgess L, Clarke L & Cronin N(1997) *Fathers and Fatherhood in Britain.* London:Family Policy Study Centre
[17]   a. ICM/Guardian Opinion Poll, August 17th 2004
        b. Patricia Hewitt at the Confederation of British Industry Conference 21.9.04
        c. London HealthObservatory (2004) *Prevalence of Mental Health Problems,* Office for National Statistics, Psychiatric Morbidity Surveys, Department of Health, UK http://www.lho.org.uk/Disease_Groups/MentalHealth_Prevalence.htm
[18]   a. WHO Report (2003) Healthy Life Expectancy for 191 Nations, *WHO/OMS*
        b. Also see Healthy People 2010 – a systematic approach to [USA] health improvement, Leading Health indicators
        http://www.health.gov/healthypeople/
        c.UK Government Actuary's Department (2004)
        http://www.statistics.gov.uk/cci/nugget.asp?id=168
[19]   a. Office for National Statistics Series DH3 Mortality statistics: Childhood,

infant and perinatal, UK
http://www.statistics.gov.uk/StatBase/Product.asp?vlnk=6305&Pos=&ColRank=1
&Rank=208)
b. Bambang S, Spencer NJ, Logna S & Gill L (2000) Cause specific perinatal
death rates,birth weight and deprivation in Westmidlands, 1991-93,*Child Care
Health Development* **26**:73-82
c. Guildea ZE et al (2001) Social deprivation and the causes of stillbirth and
Infant mortality, *Archives Diseases of Childhood* **84:**307-10.
d. Serenius F, Winbo I, Dahlquist G & Kallen B(2001) Regional differences in
stillbirth and neonatal death rate in Sweden with a cause-of-death specific
analysis, *Acta Paediatrica* **90**:1062-7

[20]   The Center for Diseases Control National Center for Health Stastistics, *US
        Department of Health & Human Services*, 2004

[21]   US Center for System Research, 2004

[22]   a. New York Times, September 25th 2004
        b. Jerusalem Post, August 12th 2004.

[23]   mashriq.hiof.no/general/300/320/327/fafo/reports/FAFO151/2]

[24]   UNAIDS statistics 2003

[25]   Report from the 15t International Aids Conference in Bancock, *San Fransisco
        Chronicle,* cited by www.vso.org/raisa, The Big Issue South Africa, Sep.2004,
        86/8:8

[26]   a. World Wide HIV & AIDS Statistics Information (2003)
        http://www.avert.org/worldstatinfo.htm
        b. *South African News* 24, August 19th 2004

[27]   WHO/UNICEF (1998) *HIV and Infant Feeding guidelines for decision makers.*

[28]   WHO Collaborative Study (2000) Effect of breastfeeding on infant and child
        mortality due to infectious diseases in less developed countries: a pooled analysis.
        Lancet **355**:451-5

[29]   DITRAME ANRS 049 Study Group (1999) 15 month efficacy of maternal
        oral zidovudine to decrease vertical transmission of HIV-1 in breast-fed
        African children *Lancet* **354**:2050-1.

[30]   Coutsoudis A, Pillay K, Kuhn L, Spooner E, Tsai WY & Coovadia HM (2001)
        Method of feeding and transmission of HIV-1 from mothers to children by 15
        months of age: prospective cohort study from Durban, South Africa *AIDS*
        15:379-87

[31]   Nakiyingi JS, Bracher M, Whitworth JAG, Ruberantwari A, Busingye J,
        Mbulaiteye SM & Zaba B (2003) Child survival in relation to mother's HIV
        infection and survival: evidence from a Ugandan cohort study *AIDS* **17**:1827-1834

[32]   a. 'Parents sue health department', *Mail & Guardian*, SA Sept.3rd, 2004,
        www.mg.co.za
        b. World Wide HIV & AIDS Statistics Information (2003) *op.cit.*

[33]   Savage W(1986) *A Savage enquiry – who controls childbirth?* London:Virago

[34]   a. *Changing Childbirth* [chairman Baroness Cumberledge, Junior Minister
        for Health & Social Services]. London: HMSO, 1993
        b. *Scottish Framework for Maternity Services*: Our National Health: a plan for
        action, a plan for change,Dec.2000

[35]   a. Full copies of *Vision 2000* are available, from RCM Publications, the Royal
        College of Midwives (Welsh Board), 4 Cathedral Road, Cardiff CF1 9LJ.
        b. *First Class Delivery:* Improving Maternity Services in England and Wales.
        London: Audit Commission, 1997

[36]   [mailto:motherandbaby.co.uk] March 2001. Also see: 'Women's Dis-
        satisfaction', John Carvel, Social Affairs Editor, *Guardian*, March 22nd,   2001

[37]   a. National Service Framework for Children's Services (including maternity services):http://www.dh.gov.uk/PolicyAndGuidance/HealthAndSocial CareTopics/ChildrenServices/ChildrenServicesInformation/fs/en
b. NICE National Institute for Clinical Effectiveness guidance on Intrapartum Care http://www.nice.org.uk/cat.asp?c=63356

[38]   Alan Milburn, health secretary reporting to the RCM annual conference in Torquay 6th June,.2002

[39]   reported by John Carvel, Guardian social affairs editor, Thursday July 24th, 2003.

[40]   Warwick C.(2004) *British Journal of Midwifery,* 12/4:'Staff shortages: whose problem?'

[41]   Hrdy SB (1999) *Mother Nature – natural selection and the female of the species,* London:Chatto & Windus [or *Mother Nature: a history of mothers, infants and natural selection,* New York: Pantheon Books

[42]   Melender HL (2002) Experiences of fears associated with pregnancy and childbirth *Birth* **29**:101-8

[43]   Sjogren & Thowassen P (1997) Obstetric outcome in 100 women with severe anxiety over childbirth, *Acta Obstetricia & Gynaecologia Scandinavica* **86**:948-52

[44]   a. Biro MA, Waldenström U, Brown S & Pannifex JH (2003) Satisfaction with Team Midwifery Care for low- and high- risk women: a randomized controlled trial, *Birth* **30**:1-15
b. Hundley V, Penney G, Fitzmaurice A et al (2002) A comparison of data obtained from service providers and service users to assess the quality of maternity care, *Midwifery* **18**:126-135

[45]   Green JM, Curtis P et al (1998) *Continuing to Care. The organization of midwifery services in the UK:a structured review of the evidence,* Hale:Books for Midwives Press

[46]   Lundgren I & Dahlberg K. (2002) Midwives' experience of the encounter with women and their pain during childbirth, *Midwifery* **18**:155-164

[47]   Soet JE, Brack GA & Dilorio C (2003) Prevalence and predictors of women's experience of psychological trauma during childbirth, *Birth* **30**:36

[48]   a. Hundley V, Rennie AM, Fitzmaurice et al (2000) A national survey of women's views of their maternity care in Scotland, *Midwifery***16**:303-13
b. Kendall-Tackett KA & Kafman Kantor G (1993) *Postpartum Depression – a comprehensive approach for nurses*, London:Sage publications

[49]   Proctor S (1998) What determines quality in maternity care? Comparing the perceptions of childbearing women and midwives, *Birth* **25**:85-93

[50]   see for instance Wolf N (2001) *Misconceptions – truth, lies and the unexpected on the journey to motherhood,* London: Chatto & Windus.

[51]   Marks MN, Hipwell A, Kumar R (2002) Implications for the infant of maternal puerperal psychiatric disorders. In: *Child and Adolescent Psychiatry.* 4th edition. M Rutter & E Taylor (eds). Blackwell Scientific Publications, pp 858-877

[52]   Chamberlain G, Wraight A & Crowley P (eds) (1997) *Home Births: the report of the1994 confidential enquiry by the National Birthday Trust Fund*, Carnforth: Parthenon Publishing Group Ltd

[53]   Green JM, Baston HA, Easton SC, McCormick F (2004) The inter-relationship between women's expectations and experiences of decision making, continuity, choice and control in labour, and psychological outcomes: Implications for NHS maternity service policies. Final report to the Nuffield Trust and the NHS Executive.

[54]   Harrison MJ, Kushner KE, Benzies K, Rempel G & Kimak C (2003) Women's satisfaction with their involvement in health care decisions during a high-risk pregnancy *Birth* **30**:109-16

[55]   Hundley et al, (2002), ibid.

[56]   Dowswell T, Renfrew MJ, Gregson B et al (2001) A review of the literature on women's views on their maternity care in the community in the UK *Midwifery* **17**:194-202

[57]   Johanson RB & Rigby C (2002) The 'ASQUAM' programme: improving the standards of maternity care, using democratic prioritisation guidelines and audit, *Clinical Governance* **7**:112-20

[58]   Emslie MJ, Campbell MK, Walker KA et al (1999) Developing consumer-led maternity services: a survey of women's views in a local healthcare setting, *Health Expectations* **2**:195-207

[59]   Gracia J, Bricker L, Henderson J, Martin AM, Mugford M, Nielson J & Robert T (2002) Women's views of pregnancy ultrasound: a systematic review *Birth* **29**:225 -33

[60]   Santalahti P, Hemminki E, Latikka AM et al(1998) Women's decision-making in prenatal screening *Social Science and Medicine* **46**:1067-76

[61]   Grewal GK, Moss HJ, Aitken Da et al (1997) Factors affecting women's knowledge of antenatal serum screening *Scottish Medical Journal* **42**:111-3

[62]   Salonen R, Kurki L & Lappalainen (1996) Experiences of mothers participating in maternal serum screening for Down's syndrome, *European Journal of Human Genetics* **4**:113-9.

[63]   Briscoe L & Street C (2003) 'Vanished twin': an exploration of women's experiences, *Birth*, **30**:47-56

[64]   Piontelli A (2000) 'Is there something wrong?': the impact of technology in pregnancy, chapter 3, pp.39-52 in *Spilt Milk - Perinatal Loss and Breakdown* (ed.) J Raphael-Leff, London: Routledge (reprinted 2001,2,4)

[65]   Mitler LK, Rizzo JA & Horowitz SM (2000) Physician gender and Caesarean Sections, *Journal of Clinical Epidemiology* **53**:1030-5, cited by Wolf, *op.cit.*

[66]   ARM, Editorial, *Midwifery Matters* 77, summer 1998.

[67]   Cochrane report

[68]   Scott K, Berkowitz G & Klaus M(1999) A comparison of intermittent and continuous support during labour: a meta-analysis, *American Journal of Obstetrics & Gynecology***180**:1054-9.

[69]   Parliamentary Office of Science and Technology, Oct.2002, no **184**, Caesarean Sections

[70]   United States National Centre for Health Statistics, 2003

[71]   Dr Foster's case notes – social class and elective caesareans in the English NHS, *British Medical Journal* **328**:1399, 12. June, 2004

[72]   a. Home Births - *The report of the 1994 Confidential Enquiry by the National Birthday Trust Fund,*. Chamberlain, G, Wraight A & Crowley, P(eds) Parthenon Publishing, 1997. [A summary of the report on home births was published in *'Midwives'*, May   1997: 'Home Births - a report of the 1994 Confidential Enquiry by the National Birthday Trust' by Ann Wraight, Project Co-Ordinator; and in *Practising Midwife* 1999 Jul-Aug;**2**(7):35-9 b. National Birth Alliance press release, 23.10.04

[73]   a. see *The Sun*, July 22nd 2004.
        b. www.miscarriageassociation.org.uk

[74]   Harper J.(2003) Midwives and miscarriage: the development of an early pregnancy unit *MIDIRS Midwifery Digest* **13**:183-5

[75]   Hughes PM, Turton P, Evans CDH (1999) Stillbirth as a risk factor for

anxiety and depression in the next pregnancy: does time since loss make a difference: cohort study. *British Medical Journal* **318**: 1721–24

[76] Turton P, Hughes P, Evans CDH, Fainman D. The incidence and significance of post traumatic stress disorder in the pregnancy after stillbirth. *British Journal of Psychiatry* 2001; **178**: 556–60.

[77] Lundqvist A, Nilstun T, Dykes A-K (2002) Both empowered and powerless: mothers' experiences of professional care when their newborn dies, *Birth* **29**:192-9

[78] Allen NB, Lewinsohn PM, Seeley JR (1998) Prenatal and perinatal influences on risk factors for psychopathology in childhood and adolescence. *Development and Psychopathology*; **10**: 513–29.

[79] a. Van Izendoorn MH, Schuengel C, Bakermans-Kranenburg MJ (1999) Disorganised attachment in early childhood: meta-analysis of precursors, concomitants and sequelae. *Development and Psychopathology* **11**: 225–49
b. Hughes P, Turton P, Hopper E, McGauley GA, Fonagy P. (2001) Disorganised attachment behaviour among infants born subsequent to stillbirth. *Journal of Child Psychology and Psychiatry* **42**: 791–801

[80] Bourne S & Lewis E (2003) Pregnancy after stillbirth or neonatal death: psychological risks, chapter 22 in *Parent-Infant Psychodynamics – wild things, mirrors and ghosts*, J Raphael-Leff (ed), London:Whurr. Originally in *Lancet* 1984 339:31-3 Also see: Bourne S & Lewis E (1992). *Psychological aspects of stillbirth and neonatal death: An annotated bibliography*. London: Tavistock Clinic.

[81] Hughes P & Riches S (2003). Psychological Aspects of Perinatal loss. *Current Opinion in Obstetrics and Gynecology*, **15**:107-111

[82] Leon IG (1996). Revising Psychoanalytic Understandings of Perinatal Loss. *Psychoanalytic Psychology*, **13**:161-176

[83] a. Lanham CC (2004) *Pregnancy after a loss: a guide to pregnancy after a miscarriage, stillbirth or infant death*, Berkley Publication Group
b. Davies R (2004) New Understanding of Parental grief: Literature Review *Journal of Advanced Nursing* **46**:506-13]

[84] Caelli K, Downie J & Letendre A (2002) Parent's experience of midwife-managed care following the loss of a baby in a previous pregnancy *Journal of Advanced Nursing* **39**:127-36

[85] see Cohen M (2003) *Sent Before My Time – a child psychotherapist's view of life on a Neonatal Intensive Care Unit*, London:Karnac

[86] see pp206-7 in Shonkoff JP & Phillips DA (eds) (2000) *From Neurons to Neighborhoods – the science of early childhood development*, Washington DC:National Academy Press

[87] Bergman NJ, Linley LL & Fawcus SR (2004) Randomized controlled trial of skin-to-skin contact from birth versus conventional incubator for physiological stabilization in 1200g to 2199g newborns, *Acta Pediatrica*, **93**:779-785

[88] Francke LS & Spencer C (2003) Parent visiting and participation in infant caregiving activities in a Neonatal Unit, *Birth* **30**:31-6

[89] Kramer MS and Kakuma R (2002) Optimal duration of exclusive breastfeeding, *Cochrane Library issue 1*, Oxford:update software.

[90] *One World*, South Asia, 19.8.04

[91] *Department of Health, Report on Infant Feeding, 2000* www.[dh.govt.uk/assetroot/04/05/97/63/04039765.pd/-

[92] Blyth R, Creedy DK, Dennis CL, Moyle W, Pratt J & De Vries, SM (2002) Effect of maternal confidence on breastfeeding duration: an application of breastfeeding self-efficacy, *Birth* **29**:278 -84

[93] Li R & Grummer-Strawn,L (2002) Racial and ethnic disparities in breast-feeding among United States infants :Third National Health and Nutrition Examination Survey, 1988-1994, *Birth*, **29**:251-9

[94] DiGirolamo AM, Grummer-Strawn LM & Fein SB (2003) Do perceived attitudes of physicians and hospital staff affect breastfeeding decisions? *Birth* **30**:94-106

[95] McKeever PP, Stevens B, Miller KL, MacDonell JW, Gibbins S, Guerriere D, Dunn MS &Coyte PC (2002) *Birth* **29**:258-67

[96] Pugh LC, Milligan RA, Frick KD, Spatz D & Bronner Y (2002) Breastfeeding duration, costs and benefits of a support program for low-income breasfeeding women, *Birth* **29**:95-106

[97] [McConnachie A et al (2004) Modelling consultation rates in infancy:influence of maternal and infant characteristics, feeding type and consultation history, *British Journal of General Practice* **54**:598-603

[98] Raphael-Leff, J (2003)'Cannibalism and Succour: is breast always best?' Chapter 17 in *Parent-Infant Psychodynamics – wild things, mirrors and ghost,* (pp 231-240), London: Whurr publications

[99] Census 2001: the composition of origins of the British population, Office for National Statistics, UK

[100] House of Commons Health Committee report: *Inequalities in access to maternity services*: Eighth report of session 2002-03 http://www.publications.parliament.uk/pa/cm200203/cmselect/cmhealth/696/696.

[101] *Choice in Maternity Services*: Ninth report of session 2002-03 http://www.parliament.the-tationeryoffice.co.uk/pa/cm200203/cmselect/cmhealth/796/796.pdf

[102] WHO making pregnancy safer – mediacentre factsheet No. 276, Feb. 2004

[103] Itano N (2004) Us anti-abortion policies take heavy toll, Global Policy Forum, www.globalpolicy.org/socecon/develop/oda/2004/0128antiabortion.htm

[104] Ekanem Oyo-Ita, A., Ekott, M., Adaonu Chiazor, H., & M adu Meremikwu, M.(2001) Calabar project - Nigeria Better Birth Initiative. University of Calabar Poster Presentation: Session B, 9th *Cochrane* conference, Lyon, France, October 2001

[105] Brown, Hoffmayer D & Garner P (2004) Evidence based obstetric care in South Africa influencing the BBI, *South African Medical Journal* **94**:117

[106] WHO making pregnancy safer – mediacentre factsheet No. 276, Feb. 2004

[107] for some of the challenging life-changes in intimate relationships see the various contributions to Clulow, C. [ed] (1996) *Partners Becoming Parents – talks from the Tavistock Marital Studies Institute,* London:Sheldon.

[108] Cox JL, Murray D & Chapman G (1993) A controlled study of onset, duration and prevalence of postnatal depression. *British Journal of Psychiatry* 163:27-31

[109] a. Lee DTS, Yip ASK, Leung TYS & Chung TKH (2004) Ethnoepidemiology of postnatal depression. Prospective multivariate study of sociocultural risk factors in a Chinese population in Hong Kong, *British Journal of Psychiatry*, **184**:34-40
b. Danaci, et al (2002 Postnatal depression in Turkey: epidemiological and cultural aspects, *Social Psychiatry &Epidemiology,***37**:125-9

[110] a. see Raphael-Leff J (2000) 'Climbing the walls':therapeutic intervention for post-partum disturbance', chapter 5 in *'Spilt Milk' – perinatal loss & Breakdown,* J.Raphael-Leff (ed), pp 60-81, London: Routledge for a detailed case history.
b.Wolf N (2001) *op.cit.* for examples of postnatal couple dynamics based on personal interviews.

[111] Smith, C (1996) *Developing Parenting Programmes*, London:National Children's Bureau, UK

[112] Oates, MR. et al (2004) Postnatal depression across countries and cultures: a qualitative study, *Briish Journal of Psychiatry*, (supplement 46), **184**:10-16

[113] James, K. (1998) The Depresed Mother - a practical guide to treatment and support, London:Cassell.

[114] a. Ballard, C & Davies, R (1996) Postnatal depression in fathers, *International Review of Psychiatry* **8**:65-71
b. Dudley M et al (2001) Psychological correlates of depression in fathers and mothers in the first postnatal year. *Journal of Reproductive & Infant Psychology* **19**:187-202

[115] Connell A & Goodman S (2002) The association between psychopathology in fathers versus mother and children's internalising and externalising behaviour problems: a meta analysis. *Psychological Bulletin* 128:746-73

[116] Da Costa D, Larouche J, Drista M & Brender W (2000) Psychosocial correlates of prepartum and postpartum depressed mood. *Journal of Affective Disorders* **59**:31-40

[117] Bolton HL, Hughes PM, Turton P & Sedgwick P (1998) Incidence and demographic correlates of depressive symptoms during pregnancy in an inner London population *Abstracts* **19**:4.Dec.

[118] Copper RI, et al (1996) The preterm prediction study: maternal stress is associated with spontaneous pre-term birth at less than 35 weeks gestation, *American Journal of Obstetrics & Gynecology* **175**:1286-92]

[119] Evans J, Heron J, Francomb H, Oke S & Golding J (2001) Cohort study of de-pressed mood during and after childbirth *British Medical Journal* **323**:257-60

[120] Oates MR (2002) Adverse effects of maternal antenatal anxiety on children: causal effect or Developmental continuum? *British Journal of Psychiatry* **180**:478-9

[121] O'Connor TG, Heron J, Glover V & the Alspac Study Team (2002) Antenatal anxiety predicts child behavioural/emotional problems independently of postnatal depression *Journal of American Academy of Child and Adolescent Psychiatry* **41**:1470-77 122

[122] Susman EJ, Scheelk KH, Ponirakis A & Gariepy JL (2001) Maternal prenatal, postpartum and concurrent stressors and temperament in 3-year-olds: a person and variable analysis, *Developmental Psychopathology,* **13**:629

[123] Murray, L & Cooper, PJ (1997) Editorial: postpartum depression and child development, *Psychological Medicine* 27:253-260

[124] a. Raphael-Leff, J (1997) The casket and the Key: thoughts on gender and generativity, chapter 13,pp.237-257 in Female Experience: three generations of British Female Psychoanalysts on work with women (eds. J.Raphael-Leff, & R.Jozef Perelberg), London, New York:Routledge
b. Raphael-Leff, J (2000) 'Behind the shut door' - a psychoanalytical approach to premature menopause, in Premature Menopause - a multidisciplinary approach (eds) D.Singer & M. Hunter, London:Whurr publishers

[125] Gorman LL et al (2004) Adaptation of the Structured Clinical Interview for DSM -IV Disorders for assessing depression in women during pregnancy and post-partum across countries and cultures *British Journal of Psychiatry,* (supplement 46) **184**:17-23

[126] O'Hara MW & Swain AM (1996) Rates and risk of postpartum depression – a meta-analysis. *International Review of Psychiatry* **8**, 37–54.

[127] Lovestone S & Kumar R (1993) Postnatal psychiatric illness: the impact on partners, *British Journal of Psychiatry* **163**, 210–216.

[128] Confidential enquiries into maternal death (2001), *Why mothers die* 1997-1999.London:RCOG

[129] a. Bernazzi O(2004) Contextual Assessment of the Maternity Experience: development of an instrument for cross-cultural research, *British Journal of Psychiatry*, supplement 46, **184**:24-30
b. Chisholm et al (2004) Health Services research into postnatal depression: results from a preliminary cross-cultural study, *British Journey of Psychiatry* (supplement 46) **184**:45-52.

[130] a. Astbury J, Cabral M. *Women's mental health: an evidence based review.* Geneva: World Health Organization, 2000.
b. Brown GW, Harris TO & Hepworth C (1995) Loss, humiliation and entrapment among women developing depression: a patient and non-patient comparison, *Psychological Medicine* 25:7-21

[131] Royal College of Psychiatrists(1968) *Men Behaving Sadly*, http:///www.rcpsych.ac.uk

[132] Raphael-Leff J (1996) Procreative Process, Placental Paradigm and Perinatal Psychotherapy ,*Journal American Psychoanalyic Association, **44**:373-399, Supplement the Psychology of Women: psychoanalytic perspectives

[133] Wisner KL, Peindl KS, Gigliotti T & Hanusa BH (1999) Obsessions and compulsions in women with postpartum depression, *Journal of Clinical Psychiatry* **60**:176-180

[134] Cooper PJ, Tomlinson M, Swartz L, Woolger M, Murray L & Molteno, C (1999) Postpartum depression and the mother-infant relationship in a South African peri-urban settlement, *British Journal of Psychiatry*, **175**:554-8

[135] Jadresic E & Araya R (1995) Prevalence of postpartum depression and associated factors in Santiago, Chile *Review Medicine Chile* **123**:694-9 [cited by Danaci, op cit]

[136] Patel V, Rahman A, Jacob KS & Hughes M (2004) Effect of maternal mental health on infant growth in low income countries: new evidence from South Asia, *British Medicine Journal* **928**:8204, April.

[137] Glasser S, Barel V & Shoham A, et al (1998) Prospective study of postpartum depression in an Israeli cohort: prevalence, incidence and demographic risk factors, *Journal of Psychosomatic Obstetrics & Gynaecology* **19**:154-64

[138] a. Ray KL & Hodnett ED (2001) Caregiver support for postpartum depression, *Cochrane Database Systematic Review,* CD000946
Wickberg B & Hwang CP (1996) Counseling of postnatal depression: a controlled study on a population based Swedish sample, *Journal of Affective Disorders,* 39:209-16
c. the *Solihull Approach Resource Pack*, School of Primary Health Care, University of Central England Birmingham, 2001
d. Heinicke, CM., Fineman, NR, Ponce, VA & Guthrie, D (2001)Relation-based intervention with at-risk mothers: outcome in the second year of life, *Infant Mental Health Journal* 22:431

[139] McDonald Culp et al (2004)First-time mothers in home visitation services utilizing child development specialists, *Infant Mental Health Journal,* 25:1-15

[140] a.Puckering C, Rogers J, Mills M et al (1994) Process and evaluation of a group intervention for mothers with parenting difficulties *Child Abuse Review* 3:299-310
b. Boathe EB, Barnett, et al (1995) When the bough breaks: Charles Street Parents and Baby Unit, *Journal of Reproductive and Infant Psychology* 13:237-240
c. Karlsson K, Malmquist Saracino A & Bergdahl EN (2004) Relationship treatment at a baby -parent unit, Maskan, Stockholm, *The Signal – Newsletter of the World Association for Infant Mental Health,* 12/2: 1-8.

[141]   a. Sackler Lefcourt, I 1997) Mother-infant intervention: an application of
        psychoanalytic theory and technique, *Psychoanalysis and Psychotherapy*
        14:267-287
        b. Hanna Perkins Centre, Cleveland Ohio http://www.hannaperkins.org
        c. Zaphiriou-Woods M (2000) Preventive work on a toddler group and nursery,
        Journal of Child Psychotherapy **26**:209-33, also see www.annafreud.org
[142]   a. Kennedy, R(1997) *Child Abuse, Psychotherapy and the Law,* London: Free
        Association Books
        b. Asen E (2001) *Multiple Family Therapy: The Marlborough model and its
        wider applications,* London:Karnac
[143]   Siney C (ed) (1999) *Pregnancy and Drug Misuse,* 2nd edition. Hale: Books
        for midwives
[144]   Jones H, Svikis DS & Tran G(2002) Patient compliance and maternal/
        infant outcomes in pregnant drug-using women, *Substances Use & Misuse*
        37:1411-22
[145]   Stevens-Simon C &Orleans M (1999) low-birthweight prevention programs:
        the enigma of failure, *Birth* **26**:184-191
[146]   Rubovits P (1996) Project CHILD: an intervention programme for psychotic
        mothers and their young children, in *Parental psychiatric disorder:distressed
        parents and their families*.(eds) M Goepfert, J Webster & MV Seeman,
        Cambridge University Press, pp.161-170
[147]   Matthey S, Barnett B, Ungerer J & Waters B (2000) Paternal and maternal
        depressed mood during the transition to parenthood. *Journal of Affective
        Disorders* **60**, 75–85.
[148]   Deater-Deckard K, Pickering K, Dunn JF & Golding J (1998) Family
        structure and depressive symptoms in men preceding and following the birth
        of a child. The Avon longitudinal study of pregnancy and childhood study
        team. *American Journal of Psychiatry* **155**, 818–823.
[149]   Areias MEG, Kumar R, Barros H & Figueiredo E (1996) Correlates of postnatal
        depression in mothers and fathers. *British Journal of Psychiatry* **169**: 36–41.
[150]   Lovestone S & Kumar R (1993) Postnatal psychiatric illness: the impact on
        partners, *British Journal of Psychiatry,* **163**:210-6
[151]   Ballard C & Davies R (1996) Postnatal depression in fathers, *International
        Review Psychiatry* **8**:65-71
[152]   a. Zelkowitz P & Milet TH (2001) The course of postpartum psychiatric
        disorders in women and their partners. *Journal of Nervous and Mental Disease*
        189, 575–582
        b. Kane P & Garber J (2004) The relations among depression in fathers, children's
        psychopathology and father-child conflict: a meta-analysis,*Clinical Psychology
        Review,***24**:339-60
        c. Lewis C & Lamb ME (2003) Fathers' influences on children's development –
        the evidence from two-parent families, *European Journal of Eductaion,*
        18:211-228.
[153]   Goodeman JH (2004) Paternal postpartum depression, its relationship to
        maternal postpartum depression, and implications for family health.
        Integrative literature reviews and meta-analyses, *Journal of .Advanced Nursing*
        45:26-31
[154]   a. Field T (1998) Maternal depression: effects on infants and early interventions.
        Preventive Medicine **27**, 200–203.
        b.Hossain Z et al (1994) Infants of depressed mothers interaction better with their
        non-depressed fathers, *Infant Mental Health Journal,* **15**:348-57
[155]   Butterworth P (2004) Lone mothers' experience of physical and sexual

violence: association with mental disorders, *The British journal of Psychiary,* **184**:21-7

[155b] Groves BM, Lieberman AF, Osofsky JD & Fenichel E (2000) Protecting young children in violent environments - a framework to build on, *Zero to Three,***20**:9-13

[156] Huth-Bocks AC, Levendosky AA, Theran SA & Bogat GA (2004) The impact of domestic violence on mothers' prenatal representations of their infants, *Infant Mental Health Journal* **25**:79-98.

[157] for clinical examples see Raphael-Leff J (2002) 'Presence of Absence' in *Journey to Motherhood,* F Thomson-Salo (ed), Melbourne: Stonningt on Press

[158] Coates S & Moore MS1997) The Complexity of Early Trauma: Representation and Transformation *Psychoanaltic Inquiry,* **17**:286-311

[159] Crawford TA & Lipsedge M (2004) Seeking help for psychological distress: the interface of Zulu traditional healing and Western biomedicine, *Mental Health, Religion & Culture,* 7:131-148

[160] a. Oates at al, 2004, *op.cit.*
b. Editorial (2003) Treatment of postnatal depression *British Medical Journal* **327**:1003-4

[161] a. Spielvogel, AM (1997) Psychiatric aspects of pregnncy and the postpartum, *International Medical Journal,* **4**:87-92
b. Cott AD & Wisner KL (2003) Psychiatric disorders during pregnancy *International Review of Psychiatry* 15:217-230

[162] McIntosh J(1993) Postpartum depression: women's help-seeking behaviour and perceptions of cause .*Journal of Advanced Nursing* 18:178-184

[163] Asten P, Marks MN, Oates MR & the TCS-PND Group (2004) Aims, measures, study sites and participant samples of the Transcultural Study of Postnatal Depression *British Journal of Psychiatry* (supplement 46) **184**:3-9

[164] Heneghan AM, Silver EJ, Bauman LJ & Stein REK (2000) Do pediatricians recognise mothers with depressive symptoms, *Pediatrics* **106**:1367-73

[165] Hendrick, V (2003) Editorial: Treatment of postnatal depression – effective interventions are available but the condition remains underdiagnosed, *British Medical Journal,* **327**:1003-4

[166] Richter-Rössler A & Hofecker Fallahpour M (2003) Postpartum depression: do we still need this diagnostic term? *Acta Psychiatrica Scandanavica***108**:51-6

[167] Gorell Barnes J (1998) *Family Therapy in Changing Times* Basic Texts in Counselling and Psychotherapy, London:MacMillan.

[168] Heinicke CM et al (2001) *op.cit.*

[169] Daws D (2003) Sleep Problems in babies and young children, chapter 10 in *Infant-Parent* Psychodynamics – wild things, mirrors and ghosts, (ed). J Raphael-Leff, London: Whurr, 2003

[170] Hopkins J (2003) Therapeutic interventions in infancy: two contrasting cases of persistent crying in *Infant-Parent Psychodynamics – wild things, mirrors and ghosts,* (ed). J Raphael-Leff, London: Whurr

[171] Aquarone S (2003) Feeding disorders, chapter 23 in *Infant-Parent Psycho- dynamics – wild things, mirrors and ghosts,* (ed). J.Raphael-Leff, London: Whurr

[172] Baradon T (2002) Issues from the Floor - some dilemmas for the therapist In Parent-Infant Psychotherapy, pp.80-82 in *Between Sessions and Beyond the Couch* (ed.) J Raphael-Leff, University of Essex

[173] Norman J (2002) The Experience of Infant Psychoanalysis is a surprise, pp.94-6, in *Between Sessions and Beyond the Couch,* ibid

[174] Thomson-Salo F (2002) Working Psychoanalytically with the infant in the

consulting room, pp. 77-9 in *Between Sessions and Beyond the Couch,* ibid

[175] Watanabe H (2002) Treating Anorexia Nevrosa: Ghosts in the Paediatric Ward or fetus in a new womb, pp.83-4 in *Between Sessions and Beyond the Couch,* ibid

[176] Berg A (2002) Ubuntu – from the consulting room to the vegetable garden, pp.102-7, in *Between Sessions and Beyond the Couch,* ibid

[177] Cohen NJ et al (2002) Six-month follow-up of two mother-infant psychotherapies: convergence of therapeutic outcomes, *Infant Mental Health Journal,* 23:361-380. [For detailed exposition of this method of therapeutic work see Tuters (2002) Infant-Parent Psychotherapy: Creating an Optimal Relational Space pp. 88-91, in *Between Sessions and Beyond the Couch,* ibid].
b. Zilbowitz M (2004) Watch, Wait and Wonder: A Parent-Child Attachment Intervention, *Infant Mental Health Journal,* **24**:5 *supplement 6A* 9th World Congress, Melbourne, Australia

[178] a. Ben-Aaron, M., Harel, J, Kaplan, H & Patt, R(2001) *Mother-Child and Father-Child Psychotherapy - a manual for the treatment of relational disturbances in childhood,* London:Whurr publishers
b. Acquarone, S.(2004) *Infant-Parent Psychotherapy – a Handbook,* London: Karnac
c. Baradon, T et al(2005) *Parent-Infant Therapy Manual* London:Brunner-Routledge

[179] a. Fivaz-Depeursinge (2004) The Primary Triangle: treating infants in their families *Infant Mental Health Journal,* **24**:223, *supplement 6A* 9th World Congress, Melbourne, Australia

[180] Lieberman A(2002) Treatment of attachment disorders in infant-parent psychotherapy. Chapter in Maldonado-Duran, JM (ed) *Infant and toddler mental health:Models of clinical intervention with infants and their families,* pp.105-128. Washington DC:American Psychiatric Publishing

[181] Trevarthen C (2003/1974) 'Conversations with a two-month old' *New Scientist,* May 2nd 1974, with 2003 updating preface, Chapter 3, pp.25-34 in *Parent-Infant Psychodynamics – wild things, mirrors and ghosts,* (ed). J Raphael-Leff, London: Whurr

[182] Trevarthen C (2001) Intrinsic motives for companionship in understanding: their origin, development, and significance for infant mental health. *Infant Mental Health Journal,* special issue – contributions from the Decade of the Brain to infant mental health, **22**:95-131

[183] Trevarthen C (1999) Intersubjectivity. In R Wison & F Keil (eds) *The MIT Encyclopedia of Cognitive Sciences* (pp.413-6) Cambridge, MA :MIT Press

[184] Beebe B, Rustin J, Sorter D & Knoblauch S(2003) An expanded view of Intersubjectivity in infancy and its application to psychoanalysis, *Psycho-analytic Dialogues,* **13**:805-841

[185] Gergely G & Watson S(1996): 'The social biofeedback theory of parental affect-mirroring', *International Journal Psychoanalysis* 77:1181-1212.

[186] Target M & Fonagy P(1996) Playing With Reality: II. The development of psychic reality from a theoretical perspective. *International Journal of Psychoanalysis* **77**:459-479

[187] Hobson P (2002) *The Cradle of Thought – exploring the origins of thinking,* London:Macmillan

[188] ibid, p. 43

[189] Trevarthen C (1999), *op.cit.*

[190] Stern D (1995) *The Motherhood Constellation – a unified view of parent-infant psychotherapy,* New York: Basic Books

[191] Tronick EZ (2003)"Of course all relationships are unique": How co-creative processes generate unique mother-infant and patient-therapist relationships and change other relationships *Psychoanalytic Inquiry* 23:475-491

[192] Tronick EZ (1989/2003) Emotions and emotional communication in infants, *American Psychologist*, 1989, **44**:112-9 with updating preface Chapter 4, pp.35-53 in *Infant-Parent Psychodynamics – wild things, mirrors and ghosts*, (ed). J Raphael-Leff, London: Whurr, 2003, p.36

[193] For instance Proner K (2000) Protomental synchrony:some thoughts on the earliest identification processes in a neonate, *The International Journal of Infant Observation*, **3**:55-63

[194] Raphael-Leff J (1985) Facilitators and Regulators: vulnerability to postnatal disturbance *Journal of Psychosomatic Obstetrics and Gynaecology*, **4**:151-68

[195] a. Schore AN (2003) *Affect Dysregulation and Disorders of the Self*, New York:Norton
b. Schore AN (1996) The experience dependent maturation of a regulatory system in the orbital prefrontal cortext and the origin if developmental 'psychopathology, *Development & Psychopathology*, **8**:59-87
c. Schore AN (2001a) Effects of a secure attachment relationship on right brain development, affect regulation, and infant mental health, *Infant Mental Health Journal* **22**:7-66 Special Issue – Contributions from the Decade of the Brain. For an accessible presentation of recent neuropsychological findings see Gerhardt, S (2004)*Why Love Matters – how affection shapes a baby's brain*, London: Brunner-Routledge

[196] Siegel DJ (2001) Toward an interpersonal neurobiology of the developing mind: attachment relationships, 'mindsight' and neural integration, *Infant Mental Health Journal* **22**:67-94

[197] Beebe B, Jaffe J, Lachman F, Feldstein S, Crown C & Jasnow M (2000) Systems models in development and psychoanalysis: the case of vocal rhythm coordination and attachment. *Infant Mental Health Journal* **21**:99-122

[198] Fonagy P. & Target M. (1996): 'Playing With Reality: I. Theory of Mind and the normal development of psychic reality'. *International Journal of Psychanalysis* **77**:217-233

[199] a. Schore AN.(2001b) The effects of early relational trauma on right brain development, and affect regulation *Infant Mental Health Journal* **22**:201-69 Special Issue – Contributions from the Decade of the Brain
b. Damasio A.R(1999) *The Feeling of what Happens: Body and emotion in the making of consciousness*, New York: Harcourt Brace

[200] Panksepp J (2001) The long-term psychobiological consequences of infant emotions: prescriptions for the twenty-first century, *Infant Mental Health Journal* **22**:132-173

[201] Damasio AR (1999) *op.cit.*

[202] Freud S (1920) Beyond the Pleasure Principle London: Hogarth Press, 1948 pp. 33-341.

[203] O'Connor TG, Bredenkamp D & Rutter M(2000) Attachment disturbances and disorders in children exposed to early severe deprivation, *Infant Mental Health Journal* **20**:10-29

[204] Beebe B (2004) Faces in Relation, *Psychoanalytic Dialogues*, **14**:1-15

[205] Schore AN (2001a,b) *op.cit.*

[206] Hugdahl K (1995) Classical conditioning and implicit learning: the right hemisphere hypothesis. In RJ Davidson & K Hugdahl (eds), *Brain Asymmetry* (pp.235-267), Cambridge, MA:MIT Press. [Cited in Schore (2001a), pp.41-2].

[207] Raphael-Leff J (2001) 'Primary Maternal Persecution', Chapter 3 in *Forensic Psychotherapy and Psychopathology Winnicottian Perspectives* (ed.) B.Kahr, London: Karnac

[208] Raphael-Leff J (2000) 'Climbing the walls': puerperal disturbance and perinatal therapy in *Spilt Milk - perinatal loss and breakdown* (ed). J Raphael-Leff, London: Institute of Psychoanalysis & Routledge

[209] Stern D(1995) *op.cit.*

[210] a. Bowlby J (1969) *Attachment and Loss*, Vol. 1: *Attachment*, New York: Basic Books
b. Bowlby J (1973) *Attachment and Loss*, Vol. 2: *Separation* New York: Basic Books
c. Bowlby J (1980) *Attachment and Loss*, Vol. 3: *Loss* New York: Basic Books

[211] Main M (1991) Metacognitive knowledge, metacognitive monitoring, and singular (coherent) vs. multiple (incoherent) models of attachment . In: *Attachment Across the Life-Cycle*, CM Parkes, J Stevenson-Hinde & P Marris, (eds). London: Routledge, pp. 127-159

[212] a. Fonagy P, Steele M, Moran G, Steele H & Higgitt A (1993) Measuring the Ghost in the Nursery: An Empirical Study of the Relation Between Parents' Mental Representations of Childhood Experiences and their Infants' Security of Attachment. *Journal of American Psychoanalytical Association* **41**:957-89
b. Steele H, Steel M & Fonagy P (1996) Associations among attachment classifications of mothers, fathers, and their infants, *Child Development* **67**:541-55

[213] Scher A (2001) Facilitators and Regulators: maternal orientation as an antecedent of attachment security. *Journal of Reproductive and Infant Psychology*, **19**:325-333

[214] a. Cassidy J & Shaver PR (eds)(2002) *Handbook of Attachment*, New York: Guilford Press
b. Holmes J(2001) *The Search for a Secure Base: Attachment Theory and Psychotherapy*, Brunner-Routledge.
c. Carlson EA & Stroufe LA (1995) Contributions of attachment theory to developmental psychopathology, in D.Cicchetti & DJ Cohen (eds) *Developmental Psychopathology*, vol 1, New York:Wiley

[215] Zeanah CH, Brois NW & Larrier JA (2000) Infant development and developmental risk: A review of the past 10 years. *Journal of the American Academy of Child and Adolescent psychiatry*, **36**:165-178

[216] Murray L & Cooper P (eds) (1997) *Post Partum Depression and Child Development*, London: Guilford

[217] Cooper PJ, Murray L, Wilson A & Romaniuk H (2003) Controlled trial of short- and long-term effect of psychological treatment of post-partum depression, *British Journal of Psychiatry*, **182**:412-9

[218] O'Hara M, Stuart S, Gorman LL & Wenzel A (2000) Efficacy of interpersonal psychotherapy for postpartum depression, *Archives of GeneralPsychiatry* 57:1039-45

[219] Sharp D & Hay D (1992) Susceptibility of infants to maternal depression: effect of timing and differential impact in males and females *Infant Behaviour & Developmen,*17 (special ICIS issue)

[220] Burke L (2003) The impact of maternal depression on familial relationships, *International Review of Psychiatry* **15**:243-55

[221] see Schore, A. (2001b), *op.cit.*

[222] Gopfert M , Webster J & Seeman M (eds) (1996) *Parental Psychiatric Disorder* – distressed parents and their families, Cambridge: Cambridge University Press

[223] Sharp HM & Bramwell R (2004) An empirical evaluation of a psycho-analytic theory of mothering orientation: implications for the antenatal prediction of postnatal depression. *Journal of Reproductive and Infant Psychology,* **22**:71-89

[224] Moore MS (1997) How can we remember but be unable to recall? The complex function of multimodular memory . In: *Memory in Dispute,* V. Sinason (ed). London: Karnac.

[225] see Sinason V (ed) (1994) *Treating Survivors of Satanist Abuse* London: Routledge

[226] *Child Physical and Sexual Abuse: Guidelines for treatment,* April, 2004 National Crime Victims Research & Treatment Centre, Medical University, Charleston, South Carolina, and Centre for Sexual Assault and Traumatic Stress, Harborview Medical Center, Seattle, Washington

[227] United States Department of Health (2003) Third National Incidence Study of Child Abuse and Neglect (NIS-3)

[228] Royal College of Psychiatrists (2002) The Mental Health & Growing Up series fact sheet 20 *Child abuse and neglect - the emotional effects*

[229] Shonkoff, JP & Phillips, DA (Eds) (2000) *From Neurons to Neighborhoods – the science of early childhood development,* Washington DC:National Academy Press

[230] Ekstrom A, Matthiesen AS, Widstrom AM & Nissen E (2005) Breastfeeding attitudes among counselling caregivers, *Scandinavian Journal of Public Health,* **33**

[231] Sharp HM. (1995). Women's expectations of childbirth and early motherhood: their relation to preferred mothering orientation, subsequent experience, satisfaction and postpartum depression. *Doctoral thesis*, University of Leicester.

[232] Sharp HM and Bramwell R (2004) *op.cit.*

[233] Scher A & Blumberg O (1992). Facilitators and Regulators: cross-cultural and Methodological considerations. *British Journal of Medical Psychology,* **65**, 327-331

[234] Scher A & Blumberg O (2000) Night-waking among one year-olds: a study of maternal separation anxiety *Child: Care, Health & Development* **26**:323-334

[235] McBride S & Belsky J(1988) Characteristics, determinants and consequences of maternal separation anxiety, *Developmental Psychology,* **24**:407-414

[236] Scher A (2001) Facilitators and Regulators: maternal orientation as an antecedent of attachment security. *Journal of Reproductive and Infant Psychology,* **19:** 325-333

[237] Lulav-Greenwald D (1994) Attachment p atterns of Kibbutz mothers, their attitudes towards raising children and adjustment of their children in different sleeping arrangements. Unpublished MA thesis, Department of Psychology, University of Haifa, Israel.

[238] Van Bussel J (2003) Unpublished MA thesis, Family and Sexuality Studies, Faculty of Medicine, KU University Leuven, Belgium

[239] Charles L (2001) Development of the PPP (Placental Paradigm) measure, Unpublished doctoral thesis, University of East Anglia

Preface

We are each trapped inside our own conscious experience. This makes us solitary prisoners unless we can stretch that inner space like a membrane to envelop a wider experience. We expand personal boundaries by extending a mental 'antenna' outwards and fine-tuning our receivers, by verbally articulating our own undefined impressions and by courageously reaching inwards into the dark interior of our unknown selves. In this book, all I can do is provide a vocabulary of experience as it has been shared with me. The degree to which it can be heard is up to the reader's receptivity to his or her own experience. Much of it is disturbing, dwelling as it does on the basic, universal, age-old questions of mankind: 'Where do babies come from?'; 'How are they made?'; 'What are the differences between the sexes?'.

Ovum meets sperm and the reproductive process begins. So it has been since the beginning of human life. Yet suddenly, in our day, not only is sex possible without conception, conception is possible without sex. We live in exciting times. Readers engaged in the process of childbearing and professionals working in this field are privileged in having direct access to some of the most primitive human experiences and some of the most novel and profound psychosocial and ethical controversies of all time. In our experience, we become intensely aware of the raw ingredients of emotion and society – the biological male/female division that lies at the crux of many social structures; elemental passions of pain, love, envy and longing; the eternal repetition of 'birth-copulation and death'-cycles in each generation in which an individual is simultaneously both a cipher in the human chain between past and future and the unique centre of his or her own world.

Conception physically activates potentialities for procreation inherent since the emergence of reproductive organs in the male and female fetus. Similarly, maturity vitalizes the psychological processes of procreativity which have been evolving since infancy, however, these are triggered not by conception but by the idea of having a baby. Thus, psychosocial influences leading to reproduction are initiated not when woman meets man or ovum sperm, but commence decades earlier from the moment the newborn baby is introduced to the world of parent(s), caring professionals (be they obstetricians, midwives, paediatricians, nurses, GPs, health visitors or others), relatives and friends. The process may even begin prenatally, in fetal encounters with the sound/touch of his or her pregnant mother and her familiars. Unwittingly, we adults, in our professional roles or social capacities all help shape the young child's ideas about future childbearing. Even as the person who assisted each of our own mothers in her delivery, influenced not only the course of that birth but set the tone for our early encounters with that all-important parturient woman.

You, the reader, who share common psychosocial surroundings with me, the writer, and the same fundamentally human emotions as the human subjects of this book, may find much that is familiar and known from within. However, some ideas may seem far-fetched or strange, others disturbing, stirring flurries of long forgotten dim memories or evoking faint echoes of feelings that have been buried or banished. Rather than dwelling on what is rational and socially acceptable, we shall be exploring the human emotions that lie behind the facade. Listen to what is not being said in the interview; glimpse the experiences that cannot be shared with strangers, professionals or even confidantes; grasp fleeting unrevealed thoughts and dreams that fade in daylight only to return unbidden in the dead of night. You, the reader, may have to suspend judgement at times in hearing what is not usually spoken, trying to remain receptive despite an urge to flee to reassuring solid ground. Perceptiveness is not easy, but the reward lies in glimpses into others which can enrich understanding not only of them, but of one's own responses to them. To understand each other, I will set out several basic assumptions.

1. That our adult behaviour is rooted in earlier experiences and that different levels of conscious and unconscious experience coexist in each of us.
2. That consciousness flows like a stream, yet in our conscious life, we attend largely to the surface level, censoring out the myriad associations and network of images that lie in the 'depths', the whirlpools and undercurrents of which nevertheless affect the stream's flow. During sleep and in times of greater permeability, unconscious material from the deeper 'waters' and 'river-bed' are dredged up in the form of fantasies and dreams.
3. Thus, that latent fantasy accompanies ongoing experiences, and 'inner reality' can be as real and influential as external reality, and overspill into it.
4. That at times of greater vulnerability and during the upheaval of 'transitional' phases in our lives such as adolescence or pregnancy, earlier modes of functioning are reinstated and unresolved conflicts are reactivated.

A book is the sum total of cumulative multifactorial growth. The main fabric of this book is woven both from my clinical experience as a psychoanalyst and from studies I have conducted as a social psychologist. I have drawn on thousands of hours of being with patients, day after day for several years with each, working through deep emotional processes, in psychoanalysis or psychotherapy within a practice dedicated to issues of reproductivity. In addition to therapeutic work with individuals, couples and groups, I have utilized many reams of tape-recorded in-depth discussions over the past 15 years with pregnant and parturient childbirth education group and workshop participants, pregnant couples, colleagues, and playgroup mothers and fathers talking about their feelings. Although I do not present case histories in this book, I have inserted illustrative quotations (in brackets) where these could enliven relevant txts. This interactive work has been supplemented by three modest surveys and disciplined observation of 23 mother-baby pairs on a thrice-weekly basis in a very large Community Centre PACT (Parents and Children Together) Playgroup over a period of the eight years I spent there. Larger studies are being conducted to replicate this model.

Above all, being part of the culture I study, my work is inevitably grounded in and informed by the matrix of my own pregnancies, babies and motherhood. Finally, to enrich the tapestry of internal and external human realities, I have attempted to bridge the gaps in my experience by drawing (albeit selectively) from the vast pool of research findings and work of colleagues in many different disciplines — psychoanalysis, social and experimental psychology, anthropology, ethology and neonatology. Reproductive research is a rapidly expanding field and by the time this book goes to press a great deal of new and relevant data will have been published. I have only been able to cover a small proportion of studies in the many areas of interest, but hope this will whet the reader's appetite to explore the current literature further.

JRL/1991

Acknowledgements

In gratitude to my family of origin and the extended 'clan' in which I grew up; to my husband, daughter and sons, and to the many people who have shared their sorrow, and joyful experiences of childbearing with me.

2005 Addendum: dedicated to all our grandchildren

Foreword

Over a quarter of a century ago Bibring (1959) and Brazelton (1973) first described, from prenatal psychoanalytic interviews of normal pregnant women, the turmoil and anxiety that is contained just below the surface. Initially these observations were cause for much concern. Over time, however, Brazelton and others began to view the prenatal anxiety and distortion of fantasy as a healthy process that helps a woman's emotional homeostasis to re-organize and ready her circuits for new adaptation. The process also helps make her unusually sensitive to the infant's individual needs and requirements. As he noted, 'This very emotional turmoil of pregnancy and that in the neonatal period can be seen as a positive force for the mother's adjustment'. About the same time, Winnicott (1958) described a unique state a mother reaches shortly before delivery which he termed 'Primary Maternal Preoccupation' and noted: 'The state lasts for a few weeks after the birth of the child. Only if the mother is sensitized in the way I am describing can she feel herself in to her infant's place and so meet the infant's needs'.

Following in the creative traditions of Bibring, Brazelton and Winnicott, Joan Raphael-Leff brings their concepts several steps forward as well as adding original crucial elements. For instance, she supplements the concept above with another of 'Primary Maternal Persecution', similarly experienced by a mother in the early weeks after the birth of a baby, but one with whom she feels unable to empathize. The author has written this unique and valuable book after a prolonged (15 years) and in-depth immersion as a psychoanalyst and social psychologist working mainly with problems around childbearing. Her own life experiences in pregnancies and mothering clearly helped her develop a special sensitivity and profound understanding of the diverse reactions to childbearing, as observed throughout the text. Also exceptional in her work is the integration of unconscious material from her many years of clinical work with patients, with empirical data from surveys and controlled observation of ordinary mothers and babies. The book covers all areas of childbearing including roots of the early wish to have a baby, the sorrows of infertility, the experiences of lesbian partners, birth practices, beliefs and the setting of birthplace in different cultures, emotional reactions of siblings, adoption, postnatal depression and even aspects of caring for families following the birth of a malformed or sick infant.

Major innovative sections of the book follow when Joan Raphael-Leff notes that a woman's motivation for accepting help during pregnancy is not only to alleviate suffering from her present symptoms but 'it rides on a tide of emotional resurgence which both awakens forgotten feelings and strives for reappraisal of identity'. She also observes and confirms that pregnancy is accompanied by 'permeability of the psychological boundaries between conscious thought and hitherto unconscious fantasies resulting in an accessibility of buried emotions and earlier modes of symbolic thinking and irrational ideas', and she continues 'the pregnant womb serves as a receptacle for pregnancy projections and fantasies about the fetus'.

Within the family, the crisis of childbirth provides a unique window of exploration and an opportunity to rework fantasies that are usually deeply submerged. Due to the intrapsychic reorganization necessary to make space for the infant as a new member of the family system, these are churned up in siblings and parents and are for a brief period accessible near the surface. Joan Raphael-Leff has recognized the therapeutic implications and unusual advantages of this short period of openness and she describes how to use it most effectively. She is also acutely aware of how each person's past, including very early experiences, alter, modify and direct their care of the infant. She notes; 'The pregnant woman undergoes profound psychological and physical upheavals condensed into a relatively short period of time, which may necessitate some external therapeutic intervention to prevent her becoming overwhelmed. While brief psychotherapy during pregnancy offers a form of crisis intervention, long lasting changes may arise out of the experience of therapy, such as an inhanced capacity for tolerating uncertainty, ameliorated prenatal bonding, ongoing increments from the retrieval of a greater array of positive moments and figures in the internal world, and receptivity to the repeated affirmation of self-growth in positive labour and mothering experiences.'

Her observations cover a variety of perspectives – dwelling on too overt attitudes and underlying unconscious pressures in caretakers. As an example, 'The non-pregnant therapist inevitably experiences disturbing twinges of envy and awesome appreciation of the powerhouse of tangible creativity. Access to particularly primitive emotions may re-evoke repressed elements from a female therapist's own previous pregnancies arousing empathy, protectiveness, defensiveness or aversion.' Equally helpful are the many observations about clients' transferential feelings and the counter-transference responses and defences of medical and paramedical carers.

She has, in her beautiful writing, the capacity to encourage the reader to sense and evoke many subjective experiences, such as that of the pregnant woman herself; 'all she knows is that somebody else, living with her under her skin, is growing larger and expanding inside her body and feels she will burst at the seams. Her boundaries seem too tight to contain them both and clearly one of them must go! However, in the deepest recesses of her mind lurks a primitive dread that the wrong one will be expelled. In her unspeakable fantasy she fears that she might just vanish during the transition of childbirth and the baby will retain her body.' This tallies with my clinical observation when as a physician I have noted that many women immediately after delivering a baby have to wait a moment before taking on their own infant until they are sure that they themselves are all in one piece.

We owe an extended gratitude to Joan Raphael-Leff for both the thoroughness of the work which includes the complete range of child-bearing problems and a review of research in the field and for her own original formulations and observations, models and schematic concep-tualizations. We are fortunate that the author is deeply immersed in clinical practice. This comes through on every page from her insights and from the literature that she has discussed. We owe the author thanks for what is probably the first complete, and certainly innovative, book on the psychology of childbearing . . . a must for all caregivers working in this field. Coming at a time when we are now questioning present practices in all areas of childbearing, this book will serve as a handbook for the care of the family at this period of life.

REFERENCES

Bibring, B.L. (1959) Some considerations of the psychologic processes in pregnancy. *Psychoanalytic Study of the Child*, 14: 113–121.

Brazelton, T.B. (1973) Effect of maternal expectations on early infant behaviour, *Early Child Development and Care*, 2: 259–273.

Winnicott, D.W. (1958) Collected Papers: *Through Paediatrics to Psycho-Analysis*, Basic Books, Inc.

Marshall Klaus 1990
Professor of Paediatrics

Part One

PREGNANCY EXPECTATION

Chapter 1

The wish for a baby: psychosocial and cultural factors

1.1 INTRODUCTION

This chapter locates the wish for a baby in the contexts of cultural, social and personal motivation to reproduce. It also presents an extended exposition of unconscious intrapsychic (within the psyche) factors based on a psychoanalytical understanding of early human relationships. This material may be completely novel to some readers and consequently difficult to absorb at first reading without reference to the clinical situation with which they are familiar.

Here and elsewhere, you are advised to follow your interests. If you wish, omit this chapter and move on to Chapter 2 which deals with the decision to become parents (paying special attention to ethnic minorities, and lesbians) or if you prefer to get directly to the psychological aspects of infertility or pregnancy, go to Chapters 3 or 4 and return to the beginning when you have completed reading the clinical application of the theory. The summary of key points at the end of each section map the terrain and can serve as a guide on your journey through this volume.

1.2 MOTIVATION FOR REPRODUCTION

Why do we have babies? In this era of rapid social and technological change our accepted view of reality has been undermined. Whereas previously sex and pregnancy were inextricably linked, efficient contraception, artificial insemination and free access to abortion have created a new climate in which female sexuality is potentially freed from reproduction and both sex and childbearing can be unhitched from the social institution of marriage. Recent developments in western society have revealed that the human desire to reproduce is not inbuilt as we have been led to believe but has both conscious and unconscious roots embedded in the particular origins of each individual – the family in which one was brought up, the culture into which one was born and the society in which one lives as an adult. Today, we can no longer cling to myths of 'maternal instinct' or beliefs that 'anatomy is destiny' or even teleological assumptions that we are governed by a purely biological drive of 'selfish' genes but we have to account for pregnancy in terms of a complex psychosocial wish to reproduce. Although motivation for reproduction is complex and highly personal, there are a few constant factors:

1. **Genetic immortality**. Faced with the uniquely human fore-knowledge of death, individuals wish to prolong their existence by casting their genes into the future to survive after their death.
2. **Becoming 'adult'**. Since our earliest interaction is with people who are parents, 'mummies and daddies' become synonymous with adults. Even when we grow up, irrationally it may seem to us that we never finally achieve true adulthood until we parent our own children.
3. **Emulating the parent(s)**. While growing up, children are aware of the difference between their own limited abilities and those of the mother and father. This discrepancy is most marked in the fertile parents' capacity to 'make babies' in contrast to the child's pre-nubile infertility and pubertal postponement of procreation. Having a baby erases this primal dividing-line and enables the 'child' to assume the productive sexual identity of a parent finally engaging in all the hitherto prohibited or withheld activities, emulating the admired parent with whom they have identified.
4. **Reciprocating parental care**. Human babies are born dependent. In fact, a British psychoanalyst once went so far as to suggest that 'there is no such thing as a baby'[1], since no infant can survive on its own without a caregiver. One way of repaying all the caring love and attention received is to lavish it on an equally dependent being, the previously needy child now occupying the position of a generous parent.
5. **Second chance**. No parent can be perfect. We all suffer from recollection of frustrating times when the quality of care did not meet our exact needs. To some, these were not rare occasional lapses but the ongoing stuff of infancy. Having a baby offers a rare opportunity actively to correct that experience by vicariously giving the infant all one would have wished to have had. Being in control this time helps master old anxieties. Close contact with a growing baby can enable some parents to relive painful passages of their own infancy, resolve, repair and reintegrate them. Others may abuse their position of power.
6. **Love object**. The indulged baby can thus represent one's own ideal or brutalized baby-self. But babies also reciprocate in a unique way, loving the mother or father despite their lapses and failures, making them feel lovable and invested with a special warmth. This loving response may be sought as a novel variation of that early

unconditional love which we all unconsciously continue to crave.
7. **Cultural transmission.** The point at which individual and societal goals intertwine is the parent's wish to pass on a fund of experience, knowledge, skills and personal-lore accumulated in one's lifetime.

1.3 CULTURAL EXPECTATIONS OF CHILDBEARING

'Culture consists of abstract patterns of and for living and dying' Samuel Johnson.

Pregnancy and birth are social as well as biological events. With our new technologies a fundamental discrepancy has been revealed: for society procreation is survival; for the individual it is a choice. In any particular society, should women cease to become pregnant, that society would die out. Thus, all cultures develop means to ensure that women will continue to reproduce. Virtually all known human societies have organized around a social division into two genders with woman defined by her biological role of reproduction of the species.[2]

To begin at the beginning. Ethological, archaeological and anthropological evidence suggest it is likely that the original social unit was that of the foraging mother and her suckling [3, 4]. Upright posture and consequent reshaping of the pelvis reduced the diameter of the birth canal, with natural selection for small-headed premature babies [5] necessitating ongoing maternal care. How human social networks evolved is open to speculation. One possibility is that the invention of containers (mimicking that first container, the womb?) permitted food-gathering, storage and, hence, mobility, sharing and cooperation. These contributed to the formation of small social groups, enabling individuals to gain access to a greater variety of materials and services [6]. It has been argued that the loss of oestrus in human females cemented heterosexual pair-bonding [7], and although it is not known when man's role in procreation was recognized, we may assume that acknowledgement of paternity provoked patrilineal (father-line) kinship bonds [8]. To this day, fatherhood remains a social construct. Whereas the mother-infant connection is unquestioningly demonstrated by pregnancy and birth, paternity is based on trust, and in all societies the social father is marked by declaration (such as *couvade* or naming) and need not coincide with the biological impregnator.

Patriarchal societies thus need to grapple with the problem of male genetic immortality. To this end they elaborate rules and regulations which prescribe, restrict and organize female sexuality and procreation. In other words, (male) authorities define social mores which determine which women can become mothers and at what age, the context in which pregnancy is permissible ('legitimate') and even the interval between babies is regulated by social taboos on intercourse after a birth. Woman's

identity in most societies is defined by her procreativity, whereas man
has to define his role in cultural terms. Male elders exert control over
female fecundity by ideological and magico-religious means, through
monopoly over communication with ancestors and the spirit world and
rituals which regulate fertility. On an unconscious level, woman is
associated with Nature. Pregnant and lactating, she is regarded as closer
to natural functions unavailable to men who deem themselves superior.
They, in turn, create artefacts in their attempt to transcend natural
conditions by evolving 'Culture' [9] from which women are excluded,
confined as they are to domestic intimate childrearing rather than public
realms [10]. Reproductive obedience and female subordination are thus
ensured by the exclusion of women from political, religious and public
organizations; psychosocial, medical and sometimes legal non-ownership
of their bodies; confinement to childbearing and rearing and lack of
economic control over the material surplus when they help create it, even
though in many traditional societies women make the bulk of produce.
(WHO statistics show that women do two-thirds of the world's work;
provide 45% of its food; earn 10% of its income and own 1% of its
property [11].)

Moreover, children not only signify survival and continuity; they can
constitute wealth. In horticultural and agricultural societies, successful
men can increase production of a surplus by having many labouring
children, who also provide heirs, ensure property succession and security
in their father's old age. In societies in which a wife is vulnerable because
marriage uproots her from her home, by having a male baby she may
enhance her status and secure her precarious position as a stranger to
her husband's tribe.

I am suggesting here that cultural transmission of the vital wish for
a baby across generations and within a caring family unit has so far been
ensured by limiting the social definition of women's role to childbearing
and childrearing and by promoting economic and political advantages
to men who produce offspring. However, today, western societies are
facing an unprecedented reproductive upheaval as women claim a right
to control their own fertility and be non-breeders if they wish, and to
occupy public roles in non-domestic cultural institutions and in the
workforce as automation reduces the excuse of physical differentiation
of the sexes in division of labour. Social and political pressures have
emphasized maternal exclusivity as primary caregiver. However, as more
fathers are included in the birth process and infant survival no longer
depends on a lactating woman, the importance of the father for the
infant's well-being is becoming apparent and some men are claiming
their right to 'mother'. Concurrently, a multidisciplinary approach is
contributing ever refined understanding of the complex psycho-bio-social
(as opposed to purely biological, psychological or sociological) roots of

the wish to reproduce, and it is to these that we now turn.

1.4 EARLY EXPERIENCE AND EXPECTATIONS OF CHILDBEARING

'The Child is father of the Man'. Wordsworth

We cannot generalize about early experience. Although in traditional societies the lore of baby-care is passed on from mother to daughter (or to son's wife) thereby remaining fairly constant over time, the way babies are nurtured, the tenor, style and quality of maternal care varies across societies and in industrial societies across and even within classes. In the West, changing beliefs about babies have engendered different childcare patterns between generations of mothers and daughters [12] and it is also possible to note variations in the same mother with different babies. Clearly, since some extended families practise surrogate mothering and in certain households in our own society mothers share childcare with nannies and au pairs, exclusive mothering is neither inevitable nor biologically determined by pregnancy. Furthermore, a variety of constellations occur – we encounter adoptive parents, lesbian couples, group parenting, single fathers and older siblings rearing their brothers or sisters. Nevertheless, tracing the intergenerational development of my theme of the 'wish for a baby', I shall focus here mainly on the heterosexual progenitors, present or absent, embedded in the generative matrix, and within it on the basic triangle of mother–father–child. I do so advisedly, since psychological processes do not always deal with the objective external reality that a child actually encounters, but are concerned with the internal reality – what each individual subjectively makes of the world s/he experiences.

To begin again at the beginning. At birth, each baby differs in its innate endowment of sensory-motor, cognitive and proprioceptive capacities. Research findings suggest that newborns already display 'personality' characteristics which are genetically determined and affected by gestational factors. Each infant also encounters particular nurturers through which his/her world is filtered. These parenting figures both display idiosyncratic features of their own and also convey prevalent ideas and features of their culture. As infants take in milk, so they also imbibe aspects of the social environment with which they interact in an ever widening circle, initially containing only the parent(s) and/or other significant figures. This interplay is gradually internalized becoming an unconscious substratum which persists in the internal psychic world independently of the relationships in which it originated.

Traditionally, not only have women given birth, they have also been allocated main responsibility for infant care. In any society where the mother is the primary caregiver, she will form the foundation of her infant's emotional self-image. The baby absorbs not only her milk but

her smell, warmth, touch, sound of her voice, her gaze and her disappointments and desires, her social status and self-image and her concept of her newborn baby. Inevitably, the mother relates differently to
her son and daughter. However, both male and female babies form
identifications with their early intimates, and when the primary caregiver
is the mother, both boy and girl baby learn to 'mother'.

The composition of the household is very important in determining
the experience of those early years: whereas extended family households
may include a variety of influences from several consecutive generations,
and/or different parallel groups related by blood or marriage (such as
brothers and their wives and children all living under the same roof,
or one man and several wives) industrialized societies (and hunter-
gatherers living at subsistence level) have evolved an insulated separate
household for the nuclear family, composed of a triangle of (present or
absent) father, mother and her child(ren). Thus, in western societies
where often each mother is isolated in her own home and exclusively
responsible for care of her infant, the baby will develop an intensely
specific 'monotropic' attachment to her [13] unmitigated by other
influences. In such 'mother-care' societies, at some point the growing
boy is required to 'dis-identify' from his nurturing female [14], by
emulating males instead and being socially initiated into the rites of
masculinity. In our culture, male identification with an often absent father
has been found to pose particular problems for the little boy, who has
been exposed to the minutiae of the feminine daily routine at home, and
later to a female teacher at nursery school. Lacking direct access to male
caregiving and enterprise, a western boy has had to construct a masculine
identity on his father's elusive and often idealized non-domestic role,
which some feminists regard as one root of female denigration, and which
many men are now trying to rectify by becoming nurturing fathers.

1.5 PSYCHOSEXUAL DEFINITIONS AND THE WISH FOR A BABY

In exploring the complex area of psychosexual identity it may be helpful
to examine three components separately:

1. Core gender identity – the sense of being male or female.
2. Gender role identity – establishing oneself as masculine or feminine
   in terms of social definitions.
3. Sexual partner orientation – choice of a heterosexual or homosexual
   love relationship [15].

Core gender identity begins very early, with sex-specific hormonal
influences [16], innate anatomical and biological factors, parental and
self physical-handling [17], growing male or female body image [18] and
sex assignment at birth leading to a sense of belonging to one sex and not

the other [19]. From very early on, parental attitudes towards their child's biological sex will be subtly conveyed in the quality of their differing interactions with boys and girls, the roughness or gentleness of touch and tone, the encouragement of some aspects of behaviour but discouragement of others. However, the picture is further complicated by differences between male and female parents in their own patterns of interaction with the newborn. Micro-analysis of parental behaviour reveals that in general, fathers provide more auditory and arousing physical stimulation than soothing maternal rhythms [20].

Gradually, the infant has to realize that being male or female will also define what is allowed. Thus, the growing infant develops a complex unconscious understanding of gender role expectations, which as discrimination increases, is supplemented by imitation of admired behaviours, conscious learning and practice. In the first year or two, before such limitations are acknowledged, both little girls and boys may wish to have a baby, too, like their mothers, or, in the irrational logic of the unconscious, even wish to have the mother herself turn into a baby, so that the child can nurture her in turn. It is not uncommon to see a baby feeding his/her mother reciprocally, or nursing a doll or pet, in imitation of and identification with the parent. Such games of becoming the mother reflect a host of different and ambivalent wishes; emulation of her power; angry revenge on her for frustrations; mastery of the situation of dependent helplessness; active learning through practice; gratitude and a desire to repay this debt of nurturing; a vicarious re-experiencing of earlier modes of babying or compensation for having missed out on gratification. Despite increasingly rational thought all these and other complex and irrational emotions, continue to surface in the individual at various times in his/her development and in adulthood combine to constitute a wish for a child. At first, little girls and boys of about 3 years old will each declare a wish to be like *both* their mummies and daddies, and although not yet interested in how babies are made and the father's role in procreation, will want to know how and where they came out [21].

As little boys and girls grow older and more aware of sexual male and female differences, each society dictates that they accept definition of themselves as either masculine or feminine according to that culture's strictures. They can no longer indulge in the fantasy of being omnipotent and sexually multifarious. A boy is expected to identify with the gender role of his father (or uncle or male head of the household) and a girl with her mother's. Their earlier experiences are now 'recategorized' in gender terms, relating to each parent in terms of their sex [22]. This means that the little girl now learns to relate to her mother as a 'same-sex person' and to her father as specifically male in relation to herself as female. Like her, the boy also has to give up his initial assumption of having unlimited gender potential. He has to exchange his desire to be pregnant, give birth and suckle a baby like his mother, for a wish to become like his father, whose penis is said mysteriously to provide the seed for the baby and whose job happens 'out there' in the unknown public world. The little girl may wish to be like her father too, and envies her brother not only his visible physical equipment, but greater independence and esteem, wider sphere of action outside the home and degrees of freedom within it. However, traditionally, she was usually dissuaded by family and friends who encouraged her to develop a gender role appropriate to females, and be satisfied with less adventurous domestic games and with the promise of becoming a future mother.

1.6 INCESTUOUS AND BISEXUAL CONFLICTS IN THE MALE

Our human capacity to identify with early caregivers across the gender boundary is the source of empathy and subtle understanding of each other. However, with the discovery of anatomical differences and their gender role corollaries, some of this extraordinary fluidity is lost. Understanding sexual restrictions brings about a sobering loss of omnipotence and, in the boy, an envy of breasts and womb that are the counterpart to the little girl's penis-envy. If his father is self-assured and encourages self-esteem in masculinity, the boy can relinquish these unrealized feminine wishes.

All his energies will now be invested in discovering what males do. He compensates by heightened phallic pride, identifying with his 'seed sowing' phallic father. At first, being like father means possessing the mother, and the esteemed father is also therefore a rival, since he is the one who impregnates and is husband to the mother, and what is more has an enviably larger penis. In his childish imagination the murderously competitive boy fears his father's retaliation, a fitting punishment of castration. Genital masturbation increases to reassure himself of his intact penis and its erectability. Eventually, given reassurance of a loving relationship with his father, the boy can transfer his desires from his mother to a future love of his own and allows these thoughts to subside until they are rearoused during adolescence.

If he resolves this problem it is likely that when the desire for a baby surfaces in adulthood, the man will wish to impregnate a woman with his child as his potent father did. However, a man who as a boy retained the unconscious and unsublimated wish to 'grow' a baby rather than 'give' one (particularly if a younger sibling was born at the peak of his castration fears [23]) may regard marriage only as a means of begetting children or view his wife as a mother.

If his wish for a baby remains based on unresolved envy, unsublimated rivalry and feminine identification with the woman throughout her pregnancy, he may sabotage its completion or try and control or upstage the birth, or compete in mothering.

If his father has been unsure of his own masculinity and unavailable to present a secure model and mentor, the sexually differentiating boy may have begun by defining his maleness negatively, repudiating his earlier nurturing experience, being not-feminine, not-dependent and macho in his dis-identification from the baby-creating/mothering female.

If his father was actually sadistic and punitive, the boy may grow up afraid to pursue his masculine role at all.

If his father has been too idealized, emotionally unavailable or seductive, he may remain fixed in yearning for his father, wishing to be feminine and loved or impregnated by his father as his mother is.

Alternatively, if his mother has been too babying and gratifying and/or father has been passive, unable to protect the boy from maternal overinvolvement or her domination, the boy may wish to remain merged with and cared for by his mother and fear assuming a masculine role.

On the other hand, a boy who has had a close relationship with a caring, emotionally present father, can experience a continuity, and will not have to repudiate his early nurturing capacities or label them as foreignly feminine. He can grow up wishing to care for a baby in full identification with both his father and early nurturing mother.

1.7 FEMALE GENDER IDENTITY AND SEXUAL PARTNER ORIENTATION

Nuclear families, where a female is the primary caregiver, promote particular patterns. For a woman, having a baby completes the original triangular family relationship of mother–father–baby. In the absence of early paternal nurturing, the early highly charged loving relationship is focused on a woman, the mother. However, unlike the heterosexual man who marries a woman (female like his original love, his mother), the heterosexual woman has had to change her first love-relationship from that with a female, her mother, to a male, like her father. One theory suggests that this enforces the female need for a baby to recreate the early twosome experienced with her mother, this time with herself in the maternal role. Men who have had a woman both as primary caretaker-mother and, later, as wife have not had to make this dramatic transition and therefore, in marriage, do not seem to have the same driving need for a third 'corner' to complete the relational triangle [24].

The little girl who identifies with her mother's female role as childbearer will wish to have a baby of her own, like mother's, from her father. If love for her mother triumphs over her jealous desire to get rid of her, she can continue to build her relationship with both parents, content to come to terms with postponement of her wishes and the promise of a future baby and man of her own. Meanwhile, until reactivation of these issues in adolescence, her life may be spent in consolidation of her identity and extension of her 'non-gendered' capacities. Having both a nurturing mother and a caring appreciative father she can grow up without the unfulfilled craving that drives women into seeking solace and compensation rather than a human relationship with her baby.

However, if her father has been emotionally or physically too seductive, ambivalence and a disturbing sense of disloyalty may disrupt her earlier positive relationship towards the mother who does not intervene to establish her rightful place and protect her daughter from precocious sexual arousal (Chapter 33).

Likewise, a little girl whose mother is not comfortable with her own feminity and cannot encourage her daughter's female self-esteem, may be unable to overcome her envy of male power and the sexual organ she was not endowed with, and denying the importance of her inner creative space and feminine qualities, may spend her life defiantly engaging in what is socially defined as 'masculine' [25].

Or else she might compromise, promising herself not a maternal vocation liker her mother's, but a (male) baby who will substitute for the absent penis [26]. (Such a woman might wish for an infant to renew her early sense of omnipotent completeness, thus expecting the baby to produce miracles or be perfect, or wanting to keep her child as an 'appendage' rather than a person in its own right [27]).

She might find it difficult to identify with her mother given the vast differences between her own skinny little body and mother's full breasted one. In a stratified society she may not see the full range of female bodies from childhood through puberty to adulthood. And in a culture which, like our own until very recently, delegates to females the roles of wife, baby-incubator, mother and little else, postponement of her feminine definition until maturity may mean living out years of 'limbo', waiting to be awakened by The Man and A Baby.

A woman for whom childhood envy of the mother's fertility has been intense, or whose mother devalued the daughter's sexuality, may become unconsciously fearful that the powerful mother might retaliate against her daughter's envious attacks, by magically damaging her ability to have a baby [28]. Pregnancies for such a woman might perform the function of ratifying her undamaged fertility, proving she is reproductively intact, and/or mistress of her own body. In such cases conception may be followed by repeated abortions rather than a baby [29].

A woman whose father was (emotionally or physically) absent in childhood might yearn to recreate the early exclusive merging with her mother, particularly if the socially isolated, intellectually and sexually unfulfilled mother was herself emotionally overinvolved in this exclusive relationship too. In adulthood, she might choose as her partner an effeminate man, or no man at all but artificial insemination and/or a female partner.

Alternatively, if mother selectively spurned her daughter and drew emotional sustenance from her son, such a woman when grown up might wish for a baby of her own to represent her own neglected baby-self in a new symbiotic fusion in which she is now the mother and can lavish attention on her infant or punitively deprive him/her.

In the sections on infertility, conception, pregnancy and early parenthood, people will be encountered who have chosen any one of these solutions. What I wish to emphasize here is Freud's discovery that adult sexuality is defined by the child's early emotional experiences within his/her own specific family. And that these primitive influences persist and are involuntarily re-enacted in later life.

Clearly, the wish for a baby stems from many complex and varied sources, bio-socio-cultural and conscious as well as unconscious intrapsychic experiences. Although for many centuries it was assumed to be innate, modern technological developments and theories enable us to tease out a variety of socioeconomic and psychological factors contributing to the desire to become pregnant. The decision to become a parent in our modern-day western industrial civilization poses new complexities and ethical connotations previously unknown in the fulfilment of the wish to have a child. The psychological implications of some of these will be explored in the next chapters.

KEY POINTS

*Cultural transmission of the vital wish for a baby across generations and within a caring family unit has thus far been ensured both in traditional and western societies by limiting the social definition of women's role to childbearing and childrearing and by promoting economic and political advantages to men who produce offspring.

*With modern innovations, the psychosocial origins of the wish for a baby can be seen to be separate from biological urges towards copulation.

*Common motivations for having a child are the wish for genetic immortality, the desire to achieve 'true' adulthood by finally erasing the dividing line between sexual maturity and actual reproductivity;

the need to emulate and reciprocate parental care, actively to master early experiences and to find a new object and/or source of love.

*Early psychological origins and social expectations of having a baby are considered as functions of the interchange between each individual's intrapsychic wishes and each culture's psychosocial gender definitions.

Chapter 2

Considering parenthood: cultural, sexual and ethnic variations

'Your children are not your children.
They are the sons and daughters of Life's longing for itself.
They come through you but not from you.
And though they are with you yet they belong not to you.

You may give them your love but not your thoughts.
You may house their bodies but not their souls.
For their souls dwell in the house of to-morrow, which you cannot visit,
not even in your dreams.
You may strive to be like them, but seek not to make them like you.
For life goes not backward nor tarries with yesterday.
You are the bow from which your children as living arrows are sent forth.'
Kahlil Gibran (*The Prophet*)

2.1 DECIDING WHETHER TO BECOME PARENTS

2.1.1 Recent developments and their psychosocial effect on childbearing

Becoming a parent is a long-term commitment with irreversible effects. In western society, it means inviting a stranger to come into your life and inhabit your home for a minimum of 16 years. There are few economic gains to be had from such a decision and many costs in terms of time, space, emotional investment, sleep loss, space restrictions, decreased mobility and freedom. Nevertheless, until recently, becoming a parent was not considered to be a decision to be pondered. However, today, in many parts of the world, having a child is an option not an inevitability.

If more permissive social mores and efficient contraception have meant that western women can choose to be sexually active with less fear of social disapproval or unwanted pregnancy, then theoretically it is possible to postulate that in most cases pregnancy is voluntary and based on a conscious wish for a child. Unmarried pregnant women can no longer

be ostracized on the ground that they have 'fallen' since it is likely that
they have chosen to conceive or at least not to interrupt the pregnancy.
Needless to say, having the choice does not necessarily mean that choice
has been exercised, or even if it has, that it is non-conflictual. 'Accidents'
continue to happen, contraceptive failure is not uncommon, misconceptions and unconscious motivation still determine conception. In addition,
all pregnancy involves loss. For the woman having a child entails loss
of unquestioned singleness in her body, loss of her physical well-being,
loss of her figure, her carefree social life, postponement of her career
or occupation, and for the couple, loss of their intimate twosome,
diversion of emotional resources and threat of financial drain in addition
to the inevitable risk of producing an abnormal baby or losing it. In effect,
many pregnant women have mixed feelings about pregnancy at this time.

Contraception now means that motherhood is no longer inevitable.
Indeed, there are powerful social forces militating against it. Lower infant
mortality rates and longer life expectancy have created a population crisis.
'Zero Population Growth' policies still exert moral influence to have few
or no children, as in China. The nuclear threat, too, has acted as a
deterrent to would-be-parents. Legal and educational rights fought for
by the Women's Movement have enabled women to utilize their greater
freedom to participate actively in the public sphere. To some, maternity
and confinement to domesticity might seem a politically retrogressive
step, or an interruption of their 'real' lives. Socioeconomic factors still
operate detrimentally to women who wish to combine career and
motherhood. Greater flexibility of social expectations and emphasis on
individual achievement offer a large variety of sublimations and choices
for both men and women for whom it has become socially acceptable
to lead 'child-free' lives. In addition, in our society, we have all but
severed the close generational kinship ties of traditional societies.
Although parents may exert some emotional pressure on a couple to
have a baby, the ultimate decision and main parenting burden rest with
the young people themselves.

However, contraception itself has posed new dilemmas. To become
pregnant, a sexually active woman or couple must decide to stop
contraception. And even non-contracepted childbearing is no longer a
matter of 'leaving it to Fate', since pregnancy can be terminated by
abortion without physical or law-breaking risk to the mother; and
even in the unfortunate case of infertility it can often be combatted
with new methods of reproductive technology and surgical treatments
such as artificial insemination, *in vitro* fertilization, embryo transfer,
surrogacy or even donor ovum. Thus, sterility too no longer entails
resignation to a barren 'destiny' but involves the couple in choice of
childlessness or a new round of pressures to dedicate their lives to
conceiving. Ironically, it is possible that factors specific to the hi-tech

modern world such as radiation, chemical pollution and resistant strains of venereal disease have contributed to the rise in infertility. And, para-doxically, technological innovations in keeping ever-younger premature babies alive are now encroaching on freedom of abortion [1].

2.1.2 Deliberating

Increasingly, women, men and couples engage in making informed choices allowing them to take conscious personal responsibility for what society has decreed to be their social duty and obligation. In traditional societies, the social sequences from menarche to childbearing are ritually determined and the extended family or group collectively welcome a new baby and insert him or her into a social order of peers who share the trials and tribulations of growing up. Whereas in most modern industrial societies the decision to begin a family rests with the couple. Their child will belong to a nuclear family, and although education is taken over by the State, responsibility for upbringing is on the parents(s).

Parenthood has thus become a serious and demanding task not to be embarked upon without deliberation as autobiographical accounts testify [2]. Postponement of pregnancy until the 'right time' is an option many couples take for granted. In the absence of marriage, the decision to have a child may signify the crucial form of emotional commitment. In many cases, it marks the end of curtailing their reproductive fecundity, an active testing out of fertility which has been postponed since their bodies attained sexual maturity many years previously. In recent years, discussion groups have sprung into existence for people considering parenthood. Individuals or couples can attend these groups to explore their conflictual feelings with other would-be-parents and/or a counsellor or marital-therapist. Women's groups may focus on the dilemma of whether to mother at all, and/or the practical issues and additional hardships for single heterosexual women wishing to become pregnant but lacking a suitable companion and, as will be discussed later, lesbian women on their own or in a partnership. In some cases, women attend these groups having found themselves pregnant, and needing to decide retrospectively whether to keep the baby or abort. Many couples engage in less formal discussions with friends and relatives, or a reciprocal deliberation occurs within the relationship.

2.1.3 Time will decide

Most commonly a heterosexual couple will simply reach a point in their relationship when they mutually feel the need to face the future. Often, it is the 'biological clock' that sets the pace. The average primagravida is no longer a woman in her early twenties or late teens. Childbearing, particularly in professional women, may be put off until she has completed her training, and is often postponed as she climbs the professional ladder. For many women, 35 is a 'conceptual boundary', and as she passes her 30th birthday, whether single or in a partnership, she becomes aware of time passing. ('Life is rushing by, days pass like stitches on a sewing machine and suddenly my prime time is almost over.') For many, there is the image of the 'little old lady' at the end of her life who will look back with regret at the childless years. For some people, illness, ageing or death of their own parents act as a catalyst to the decision to conceive. In our society, where families have fewer children, would-be parents have a sense of obligation to be able to provide what each couple deems necessary for their upbringing. This might mean space (a room for the baby), or equipment (pram, cot, high-chair, bouncer, stroller), education (the dearth of State-run nursery schools make this an early feature), or just care-giving time. Hence, a specific life event, such as achieving a particular career goal, moving house, getting a long-awaited raise, can contribute to the timing of the decision to begin a family or have another child. On the other hand, an event beyond one's control such as involuntary redundancy, a death in the family, threat posed by a severe illness, conscription or being posted abroad, may activate the wish to reassert personal control and redress the balance – to compensate oneself or 'duplicate' oneself, particularly in life-threatening situations.

2.1.4 The toll on women

Many women have spent years of their lives effortfully achieving and maintaining their place in a world that still favours men. The desire to have a baby is often relegated to the 'back burner' while jockeying for social and professional positions and, in the course of the struggle, the inner little girl who wanted to be like mummy may be neglected or despised. To allow herself to want a child and realistically engage in getting pregnant, a woman must weigh up the consequences of becoming a mother.

The desire to have a baby can herald a complex internal need to recapture an old familiar dream, to repeat her own babyhood and heal her mother and/or to fill an empty space inside and out, and to fling out into the unknown. The wish to be pregnant (which does not always coincide with the wish to have a child) may represent a desire to prove her feminine fertility or to assume physical maturity or bodily ownership while separating emotionally from her mother [3]. Allowing the wish for a child to resurface can reactivate painful doubts: ('I desperately want to have a baby but fear something won't allow me to have it. Since I was little I've often felt incapable of having something good without spoiling it. Do I deserve to be a mother?')

In addition to the emotional toll exacted, motherhood may be sub-divided into three components: a biological one, involving gestation, procreation and lactation; a social one involving childrearing; and an ideological one, involving the value of mothering [4]. With changing expectations of women's roles, the primacy of female mothering as woman's sole destiny and source of adult feminine identity is being questioned. Voluntary childlessness is compatible with female role definitions and westernized women may wonder whether mothering will clash with career expectations: how best to combine employment with the quality of mothering she wishes to bestow on a baby, and whether she can afford to take several years out of a professional career. To teenagers, pregnancy might imply having to drop out of the educational system with few alternative provisions. Many women are rightly concerned with the lack of social support, the devalued status of mothers, the private isolation and public hardships (meagre financial support, inadequate breastfeeding facilities, lack of childcare resources, anti-pram restrictions such as high pavement curbs and narrow aisles, public transport obstacles, etc.). To many women, the drastic physical changes of pregnancy and possible irreversible loss of figure postnatally arouse deep-seated anxieties about bodily integrity and body image. Other women fear the unrelieved, unsupported repetitive drudgery, mess, , noise and emotional involvement of raising an infant as a single parent or in a nuclear household. Many feel at sea not having been prepared by society for parenthood, often having lived an 'age-segregated' life, rarely exposed to newborns, pregnant women, birth or breastfeeding ('I've had nothing to do with baby-stuff. I've been like an alien in the land of the parents'). With few traditional values to fall back on and little continuity between generations, each individual woman almost has to 're-invent' parenting – a daunting prospect riddled with uncertainties and anxiety.

2.1.5 Couples

Deliberating couples usually weigh up the rewards and losses of becoming parents: the opportunity to relive tender experiences from their own infantile past; an exciting chance to cherish, cuddle, teach, have fun with a little person of their own joint making, and to bestow some of the treasures they have stored up and long to pass on. Some see it as the next phase in their relationship, a mark of commitment, moving from a pair to a family, creating a live reflection of their mutuality; confirming hope in the future and becoming a link in the long chain of parents since time immemorial ('Now that we've found each other we feel we could fulfil all our childhood dreams together'). To some, a child ensures genetic immortality, a means of passing on some-thing of themselves to future generations or leaving something behind when death looms. Marital crisis or dissatisfaction with a 'stuck' relationship may trigger a desire for a baby, 'to bridge the gap', start things moving, cement the partnership or serve as an outlet for unrequited feelings. Conversely, the desire to have a baby might in itself engender a marital crisis in a couple whose needs differ ('He could happily live his life in a relatively autonomous and self-sufficient way. I need to be loved, I want to be needed, to be at the hub of things and to have a sense of connectedness'). One partner may be afraid of the intrusion of another into their cosy twosome; or that the marital resources cannot stretch to include a third or that the nurturing he or she now receives will be redirected towards the real baby ('I'm afraid I'll feel excluded, neglected, and pushed out into second place'). Some fear a change in life style, restricted mobility or curtailed social and academic freedom; others may have negative personal memories of their own childhood and be loath to relive them with a child of their own; some may question their own parenting capacities, or those of the spouse ('What kind of a mother could I be when there's a baby inside me screaming for help?'). Some people feel it is immoral to overpopulate the world, or bring babies into an age of disasters or into a bad marriage (How could I subject a child to the emotional landscape of him and me?'). Others wish to dedicate their energies to society or channel them into scientific projects or art while yet others feel they cannot do justice to an ideal of parenting. On the other hand, when considering parenthood, a child may represent their contribution to society, or a way of re-balancing the 'family ledger', of repaying debts to one's parents or compensating oneself vicariously for the parenting one wished had been available.

2.1.6 Risky reasons for parenthood

In some cases, the latter might reflect pathogenic motivation to recapture the past, which taken to extremes can have adverse effects on the relationship with the real baby who comes along. Similar perils foreshadow a decision to have a baby as a means of patching up a marriage or to compensate for a loss. Likewise the seemingly positive hope that the birth will be a 'rebirth', or the baby's coming will 'make it all different', change a drab world or provide the parent with all the love craved. A deprived woman might desire the baby as a possession ('something of my very own'), a teenage girl may use the baby as an excuse to leave home, or as a magical means of achieving adulthood or allow it to be born because of the fear of an abortion, or to make up for a break up. In some sub-cultures, social pressures to conform with one's contemporaries can induce couples to parent before they are emotionally ready. Likewise, socially ingrained romanticized notions, reinforced by soap operas and well-meaning childcare experts, may lead to bitter disillusionment after the birth ('I expected to love every blissful moment instead I find it all so hard and feel trapped. What is the matter with me?'). People suffering from persistent psychological uneasiness about having a baby or partners who cannot agree ('He makes me feel so monstrous for wanting a baby'), may benefit from undertaking psychotherapy to resolve unconscious conflicts underlying the decision. Other factors complicating the decision-making process, such as fear of being a carrier of hereditary disease or excessive worrying about having an abnormal baby may be aided by genetic counselling.

2.1.7 Remaining childless

After soul-searching deliberations, in which at times each member of the pair highlights one extreme position on this multifaceted dilemma, some partners decide together or unilaterally not to have a baby. While some couples still leave the outcome to 'Fate' others may continue with contraception and postpone the final decision to a later time; alternatively, one of them may choose to become sterilized. Where a mutual decision has been made, the partners may wish to discuss their crucial resolution with other 'child-free' couples or socialize with like-minded people. In England BON (British Organization of Non-Parents) and in North America NON (National Organization of Non-Parents) offer such support.

In cases of divergent partners where one imposes his or her rejection of parenthood on the other, particularly by means of irreversible sterilization or a prohibition on conception, the marriage/relationship may continue apparently as before. However, an emotional rift inevitably develops around the taboo subject, bitterness often seeping into other areas of the relationship in the form of unconscious retaliative sabotage or mistrust ('Every period I feel cheated, furious that he stole my babies away'). Even postponement of childbearing by one partner against the wishes of the other will reflect discord and lack of mutuality in the relationship ('I can never forgive her for not recognizing my urgency to have a child'), and can have long-term repercussions particularly if fertility problems are later incurred.

2.1.8 Some specific considerations about lesbian parenthood

Lesbian women cannot slip into parenthood in the manner of heterosexuals or bisexual women. The decision to have a baby, either in a lesbian couple or as a single woman, involves foresight, planning and a conscious decision and, in some cases, ideological commitment [5–7]. In some communities, particularly in North America, special women's groups have been set up in community health centres as self-help projects or run by 'educators' or counsellors [8]. The proclaimed purpose of such groups is to identify and explore issues necessary to making the decision of whether to have a baby or not, to obtain information and resources and prepare lesbians for the trials of such parenting.

Some specific considerations of lesbians are those of identifying the options and procuring the means for parenting. First, there is a question of whether a couple equally shares a wish for a baby, whether this is a biological venture or a social one, and if the former there may be an issue as to which woman in a couple is to have the baby and/or whether one of them will be 'mother' or whether nurturing will be equally shared. Once these often stressful and conflicted emotional issues are settled, there are the practicalities to be considered:

1. Alternative fertilization (known or unknown donor).
2. Sexual intercourse with a man (known or unknown partner).
3. Adoption (public, private, foreign).
4. Foster parenting.
5. Non-biological parenting (alone, with friend, lover, nuclear-family or collective.
6. Legal guardianship.

Where a woman decides to bear the child herself, alone or with a partner, she is faced with further decisions. If insemination is to be by donor, dilemmas abound as to whether her source should be a gay or 'straight' man; whether to obtain the semen from a sperm bank or rely on a discrete go-between; whether to use fresh or frozen sperm given that each method has drawbacks, such as lack of medical screening for AIDS and gonorrhoea with fresh semen, and lower birth-defect rate but also fewer motile sperm and possibly higher cost and less information about the donor with frozen semen. She may decide to be artificially inseminated by a doctor in a clinic or use a self-insemination kit (or diaphragm cup or even turkey baster!). She may wish to include her lover in this operation or decide to become a single mother. Whatever path she chooses, a lesbian woman deciding to become a mother will have to contend not only with the emotional issues of pregnancy and motherhood, but with additional stresses related to the social prejudice she will no doubt encounter, the queries her child will raise ('Why don't I have a daddy?' 'How did I get into your tummy?'), and longer-term issues such as what she might feel if her fetus is male or her child grows up heterosexual.

2.1.9 Ethnic minorities

In discussing notions of conception, antenatal care and childbirth patterns, the USA for a very long time, and Britain in the last decade, must be considered multicultural societies. We can no longer afford to overlook the demographic patterns of our population and the variety of different customs, religious practices, folk beliefs influencing concepts of illness and health and diverse experiences of everyday living in our society. The following summary is offered merely as a background to some of these variations in Britain today. Essential to health care is an understanding that individual differences always exist, within ethnic minority groups as within any other group of people. It is as crucial to avoid prior assumptions about any group as a whole as it is to cultivate an awareness that one's own culture is merely one of many.

In total, about 43% of the British ethnic minority population were born in the United Kingdom [9]. Half originate in the Indian subcontinent; black Caribbeans constitute a $^{1/6}$; black African constitute an ? and Chinese a $^{1/20}$ [detailed breakdown in 0.2.10]. Surveys reveal a very young age structure for most ethnic minority groups reflecting patterns of both immigration and fertility [10]. One estimate holds that the ethnic minority population is growing by 90 000 per year, two-thirds of which is by natural growth and one-third by immigration [11]. Estimates based on the Labour Force Survey show a rise in ethnic minorities within the population from 3.9% in 1981, to 5.7% in 1994 to 6.4% in 1997. Similarly, marital status differs, with South Asians in particular showing a very high proportion of marriages compared with white counterparts. According to the total population survey, persons of West Indian or African origin are roughly twice as likely to be in mixed marriages as their South Asian counterparts, and unlike all other groups Chinese women are more likely to be in mixed marriages than Chinese men [12] Today (as in the late 80's [13]) people of Indian origin form the largest ethnic group (over a quarter) mainly Sikhs from the Punjab and Hindus from Gujarat. Another large group (about a sixth) originate in Mirpur in Pakastan and the Northwest Frontier province, mostly Muslim and Urdu-speaking or Pushto-speaking Pathans. About one in 20 originate in Bangladesh. In addition, a large group who are ethnically Indian came here from urban East Africa as a result of political persecution (60% of whom arrived between 1965 and 1974) [14]. As well as originating from different areas, the Asian communities have settled in different regions. Many Pakistanis live in the midlands and north of England, whereas the majority of those from India live in the London area; the Bengali community centred in east London, the Sikh community concentrated in southwest London, and more Gujarati-speaking Hindus have settled in north London [15]. Different ethnic groups experience diverse living and working conditions. In the 21st century, the highest group of unemployed men originate in the West Indies. This is a shift since the Labour Force Survey in the mid 1980's which found showed that although a higher proportion of Indian men than white men are in professional jobs; that the highest level of unemployment is found among Pakistani or Bangladeshi population; that approximately 60% of households amongst these two minorities contain five or more persons (vs. national average size of 2.6), and that almost 30% of the Bangladeshi population are under 16 years old [16].

Sensitive issues such as contraception, menstruation, fertility and sexuality are clearly influenced by different local religious beliefs and cultural practices. However, in general, cultures in which female modesty is cherished and/or Purdah practised, dictate a need for same-sex health care, strict privacy and sensitivity regarding choice of interpreters when intimate physical matters are discussed. In many households, a closeknit extended family structure is maintained. Intergenerational clashes of traditional vs. 'Modern' non-domestic values may permeate the inner sanctum, particularly between overseas-born and second-generation UK-born family members. These include milder conflicts about school co-ed-friendships, 'unsuitable' activities and girls' demands to work outside the home and in some families full-scale rebellion against religious observances and arranged marriage.

Changes are also occurring in traditional cultures. Hindu beliefs see the conjunction of man and woman as sacramental, a combination of the male 'cool' transcendental principles and the female one of 'heat' and energy, to be contained and controlled as a balanced unity [17]. Chastity and self-regulation, therefore, had been the major means of birth control until the national policy of family planning was adopted in India in 1951, with IUD in the 1960s, sterilization and a vasectomy drive in the 1970s, and injectable contraceptives in the 1980s [18]. In some Muslim societies, although children are seen as the 'gift of Allah' Islamic scholars regard contraception as justified to save the mother's life or enhance the child's quality of life [19]. Thus, today, the decision of whether and when to have a child may also apply to some ethnic subcultural groups.

In Britain the next largest ethnic minority is the Afro-Caribbean (West Indian and Guyanese community), with about half a million people either from those many islands (63% of whom entered the UK between 1955 and 1964) or born here of immigrant parents. About 60% live in Greater London (as do 60% of the African population) and as 90% of this ethnic group are of working age, in the Labour Force Survey they have the highest economic activity rates of any group including whites, although it has been found that white men and women are more likely to be in employment than ethnic minority counterparts and 77% of West Indian men are in manual jobs as opposed to 54% of white men [20]. On the islands, Caribbean family structure usually revolves around the woman, brought up to be independent and self-sufficient although reliant on her mother and other females in a common 'yard', particularly for help with childrearing. Couples tend to live together only when they can purchase their own property and then the man will take responsibility for bringing up children, regardless of whether he is the biological father [21]. Inevitably, hardships occur in the absence of such support structures in Britain and when discrimination and prejudice are encountered. Where families were split as a result of emigration, older children, often left in the West Indies with a grandmother, may, on arrival in England, be in conflict with the mother's newly established family. In middle-class families, unmarried pregnancy may cause a family crisis of 'respectability' conflicts.

A large number (115 000) of Chinese immigrants, largely from Hong Kong, live scattered in Britain, often thinly spread, with men usually working in the restaurant trade and women largely isolated from support networks. Most recently, many Vietnamese refugees arrived here after considerable hardships to avoid racial and political discrimination in their country of origin, but then have been further dislocated in Britain by the official dispersal policy.

Although a religious rather than ethnic group, Rastafarians, whether of African or Afro-Caribbean origin, share in common a belief in preservation of virility and black pride, of which their uncut dreadlocks are a symbol. Only 'live' foods are eaten in a strict vegan diet. Contraception and abortion are often unacceptable, being seen as white means of black-fertility control [22].

Women of African descent may occupy a paradoxical position. In their original cultures, although often trained to become economically independent by craft or garden produce, they are nevertheless subordinate to dominant husbands, some of whom are polygamous as co-wives are needed to share the burden of childrearing and agricultural work. This is at variance with cultures where market trade is dominated by men, as in the Arab, Hindu or Chinese cultures, where men also do most of the agricultural work [23]. In most African cultures many children are regarded as an achievement and all are acknowledged by the father, both legitimate and otherwise. However, in the traditional community some children might have been lodged with relatives for educational reasons or to meet the needs of the kin-foster parent [24]. In Britain, in the absence of these female networks, lack of family support links and a high divorce rate mean that many mothers feel overburdened and isolated. A common belief that semen makes women strong decreases popularity of barrier methods of contraception and male sterilization.

As well as groups defined by different religions (such as a range of Christian, Jewish, Muslim, Hindu and Bhuddist sects) many other smaller immigrant groups exist, originating in Ireland, the Mediterranean, middle-Europe, Australia, South America, etc., each of whom have customs that were brought with them, other practices that have been abandoned and new ones created. This means that in addition to old traditions, some structures, such as the extended family may have had to be relinquished in the host country and replaced by other improvised customs, grounded in local subcultural structures growing around their minority status. In each of these groups, pregnancy and parenthood has a different meaning and young individuals or couples considering parenthood often experience conflict – motivated not only by the traditional influences of their parental families but also by those of the dominant white culture as well as their specific local subculture. If this is complicated for each minority, couples of mixed heritage have to contend with additional complexities. Clearly, given this diversity, professionals cannot be expected to be knowledgeable about each ethnic group. Furthermore, such an approach can lead to overgeneralizing and subtle prejudice. All we can do is to be aware of the heterogeneity of our society and that many members of ethnic minorities suffer daily experiences of inequality and discrimination in ordinary encounters and at the hands of professionals in education, housing, social services and law-enforcing agencies [25]. In the areas of caring professions which deal with procreative issues common to all people, we must strive towards greater sensitivity to individual differences and needs. Intercultural awareness of professionals can be increased through seminars, workshops and multidisciplinary courses run by a variety of bodies such as Nafsiyat [26], Health Education Council Extension College for Training in Health and Race [27] and, in some areas, the Commission for Racial Equality.

2.2 TRYING TO CONCEIVE

Often pregnancies occur without the partners having made a conscious decision, whereas other couples, after deliberation, decide to take the leap. For these, the period awaiting conception takes on special significance.

2.2.1 Baby-making magic

In many cultures a marriage is not ratified until the woman conceives. Pregnancy is tangible proof of the couple's sexual union and signifies a mutual achievement. Indeed, in many folk beliefs, both partners have to desire the pregnancy for conception to occur. Thus, the Tamil-speaking Sri Lankans attribute conception to the united orgasmic ejaculation of male and female seminal fluids in the uterus coming together to form a 'sprout' [28]. Superstitious beliefs, purification and offerings, special dietary restrictions ('hot'/'cold' or 'fertile' foods), aphrodisiacs and specific sexual practices or lovemaking conditions (full moon, beach-house, scent of lilies, etc.) may be deemed to promote the optimal conditions for inducing conception. In some cultures, ancient rites and rituals exist for securing a male pregnancy [29]. In industrial societies too, as many sex-therapists and family doctors find out, despite widespread media education about the biological facts, old wives' tales and folk beliefs prevail and adults often imagine conception taking place in ways which reflect their unconscious ideas and primitive schemata of the body and its processes rather than being based on a scientific model.

A couple trying to conceive may find themselves indulging in 'love magic' surrounding the sexual act now released from its imposed contraceptive boundaries. Intercourse, with the artificial barrier of contraception removed, often acquires added erotic excitement and a new dimension of freedom as the couple engage in intentional, previously 'forbidden', deliberate impregnation. Some partners go to some lengths to ensure 'perfect' atmosphere during love-making reflecting a semiconscious belief that the circumstances of conception can influence the future perfection of the baby or its gender. A romantic scene, an auspicious date, a protein-rich diet, specific background music, exuberant dancing, beatific thoughts, pre-intercourse dinner by candlelight, a 'receptive' position, all might be magically employed to call forth a special union between a particular sperm and the ovum. During this period of heightened excitement and waiting, the couple may 'fall in love' all over again while yet others are thrown off balance by the increased tension and begin to feel uneasy.

2.2.2 She and he

As at no other time during the life-cycle, the heterosexual couple trying to conceive become aware of their differences of gender, and the sudden release of unconscious fantasies underlying this male/female division are played out in their daily (and nocturnal) lives. The inactive ovum, awaiting a fertilizing sperm-'suitor' can come to life and be lovingly or angrily enacted in the couple's own relationship – the woman may have a sense of passively awaiting fertilization or being relegated to a dependent state like her egg, or the man may experience pleasure and pride in his role as sole impregnator, or have a sense of exploited post-coital redundancy. In cultures where semen is cherished as a source of strength (there is a Hindu belief that it takes 40 days and 40 drops of blood to make one drop of semen) the male partner may feel drained and enfeebled by prolonged baby-making. Another may come to dread being engulfed in his wife's body like a sperm encompassed by the egg, or she may begin to feel penetrated and pierced like her counterpart ovum. Intercourse may no longer seem to be the private affair of their previous relationship, but now tend to involve their encouraging or disapproving real and internalized parents, while they may each be aware of emulating their own preconceptual love-making mother and father.

Time now takes on a cyclical dimension, repetitively peaking in excitement around the expected menstrual phase, and sadly greeting the disappointment of a period. Then, with rising hopes as the amenorrhoea persists, the thrill of inner certainty or eventual decision to test for pregnancy with home-kit or via the GP or clinic. If conception is felt to have occurred or the test is positive, a whole further surge of psychological processes are inaugurated in both partners, as will be shown in later chapters.

However, in about one in five couples, the cycles of hope and disappointment accumulate. Amid denial of worry, fleeting anxiety, increasing concern and, often, evasive silence, there is a gradual dawning or realization that something is wrong. The psychological processes and reactions to infertility will be explored in the next chapter.

KEY POINTS:

*Recent biochemical and technological innovations create new expectations and necessitate new approaches to old issues of conception, pregnancy and birth.

*Psychosocial motives and implications of considering parenthood for heterosexuals include whether and when to become parents, what resources each will bring to parenting and repercussions of these decisions on each partner and on the couple's relationship.

*Additional questions need to be answered by lesbians wishing to parent, including who will conceive, how, by whom, and how to parent.

*Ethnic minorities, now a substantial part of our multicultural societies, vary in their approach to issues of fertility, contraception and conception. Decisions are affected by individual differences, regional variations, traditional practices, media and dominant cultural pressures and local sub-cultures.

*Unconscious fantasies fuel magical activities during the attempt to conceive, reflecting folk beliefs and private ideas that conditions surrounding conception will determine the nature or gender of the baby, with heightened awareness of the irreducible male/female basic differences between the partners.

Chapter 3

Prolonged infertility: psycho-dynamics and psychological impact of diagnosis and treatment

The biblical matriarch Rachel envied her fertile sister Leah and reproached their mutual husband Jacob, saying: 'Give me children or I shall die!' He angrily retorted: 'Am I in the place of God, who has withheld from you the fruit of the womb?'
In desperation, Rachel gave Jacob her maid Bilha and adopted the two sons, Dan and Naphtali, from this surrogacy. At long last 'God remembered Rachel' and she conceived and gave birth to Joseph, and later Benjamin but died in childbirth (see Genesis 30). This brief account captures in essence a tragic saga of infertility.

3.1 PSYCHOLOGICAL ROOTS OF UNEXPLAINED INFERTILITY

Today, infertility is defined as inability to conceive after a year of uncontracepted normal intercourse. The actual diagnosis may follow the couple's decision to seek medical help and investigations, or be the outcome of a medical emergency such as an ectopic pregnancy. Distinction is made between sterility resulting from irreversible damage or defect, infertility and subfertility. Until fairly recently no known physical explanation could be found for some 40% of infertility, and as a result it was attributed to emotional factors. With modern technology and diagnostic refinements, the causes of many cases of infertility may now be clearly attributed to a single problem or a combination of physical factors in either or both partners at any stage between successful meeting of sperm and egg, such as ovarian failure, tubal damage or disease, cervical mucus incompatibility, sperm production deficiencies, etc. However, there are still some 5–10% of couples for whom no abnormality or functional pathology can be found to explain their failure to conceive, implying either current diagnostic shortcomings or the possible contribution of psychosomatic or psychosocial emotional factors. (A more recent study of the Bristol Health District puts the incidence of unexplained infertility as high as 28% of couples.) A review of 30 research publications has found convincing evidence that patients treated in infertility clinics show significantly higher levels of psychosocial distress, and, among them, females score higher than males [1]. How should these findings be interpreted? Three hypotheses have been cited: (a) that psychosocial problems trigger infertility; (b) that infertility triggers psychosocial distress; (c) that there is an interactive causal relationship between the two. If it is the case that psychogenic factors are responsible for some infertility we would expect to find differences on personality measures or emotional states between individuals with unexplained fertility and those with organically based infertility. However, a recent review of studies conducted between 1972 and 1983 found no such personality differences although there was some evidence of heightened anxiety in the former group [2], possibly attributable to the effect of the non-specific nature and hence uncertain treatability of their diagnosis. Similarly increased psychological stress factors have been cited and these, with raised anxiety levels, may indicate different ways of responding to stressors rather than personality variables. Exploration of the inter-connections between reproductive failure, prolactin concentration, anxiety and stress suggest there is some evidence for the effect of psychological factors on hormonal mechanisms contributing to infert-ility [3]. Similarly it has been suggested that psychogenic infertility may result from emotional tension, chronic anxiety and unconscious fear of pregnancy altering hypothalmic–pituitary pathways or by causing spasm of uterotubal musculature [4] or interference with implantation, all of which may be responsive to biofeedback and relaxation techniques or psychotherapeutic intervention. Some psychoanalysts have stressed psychic conflicts, repressed anger and depression contributing to infer-tility, ambivalence about femininity or the woman's envious incapacity to identify with her fertile mother inhibiting fecundity through complex psychophysiological pathways and sexual dysfunction [5–8]. Indeed, there is convincing evidence of psychogenic factors from accounts of suc-cessful psychotherapy with infertile individuals or couples resulting in conception. It seems then that there is a subgroup whose unexplained infertility is triggered by conscious or unconscious psychosocial factors which interact with biological ones to prevent or interfere with concep-tion, and who may benefit from psychotherapy.

3.2 PSYCHOLOGICAL TOLL OF PROLONGED INFERTILITY

However, in addition to the cause of infertility, in all cases it is also necessary to consider the psychological impact of involuntary childlessness on couples who are unable to fulfil their wish for a baby. In my clinical experience, the repeated trauma of prolonged failure to conceive arouses self-doubts, erodes the couple's sexual and emotional resources (thereby constituting a destabilizing danger to the current stability of the marriage/relationship), and poses a threat to each partner's personal and gender identity and to their mutual future legacy.

A comparison was made among women with organic and unexplained infertility, mothers and women childless by choice. No differences were found in terms of psychological variables between the two groups of infertile women; however, they both differed from the others in having higher expectations about being loved and needed by other people, and more exaggerated traditional 'feminine' role beliefs [9]. These findings highlight the poignant deprivation experienced by women who wish to define themselves as mothers without having the control to achieve this status. In addition to helping infertile couples work through their anger and grief at their deprivation, psychotherapeutic intervention also aims to help such women achieve greater freedom, satisfaction and personal pride by channelling and sublimating their caring needs and achieving a redefinition of feminine identity, rooted in personal creative capacities rather than restricted to procreative and mothering ones.

In the past, the diagnosis of infertility culminated either in acceptance of childlessness or adoption. Nowadays, the adoption option is curtailed. With reduced social stigma of illegitimacy and easier access to abortion, fewer babies are now available for adoption (1987 figures from the Central Statistical Office show that 74% of children adopted in 1984 in the UK were over 2 years old). Conversely, recent interventive technologies offer new hopes, yet bring in their wake long periods of often intrusive treatment, years of waiting, wishing and wanting sometimes extending into menopause. The treatment period is undefined, with few boundaries to determine final failure as promising new techniques seem always just around the corner. Treatment itself is invasive, disruptive to everyday life and, at times, physically painful and painfully disappointing. For instance, a recent worldwide assessment of 58 IVF (*in vitro* fertilization) programmes revealed a pregnancy rate of only 13% per IVF cycle [10]. Research findings demonstrate that the emotional well-being and marital relationship of infertile couples is affected by prolonged periods of clinical investigation [11, 12]. Psychotherapy with individuals who subsequently undergo treatment for infertility reveals treatment-related psychological disturbances [13]. These may be found to include symptoms of derealization, depersonalization, defensive denial, hypochondria, low self-esteem, paranoid states and neurotic depression, anxiety reactions and defensive manoeuvres such as phobic avoidances and obsessional reactions with rumination, magical thinking and compulsive rituals.

3.3 IMPACT OF DIAGNOSIS

The diagnosis of infertility, sterility or subfertility may come as a long-awaited verdict following a prolonged period of medical investigations or it may come abruptly, after a medical procedure or complications. In an emergency situation (such as an ectopic pregnancy), particularly if life-threatening, doctors may not be aware of the impact of their message – the implications of which in one fell swoop render an ordinary adult powerless, marginal and dependent. Suddenly (and at a time of physical vulnerability) the person is made bereft of hopes and plans, at odds with past taken-for-granted expectations. In the case of a previously pregnant woman, now told of tubal damage or internal complications, she experiences a devastating fall from expectant grace into the limbo of possible infecundity.

In contrast to this sudden disillusioning loss of faith in the body's natural functioning, gradual realization of the existence of a problem is often followed by defensive denial, with each partner clinging to their childhood confidence in reproductive capacity. However, as the months go by without conceiving, doubts arise, the couple may resort to blaming each other, each disowning their share of 'failure'. Once responsibility for coping with the problem is acknowledged, the third line of defence arises: 'if a problem exists a cure must exist'. The expert is sought to bring the problem under control. However, seeking help confirms reality; 'infertility cannot be denied, or avoided and may not be solvable'. With this realization, old assumptions have to be relinquished by degrees, until mourning can ensue resulting in acceptance of helpful alternatives [14]. Thus, the emotional stages of discovering infertility follow the pattern of acceptance of all loss. Grief reaches its height each month, as menstruation reconfirms the lack of personal choice when the combination of two bodies are incapable of producing a third. Whatever form it takes, the diagnosis of infertility shakes the very roots of human self-image, constituting an existential blow that has repercussions on all levels, intrapsychic, interpersonal, psychosexual and occupational [15].

3.4 INITIAL REPERCUSSIONS

Research suggests that the intensity of initial disappointment is greater in women and they take longer than their husbands to come to terms with the problem [16]. It has also been suggested that greater emotional and marital difficulties are experienced by both sexes when the cause of infertility lies with the man [17].

My clinical experience reveals that whether one-sided or shared, initially, following the diagnosis of infertility, a painful emotional inhibitedness often emerges in the couple as each partner initially retreats inward, bottling up shocked hurt and searching for ways to deal with the anger and growing frustration, trying to be sensible and appear 'grown-up' in this unproductive situation that makes them feel so disempowered. Behind the controlled exteriors, professionals often find two very frightened people hiding behind their respective barriers – a chasm yawning between them which they feel helpless to bridge [18]. They may become ultra-careful with each other, groping for neutral topics as the internal pressure rises. Each may feel s/he contains a lot of painful upset and 'messy', nasty, intolerable feelings which are dangerous to share. Each may be protectively holding onto these inside him/herself, believing that if such feelings spill out she or he would go mad or wreak havoc in the relationship which would 'crack under the strain'. Each also may be holding on deep inside to a cherished spark of hope, erecting barriers to prevent the other partner's sense of loss, anger, grief and disappointment from flooding in and extinguishing it – thus even hope can increase the insularity and isolation. ('What I feel I want is non-negotiable. The words come out so stark but I cannot supress it – the alternative is like having an arm and a leg taken away. How can I keep the hope alive in the face of such resignation, and the hospital's views? All I can do is look after my own needs'.)

However, raw and primitive feelings abound and anger may erupt against the expert as well as the partner. Since infertility is often irrationally interpreted as a punishment for past sexual transgressions it stirs up remorse or recriminations about masturbation, promiscuity, abortions, VD or celibacy. Not only is each individual's sexual identity thus undermined, but a deep narcissistic wound is experienced in relation to the core gender identity as a physically mature man or woman capable of reproducing. I have found that this diminished confidence in one's own creative capacities spills over into all realms of life as the ability to work is impaired by doubts about productivity and mental resources become absorbed in internal conflicts, preoccupations and defensive secrecy. Furthermore, work schedules get disrupted by cycles of monthly elation-deflation and frequent time-off for examinations or treatment.

3.5 TENSIONS WITHIN THE INFERTILE COUPLE

Several studies have reported emotional, marital and sexual difficulties following discovery of infertility [19]. A prospective study of infertile couples undergoing treatment states in its preliminary conclusions that although it is unlikely that infertile couples differ from fertile ones on personality variables, psychopathology and patterns of marital interaction and social support, nevertheless investigative procedures themselves provoke distress and potential marital disharmony [20]. However, a recent study has found that of the 71% women and 53% men in IVF or AID treatment who reported that infertility had affected their marital relationship, over half also reported some positive effect [21]. This tallies with clinical findings that couples wishing to undergo extensive and often selective treatment have to tackle difficult issues together which may strengthen the relationship.

Reproductive failure forces a couple to question what others take for granted. Having been raised with ordinary trust in natural processes and tacit expectations of growing up to become parents, they are faced with profound disillusionment as infertility violates the promise of adult fecundity. Poignantly, they are unable to become parents at the very point at which they have resolved to exchange their pair-relationship for a family. Having felt adult and ready to realign loyalties from their respective childhood families of origin to a new family of their own making, they find themselves relegated to the position of perpetual 'non-adults' lacking control over their bodies and plans. The prospect of an involuntary childless union invariably forces the pair to reassess their marital contract, and while the common heartache can draw some couples closer, there are periods, both before engaging in treatment and at decision points within it, when the continuation of a joint future must be questioned. ('I have the sense of being "driven", driving us towards parenthood, driven by my need for a baby which he doesn't share. He is content with being a couple but that leaves me feeling stranded and hollow.')

One formulation suggests that during the 'crisis of infertility' couples experience a problem of 'boundary ambiguity' on three levels:

1. The fantasy child is a psychologically present yet physically absent member of the infertile marriage.
2. One or both partners has divided loyalties between the marriage and their family of origin.
3. Family ties of continuity are obscured in the biological/hereditary ambiguity of infertility [22].

Within the duality of the couple, each partner has a heightened awareness of his/her own male or female gender and state of fertility. When the problem is unilateral, the infertile partner will identify the pain of the problem as his/her own, experiencing a continuous lonely core of distress that is unshareable. Whatever the sympathetic other is feeling, ultimately there is a deep sense of separateness which nothing can assuage. Indeed the other may be openly, covertly or unconsciously contemptuous of the infertile partner who is unable to achieve what any animal can, seemingly the most basic feat of all. Within such couples tensions rise as guilt, blame, dissatisfaction, resentment and derision fester below the surface or erupt in desperate attempts to regain personal or marital equilibrium. In less robust individuals, distress may be manifested in symptoms of alcoholism, compulsive eating, extramarital affairs, self-sacrificial separation or even suicide.

In some couples, there is a painful irony: belated stopping of contraception because of a decision to conceive has led to discovery of their infertility and further emphasizes the wasted dormant years of trying to prevent conception. ('I can never forgive him for having wasted my youth, all that time when I offered to share my fertility with him – he just wasted the chance and used the time for himself to feed off me.') Particularly guilt-ridden are individuals who elected in the past to be sterilized and are now seeking reversal or treatment in a second marriage or renewed relationship. Women who have postponed having children until early to mid-thirties retrospectively blame themselves or their partner when advanced age is decreed responsible for decreased fecundability (currently peak fertility occurs at age 26). And while evidence from semen analysis in infertility clinics and sperm banks indicate that possibly due to environmental or occupational factors, the general quality of semen has declined in recent years [23], nevertheless, infertile men tend to feel acutely ashamed of a low sperm count or abnormality, as if it were a personal indictment of their general creative capacity. Indeed, virility is unconsciously confused with potency. One study has found a 63% incidence of transient impotence (lasting one to three months) following the discovery of male infertility [24].

3.6 SOCIAL REPERCUSSIONS

On a social level, feeling singled out for barrenness, the infertile couple may be so shamefully conscious of the differences between themselves and their fertile friends that the similarities and shared experiences are no longer sufficient to keep friendships alive. Ironically, even their own parents are envied for having had children in a world unfairly divided into haves and have-nots. Shame at being unable to achieve what many people have to prevent happening may result in them feeling inferior, cheated, excluded, stigmatized or even ostracized.

Some subfertile couples retreat into reticence, withdrawing into a social 'reservation' to protect themselves from well-meaning inquisitive relatives and friends as pressures and taboo subjects accumulate. Some may avoid going out for fear of seeing a pregnant woman or a pram-pushing dad. Even other infertile couples become threatening as exposure to news of their successful conception is a 'stab in the back' tinged with bittersweet stirrings and fear of being left behind. ('It's difficult when friends conceive but even harder when people have had difficulties – our bond is broken and I feel left behind, the door shut and me left outside it with all these horrible feelings welling up, clinging to hope of a last minute reprieve.') Increasingly, birth-orientated media ('even the *Guardian* is not safe anymore') and gushing pregnant strangers rub salt into the wounds of their deprivation. With some infertile people seclusion may escalate into virtual housebound isolation as any woman with a pushchair or a bulge becomes the much envied, murderously hated enemy. Panic and paranoid feelings seethe not far below the surface as other people seem to be getting so easily what feels cruelly witheld.

3.7 TREATMENT FOR INFERTILITY

A common irrational but nonetheless real feeling among people having prolonged difficulty conceiving is that there are only a limited number of babies to go round, and that anyone else's pregnancy or birth reduces the statistical probability of the infertile couple having a baby. This unvoiced belief reverberates like electricity in the air where infertile couples meet each other. Thus, at hospital briefings for couples about to embark on treatment, such as AID (Artificial Insemination by Donor) or IVF (*in vitro* fertilization) one finds apparently civilized people secretly resentful and hostile, vying with each other in this life-and-death competition for scarce resources – 'Will those be called before us?' 'Who will be the lucky ones?' 'Will they get our share?' 'Are we destined to be the losers?' 'Will someone else get our baby?' Clearly, professionals organizing such group meetings, have to bear in mind the loss of adult autonomy these interventionary procedures entail. Grown-ups feel 'like children gone back to the classroom to be taught the facts of life by Guru-like omniscient teachers' who insist each patiently awaits their turn.

Often, couples accepted for National Health Service treatment have a predefined programme mapped out. For instance, only three attempts at IVF are allocated – which, like the three wishes of the fairy tales, are finite and awe-inspiring. Such treatments are not undertaken lightly by couples. Most are aware of the burdensome commitment in terms of discomfort, time consumption and exorbitant finances when private, and most have also deliberated the risk of the possible treatment outcome of multiple births. Couples who have applied for infertility treatments which require surgical or mechanical intervention often feel that they have an obligation to exercise their options. They have acted on the need to get specialized help rather than resigning themselves to childlessness or a hit-or-miss approach to conceiving naturally. ('IVF and the real possibility of having a baby after all is like going from a nightmare into a dream'.) To others, seeking help following failed or ectopic pregnancies entails a raw re-exposure of partly healed wounds and a revival of old hopes and fears.

3.8 FEELINGS ABOUT INFERTILITY SPECIALISTS

Inevitably, there is a strangeness in accepting a stranger's interference in the intimacy between husband and wife. Already in the diagnostic phase they are separated as he is sent off to produce a sperm sample; and she is examined in his absence. Their sexual activity is reduced to non-procreative romping while the real fertilization happens elsewhere, outside, under the control of strangers with God-like powers. In an institutional parody of the 'roulette' of conception, excitement, anxiety, apprehension and suspense accompany the process of waiting to be chosen to go on 'Red alert'. Bracing themselves for 'rejection' each cycle, the couple experience a confusing mixture of feelings towards those allocating treatment – grateful for the miracle offered them yet resentful at needing it and fiercely angry at their newly created dependence on a service they would be devastated to lose.

Ironically, dependency on the treatment increases both the sense of hopefulness and the sense of precariousness – the danger of failure always lurking in the background. The patient feels helplessly at the mercy of both impartial professionals and his/her own recalcitrant body as the biological clock ticks the months and years away. Most disruptive of all is the chronic ambiguity and uncertainty of outcome. Living with the unpredictable frustration of not knowing how long this period will extend, the infertile person seems to have to juggle bits of him/herself over the weeks and months and sometimes years, hoping against hope that dream and reality will eventually connect, trying to get on with daily life and responsibilities regardless of the constant inner grief.

When first deciding to have a child the couple's options were wide open. Increasingly, with time and awareness of the nature of their condition, those options are stripped away until, funnel shaped [25], all their efforts are focused on the last urgent option, whether it be AIH, AID, IVF or GIFT (Gamete Intra Fallopian Transfer). Paradoxically, if the battle spirit has not abated, it may enhance the sense of hope and energy all richly concentrated in one narrow area of activity. Likewise, after so long, with options falling off along the way, at this last stage, there is a powerful temptation to put all one's trust into being saved by the one magical, omnipotent specialist. Childhood's yearnings are invested in the doctor's parental power to grant or withhold, to make better, restore or forbid entry to the promised land. It is very difficult for the infertile person to hold on to the concept of the doctor's human fallibility, and all the more so if hindered by medical mystification and paternalism or distant formality. In addition, the very language of infertility used by doctors invariably arouses emotional connotations: 'incompatible' mucus, 'hostile' cervical secretions, 'low motility' or 'poor quality' sperm, 'swim-up test', 'blocked' tubes and vaginal 'antibodies' are figures of speech which evoke images in the bruised internal world of the sufferer and often become incorporated in sexual fantasies.

3.9 SEXUAL REPERCUSSIONS

Not only does infertility undermine the individual's sexual identity, but further tension is generated by the treatment situation. Where the couple is left to copulate following drug treatment or corrective surgery, passion drains away as baby-making overrides love-making and the spontaneity of the couple's sex life is now lost to temperature charts and regulated intercourse. For the subfertile husband, semen can take on symbolic properties as he resentfully feels his 'life force' ebbing, drained by his 'greedy' wife. She may resent her own dependence on his arousal while he may feel so dominated by her menstrual cycle as to become temporarily impotent or have dormant herpes flare up on 'chore' nights. Autonomy and intimacy is invaded by humiliating treatment procedures, post-coital inspection and detailed sexual reports to doctors.

The deep desire to grow a baby in one's own body or father a genetic continuity of oneself can become an all-consuming passion, impairing external concentration in its inward-looking single minded focus, taking priority over wordly events. The infertile women lives often for years in a constant tension between an inner state of readiness and anticipation – yearning, wishing and waiting to be fulfilled – yet holding back in protective preparation for external disappointment. At times it feels to her as if the awaited baby, too, is waiting, out of sight in the 'wings'. As if the child already has a reality, as did her mate before they met, and she finds herself straining, craving, asking: 'Where are you? when are you going to come into our lives?', feeling conception is just out of reach, always about to be achieved [26]. She may almost be afraid to lose sight of her wish or to give up the succession of treatments for fear that it will destroy the reality of her phantom baby. The focus is no longer what it feels like for them to be waiting for the baby, but a fantasy of the baby's experience waiting to be conceived. These magical thoughts may extend to love-making, a belief that the phantom child will be called forth by special intimacy and closeness. If one partner does not share these ideas, or scoffs at their irrationality, further barriers are built up between the couple and within the believer who protectively regards him/herself as 'guardian of the flame'.

In the case of active intervention – insemination or embryo insertion by a third person – sexuality and procreation are further separated, and fantasies may arise about the identity of the father, now seen as the intervening doctor. Sexual difficulties may arise as each partner has to build up an altered sexual bodily identity that can encompass the intervention of fertility techniques in relation to his/her own body and the body of the marriage. (Some of these emotional difficulties are examined in the section on conception following medical intervention, Chapter 7.)

3.10 OVERLAPPING PHASES IN INTRAPSYCHIC EXPERIENCE

Inside, the infertile individual feels assailed by primitive forces. Rage, despair, puzzlement, deprivation and hurt all jostle as s/he tries to adjust to a new self-image. Gone is a sense of belonging; s/he feels alone, isolated and singled out, unable to fulfil the most basic requisite of the human race. Gone is the sense of continuity, of generations inevitably succeeding one another; of oneself as a genetic link between past and future. Parents are resented and unconsciously blamed: the early childhood promise has been broken – s/he will not simply grow up to become a mummy or daddy. Either they lied or else the omnipotent parents of early childhood must have had reason to withhold fertility or even spoil it. Even eventual conception cannot make reparation for the shattered trust. No longer able to take natural fecundity for granted, the body becomes alienated, possessing a will of its own, liable to play malevolent tricks beyond its owner's knowledge or control.

Gradually, stunned anger gives way to grief as s/he mourns the lost easy optimism, the fertile self, the wished-for babies. The primal complaint of 'Why me?' pales as explanations are sought – both medical and philosophical. Even the most rational infertile person finds it hard to shake off the feeling that s/he is not being 'allowed' to have a baby, as a punishment for a past unexpiated transgression or because it is inexplicably forbidden. A frightening shadowy side of wanting to conceive is a continued vicious cycle of anxiety that the more it is wanted the more it will be witheld. This is particularly acute when there is no clear diagnosis of the problem.

Clearly, emotional conflicts and unconscious fantasies continue to operate throughout the treatment period and contribute to adjustment and resolution of the crisis. Persistent unsuccessful treatment of infertility year-in year-out can be bleakly wearisome and eroding, as gradually a deep-seated pessimism and fatalistic helpless tiredness sweep over the hope. ('My head says: you can't be pregnant, move away, move forward but images of my pregnant body come. There are lots of things in life most of us never do, but this feels such a core thing – being a woman, having a woman's body, being healthy and fit, yet it's beyond reach. . !') For some people, it is easier to give up and come to terms with childlessness. Some opt for the now remote possibility of adopting a baby. Others may decide to give up treatment and 'leave conception up to Fate' or even take up contraception again to provide themselves with a measure of dignified control. It has been suggested that optimal treatment means that from diagnostic evaluation, through the intervention phase and/or choice of alternative solutions, part of the psychological and social management of an infertile couple should include the professional's awareness of infertility as a conjugal and psychophysiological problem which needs to be addressed by collating interdisciplinary insights [27].

3.11 PSYCHOTHERAPY FOR INFERTILE INDIVIDUALS OR COUPLES

For some people the struggle continues, unabated, often for 10–15 years or more, even into menopause, of cyclical hope and despair, persistent search for further treatments, determination not to dilute their feelings or compromise the burning desire. As if s/he feels compelled to hold on to hope, deprivation and disappointment all the time, like grieving, otherwise the wish will never come true.

When individuals will go to such untold lengths to procure their pregnancy it invariably emerges that their personal identity is so enmeshed in achieving parenthood that they fear without it they would become 'invisible'. Unconsciously, the hunger is for a physical baby in which to invest all the unknown or unexpressed aspects of the self. A person may feel that having a baby is the only way to make conscious his/her own experiences of infancy and to retrieve elusive facets of one's inner being. Inhabiting a twilight world of limbo, belonging neither to the world of childless people nor those with kids, it is as if the gap of emptiness will not be filled until the actual baby arrives and yet paradoxically the pregnancy cannot occur until a place is vacated for it. ('My insides are full of shitty feelings – there is a great big lump of angry stuff where the baby should be'.) These people often benefit from psychotherapy, and the therapist's ability to 'wait out' the vigil and keep faith for him/her while the person begins to explore the inner void.

I have found that gradually with the discovery of an internal space (rather than 'hole') and of inner resources which, untrapped, can be utilized, the infertile person becomes able to cross the insurmountable gulf between themself and others, finding a way back into common humanity. This also means relaxing internal boundaries, getting in touch not only with inner creativity but also with the destructive feelings of hatred and envy, helplessness and deprivation and a sense of 'double desertion' – being vulnerable yet no-one else remembering one is different and hypersensitive. Working through these feelings also means having to accept one's own subversive, guilt-ridden and deeply corrosive resentment. The primitive outrage and poignant cry of 'What about me?' eventually subsides with psychotherapeutic help, if the individual can courageously show determination to go forward into the situation of potential hurt that such human belonging entails.

Going forward also means catching up with oneself, refinding, gathering up, owning and integrating scattered aspects of past experiences and gaining an emerging sense of self that is not a watered down version of a previous identity but is based on solid knowledge and a process of self-acceptance. Vigilant waiting for materialization of a future that might never happen and rigid fixity in past wishes gradually give way to a realization that one is missing out on life right now, in the precious present. When optimism is regained, having a baby becomes a 'bonus' rather than the sole and total raison d'être or source of fulfilment. After hard therapeutic work new found independence is accompanied by a welcome sense of creative achievement and greater awareness of realistic options and choice. It is usually at this point that conception will occur if infertility is of psychogenic origin.

Pregnancies which follow prolonged treatment for infertility often constitute special cases. Particularly problematic psychologically are IVF, GIFT 'conceptions' for women, and AID (Artificial Insemination by Donor) fertilization for men. The former will be dealt with separately in Chapter 7, the latter in Chapter 10.

KEY POINTS

*Whereas some unexplained infertility may be of psychogenic origin, the psychological impact of persistent reproductive failure and trauma of diagnosis must be considered.

*The effects of altered self-image and social status coupled with prolonged treatment may be seen in intrapsychic terms within each individual; in marital and interpersonal contact and in the sexual relationship between the partners as well as in their work situation and social interactions.

*Strategies of adjustment and coping with the vicissitudes of treatment depend on working through the fantasies and emotional reactions to the condition and to the professionals involved.

*Anxious, rigid or highly defended individuals or couples may benefit from psychotherapeutic help in accomplishing the social reframing and psychological redefinitions necessary to complete the stages of adjustment to prolonged and possibly unsuccessful treatment and, where appropriate, to resolve disturbances which may be at the root of unexplained functional disorders.

Part Two

PREGNANCY

Chapter 4

Womb and world: the mother-to-be – common experience and cultural variations

4.1 COMMON EXPERIENCE

4.1.1 Womb and world

No two pregnancies are alike. Every woman's experience of pregnancy is different from all other women and each recurrent pregnancy differs from those that preceded it even in the same woman. We are each of us unique and continue to grow and change throughout our lives. Thus, every pregnancy also takes place within the context of different emotional, psychosocial and physical circumstances. It is therefore hardly surprising that each encounter with this crucial process in a woman's life is singularly personal and, on some level, each one treats her pregnancy and expects to be treated as if she had invented the condition. Nevertheless, as with all life's universal events, it is possible to distil a number of experiences which are common to most pregnancies. The next chapters will explore psychological processes during the three stages of pregnancy and women's differing approaches to these. Here, the focus is upon aspects of pregnancy common to the majority of women, across the world, throughout time.

With conception, a male substance, a sperm has lodged itself within her, uniting with her ovum to produce a genetically foreign body living inside her. In the normal course of events such an invasion would be destroyed or rejected by the host's immune system, but, through mechanisms we do not yet fully understand, pregnancy allows for suppression of the normal response[1]. To become a mother the gravida's body has to overcome its immunological urge to abort. However much wanted, on a psychological level too, conception is a foreign body in danger of expulsion. Remnants of 'preconceptive ambivalence' are retained on that most primitive level of narcissistic exclusivity, where even a loved baby constitutes a threat even though awaited as a blessing [2]. We may say that childbearing means that the pregnant woman has to find a way of incorporating the idea and bearing the reality of another being sharing her inner space and becoming part of her internal world. In this sense her mental 'holding' experience echoes the physical experience of containing the embryo – that intimate loved/hated parasite feeding off her tissue, directing her nutrients to its own system, spewing out its waste for her to get rid of. The idea of a wanted child must be psychologically nourished and cherished in the womb of her mind to create the concept of a baby who can be held and awaited, rather than aborted physically or rejected psychically before term.

Gestation seems so mysterious a process that at times it is difficult for the pregnant woman to sustain a belief in her own natural ability to 'transform a microscopic "seed" into a real baby' [3]. Inexplorable doubts undermine her faith in her own capacity to contain, sustain and preserve the precarious little embryo. Wordlessly and whimsically she wonders if her womb is spacious, safe and roomy enough or whether the fetus will feel 'crammed in a dark, narrow horrid place' or get 'stuck' on the way. Will it be secure? Can she prepare a 'soft, warm nest' to hold him/her or is the embryo 'floating around inside' unable to become embedded? Will it cling in there or fall spiralling down the 'plug hole' of her uterus and just tumble out? Is her body 'full of poisons' which harm the baby (anxieties which in the West are located in bad foods, nicotine, chemical additives, accumulated X-ray radiation, etc., but also anger, fear and old resentments); ('Sometimes I feel my insides are all messed up, rotten, tied in knots and ripped to bits by all the stuff I swallowed-back in terrible arguments with my mother throughout my life'). At times, within herself, the woman falls into her own deep well of semi-conscious panic – feeling trapped in her pregnancy, unable to go back and yet unable to see the way forward. Can she trust her ordinary body to perform 'miracles', to convert her flat belly into a powerhouse of propagation, to produce a living breathing being from a mass of cells? How will she magically create the placenta, a new organ to feed her fetus, or find the 'amazing substance' to convert her bodily fluids into nourishing milk for the baby? Can she both shelter her baby from external and internal injury and yet also protect herself from damage inflicted from within and without? In these first weeks she feels fragile – as if the membrane within and the skin between herself and the world is 'too thin' to contain both herself and her conception without bruising or bursting ('I feel I have to physically hold my belly to protect it when I'm in a bustling market and when music is too loud or words too harsh'). Gradually, with time and familiarity the boundaries 'thicken' as she settles into her own resolution of the 'two in one' dialectic I proposed elsewhere [4].

4.1.2 Two in one

Conception heralds a quantum change. From infancy on we have all learned to accept as a basic premise a simple fact: that each individual is separate and confined to his/her own single body. Yet, in pregnancy two people actually inhabit one body. Professionals tacitly accept this duality in their care for two clients – mother and fetus – under one skin; however, for the woman in whose body the fetus resides, the idea is bizarre and often unacceptable. How she resolves this existential experience of two people cohabiting inside her body-boundary determines the psychological nature of her pregnancy.

In traditional societies, where life is seen to be made up of a succession of progressive stages, there are ceremonies and rituals which enable the individual to pass through the interim period of strangeness between one well-defined position to another. Like puberty, pregnancy is one such transition, and there are specific 'rites of passage' to facilitate the transition, particularly for the primagravida [5]. In our own society, where each pregnant woman has to find her own resources, the concept of her duality may feel too weird to contemplate and is hurriedly dismissed from awareness. If she does ponder it she may have difficulty finding the words to express it or a sympathetic ear to hear her. She risks being misunderstood or feels she may be derided for questioning what others tend to take for granted – that she is a container, a hothouse in which another life will grow. Paradoxically, therefore, at the very time of discovering her 'twosomeness' the pregnant woman also feels very lonely and irredeemably alone with an experience that cannot truly be conveyed. At the end of the day it is her body that will undergo the changes, only she who will experience them, and she who will be swept along to and have to endure the inexorable outcome when the baby leaves her body, be it by miscarriage, labour in vaginal birth or caesarean section.

4.1.3 Body image

Thus, even before the pregnancy is expressed in somatic symptoms or visible physical change, the woman's concept of her body undergoes transformation. She is no longer single and indivisible. Two people now live inside her and, no longer only a daughter, she is becoming a mother. Conception grants her a peephole back into the uterus of her mother – the woman in whose body she herself resided and grew, as she did in the womb of her own mother, and she in hers, like a human chain of Russian dolls. Becoming pregnant thus imposes recognition of a residue inside herself from the complex relationship with her archaic mother. As pregnancy progresses, her changing body serves as the visual/tangible embodiment of her new classification, signalling to others as to herself that she is a female/adult/sexually active/fertile/mother-to-be.

If the onset of menarche and the development of breasts signified crossing the threshold between childhood and mature sexuality, so conception forms another watershed, between womanhood and motherhood. As in adolescence, unfamiliar physical sensations, escalated hormonal activity, and rapid bodily change means that an ever-changing new body-image is superimposed upon and supersedes the old. Corporeal consciousness now expands to incorporate the inner reproductive space. Whereas inner genital sensations were experienced from early childhood, hinting at future maternity [6], her hitherto unexplored womb interior, her uterine emptiness now filled, belly and bust expanding from within, her inside mysteriously occupied by another – these are new and disturbing experiences. Her own familiar body becomes strange. Breasts that she has taken for granted over the years suddenly swell, developing prominent veins, changing pigmentation and oozing if squeezed. Her vagina, previously a 'gateway' to her body, now becomes a 'passage', a corridor between womb and world. No longer her own most intimate part, privileged entry to which she chooses to grant to one or some but not others. Now, she may be rudely assaulted by medical internal examinations, which brush aside her shyness and privacy in an attempt to gain access to the hidden interior and its unseen resident. Her body walls seem mere opaque obstacles, overcome by modern visualizing technology. This invasive probing serves as a further reminder that she is no longer her own person, her body is shared and 'what is in will have to come out' – a major preoccupation of every primagravida, the unknown but inevitable bodily experience of childbirth.

Thus, being impregnated stirs up in even the most assured woman a flurry of uncertainties, which necessarily entail revision of her feminine identity, relating to her fecundated body, its unseen processes and the physical, emotional and relational changes it brings about.

4.1.4 Emotional disequilibrium

Like all such turning points, the transitional phase of pregnancy reactivates dormant conflicts, revitalizing earlier emotional process now being reintegrated through current experiences. The rather sparse psychoanalytic research in this area has focused on the 'critical nature' of pregnancy, which like menarche and menopause, constitutes a change following which the woman will no longer be as she was before [7, 8]. Such a turning point has been found to engender an emotional disequilibrium, necessitating new solutions to old formulations [9–11]. In my experience, each pregnancy calls for reshuffling of internal resources, which involves finding new resolutions and reinterpretation of the past in the light of the present. If maternity constitutes personality development in adult life under the influence of reproductive physiology, pregnancy may be said to have a developmental function, allowing for reorganization of the concept of self [12]. However, I disagree with the classical view that pregnancy is a necessary feminine developmental phase in the female life-cycle [13].

What I find markedly apparent during pregnancy is an involuntary *'permeability'*, a loosening of internal barriers between levels of consciousness and within memory. Thoughts, feelings and fantasies which are usually subliminal suddenly seep into consciousness and must either be attended to or effortfully kept at bay. Different women, as we shall see, deal differently with this experience at different times – some become introspective and 'listen' to their unconscious while others turn away. Yet at some time during their pregnancy most women will experience a whole gamut of inexplicable mood swings, intense urges, heightened emotionality, altered states of consciousness, memory lapse and sudden flashes of insight that accompany pregnancy. ('When I discovered I was pregnant I looked around and thought: every person I see has been born. How did all their mothers ever manage it? How could all those women hold onto their own selves during pregnancy and yet keep their babies going too?') Psychologically, this is perhaps the eternal essence of pregnancy – the internal receptivity to strange, disturbing, uncontainable emotions which must be contained because they cannot be shared, expelled or vaporized without loss.

4.1.5 Pregnant dreams

Her increased permeability to unconscious processes is evident in the pregnant woman's abundant, unusually vivid and at times, overwhelmingly realistic dreams. Inevitably, although rich in residues of each individual woman's ordinary daily life, their themes reflect the universal preoccupations of pregnancy. These dreams are peopled by mysterious creations of each woman's own inner world, drawing up to the surface figments of her repressed procreational imagination, since childhood confined to the dark depths. My structural analysis of many pregnant women's dreams reveals some themes that recur:

(a) Working through contradictions

Past, present and future, internal and external worlds meet at the junction of pregnancy, and are reflected in dream sequences of confrontation and/or reconciliation between elemental opposites in the woman's psychic world. Female and male, birth and death, creation and destruction, order and chaos, big and little, strong and weak, self and other.

(b) The process of gestation

These are dreams depicting the inexorable course of pregnancy which the woman has to traverse alone. The dreamer often has to negotiate an unescapable one-way course such as a narrow tunnel, an irreversible passage, a strongly currented stream or an upright ladder – the end of which must be reached after a lone journey fraught with hazard.

(c) Identity reappraisal

These dreams reflect old grievances reawakened and fond hopes rediscovered. The pregnant woman's corporeal marginality is explored – no longer single, not yet divisible, caught between being a fertile female and becoming a parturient woman. Likewise her emotional marginality is revealed, poised as she is between wishing, and actually seeing the materialization of archaic wishes.

(d) Triangular tales of mother, father and self

Old sagas are spread out again and again, retold in this phase of transition between being somebody's daughter and becoming somebody's mother. Key early relationships with parents, caregivers and siblings find outlets in the guise of current personae (her lover, friends, acquaintances, strangers, Royalty and TV or film characters) as the drama unfolds enacting facets of the highly emotive experience of finally being the one to 'get the baby' – a forbidden function reserved during childhood and adolescence for 'them', the grown-up parents.

(e) Identity of the infant-to-be

Often depicted as a fledgling, animal cub or fully grown child, the mother 'plays' with a variety of images of babies in her mind's eye. Sometimes, the dream baby is a disguise for a child-aspect of the dreamer, a little girl part of the woman herself that she unconsciously equates with or hopes to transpose onto the baby she is carrying. The imagined sex of the baby may be signified overtly or in subtle symbols (such as a plant with an aerial root, a bird's crest or colouring).

(f) Anxiety dreams

Anxiety dreams (at times resulting in sleep disturbances) both express fears and attempt to master the unconscious apprehension prevalent in all pregnancies. Dreams of internal bleeding, menstruation and overt miscarriage reflect preoccupations with precariousness, retention and loss or fears of unseen damage to self or fetus. Anxieties about the baby's normality and her own capacity to grow a viable baby may be reflected in visual monstrosities or a 'forgotten' baby, lost, neglected, starved or dead.

Towards the end of pregnancy in particular, dreams concentrate on child-birth and related anxieties about bodily damage, excessive pain, exposure of hidden aspects of herself, loss of internal organs in birth, wish-fulfilling alternative options (paternal childbirth; springing forth without puncturing the skin; being vomited out, etc.). Birth nightmares are common in the third trimester.

4.1.6 Dream interpretation

The meaning of these dreams, as of all dreams, is highly individual since personal connotations and symbolic disguises vary from dream to dream and dreamer to dreamer. However, in pregnancy, due to the unusual accessibility of unconscious processes during waking hours as well as sleep, the expectant mother has a less arduous task of linking conscious associations to symbols in her dream.

Seemingly a less stringent censorship is at work in distorting the dreams themselves. Thus, many dreams during pregnancy have an undisguised sexual, infantile or sadistic content.

Often, substitutions which do occur are easily intelligible, such as containers, houses or rooms representing the body; doors or openings – the body orifices, with new tenants or newly built extensions and excavated cellars concretely reflecting the pregnancy within her uterus (as well as realistic preoccupations with the need for more domestic space to accommodate her growing family).

The mobile fetus is often represented by a lively fish, tadpole or frog swimming in a watery medium; a barely glimpsed kingfisher or hummingbird darting, unseen in a secret world, or in our times, an astronaut floating in space, linked by umbilical cord to the mother craft.

High tech medical tests like ultrasound or amniocentesis, may be symbolized in dream images, as deep-sea diving, a glimpse of a hidden world or an expedition to a remote mysterious territory, while a wish to know might be reflected in dreams of exploration of the unknown.

Sometimes, a pregnant woman may feel herself to be on the verge of self-discovery, about to grasp an enigmatic insight regarding her inner life. This could be signified in dreams by a tangible symbol like finding a key or decoding a message, or giving birth not to a baby but some vital aspect of herself. At such times, waking may be experienced as a continuation of the dream reality, more real at times than that around her, a factor which contributes to the 'introspective' air of many pregnant women engaged in contemplating psychic rather than external reality.

4.1.7 Psychosocial rebirth

In waking life too, a pregnant woman may relate more keenly to her environment: 'I experience such intense peaceful sensations: it is as if I'd never seen colours before, all so clear and miraculous, it makes even mundane things beautiful'. On the brink of taking her place among society's mothers, she may at times feel close to revelations about hidden capacities in herself. She may feel that apart from her fetus, she harbours inside her an unborn self, some unrevealed aspects of her personality which are maturing inside her and about to be released. In fact, she is pregnant with herself – herself as a mother, a fully mature woman, the person she had imagined as a child she would become when adult. There may be some trepidation at the psychic changes occurring within her, or excitement and wonder at her new sense of powerful untapped resources. She may consciously recognize this potential as her own or else attribute it to the baby. A woman unconsciously wishing to free hitherto atrophied 'masculine' aspects of herself forbidden expression by society or by her own inhibitions, may imagine the baby as a male 'soul mate' to her female self, the 'hero' who will express it for her. Another may envisage giving birth to a baby girl as the ideal wished-for components of herself reborn in a daughter, who will be everything she herself has secretly wished to be. Equally, she may feel susceptible to earlier modes of being, experiencing a regressive shift that enables her to delve down into her own dormant infantile memories to retrieve souvenirs from her own experience of being mothered for future use in an active capacity as mother. Other women may find pregnancy and motherhood often the means of reenacting in reality non-verbal emotional and bodily experiences which have found no other outlet.

Clearly, pregnancy can be utilized as a time of personal growth and emotional 'rebirth', enriching the woman, fostering the integration of disparate parts of herself, her past and personality by re-incorporating facets of herself that have been split off, neglected or disowned.

As we shall see, much of this growth stems from a re-evaluation of herself, both as her mother's baby and as her future baby's mother. While becoming essentially herself in a new way she is paradoxically also joining forces with an age-old collective of women. Suffice to say here that a common theme for many pregnant women is the sense of continuity, becoming a link in a chain of mothers since time immemorial. Dreams may reflect this in family trees, intricate webs and weaving or genealogical charts of kings and queens. At times, this might become a rather frightening concept, a 'Hall of Mirrors' effect with confusion of identity and blurring of generations. However, this experience also restores to the modern expectant mother a glimpse of the sense of maternal continuity taken for granted in traditional societies. The pregnant western woman may feel an unusual simple sense of belonging and kinship with other women. Her own mother might be far away, estranged or even dead, yet through her pregnancy she automatically gains 'associate membership' in the historical line of mothers. In imagination, she is as encircled by timeless matriarchy as her womb envelops her child-to-be.

4.1.8 Single mothers-to-be

The experience of pregnancy for the single woman may be very enjoyable if she has sought conception or whole-heartedly wants a baby despite the absence of a steady partner. It is different for the woman who has found herself pregnant, has deep qualms about the father, and worries about her own capacity to juggle life as a mother and as a supporter, particularly if she has been ambivalent about having a baby at all. Although looking forward to the birth she may regret not having had an abortion before forming an attachment to the fetus. She may relish pregnancy but fears future hardships and entrapment, frightened that she will 'ruin the infant's life' or the baby, hers.

The entire first trimester or even beyond may be filled with doubts and uncertainty or even hopes of miscarriage ('I am so afraid to let go of the whole dilemma, afraid to have an abortion although I tell myself that just because I'm pregnant doesn't mean I have to have the baby – I should treat it like a mastectomy. In my heart of hearts I feel it's crazy to put my life and the child's in jeopardy, but I'm terrified of having an abortion, of letting go of hope, of being pregnant, I don't want to return to my ordinary life and let this door slam shut. Part of me says I'm worthy of more, I'm selling myself short but the biological clock keeps ticking away and I can't risk waiting'). In her anguished deliberations about whether to keep the baby or abort, the single woman undergoes an accelerated process of sorting out her priorities, weighing up the basic values of her life ('I have had to stop lying to myself and review the pattern of my existence – see it not as isolated incidents but stuff that keeps repeating over and again – I start something good, then rubbish it and blame someone else. This time I'm seeing it through'). She may recognize herself in her fetus; a sense of being on the verge of harsh judgement and rejection. The decision to retain the pregnancy may constitute a first step in integration of hitherto fragmented aspects of herself ('I was raised to see black and white, scorn, disgust and rejection with no tolerance or acceptance of who you are. The abortion would have been a way of cutting out the bad, but here I am pregnant, realizing there never is perfection, just a mixture'). Exercising the choice to have the baby despite a realistic evaluation of the hardships involved may signify a healthy decision or an act of desperate hope ('I'll never forget these weeks – the biggest ordeal of my life. I'm so accustomed to being a survivor, brazening it out on the dangerous edge of things, I'm having this baby out of fear that I'll collapse, just relapse into more of the same; this is a chance of starting over'). As in all pregnancies, it may be seen as a testing ground of internal capacities ('If this fetus is receptive, at least I have been honest; not given the baby any false assurances, yet it's still there – I must have something good inside').

Unlike the supported woman in a couple, a single woman is unable to indulge herself in full identification with her fetus during the pregnancy without feeling guilty, because no-one is there to 'hold the fort' while she regresses. There may be a man around, even one who is keen to play the paternal role for the baby, but if he is unsuitable in her mind as a father, he adds to her burden of already having responsibly to map out her future child's life ('It's such a relief to have realized I don't have to marry him for the sake of his child. On the contrary, the most important thing in his life is drink – he's fun and games, exotic, exciting but erratic and totally irresponsible and his life is full of confusion and pazzaz. Now that I've put away daydreams of his changing, I've come to realize that I must be on my own to be reliable for the baby, and he can come and go if he pleases').

Her self-image may change more rapidly than that of the pregnant woman in a safe couple, having to accommodate to her new pregnant condition and future state as single mother without the hothouse protection of a familiar enveloping presence or the constancy of her own sense of self ('It is upsetting to see my sister in her domestic bliss. Where did I go wrong? I felt destined to be a shrivelled up career woman resigned to not having a good relationship with a man but suddenly there's more purpose in life, a sense of direction, goals I've never had before, wanting to provide for someone else, having something I want inside, not far off and intangible'). In sum, I have brought quotations from single women in doubt, to illustrate some of the painful deliberations this decision may entail during pregnancy and how much internal work a woman may have to do in coming to terms with an unplanned or ambivalently maintained pregnancy on her own. Brief psychotherapeutic intervention or crisis counselling can help her accomplish the task before the birth. It is needless to reiterate that many single mothers have completed these deliberations before conceiving and, in their case, psychological processes follow the more common, unimpeded pattern.

4.1.9 The older woman

'Elderly primagravidae' or 'mature multips' may experience additional physiological and psychosocial stresses. Their greater age and life-experience also prime them to deeper awareness of both the risks and the miraculousness of pregnancy. A 'surprise' pregnancy in the mother of older children means having to contend with the shocked responses of her offspring (and all and sundry) who treat her as irresponsible and frivolous. However, with adjustment to this new perspective on their mother, even teenagers may become excited at the prospect of an addition to the family, and show responsibility and tenderness towards the fetus and their mother, too. Adolescent daughters, while initially embarrassed by the overlap of generations, can find womanly closeness with their fertile mothers, if competitiveness is not an issue. In a stormy and empoverished relationship between mother and daughter, the elder's pregnancy might serve as 'the last selfish straw' following which the latter may leave home.

The mother herself may feel this belated return to reproductivity offers a rejuvenating 'new lease on life', or alternatively, she may dread the idea of pregnant discomfort, pram-pushing bondage and sleepless nights at her 'advanced' age of 'decrepitude'. On the other hand, aware with experienced hindsight that babyhood passes 'like a flash', she may relish every moment of this last autumnal pregnancy (once the anxious suspense of amniocentesis is over) and plan to devote herself wholeheartedly to enjoying her baby. ('I am pregnant. Everything I know about my body told me I was – but although delighted, shocked and surprised I am frightened about being excited. I'm so aware of forces in my body that could go wrong – aware of my limitations and it's quite an awakening how fatigued I've been. It hits me forcibly how this need of mine for another child is going to disturb all our lives although my boys are very happy and solicitous of me'.)

A first time mother over 35 years old may have waited and worked long towards this pregnancy. It may follow on infertility, or repeated miscarriages or just postponement while she built up her career or life style, or she may have awaited suitable circumstances or a compatible man. Her maturity inevitably engenders mixed feelings as she is aware of the increased risk of complications and malformations, the obligations of being responsible for another human being and the losses involved in giving up her personal space, income and professional achievements, particularly if she has no partner. ('It is so hard to have a baby this way but the option of not having a baby is harder'.) In late pregnancy, fatigue is a real problem for the older woman, especially one who has led a relatively sedentary life. She may be anxious, having read the statistics about increased chances of miscarriage, premature labour, caesarian section and perinatal mortality in older women. However, if she is emotionally mature, her confidence may enable her to be on more equal terms with the white-coated medical authorities who are experienced as intimidating by younger or less secure women, and she is likely to make better use of antenatal advice available. Likewise, she is often also aware of the greater resources she herself has to offer, as a result of her own stocktaking and having thought long about the needs of fetuses, newborns and ideas about mothering. She may also have reached that philosophical understanding that life and death, happiness and suffering, strength and weakness and frailty are all inextricably linked up to each other in our human condition. The older mother who can share her experience with others, thus may be an asset in antenatal care, capable of supporting and befriending anxious first-timers in her deep-seated awareness that processes must run their course, that all things pass and that we all have 'spare-tanks' of resources to draw on beyond the imagined limit.

4.2 CULTURAL VARIATIONS

The psychosocial processes of pregnancy are very complex. Not only does each woman respond in her own individual fashion, but each culture shapes the range of responses at her disposal. This can be clearly demonstrated in the distinction between western and traditional societies. In the latter, extended families of several generations and various degrees of kinship tend to live in close proximity unlike our own isolated nuclear family, which consists of the cohabiting couple and their step or natural offspring or a single parent and child/ren. Unlike our stratified social relationships and compartmentalized activities, in traditional societies a whole framework of folklore and ancestral customs are handed down from one generation to the next so that daily life is punctuated by numerous common rites and beliefs. During periods of transition in a person's life, such as puberty, marriage, pregnancy and birth, these cultural traditions assume particular importance, guiding the individual across from one social category into another. Ritualistic ceremonies accompany various beliefs during pregnancy.

4.2.1 Some rites and rituals during pregnancy

An overview of anthropological studies in various cultures reveals some focal areas of attention during the trajectory from coupling to birth and beyond [14–17].

(a) Conception

In some cultures, conception is believed to be the result of spirit entry, magical impregnation, ancestor intervention or reincarnation necessitating various rituals and observances to ensure inception, and the safety of the pregnancy, the woman, her baby and/or the community at large.

(b) Gestation

Many societies believe that the behaviour of the mother during gestation, and often that of the father or significant others too, will affect the outcome of the pregnancy. To ensure successful reproduction, various rituals are proscribed or certain acts forbidden, often involving dietary or activity restrictions or rituals in which the husband may or may not share.

(c) Social ratification

During pregnancy the identity of the baby's biological or social father may be emphasized and publicly proclaimed by ceremonies celebrating his sexual adequacy, the formalization of the marriage and/or the firm bonding of two families through the expected offspring. The woman's mother or mother-in-law now becomes an important link between past traditions and the future baby, instructing the pregnant woman how to behave, what to avoid, what duties to perform to ensure growth of a healthy baby and what rules to obey to prevent witchcraft or fetal malformations. As we shall see, in some societies, such maternal solicitude may be expected from other female initiates, such as midwives, who instruct the pregnant woman and help her to make radical changes in work habits and life style required by her new state.

(d) Supernatural powers

In many societies fear of magical practices or evil spirits may necessitate concealing the pregnancy for as long as possible, no mention will be made of it and her daily routine and dress will continue as before. In others, spirits may have to be appeased by specific rites and ceremonies and where pregnancy is problematic, divination may take place to discover the source of the trouble.

(e) Transitional state

In different cultures beliefs and practices vary; however, in most traditional societies, the pregnancy is recognized as a transitional state – the pregnant woman, and particularly the primagravida, being seen in a marginal position of 'not yet motherhood'. In her liminal state she might be thought to present a threat of contagion to certain vulnerable women, and conversely some people are regarded as dangerous to her and her unborn baby.

Whatever the belief, she is not on her own. Even when ceremoniously secluded in a special hut she is encircled by the initiated women, the mothers of the tribe or their midwifery representative, who protect, instruct and provide her with a framework of beliefs and rituals within which to channel and express her own unfamiliar emotions.

4.2.2 Ethnic minorities

Women who emigrate from traditional societies to industrial ones such as our own often find themselves in a doubly marginal position, during their pregnancy: not only are they deprived of the automatic apprenticeship and instruction of their own society of origin, they are often exposed to alien western assumptions without guidance or explanation.

In Britain, surveys have shown that a gap exists between services provided for white English women and those of colour, and that the latter do not always avail themselves of services available, either due to lack of information, rules of Purdah or fear of partaking. Advocacy schemes (such as Maternity Services Liaison Scheme [18] and Multi-Ethnic Woman's Health Project) [19] have been set up to encourage women from ethnic minority groups to make better use of the maternity services. Multi-ethnic projects such as these or specific ethnic minority counselling projects [20, 21] function by providing information about choices of care available. They serve to acquaint women with their welfare and health rights, help them define their needs and negotiate on their behalf with social services and other establishments and power structures. They often provide a female advocate to accompany women to antenatal clinics, hospital appointments and GPs, to act both as befriender and spokeswoman/interpreter where necessary. Racial equality campaigns aim to ensure that women belonging to such differing ethnic communities as Somali, Chinese, Bangladeshi, Nigerian, Afro-Caribbean, Polish or Turkish, each find appropriate maternity care, gain equal access to services and have their special needs met and their wishes respected.

To work, this acknowledgement must entail provision of a variety of facilities and flexibility within services, i.e. treatment by female doctors where requested, restrictions as to who is present during examinations, labour and birth, staff recognition of different nutritional habits during pregnancy and provision of varied cuisine (and in hospitals with a high proportion of ethnic minorities, vegetarian or Kosher meals and possibly Halaal meat), respect for ritual and religious customs such as circumcision, placenta or foreskin burial, naming, baptism, purging and maternal purification rites. Above all a multi-ethnic approach necessitates a broad understanding during training of doctors, midwives, nurses, health visitors and other practitioners that acknowledges the cultural diversity of consumers, provides modern treatments yet respects ancient lore and different concepts of health and illness.

KEY POINTS

*Despite individual variation, some experiences appear common to most pregnancies across cultures and generations: particularly fantasies related to conception; experiences of 'two in one body' and changes in external and internal body-image; doubts about one's capacity for gestation (mysteries of formation, preservation, nourishment and transformation); and finally, the common experience of emotional disequilibrium and unconscious accessibility. Unsupported single women and older mothers may undergo additional strain.

*It is suggested that psychologically, the eternal essence of pregnancy lies in the sensation of strange, disturbing, uncontainable emotions which must be contained because they cannot be shared, expelled or vaporized without loss.

*An analysis of major themes recurring in dreams and interpretation of dream content reveals some basic universal preoccupations: reconciling elemental opposites; process of gestation; identity reorganization; physical and emotional marginality; reappraisal of key early relationships; identity of infant; anxiety dreams about precariousness/loss/damage; viability and normality of infant; labour and delivery.

*Variations in the content and focus of cultural beliefs and practices traditionally shape the range of each individual's psychosocial responses to pregnancy, gestation and birth, focusing on conception, gestation, social transition, supernatural forces, and guidance during the pregnant woman's physical and emotional marginal state.

*Ethnic minorities are often in a doubly marginal position during pregnancy and may be disadvantaged by gaps or unquestioned presumptions in services available. Acknowledgement of our multicultural society must entail provision of a variety of facilities and flexibility within services and recognition of non-mainstream practices.

Chapter 5

Maturational phases

Pregnancy is not a 'condition' – it is a process. Not only does the fetus develop and mature within his/her mother according to a gradually unfolding plan, but she, too, undergoes a corresponding process of growth, bridging the single entity that she was before, with the mother she is about to become. Pregnancy may be divided into three maturational phases, roughly corresponding to the three trimesters: by 12 weeks the fetus is properly formed and by 25 weeks or so it is viable if born. These developments pertain to growth, not only of the fetus but of the mother-to-be. She is affected both by experiences of the pregnancy within her body and by her feelings about these. Like the fetus, the woman's body, too, undergoes dramatic time-scheduled changes – regular enlargement of her uterus from 6 weeks, tissue change and growth of her breasts from the first missed period, development of a new 'organ' – the placenta – by 14 weeks, stretching of the pelvic ligaments and the gradual formation of the lower uterine segment by 30 weeks. Unbidden, changes sweep her along as they do the fetus.

5.1 PHYSICAL SYMPTOMS – MIND AND BODY

In addition to physiological changes, the mother-to-be is affected by hormonal and metabolic processes occurring in her body to sustain the pregnancy. She experiences these as feelings of nausea, morning sickness, increased salivation, constipation, sweating, tiredness, breathlessness, feeling faint – to name but a few. Although common to many pregnant women, each individual's subjective experience of these symptoms is coloured by her emotional reaction to them, derived from her personal appraisal of this pregnancy. Conversely, the particular symbolic meaning she attributes to each symptom may in turn influence the physical phenomena. Nausea is a case in point. A woman may equate being sick with her ambivalent attitude towards the pregnancy or baby, unsure whether she wants the baby after all or is feeling 'sick and tired' of being pregnant. Alternatively, she may experience her vomiting as an involuntary bodily attempt to rid herself of the fetal 'invader' and therefore finds it distressing and anxiety provoking, and needs reassurance that the embryo is safely secured within her. One woman may resent the fetus for 'making' her feel nauseous, whereas another might welcome feeling sick as a repeated confirmation of the ongoing existence of her otherwise invisible pregnancy. Likewise, a woman who is afraid of miscarrying might feel that constipation reflects her control and vigilant retention of the insecure fetus, while a second mother-to-be might imagine the fetus as a large anal blockage obstructing her productivity. A third woman may find the full sensation agreeably satisfying, giving rise to the fantasy that the baby is utilizing all the raw materials inside her for its growth, leaving no waste products to be eliminated. Thus, physical symptoms generate psychic interpretations and, conversely, emotional feelings, such as anxiety, fear or joy may reduce or enhance the physical effects.

5.2 MATURATIONAL PHASES

Psychological experiences are related to and often rooted in the somatic processes of pregnancy. Thus, it is possible roughly to equate them with the three trimesters of pregnancy – the first phase lasting until the quickening is established; the second ending with the onset of increased preoccupation with labour. I have found this third stage to coincide with each individual woman's realization that her baby could exist outside her body. The timing of this stage therefore varies from woman to woman and depends on the age at which she believes a premature baby is viable. Elsewhere, I have described the psychological tasks during the three stages of pregnancy as a progression from belief in the pregnancy, to belief in the fetus and finally in the baby [1]. In some ways the three phases may be seen to recapitulate earlier childhood developmental stages of the woman herself and prepare her for early motherhood. In mapping the woman's psychological experience of the stages, I have suggested they act as a 'rehearsal' for her future relationship with the infant from early symbiotic merger, through differentiation and individuation to a form of separateness [2]. Some psychoanalytic researchers have described the reactivation of the woman's earliest relations with her mother, re-experienced during pregnancy in the form of regressive tendencies, wishes for dependency and fusion, and conflicts about separation [3]. Others have found a revival of sequences of regressive conflicts of a predominantly oral, anal and urethral nature in the first, second and third trimesters respectively [4] as in childhood. An early study divided pregnancy into two main periods, one typified by heightened 'narcissism' maintained by emotional unification of mother and fetus. During the second period, after quickening, the now separate unborn child was seen to be phallic, and associated with the 'ego ideal', modelled after her own father [5]. While such schematic changes are true for some women, many other variations exist. Unless otherwise specified, the observations reported here are based on findings from my own studies.

5.3 PHASE ONE – TYPICAL PSYCHOLOGICAL REACTIONS

During the first phase, women oscillate between feeling overwhelmed by the pregnancy on some days and totally unaware of it at other times. Although some women are convinced of their pregnancy almost from the moment of conception, others need the confirmation of a pregnancy test before they feel it is real enough to launch into an emotional response. This may be joy and excitement or a disbelieving stunned reaction of just standing and looking at the 'ring' of the pregnancy test thinking 'it couldn't happen to me!' or 'it has finally happened!' Yet other women, before sharing the news, wait for tangible or visual evidence of the baby in the form of a rounded abdomen, ultrasound picture or the three-month 'watershed safety-margin'. Once again, although women vary, it is possible to highlight some of the more common emotional experiences of this first phase.

5.3.1 Psychological slippage

One of the first psychological modifications experienced by many pregnant women is a kind of blurring of day and night contrast. A woman who is normally quite alert and productive during the day and sleeps well at night may now experience sleep disturbances and daytime lethargy. She might describe herself as 'half-awake', as she finds her attention wandering with semi-conscious daydreams or late-night-musing breaking through the daytime barriers of concentration ('I can't watch TV or concentrate on reading but I'm quite content to sit and look out of the window or at the wall for what seems like hours'). She may discover herself doing silly things – locking herself out, mislaying her handbag, forgetting dentist appointments, dropping her keys down the drain, overlooking essentials, leaving paraphenalia at home and generally, leaving herself cryptic 'messages' which she gradually begins to decipher. All these parapraxes as Freud called them [6] – these over-sights, memory slips, bungled actions, breakages and misplacements – are found, on reflection, to have symbolic meanings, as do dreams. Sometimes, in the pregnant woman's case, they reveal her inevitably mixed feelings towards her 'intruder' – her inner 'purse' is not her own, she feels excluded from her own body-home, locked out, no longer the sole 'owner-occupier' of her skin, no longer in control and 'at home' with her body. Similarly, her actions may indicate a hidden ambivalence about having to continue her ordinary way of life and go on working despite the monumental changes which are occurring within her. Memory lapses and slips of her tongue may obliquely express unconscious resentment of other people's demands upon her, or subtle rebukes over their well-meaning but unwanted attentions. Actions which lead to her having to be 'rescued' by others may constitute an unrecognized desire to be mothered or a dumb bid for help.

5.3.2 Freewheeling

These cognitive changes are part of the general disequilibrium and permeability described in the previous chapter. Many a pregnant woman may find herself unable to maintain the level of emotional discrimination she used to operate automatically. Overreaction to minor incidents, inappropriate oversensitivity or acute awareness of subtle gradations in other people's responses to her, are all common [7] and heightened emotionality and anxiety have been found in numerous studies [8–10]. The pregnant woman may find herself unable to contain her irritation over little niggles and feels uncharacteristically annoyed when things fail to meet her expectations. She may feel overwhelmed by having to face more than one demand at a time. Temper is volatile, tears closer to the surface and both may be triggered without warning by incidents beyond her control. She often experiences herself like 'a straw blown about in the storm' of strangely aroused feelings. At the mercy of her surroundings and flooding emotions, threatened by reawakened primitive anxieties and magical thinking, she feels in danger of losing her familiar identity. As we shall see in the next chapter, some women defend themselves against this 'overdose of feelings' by exerting their will-power and self-control. Others give in to the 'whirlwind' of emotions: they stop struggling to overcome the resurgence of 'childish' emotiveness and actually enjoy the sensation of 'freewheeling'. Yet other women revert to frenzied activity to counteract the uncertainty, seeking concrete achievements as proof of their productive efficiency or 'filling time' with busy bustling.

5.3.3 Bodily processes

During the first phase of pregnancy, most women are acutely aware of their basic physical needs. Particularly during these early months, the expectant mother may find herself frequently preoccupied with her bodily functions and sensations, at times able to maintain only a minimal or superficial interest in most external things. At first she is aware of subtle changes in the taste in her mouth, the texture of her hair, the changes in her vaginal secretions, in the trickle-flow of her urine. New hypersensitive patches of skin, changes in the appearance of her palms – in many undefinable ways the fine-tuning of her body is no longer as it

was. Her complaints of vague aches and pains are often an attempt to
pin-point her ambiguity and name the sense of physical unfamiliarity
of a body no longer solely her own. She may yearn for rest and seclusion to convalesce, drawing in on herself, rather like her imagined
embryo. Naturally, her preoccupations are exacerbated by physical
symptoms – frequent 'calls of nature' disturbing her sleep at night and
a host of oral and tactile sensations nagging at her by day.

5.3.4 Foodstuffs

Food becomes a major focus: hunger seems to escalate more rapidly ('I
suddenly feel so hungry – I just can't wait, I need to eat straight away
to satisfy the gnawing inside'). Unaccountable revulsions trigger nausea;
likes and dislikes become specific and finely discriminated yet subject
to sudden changes. Many cravings have symbolic connotations, unconsciously based on magical equations. Ideas about eating become
regressive as subconscious childhood notions about conception and
pregnancy are revived [11]. Eggs, grains and seeded fruit might be consumed in quantity to keep herself pregnant or may signify a repeated
acting-out and reaffirmation of an infantile idea of fecundation by mouth.

Unconscious equation of stomach and uterus may result in the woman
giving her baby 'treats' by eating sweets. Meanings are overdetermined
and varied and although usually not quite conscious, at other times an
expectant mother may be aware of the absurdity of her beliefs yet unable
to act against them. An otherwise sensible woman may feel irrationally
compelled to drink lots of milk, to 'whiten' the baby, to 'purify' her
insides or, through sympathetic magic, to help establish lactation.
Unconsciously she may intend to 'suckle' herself or even to replenish
her 'inner breasts' that the fetus is sucking dry. Believing that 'you
become what you eat', she may feel the need to incorporate candied foods
to make her 'nicer' or savoury ones to 'fortify' the baby or to 'pepper
up' her insides against the 'cannibalistic' fetus. She may tell herself that
salt-and-vinegar crisps alleviate her nausea, but unconsciously associates
these with purification. She may try to create the baby she wants by
eating succulent, luscious, juicy foods in the hope of making a baby that
is 'good enough to eat'. She may opt for solid, nourishing yet plain
healthy fare in the belief that her baby dictates this choice. Wholesome
or spicy foods might be seen as having strengthening properties, smooth
textures to enhance the baby's complexion, or sharp foods its intelligence.
Conversely, certain foods may be rejected because of their 'harmful'
potential. Not merely those known medically to be risky but others with
inauspicious properties. Thus, despite a craving for them she may
abstain from eating strawberries to avoid birthmarks or refuse pickles
to 'get' a girl. These superstitions may coincide with folk beliefs or be

idiosyncratically personal. Above all, these weird and magical ideas lurk in otherwise rational minds and, at this vulnerable time of great responsibility towards the unborn child, are often acted upon thereby altering feeding habits of a lifetime.

5.3.5 The function of intake

Eating and drinking provide one means of monitoring the interchange between the external world and the one inside:

1. **Contact**. Food may be used to provide a means of making contact with the fetus – of offering titbits, feeding and cosseting, actively contributing to growth; stroking or singing may be similarly employed.
2. **Control**. Intake may serve as a way of controlling a being beyond her control – regulating its intake, establishing who is 'boss'. She may withhold food spitefully, to restrict the baby's imagined pleasure or use specific items as a means of sending the fetus the 'message', that her own needs take preference – like drinking alcohol or coffee. The message may be that she is sad, or fed up or feeding herself for a change.
3. **Identification**. Often, in her identification with the baby, the expectant mother wants to be fed and cherished while she sustains her embryo. In reality she may achieve this by encouraging others to look after her. Her husband may be sent to obtain special foods to satisfy her cravings or induced to bring her cups of tea or little gifts. She may have dreams about discovering and feeding herself off some amazing placenta-like fruit or vegetable, with magical capacities to filter out noxious stimuli or to serve as a bountiful, never-ending supply of goodies, or may spend hours luxuriating in the bath like her ambiotic-bathed fetus or absorbing sights, sounds and smells.
4. **Pathological intake**. If the woman feels unmothered, or is ambivalent about the child's father, she may act out her resentments in her eating, smoking or drinking behaviours. Poor dietary background is known to increase the risk of spontaneous abortion and severe handicap. Therapeutic help may be necessary to enable the woman to implement dietary counselling.
   (a) Compulsive eating or overly rich food intake may reflect competition with the passively fed inhabitant of her womb. Even an otherwise sensible diet may be temporarily changed to enact her feelings, justified as 'cravings'. Resenting her baby's parasitic contentment, an envious mother may wish to spoil its unearned sanguinity by 'livening things up' with chilli or depriving it a bit.
   (b) If her antagonism is great enough, an angry woman might resort to punitive starving of the fetus with little regard for her own

health. Conversely, anorectic-type behaviour may reflect a depressed woman's poor self-esteem, boundary conflicts with her own mother or self-punitive measures that ignore the harmful effects of her self-destructive activity on the baby.

(c) Substance abuse. There has been widespread publicity of alcohol as a teratogen (responsible for fetal alcohol syndrome, still-birth and a broad spectrum of adverse pregnancy outcomes now well documented by over 800 studies [12],) and the detrimental effects of smoking and drug abuse. This means that few pregnant women can claim to be ignorant of the dangers involved in substance abuse during pregnancy.

Nevertheless, most studies reveal that 25–35% of pregnant women smoke throughout pregnancy, between one-half and two-thirds of women consume some alcohol (2–13% heavy consumption) and there is a strong association between drinking and smoking [13]. A distinction must be made between casual behaviour, the need for educational programmes and emotional difficulties. When fetal abuse is suspected, these, like other pathological symptoms, cannot be overlooked by professionals as they present potential physical dangers and augur badly for the future relationship between baby and mother. The need for help will be explored in more detail in Chapter 7 on antenatal psychotherapy for vulnerable women.

5.3.6 Telling

The first stage of pregnancy is dominated not only by adaptation to the new state of being pregnant, but by the question of sharing it. As mentioned, the expectant mother is both aware of sharing her body with another being and, ironically, of being locked into a private and unshareable experience. She becomes obsessed with her 'secret', hugging it to herself or imagining 'telling'. Sharing it with anyone other than her doctor may be delayed until early miscarriage has been ruled out. However, once she begins 'telling', an elaborate evaluation system may be constructed, ranking acquaintances in order of intimacy. The social network is rearranged in a series of concentric circles, those who are closest to the core will be told soonest, others, more peripheral, will get to know later. Friends' and relatives' responses are minutely scrutinized and 'unsuitable' reactions are warded off, as if magically able to spoil the experience of pregnancy. As advice begins to flow in, a 'filtering' process may similarly operate to ward off unwanted information. (Reactions of partners will be dealt with separately in the chapters on expectant partners.)

5.3.7 Real and 'internal' parents

Parents loom large at this point – when to tell them and how, is usually an important issue, signifying with first pregnancy the final transition from being a child of theirs into becoming a parent like them. Even if 'respect-ably' married, old feelings of shame and guilt and memories of parental prohibitions of sexuality may increase the difficulty in telling mother and/ or father about the pregnancy, reawakening old inhibitions about discuss-ing this delicate subject. These reactivated feelings may be so strong as to prevent even a happily awaited pregnancy being revealed for fear of her parent's reactions. ('All these years of bravado and rebellion – and here I am, whisked back by pregnancy into being my parent's daughter, afraid to tell them I'm expecting. The illusion of freedom I've held onto so tenaciously and all my defiance just dissolves at the thought of their icy silence.') In a family where sexuality was inappropriately eroticized, where it was 'sanitized' and the woman's mother was afraid of her own woman-hood, the pregnant woman might feel ashamed of 'parading' her budding fecundity. Anxieties might prevail about her joy being enviously 'nipped in the bud' or her exuberance squashed, spoiled or appropriated by 'grabby' parents. In a family experienced as invasive, or one in which the parents present a 'know-it-all invincible front' she may try and protect her privacy and right to self-discovery by keeping her pregnancy secret.

Particularly salient are the woman's feelings towards her own mother. Now that she contains a baby as her mother once contained her, she may be flooded by successive waves of interchangeable identifications of herself with both her mother and her baby. In her fantasy it is not her real mother that she evokes but her 'internal' mother, the archaic image of the mother of her own infancy, real, remembered and imagined. At times she has the strange wish to crawl back and curl up and hiber-nate in the dark warmth of her mother's interior. An overwhelming need to be mothered might alternate with her desire to protect and nurture the fetus like a seedling in need of care, until it is well established. She may also fear surrendering to her wishes, dreading re-engulfment in a regressive relationship with her mother symbolized by being sucked back into the maternal womb. ('My mother is so grasping – she's always treated me as if I was an extension of her. She wants us to be so close that if I'd let her she'd just swallow me up and keep me inside her.')

Regressive pressures may give way to revival of past memories and fantasies of her own babyhood coinciding with the progressive active urge to propel herself forward into motherhood, by reading, learning and imagining herself as a mother. Her relationship towards her father also changes during this early phase of pregnancy as she incorporates within her fetus the part-image of the baby's father, who may or may not be interchangeable with her own. If she clearly differentiates this man as separate from herself and different from her father, she can be relatively free of the guilt feelings that frequently beset women in whom old, unconscious equations are revived. For the latter, pregnancy promises to fulfil the postponed childhood wish of having her own baby in competition with her mother, who now may appear as an angry rival. During the course of her pregnancy, one of the psychological tasks will be the gradual relinquishment of her 'internal' omniscient daddy and consolidation of an equal relationship between them as adults. If she comes from a family in which incestuous undertones have coloured their emotional relationships, her own normal feelings will be exacerbated by the reality of reciprocity or seduction. She may feel confused about her entitlement to have this baby inside her and need psychotherapeutic help to establish ownership over her body and baby. ('I never could have anything that belonged to me. I'm so afraid now in having this baby – as if it isn't really my right and it will be taken from me.')

5.3.9 The wish for a baby

The idea of becoming a mother is never a neutral one. As we have seen, it hails back to early childhood, to the little girl's passionate desire to be like her mother, to 'make' babies, to take mother's place and have a baby from her father, followed by angry resignation to the necessity of having to postpone fulfilment of her wish for a real baby, which meanwhile is replaced by dolls [14]. Now, as she begins in reality to realize the old childhood wish, her archaic fantasies are reactivated together with infantile jealousy of the parent's relationship, envy of her fertile mother, and painful memories of the birth of siblings. When these revamped fantasies are woven around the expected baby, the baby's father is often unconsciously identified with her own father, with resulting guilt feelings and forebodings about maternal vengeance. A 'leading' female anxiety for some women is that her own capacity to give birth may have been damaged in retaliation for childhood destructive wishes against her fertile mother and unborn siblings [15]. Common fears are that the baby will be abnormal, that she will not be allowed to keep it or even that she will die in childbirth as punishment for engaging in forbidden desires.

5.3.9 Reactivation of the emotional past

Pregnancy brings a resurgence of time-lagged conflicts. In some women these childhood anxieties were never resolved and allowed to be gradually outgrown and to fade but have been repressed and remained encapsulated, 'trapped in a time warp' in their original form. During the transitional turbulence of pregnancy such a woman might feel the pressure of old feelings coming back with nothing to diffuse them, building up in her as if her emotions are 'about to burst open'. With reactivation of past feelings and her greater emotional permeability, memories may seem very close to the surface and extraordinarily real. Experiences from the past spill over into the present – the woman may feel inexplicable boundless rage at being frustrated, uncontrollable pangs at being left, deep mortification at minor slights, fervent fury at intrusions into her time with her partner. Generating these outbursts are newly erupted 'cold'-volcanoes of the past: sibling rivalries, unbridled aggression and jealous imaginary attacks on the parents' babies and envy of mother's creative powers mingled with anxieties about retaliation for wanting to usurp her, fears of punishment for naughtiness, masturbation, aggression, sexuality and imagined or actual hurt inflicted on caregivers, brothers and sisters.

Particularly vulnerable are those women who have experienced themselves to be unwanted or those whose siblings or mother actually fared badly and seemed to the child to be harmed by her omnipotent destructive feelings. In these and women whose turbulent and competitive relationships with their mothers during adolescence have remained unresolved, anxieties may reach such peaks as to endanger the pregnancy. Some women protect themselves against early guilt by maintaining secrecy and fierce independence of their parents. Others engage in excessive submission and dependency upon their mothers. In pregnancy, childhood fantasies about sharing a baby with mother might be revived, treating the fetus and later the baby as playthings, and herself as 'pretend' mother – handing over real responsibility, both for her own physical care during pregnancy and that of the baby postnatally to her mother, or to a maternal figure such as the nurse or health visitor. A variation of such guilt-evading infantile over-dependence takes the form of assigning protective powers, not to her mother, but to a paternal representative – the obstetrician or GP who is entrusted with 'giving' her a baby 'sealed, signed and delivered' without her active cooperation, thus alleviating personal responsibility for her state. Luckily, as we shall see, for most women, the emotional process of becoming a parent offers an opportunity for growth. Working through past emotions reactivated during pregnancy and early motherhood allows for resolution of infantile psychic conflicts relating to the internal parents, reintegration of more mature configurations and a more realistic evaluation of the real parents. The outcome of this emotional work during the next two phases of pregnancy greatly affects the capacity for future mothering.

5.3.10 Changing self-image

The hallmark of this first stage of pregnancy is a compulsion for continuous reappraisal of self-image and almost daily readjustment of

identity. Questions which have occupied philosophers over the generations and children throughout the world are now recast in a new light
by the pregnant woman: 'Who am I? Where did I come from? How are
babies made? Who will come after me? Who is this person I am becoming?
Who is the person I am creating? At the end of this maze, will I still
be the same person?'

The involuntary discovery of new facets of herself which do not coincide with her own or other people's expectations adds to the confusion.
The pregnant woman feels that in addition to its puzzling nature there
is a risk that this unfamiliar emergent identity will be rejected by her
friends. Her excitement at exploring new potential is sometimes overshadowed by fear of devaluing her own previous complacency and
untroubled acceptance of her limitations. Bewildered, she may find
herself gazing into mirrors or needing literally to 'touch home' between
excursions, using well-known places and objects as a reaffirming
'touchstone of familiarity' in the face of the many changes of pregnancy.

5.3.11 Transition

The last few weeks of the first trimester tend to be regarded as a
'dangerous' period, the time when threat of miscarriage is heightened
by the changeover to the placenta. Some women 'lie low' during this
period of tension, 'skimming the surface' until this hurdle is passed;
others monitor the fetus vigilantly, willing it to stay alive. Yet other
women become hyperactive, 'dicing with Fate' ('if it's meant to survive
it will, otherwise, better to lose it now than later'). Ultrasound scans
given at this stage may propel the women (and her mate if present)
precipitously into the next stage of pregnancy, by revealing the fetus
as a wriggling lively entity although movement has not yet been
experienced.

5.4 PHASE TWO

The second stage of pregnancy is heralded by the quickening – the first
felt movements of the baby. At first an almost imperceptible butterfly-
wing flutter is often confused with gastric 'bubbles', then rapidly escalates
to unmistakeable fetal activity.

5.4.1 Womb vs. world

Although she feels physically more like her 'old self', the new weird
experience of a mobile independent being within her takes precedence
over her sense of bodily well-being. The expectant mother now finds
her concentration divided between the demands of the external world and

bids for attention from within. At times she eagerly awaits signs of liveliness, while at other times she may deeply resent these unsolicited reminders that she is no longer her own person. She may feel perplexed by the fetus who paradoxically seems to insist on keeping her awake at night although needing her energy and devotion during the day. She may experience the baby as an uncontrollable invader, doing wilful and contrary things and provoking her to do them too – interrupting her activities and making her appear silly and incompetent by contrast to her previous cool self. On the other hand, she may find the world receding in importance as she experiences a reshuffling of priorities with her interest now primarily focused on her inner 'power house' and its communicating inhabitant.

5.4.2 The imaginary friend

Emphasis in the second stage thus shifts from pregnancy to fetus, highlighting the absence of information about her baby. Many a pregnant woman now begins using her imagination to fill the gap: elaborating fantasies about the fetus, ascribing characteristics, features, likes and dislikes to the little being inside her. She may communicate with her imaginary baby by talking aloud, or have 'mental' conversations while cuddling, stroking and soothing it. She may also experience it equally trying to 'caress' her from within – stroking her tenderly or communicatively responding to her chat with little kicks and jerks. The mother-to-be may now actually welcome opportunities to be alone with her baby, resenting those social occasions when the baby merely 'tags along' rather than being the centre of attention. Equally, she may resist work situations which siphon off her concentration and prevent her from directing full undivided attention to her belly. At other times, alarmed by the sense of 'drowning' in her pregnancy, she may feel the need for increased social stimulation and external involvement to counteract the inward pull and divert her from the calls from within. Most of all, there is a sense that she is no longer alone: wherever she might be, by herself or with others, the baby is there too, inside her, seemingly listening to her thoughts, watching her dreams or 'eavesdropping' on her conversations.

5.4.3 Sexuality

As the pregnancy begins to show, 'telling' is no longer within her control. Her swelling body now betrays her secret. Pregnancy becomes a declaration of fecundity disclosing her sexual relationship to the world. She sees teenage boys glance at her with 'I know what you've been up to' showing in their eyes. Even casual acquaintances offer unsolicited

advice or become involved in her intimate condition, swapping horror
stories or prying into her experience. Hypersensitive to minute changes,
she senses that she is now being treated as 'a pregnancy' rather than
a person and may resent this myth of impregnation as the great leveller,
when to her it merely highlights the great variability of gestations and
the uniqueness of her own. Some women revel in new-found pregnant
sensuality, feeling released from sexual inhibitions of the past. Others
may have the sense of shame about sexuality during pregnancy, feeling
that it is slightly immoral. As the inner sensations become stronger, the
baby's movements may add a further dimension to her sexual life – either
as an exciting participant or a dampening voyeur. She may feel increasingly 'beleagured', shut into her own body with the fetus and unable
to allow her husband in. Alternatively she may feel a sense of 'cosy union'
or 'communion' with her inmate and resent any external intrusions into
the internal intimacy. At other times, she may wish to share her 'womb'
by allowing her partner access to his baby through intercourse. As we
shall see in further sections on sexuality, making love during pregnancy
is affected by the respective fantasies of each partner.

5.4.4 Real or role

Pregnancy offers a special social perspective. Many a mother-to-be
becomes emotionally very discerning, able to differentiate intuitively
between authentic concern and self-interested contact. She feels in
possession of a useful 'sixth sense' as her sense of potency is heightened
by an awareness of her own subtle appreciation of other people's unconscious motivations in relation to her. However her loneliness also
increases with the experience of dissimilarity and distance from non-
pregnant friends. Altered interaction is due to various factors:

a. Faced with the uninitiated, she may discern concealed signs of resent-
    ment or envy of her special state. Men and childless women treat
    her differently now. She may become aware of a tension in com-
    munication, a non-verbal barrier cutting across the conversation, as
    if they feel she inhabits a world that they cannot enter or as if they
    experience an 'impenetrable aura' surrounding her like that of a bride
    or dying person.
b. At other times the source of tension lies not in her marginality but
    comes from the other person's suspended desire to feel her live belly
    – a tension that she may rapidly dispel by spelling out the unspoken
    wish, of letting them 'have a go'.
c. Non-pregnant women friends sometimes display excessive identifica-
    tion with her pregnancy, as if wanting to use it as a vehicle to relive
    their own experience and come to terms with it. She feels used at

times; as if they do not hear her account but skirt over it to turn the conversation to their own prenatal experience or try to reconstruct their own pregnancies by moulding hers in the light of their own. Often, they seem reproachful and deflated, feeling invalidated when she disregards their advice which she, in turn, may consider oppressive, denying her own individuality.

d. At other times, needing to de-fuse her own anxiety or fuel the positive pole of her feelings, she may actively seek out advice and welcome caring attention and reassurance, particularly from motherly, non-envious women, her own mother or maternal substitutes, including professionals.

5.4.5 Expanding and contracting

As she becomes larger, more rotund and less comfortable, demands outside home may feel more stressing. The expectant mother often begins to rely more heavily (!) on her partner or a woman friend to protect her from unnecessary strains by taking over some of the cumbersome practicalities of her life. Early evenings tend to be a particular arduous time as she feels about to wilt just as others are girding themselves for an evening of fun. In an attempt to conserve and replenish her resources, she may restrict relationships to a central 'core group', often a family-like nexus of close caring friends while more dispensable contacts are relegated to the periphery. She may then focus on this circle of close friends, seeing them in her own home or close by, contracting her sphere of action both socially and geographically. However, driven by thoughts of the future another pregnant woman may become gregarious, seeking to expand her network of social engagements and range of activities before restrictions are imposed by the birth. During the second phase, the couple's own relationship begins to settle into the pregnancy after dramatic upheavals of the earlier months. Slowing the pace towards the end of this stage may allow them time to share the intimate minutiae of the emotional gestation. Couples vary and some of their vicissitudes will be discussed in Chapter 14.

5.4.6 Mother and me

Increasingly, as the fetus becomes differentiated from herself and more familiar through its fine movements and active responses, the mother-to-be also begins to disentangle herself from her 'internal' mother. One detailed study of psychological vicissitudes during pregnancy found a pattern of reconciliation with the mother in all but extremely ambivalent women [16]. Most studies also emphasize the centrality of pregnant women's relationship to their mothers. An important distinction has been made between those who idealize them and those who see them realistically [17].

Now that she is grappling with her own potential motherliness, the mother-to-be may become more capable of regarding her own mother as a person in her own right, no longer the internally held version coloured by infantile emotions. From being seen as benevolently omnipotent or malevolently responsible for all ills she may now allow her mother to seem simply human – fallible, a woman like herself. In my experience, this often painful realization that 'there are no Supermums' enables the expectant mother gradually and selectively to internalize the mothering qualities she has valued in her mother, making these her own while discarding other maternal attributes alien to her nature. A spin off of such growth is new receptivity and the chance for enrichment by being tuned in to 'mothering lore'. Like a honey-bee with sensitive 'antennae' quivering, she gleans expertise from others around her and stores away information without even noticing it. Thus, progressively, she locates the source of nurturance inside herself, drawn in and encapsulated within the supportive system of fetus/self (and in some cases, her partner, too).

Women who lack these positive resources either in their internal or external worlds find it more difficult to strike an authentic balance between identification with the fetus and mother. If a woman rejects identification with her fetus, she is likely to experience it as a parasitic invader; if she spurns identification with her mother and the maternal role, she may fail to mother herself and her own baby. Conversely, if she over-identifies with her fetus, she is in danger of being sucked back into a passive state of womb-like dependence which negates active mothering, whereas if she overidentifies with her own mother, idealized comparisons or mechanical imitation will counteract her real relationship with the baby.

During this second phase of pregnancy differentiation is thus used as a means of traversing the distance between identification of herself as fetus (her mother's and her own) and as mother (her own and her baby's), through the medium of fantasies rooted in her own bodily and emotional experience.

5.5 PHASE THREE

Perspective changes dramatically with the advent of the third stage of gestation. This phase begins when the incubating mother believes that her baby could now survive outside her body if born prematurely.

5.5.1 Growing concerns

Time now becomes a precious commodity: some women are reluctant to have the pregnancy end, relishing every magical moment that the fetus is safely enveloped inside. A woman whose last baby this is to be may be poignantly aware of the transience of her special state. Primagravidae avidly use the short time left to them to prepare and to enjoy the world as a non-parent. Those on maternity-leave bask in the luxurious oasis of personal space, free of work demands and as yet unencumbered by babies.

Although primiparous women differ from those with first-hand practical experience, all (except the most highly defended) are aware of the momentous change about to occur in their lives and the brief time remaining to prepare for the birth and the baby. Preoccupation now shifts from the imaginary fetus-baby to the real 'unreturnable' baby about to emerge. As the 'moment of truth' approaches, the prospective mother is obsessed by the compelling idea that this is a lifetime commitment to a lifelong relationship with a faceless person of unknown sex and as yet undetermined qualities. Likewise, the couple too, as parents, are an unknown quality and the expectant woman is consumed with questions about her own ability to produce something live, good and valuable, her capacity to mother, the metamorphosis of her partner into a father, her parents into grandparents of her child, and the bulge into a baby. ('You can sell your house, marriages can be dissolved but once a person is born you're stuck with them and can't shove them back or send them off in a box with holes in the lid: "Dear Mum and Dad, we can't cope – you have him". Its forever and we'll be the mum and dad. That scares the hell out of me.')

5.5.2 Labour and birth worries

The end of pregnancy looms large. Even the multiparous woman wonders whether the baby will just drop out unheralded, slide out like a slithery baby seal or whether she will have to endure a lengthy and painful labour. The primagravida worries how she will fare in this unprecedented situation, whether her body will be damaged or damaging or prove trustworthy and know what to do; how she will cope with pain and the explosive build-up of excitement. At times it may seem that these fears are consuming life but nobody will save her by saying what it is really like to have a baby. She feels there is 'a conspiracy of silence and confusion' about the reality of birth with some people reiterating that 'it does not hurt one little bit' while simultaneously she is hounded by horror stories about excruciating agony and 'the worst pain ever'.

Many primitive anxieties are reactivated by the imminence of birth. One archaic concept I have encountered revitalized at this time in numerous women is the childish notion of a *single internal cavity* within the body, housing all the internal organs and a confusion of food, faeces, flatus, urine, amniotic fluid as well as the fetus. Many pregnant women have a secret fear that as it emerges the baby will draw everything else out with it – all the internal stuff will come spilling out, revealing all the mess inside and depriving the mother of her vital organs. She may also be afraid of revealing her untold thoughts and hidden bad or mad aspects of herself which she fears will tumble out too, like faeces, during the turbulence of labour [18]. If she is planning to give birth in hospital these anxieties are exacerbated by the thought of strangers attending the birth, voyeurs to an intimate almost-sexual experience. Forebodings such as these are difficult to formulate to herself and very difficult to express to another. Whether she contains or voices them or not depends on her tolerance threshhold and availability of internal and external emotional resources. A wide range of negative life experiences during childhood and regarding sexuality while growing up have been found to be associated with fear of childbirth [19]. Numerous studies have been conducted on fear of childbirth and the relationship between such anxiety and 'psychogenic' obstetric complications, however results are conflicting [20–22].

Some fears are clearly irrational but nevertheless potent, whereas others have a good basis in reality. The latter realistic worries can usually benefit by confrontation in childbirth preparation classes. The pregnant woman is then given a chance to find ways of coming to terms with the discrepancy between her own wishes and hospital system shortcomings or endeavour to change these before confinement. She will at least be prepared for what she fears and will have benefited from working through some of her worries. However, the more irrational and less conscious anxieties cannot be alleviated by rational approach. Further fears and fantasies related to childbirth will be covered more fully in Chapter 17 devoted to this topic.

5.5.3 Professional monitoring and self-observation

Contact with professionals becomes more frequent now, and the expectant mother looks to them to supply her with vital information about the state of the baby, the timing and type of birth. Conversely, she feels herself to be the baby's interpreter – a mediator between these external authorities and the baby within. She listens for signs and signals inside herself, monitors the hardening of her stomach walls with the strengthening 'practice' contractions; she scans the changing vigorousness of fetal movements, keeps track of the lightening of pressure on her ribs and investigates the new twinges in her groin as the baby's head engages and relieves her heartburn. She may observe subtle changes in her complexion, appetite, posture or sleep patterns.

Nevertheless despite this acuity of self-observation, in some antenatal clinics, she is still treated merely as a vehicle, a witless container for her growing baby. She may have to plead with ultrasound technicians to move out of the way of the screen to enable her to get a glimpse of her own baby. She might find herself having to remind a fumbling doctor that she does actually know which way the baby is lying and where the heart beat may be heard. Despite the often casually insulting 'off with your pants' atmosphere in some clinics, most women in the third phase are now more confident of their own expertise – their own intimate knowledge of this one particular pregnancy – and hopefully can put this to good use. Precarious lives of babies have been saved by women's insistence on reporting an altered pattern of movements. Many professionals accept that women are usually very good judges of changes taking place in their own bodies, particularly if they are told what to look out for. However, some professionals still hold an unfounded fearful counter-fantasy of clinics being swamped by hypochondriacal, overanxious neurotic women. As a result, even blatant symptoms such as severe headaches or amniotic leakage may not be reported by a conscientious woman determined 'not to be a bother'. In Chapters 9 and 16 on health care professionals we shall explore their special significance in the pregnant woman's life.

5.5.4 'Signs' and signals of imminent labour

An alert woman can pick up subtle signs of the approaching end of pregnancy, sometimes earning a few days warning before the actual labour: pressure on the bowels for two weeks before, constipation for 2–3 days before, natural abstinence from food the evening before, a sudden urge to clean the oven or scrub the floor, changes in the quality of her hair (less curly, or silkier) and violent movements particularly on sitting, are signs retrospectively reported by many women. Some claim their faces looked different in the mirror, but their description of 'mask-like' gives few objective clues to what the prelabour facial change is. On the other hand, suggestibility is rife at this apprehensive time, and superstitions are revived to compensate for lack of secure knowledge. Some women find they are living from one 'auspicious' birth date to another, defined by mystical means – 'good' numbers, red-letter dates of special significance or preferred days of the week. This is a magical attempt to put some order and predictability into an uncertain period of time that stretches on indefinitely but beyond which all current plans are suddenly defunct. Most women find they are increasingly susceptible to overblown emotiveness, dreading the retributive 'wrath of the gods' who will demand payment for her happiness to date.

Each twinge is regarded as the potential beginning of an unstoppable avalanche of pain; at the dead of night she muses on horror stories she has heard about birth, imagining that they all will come true for her and most certainly those experienced by members of her close family. She is nightmarishly afraid that it is she who will 'get' the monster, morbidly anxious about surviving childbirth, doubting she will be allowed to produce and keep a whole, live baby. When all is quiet she may find herself prodding the fetus, or knocking against the edge of the bath in which she soaks, to gain a sign of life within.

Once again, all these irrational yet salient fantasies cannot be dismissed by logical reassurances peppered with statistics. Most human beings can cope with only a limited number of unknowns at one time. Too many uncertainties, like those surrounding the event of birth, engender unfocused panic feelings, with which many women come to grips by focusing the fear – anchoring free-floating anxiety into specific worries. In some ways, the more unlikely these are to come true, the better they serve their purpose. Other women solve the dilemma by making certain they do know and can control – convincing the doctor they need to be induced, planning an epidural or carefully rehearsing their breathing techniques.

Another form of 'certainty' is the result of identificatory imitation. Sometimes the end of pregnancy, like its beginning, takes on an unreality for the woman who feels she is merely a link in the chain of females stretching back to her great-grandmother and forward through her unborn daughter into the future. Unless resolved through recognition of her own individuality, she is in danger of repeating her mother's labour and birth experiences, particularly her own birth or that of her sibling in equivalent position to the birth order of this baby. As noted in the section on psychotherapy and vulnerable pregnancies, most at risk are women with historical sensitization to guilt which may precipitate repetition of their mother's conditions.

5.5.5 Inside out

As the end approaches, hitherto postponed nest-feathering activities are stepped up in a race against the clock, to create an external womb-like nursery or cradle to replace the inner containment of the body. The thought of giving up the status of pregnancy arouses the woman's regret and some sheepish envy that attention will be diverted from herself to be lavished on the baby. Anticipatory joy mingles with grief, as the ripe woman begins mourning the passing of her pregnancy (particularly if it is to be her last), with a foreboding of feeling flat, empty and denuded after the birth. Eager to encircle the real baby in her arms, nevertheless, she is aware of the passing away of a dream-baby.

Gradually the previous erratic ebb and flow of energies stabilizes into an inactivity of conservation – holding herself in abeyance, poised between the lingering present and a tardy future. Time running out imperceptibly lapses into slow-motion waiting, an abstract stand-still watchful waiting, yearning for something to happen and fearing what will happen. Waiting for the curtain to be drawn aside, and another life to begin. She gradually pares down until only a question mark remains – when and how and who will be born. . . .

KEY POINTS

*The three maturational phases of pregnancy are marked by each woman's individual experience – the first phasing lasting until movement is felt, the second ending with the belief that the baby would be viable if born.

*Physical symptoms generate psychic interpretations and, conversely, emotions may reduce or enhance bodily experiences.

*The emphasis in phase one is on the pregnancy; psychological manifestations are emotional disequilibrium, parapraxes, 'free-wheeling', preoccupations with body-image, food, 'telling' and reactivation of old conflicts, particularly in relation to the mother.

*During the second phase the emphasis shifts from the pregnancy to the fetus, now experienced as separate. In the absence of objective information about the baby the mother elaborates fantasy babies, often identified with aspects of her own infantile self. Through the duel processes of identification and differentiation with both the baby and her own mother, maternal capacities and empathy evolve.

*With viability of the baby the mother becomes increasingly preoccupied with emotional and physical preparation for the birth and baby and a shift occurs from the imaginary infant to the real one, soon to be born. During this third phase primitive bodily anxieties are revived which if unresolved may affect labour.

Chapter 6

Facilitators, Regulators and Reciprocators: different approaches to pregnancy

6.1 MATERNAL ORIENTATIONS DURING PREGNANCY

There are as many approaches to pregnancy as there are pregnant women. Having examined the experiences, which are fairly common to all women, we may now focus on differences. In the course of my studies of expectant mothers I have found it possible to delineate three general orientations towards maternity, babies and motherhood, which diverge considerably from each other during pregnancy and appear to follow a predictable pattern of mothering after the birth. Although there are few 'pure types' who fit the model perfectly most women tend to gravitate towards one or another of the orientations. The divergent types described here may make sense of puzzling inconsistencies among pregnant women and serve to highlight the need for a variety of service provisions to meet different expectations within the client group.

I have called the one orientation that of the Facilitator, who gives in to the emotional upheaval of pregnancy by contrast to the Regulator, who holds out against it. A third approach, that of the Reciprocator who has mixed reactions, will be described at the end of this chapter. Women may switch orientations with subsequent pregnancies, since each conception, as we have seen, is set in a matrix of particular circumstances which determine the woman's psychological perceptions of pregnancy and representations of the unborn baby. Barring unforeseen life-events, an unusual infant or therapeutic intervention, most women remain consistent in their approach throughout the pregnancy and mothering of that baby.

What follows is a composite picture drawn from many prospective mothers' fantasies, feelings and responses to pregnancy. To illustrate how the psychological processes of pregnancy differ in these three groups of women, this account will follow the framework of the three maturational phases described in the previous chapter.

6.2 PHASE ONE

6.1 Early pregnancy: the Facilitator

The Facilitator greets pregnancy as the consolidation of her feminine identity. For her, childbearing promises to fulfil and realize childhood wishes which she now re-experiences in an upsurge of emotional intensity. Finally, or once again, it is she and not the others who is pregnant. She contains within herself the baby she so passionately desired as a little girl caring for her dolls. To the primagravida, this conception feels like the culmination of all those years of waiting. At long last, she can now let go and give in to gratification so long withheld – being introduced to mysteries of procreation and complete implementation of fecund psychosexual powers curtailed since she began menstruating.

In glowing terms, she feels she is consummating her womanhood: she too can now join the long line of truly 'grown-up' women, becoming a link in the great chain of mothers since time immemorial. Trustingly, she submits herself to the psychological and physiological processes, allowing herself to drift on a sea of emotions as old as time and as new as conception. She experiences herself merging her own identity with countless generations of pregnant women, and the past becomes active in the present as simultaneously she finds herself living in the burgeoning impregnated body of a mother-to-be and imagines herself as an embryo identical to the one she is carrying, in a series of interchangeable fused identifications.

Cherishing her newly pregnant body, at times the Facilitator luxuriates in a state of inward contemplation retaining only minimal interest in the external world. It is as if she has to remove part of herself to make space for the mystery unfolding within her. Allowing her imagination free-range, even a Facilitator who has been pregnant before may encounter in herself the revival of strange irrational ideas about impregnation, regeneration and the content of her womb. In her unconscious fantasy fertilization might be associated with something unusual she ate or drank or even a vivid dream that she had. She plays with the idea of conception idealized as a miraculous event, seeming to have occurred on a special night in a special place or after a spectacular love-making. She might fondly imagine it as parthenogenesis, an 'immaculate conception' achieved all on her own without any help from her mate. Fancifully, she may treat the pregnancy as a fabricated figment of her imagination, playing with the idea that she is bearing not a baby but a sprite, or materializing the mirage of her own infant self or sprouting an internal penis from a 'semen-seed'. Above all, the Facilitator feels she possesses a secret – a wonderous change that makes her wonder-full. . . . Proverbially radiant, she basks in an internal glow of being greater than the sum of her usual self. ('Life is incredible – I feel as if I've never been truly alive before or as if giving my baby life makes me doubly alive.') Sentimentally, she feels so at one with her internal enclosure, so fused with the content of her womb, that she hails early physical symptoms as reminders of the reality of her invisible pregnancy. Indeed, symptoms serve as anchors to her fantasies – nausea and morning sickness lending poetic licence to ideas of oral insemination, replenishment of inner resources and proof that she still contains her unvomited treasure. As the weeks pass, her early experience of conception is further confirmed by external signs of her pregnancy – pigmentation of her nipples, enlargement of her breasts, gradual swelling of her belly – tangible signs which are welcomed at this amorphous time when nausea begins to vanish, yet the fetus cannot be experienced directly.

6.2.2 The Facilitator and her partner

Where a Facilitator has a like-minded partner, the couple retreat within the boundary of their womb-like support system, fearing that outsiders will interrupt the emotional flow between them or envy their creative intimacy. Previously welcomed engagements now feel like a hassle as the parents-to-be become increasingly home-based and localized, sharing feelings with each other rather than seeking stimulation in a wider network of friends. As she herself draws inwards, so she and her partner tuck their heads together, marvelling at their united creative cleverness, enjoying an intimacy of mutual fantasizing and futuristic story-telling. (Only rarely does a woman on her own become a Facilitator, since it is this sense of being enveloped by a caring Other that enables her to submit to the luxury of introspection as she does). Friends expect the couple to be as before, but the Facilitator finds that her priorities have changed and she feels entitled to change the 'guidelines' of her friendships. Eager to remain undefined she wants no expectations thrust upon her as she experiences this new and unknown happening. Not knowing what she will feel, she refuses to anticipate situations and hopes her partner will back her up and protect her from adverse surprises. During her pregnancy, the Facilitator craves the freedom to react spontaneously and make her own unique personal choices; she abhors predetermined situations. She wishes to remain receptive and fluid, to respond flexibly and intuitively in her own pregnant way, without being instructed or restricted, and often maintains secrecy about more 'sacred' feelings.

Trusting herself to her flooding emotions and suspending all critical decisions, the Facilitator feels fulfilled and enriched by early pregnancy. Each new discovery during this first phase fills her with excitement as she curiously anticipates the unfurling of her new pregnant self.

6.2.3 The Regulator in early pregnancy

The Regulator approaches pregnancy differently. To her it is a rather tedious means of having a baby. She dislikes the pressure for continuous reappraisal of her self and body images and resolves to preserve her 'ordinary persona' for as long as possible ('I just carry on as usual. Feel fine and could not have been pregnant at all for all the difference its made to my life – I've only given up horse riding because I'm worried about falling'). She requires external verification of conception, and treats the outcome as uncertain until symptoms confirm its continuity. Hoping to prolong her familiar identity and life style and to protect herself from disappointment if the pregnancy fails, she tells few people that she is expecting a baby. Indeed, as word gets around, she rails against people who approach her with stereotyped expectations of how pregnant women behave, and becomes angry at herself for lapsing into unaccustomed moodiness or if she finds herself wearing two odd shoes. The Regulator intends to hold out against regressive tugs and to avoid emotionality which she regards as self-indulgent 'mushiness'. Strengthening her defences against the emotional upheaval of pregnancy, she resists senti- mentality and foregoes fusion with her dormant fetus, who seems at times a parasitic intruder, draining her resources and disrupting her regular pursuits. Determined to regulate demands made upon her from within, she tries to remain vigilant and keep her feelings under strict control.

Nevertheless, at times she feels that her brain is 'switched onto automatic' and she is merely skimming the surface in her job or social life, fooling herself that she is continuing as normal when inside she feels 'threatened by a landslide' of primitive emotions. Although rigorously avoiding small talk, she often finds herself eavesdropping on 'baby-centred conversations' or is surprised to find herself a bystander in social situations or political discussions, less able to get heatedly involved and/or sensing the weight or flimsiness of opponents' pessimism and intellectualizations. Whereas once she would have been 'right in there' with the others, now she seems out of it all.

Unlike the Facilitator, to the Regulator introspection appears to be the ultimate laxity, negating out-going assertive qualities she has cultivated in herself. To her, embracing a new pregnant identity seems to imply devaluation of her previous unpregnant life style, as if it entails dis- mantling an earlier self in favour of the new. Disciplining herself not to give way to the pregnancy for fear of losing her self-pride and/or running the risk of rejection by becoming a 'floppy mess', she strives to remain unchanged, her own person rather than a 'pregnant lady'.

6.3 PHASE TWO

6.3.1 Who is in there?

As we have seen in the previous chapter, during this second phase, maturational tasks focus on discovering the fetus rather than adapting to the pregnancy as in phase one.

The control exerted by the Regulator during the first stage of pregnancy is undermined in the second stage by the quickening. The strange sensation of the fetus moving around inside her body like an alien force beyond her control makes her feel invaded by a wilful, unruly being. She is flabbergasted by the bizarre idea of two people inhabiting one body and resolves to try and maintain her own separateness. She might also resentfully withdraw into separateness from the prospective father who can so easily achieve parenthood without any of the discomforts and indignities that she is suffering. Making few concessions to her pregnant state, she may step up her occupational and social activities during this stage, feeling the need for a work-challenge or a 'fling' to confirm her competence or to reinforce her attractiveness as a 'person' rather than a 'pregnancy'.

Unlike the Facilitator, the Regulator does not engage in imaginary conversations with her fetus, and tries to avoid indulging in playful fantasies or superstitious behaviour. She makes an effort to maintain an inner reserve, refusing to endow the baby with a personality or to become fond of it 'in case things go wrong'. Rather, she fixes her aim on the future and attempts to prepare sensibly for all eventualities. She enjoys being productive, crossing anticipatory chores off her list. Disconcerted by the open-endedness of pregnancy, the uncertainty and feeling of being at the mercy of things, she safeguards herself by confiding her condition only to those who will respect her 'rules'.

However, with passing time, as she resents the fetus for uncovering unknown layers of herself so she resents her body, growing out of control and divulging her secret to the world. The Regulator continues wearing her regular clothes, eventually conceding to extra-large overalls or smocks and drapes rather than abdicating her sexuality in 'twee, cute or puritanical maternity clothes'.

Not so the Facilitator. Eager to announce her pregnancy both verbally and physically, she adopts maternity wear or clothes that emphasize her bulge very early on. In her newfound voluptuousness, she chooses sparkly satins and 'glitsy' fabrics, often banishing 'sensible' corduroys and denims for the duration of the pregnancy.

For the Facilitator, the initial fusion of the first phase is interrupted by thrilling internal flutters confronting her with the existence of a separate, energetic self-willed little creature. During this second stage she becomes involved in a process of differentiation from her baby, who, no longer fused and interchangeable with herself, now begins to become a person in his/her own right. She attributes characteristics, appetites, communicated likes and dislikes, approval and disapproval. She may have a secret nickname for the baby, or several names which she tries out in succession, elaborating fantasy interactions with all the possible babies she might have, 'practising' her own capacity to mother.

6.3.2 The baby's mother

During this time the pregnant woman begins to differentiate herself not only from her baby but also from her own mother: many old conflicts are reactivated by the emotional intensity and regressive pull of pregnancy. The mother-to-be recaptures in her mind's eye details of her childhood relationship with her mother, emotionally reliving many poignant, tender and painful moments. Unconsciously, she is engaged in the difficult task of re-evaluating her own experiences of being mothered, classifying what she wishes to emulate in her mother and reintegrate, as opposed to maternal aspects with which she cannot identify (although at times of stress she will be horrified to find herself behaving just like the mother she abhors). Gradually, she gives up the idea of changing her parents to suit a fantasy-ideal, granting herself the right to differ from them and particularly her mother, and giving them, the right to be grandparents in their own imperfect way.

However, some Facilitators, unable to modify the glorified image of a nursing mother–baby dyad, retain a dangerously idealized expectation of optimal mothering of a perfect infant. Conversely, many Regulators are still engaged in a process of maternal denigration and rebellious disidentification from their own (internal) mothers, with whom they feel unable to compete or are too ambivalent to try. These unresolved exaggerations, whether overrated idealization or distortedly devaluing depreciation, are pathological constituents which uncorrected each in their own way affect orientation towards future motherhood and produce unrealistic preconceptions that interfere in the relationship with the baby.

6.3.3 Interpersonal relationships

During the second phase, many Facilitators actively change their working patterns and life style, as they have earlier altered eating and rest habits. Within the couple, the mother-to-be finds ways of encouraging her husband's bonding with the fetus, sharing tactile experience of fetal movements, divulging her fantasies and embroidering others together with him. She feels privileged in that, although the fetus is half his, she is the one who is entitled to carry the baby. She can caress it at will, has direct access to the stirrings within and can communicate effortlessly through her own physiology. In her role as mediator, the prospective Facilitator mother facilitates communication between father and fetus. Feeling increasingly energetic and outgoing, she encourages her mate to engage once more in social activities, albeit selectively; relationships which once appeared central now recede as others become important, particularly those with other expectant couples, often met through childbirth classes. The focus is on a familiar, family-like circle of friends and relatives with whom they can share and compare discoveries about the fetus as well as pooling and culling information about birth and babycare facilities and equipment.

Conversely, the Regulator at this phase is usually still actively engaged with her old friends, work colleagues and social acquaintances. She has not yet modified her life style to accommodate the baby, and is often resentful of her male partner's symptom-free acquisition of parenthood and is scornful of facilitation type 'self-indulgence'. ('I've not allowed myself to change because I've seen a lot of women lose their identities and become boring cows. I think some women use pregnancy as an excuse to be cossetted and become dependent and lazy – it's just attention seeking and self-indulgence'). This second phase when many of the unpleasant symptoms have abated and she still looks 'presentable' is the period of her pregnancy that the Regulator enjoys most.

6.4 PHASE THREE

6.4.1 The Facilitator in late pregnancy

The third stage commences at a different chronological time for each individual woman, as she believes her baby would be viable outside her body if born prematurely. It is marked by the maturational task of achieving psychological transition from a focus on the fetus to preoccupation with the baby to come. Facilitators tend to reach this stage later than Regulators.

Although still attached to her imaginary baby, the Facilitator gradually becomes consumed with curiosity about her 'real' one and eagerly 'monitors' communications from within. She has mixed feelings about the approaching end of her pregnancy: while relishing the closeness and immediacy of contact with her baby, she mourns its foreseeable ending, feeling that never again will they be as intimate. At the same time she yearns for the 'reunion' with her baby, whom she feels she knows so well. However, she worries that the eagerly awaited birth might prove unsafe for the baby tucked away so snug inside her, who might even resent being 'ejected' from his nest. Nest feathering is, therefore, gradually transferred from her internal womb to the real world, where she goes about preparing a cosy replacement habitat and hoard of postnatal resources for her infant and herself. The Facilitator, and particularly one with other children, surrounds herself with an extended 'care-circle', rooting out a network of protective people on whom she can depend for help if needed, now or after the birth, who, however, will not invade the 'inner sanctum' she aims to occupy with the baby. The working Facilitator resents the weeks of pregnancy being whisked away from her before she can truly revel in them during maternity leave. (Often, the dilemma is whether to have her leave during pregnancy or by taking it as late as possible, store it all up to prolong her time with the baby after the birth.) She aches to be at home rather than in the office, yearning to focus solely on the fetus instead of having it 'accompany' her to work. She craves space and uncluttered time by herself in which to consolidate her relationship with the unborn baby.

In the gathering excitement about the forthcoming birth, the Facilitator tries to secure her priorities: she is determined that the birth shall be spontaneous. She wishes to have as 'natural' a birth as possible and if booked into hospital is anxious that it may become overmanaged by rules and extraneous decisions not guided by the baby's movements and the sensations of her own body. Above all, whether hospital or home birth, it is deeply important to her that the twosome (or threesome) remain intact, intimate and unseparated during this very special reunion which she fears might be spoilt by unsympathetic professionals.

6.4.2 The Regulator: late pregnancy and birth plans

The Regulator finds the third stage a difficult one. She herself is larger and the bump heavier and more cumbersome. Physically she reminds herself of an unflattering 'spindly-legged ostrich' or a 'stranded beetle' unable to roll over. She craves the day when she will see her feet again, and despairs of ever returning to her pre-pregnant figure. If still working, she fears that her standard of achievement is being affected by tiredness, tension and increasingly vigorous fetal activity. Impatient for pregnancy to be over, she feels 'raw, scraped, bruised and battered' by an internal persecutor and externally hampered by ungainliness. Feeling like a detached outsider, no longer part of her usual world yet not a member of any other, she is determined to keep the interruption to her 'real life' as brief as possible. She delays giving up her job, fearing boredom at home and lack of the structure now provided by her work time table.

The Regulator, too, is worried about the birth, albeit her anxieties differ from those of the Facilitator. To her, labour represents a situation of loss of control, when she will be at the mercy of her painfully contracting uterus. Unable to foretell how she will cope with the pain, labour appears like an imposed barrier behind which she will be alone and isolated from everyone. The Regulator is afraid that under the powerful impact of prolonged pain she will be deprived of all her defences, left denuded and vulnerable, skinless and exposed 'like a snail without its shell'. She is concerned about making a fool of herself in front of strangers and fears that she may disclose closely guarded secrets and hidden aspects of herself. Labour and birth thus assume the character of a test situation, like an exam at school, for which she feels inadequately prepared. She mistrusts her body to remember what to do, afraid she will forget her breathing exercises – and fail the 'exam'. On a deeper level she fears she might damage the baby during labour or birth or be damaged herself internally as a result of it. She tries to make provisional plans, thinking around every conceivable option that may arise, involving her in a great deal of study and investigation. Losing her grip, she sometimes feels panic-stricken at the thought of the birth like a trial getting nearer. She resolves to maintain maximum control over pain and with the help of the experts to have as brief and 'civilized' a labour as drug relief and medical technology can afford her ('I have a very low pain threshold and don't like physical pain. Basically, I put it in the hands of the hospital – they'll tell me what to do – I feel very trusting of that hospital – I'll stay in a week or more if possible, but I am terrified – I've never been the sort of person who looks into prams – I think, God will it die on me? will it stop breathing? will I do the right thing?').

Beset by a terrible sense of urgency about time running out on her, the primagravida Regulator feels she must make the most of her child-free state. Having bought baby clothes and equipment, she becomes more aware both of the reality of the baby ('in a few weeks a little body will fill these tiny vests') and of trials of motherhood which await her. At home on maternity leave, the Regulator has forebodings of her future as a 'stateless non-person', fearing she will become an overlooked maternal 'blob' trapped with a repulsive infant or even 'captivated' by its power. She is concerned that the nurses in hospital will observe her inexperienced 'cackhandedness' with the infant; is terrified of the bizarre implications of a baby feeding at her breasts, sucking out her own bodily fluids. She has a horror of finding out too late that she has made a serious mistake, that parenthood will ruin her relationship with her partner, that the 'unreturnable' baby will turn out to be a monster, that she was not cut out to be a mother at all. . . .

Outside a discussion group for pregnant women, the Regulator finds few listeners for these worries. When voiced to friends, her ambivalent or hostile feelings often cannot be accepted and these embarrassing 'cracks' are papered over with facile promises of 'you'll see, it'll be alright on the day' or romantic observations about irresistible cuddlesome babies. Even other pregnant acquaintances shy away as if fearful of contamination by anxieties they themselves have held at bay. All this contributes towards confirming her view of herself as repugnant, unmotherly and only acceptable as a 'sparkling wit' or 'positive thinker' since others appear unable to tolerate her negative side. This idea makes her even angrier with the baby who threatens to undermine her familiar life style and identity so drastically. In a desperate defensive manoeuvre, the Regulator may spend the end of the last stage of pregnancy in a state of detachment, protecting herself from awareness of her anxieties. Irritated at the uncertainty of not knowing how long she has to go, she decides to use the remaining weeks for her own pleasure ('eat, drink and be merry') and resolves to treat this confinement merely as a temporary interruption before returning to ordinary life.

To conclude this section, once again a reminder that although many women fit into these categories of Facilitator and Regulator, many others belong to a third group of Reciprocators. In some ways, these women who can tolerate their naturally ambivalent feelings towards the pregnancy, the fetus, themselves and their own mothers, have a healthier and more realistic approach than either the idealized version of unadulterated joy of pure Facilitators or the wary one of Regulators. A fourth rather rarer category has emerged out of longitudinal research: 'bipolar' responses from conflicted individuals who waver between the two extremes, and may benefit from psychotherapeutic help to resolve their painful confusion. In terms of management, awareness of the need for different provisions is the main value of this model, by making sense of the confusing and seemingly contradictory demands clients make on professionals during pregnancy labour, birth and early motherhood.

6.4.3 The Reciprocator

During early pregnancy, the Reciprocator both focuses with interest on the changes occurring within and is aware that if it survives, the pregnancy and child-to-be will bring about many changes in her relationships and life style. She accommodates to living with the state of uncertainty and tries to maintain a balance between her growing need for introspective absorption and her heightened awareness of the positive and negative external world conditions in which she antici- pates bringing up her baby. During the second trimester she feels the need to consolidate her work position before relinquishing it in early motherhood, and is equally cognisant of the new demands parenting will pose and tries to envisage these. If she already has other children, she is intensely aware of the effect a new baby will have on their relationship, and feels the need to prepare her family for the changes to come, and conversely, to make space for the baby. She sees the fetus as already possessing characteristics of its own and feels curious to meet him or her.

This feeling intensifies during the third trimester and although somewhat reluctant to give up the special intimacy of pregnancy, she is equally eager to rid herself of the discomfort of the last months, looking forward to the birth with excitement tempered by trepidation. As for birth plans, she is knowledgeable about the different options but feels she will have to wait and see what the labour brings.

Although very aware during pregnancy of the sexed differences between them, male partners too may be Reciprocators in their mature ability to tolerate both mixed feelings and uncertainty of outcome. The hallmark of this orientation seems to be an ability to contain healthy ambivalence and to maintain a sense of continuity and simultaneity of different age experiences of oneself. These help the parent empathize with the baby they once were while bearing in mind their adult capacities.

Table 6.1 Emotional experiences during the three maturational phases of pregnancy:

Pregnancy	Facilitators	Regulators	Reciprocators
Phase I	**'fusion'**	**control**	**ambivalence**
Personal	blooming	depleted	changed
identity	enhanced	threatened	added dimension
Phase II	**Communion**	**Separateness**	**Differentiation**
Adaptation	surrender	resistance	Mixed experience
Achievement	communion	self-discipline	tolerance of uncertainty
fetus seen as:	benign	'parasitic'	a new being
Phase III	**Relinquishment**	**Detachment**	**Preparation**
Ideal Birth	'natural'	'civilized'	'wait-and-see'
Labour	exciting	a painful event	a mutual transition

KEY POINTS

* The model presented delineates different orientations towards pregnancy and childbirth – the Facilitator who relishes pregnancy and willingly gives in to its emotional demands; the Regulator who resists introspection and identity change; the Reciprocator who has mixed feelings.
* Psychological reactions are means of dealing with unconscious representations of the fetus as an idealized part of the Facilitator; a dangerous invader or repudiated part of the Regulator or a separate human being in the case of the Reciprocator.
* Birthplans reflect the Facilitator's desire for a 'perfect' birth minimizing intervention during the transition between the womb and extra-uterine 'nest'. Anxieties about damage she and/or the baby might inflict on the other during labour lead the Regulator to utilize medical assistance. While the Reciprocator, aware that complications may occur, wishes for a relaxed birth yet is prepared for the unexpected.
* Researchers may do well to delineate these different orientations as their contrasting responses may otherwise be swamped.

Questionnaires for use in each of the trimesters and one to tap fetal representations are available from the author.

Chapter 7

Psychotherapy during pregnancy

7.1 MENTAL HEALTH AND PREGNANCY

As I have stated elsewhere [1] in a society such as ours, where resources are becoming scarce, our mental health priorities should be:

1. Early detection of high risk groups;
2. Preventive measures, thereby reducing the cost of treating established conditions.

Pregnancy presents an ideal opportunity to meet both these requirements: widespread attendance at antenatal clinics and ongoing personalized contact with childbirth educators offer possibilities for early screening and where necessary, referral for psychotherapeutic intervention preceding postnatal distress and/or pathological mother–baby interaction.

The following formulations have been derived over the past 15 years, from a specialized clinical practice of psychoanalytic psychotherapy for female procreational problems, related to reproductivity, with a clientelle both self-selected and referred by professionals, seen individually, as cohabiting couples or in groups, 1–5 times a week, during their pregnancy and early motherhood. Psychotherapy aims to explore deep-seated irrational emotions and help resolve internal conflicts and archaic formulations which interfere with everyday life and prevent the individual from achieving new maturational growth. In my experience, pregnancy is a prime time for psychotherapy. The woman's motivation for accepting help during pregnancy differs in that not only is therapy sought to alleviate suffering and relieve the pressure of persistent symptoms, but it rides on a tide of emotional resurgence which both reawakens forgotten feelings and strives for reappraisal of identity.

Physical changes are more rapid in pregnancy than at any other time in adult life, engendering an emotional flashback to pubertal ferment. As well as the many strange bodily experiences it involves during pregnancy psychological boundaries between conscious thought and hitherto unconscious fantasies, become more permeable resulting in accessibility of buried emotions, earlier modes of symbolic thinking and irrational ideas. Heightened sensory experiences and vivid dreams, with often explicit symbolism and disturbingly undisguised content, further undermine familiar psychic equilibrium. In the absence of knowledge, the pregnant womb serves as a receptacle for projections and fantasies about the fetus which must give way to a relationship with a real baby. Previous vulnerability, deprivation and deficiencies are exacerbated and exposed. Paradoxically, at the very time of discovering she literally has two people inside her skin, the western mother-to-be is also often isolated and alone with her uncommunicated bizarre experiences. In addition to an urgent need for personal expression, stabilization and redefinition, some nulliparous women are acutely aware of the psychic growth which must be achieved to complete the trajectory from being a daughter to their own mothers to becoming a mother to a baby, while pregnant mothers may need help with the intrapsychic and interpersonal emotional changes a new baby will entail.

In short, the pregnant woman undergoes profound psychological and physical upheavals condensed into a relatively short period of time, which may necessitate some external therapeutic intervention to prevent her becoming overwhelmed. While brief psychotherapy during pregnancy offers a form of crisis-intervention, long-lasting changes can occur as a result of a greater capacity for tolerating uncertainty acquired during therapy; ameliorated prenatal bonding with the fetus; ongoing 'increments' resulting from retrieval during therapy of a greater array of positive moments and figures in the internal world as well as expression of repressed negative feelings; repeated affirmation of self-growth in adult competence, positive labour experiences and consolidation through constructive interaction with the baby. Further postnatal treatment is often indicated. Special features of psychotherapy with pregnant women will be elaborated at the end of this chapter.

7.2 INDICATORS OF INCREASED PSYCHO-SOCIO-ECONOMIC STRESS

Most pregnancies entail some degree of personal stress. Widespread disturbances have been found in normal antenatal clinic populations. Anxiety, increased introversion [2], depression [3], worry, mood lability, insomnia, impaired concentration [4], magical thinking, regressive shifts and increased dependency [5], altered spatial orientation and mild nominal aphasia have long been observed. A recent study has found 35% of women attending their first antenatal clinic in South London had high (negative) scores on the GHQ (General Health Questionnaire) while 29% were diagnosed as psychiatric 'cases', largely neurotic depression [6]. Both in this study and others, factors such as housing and financial difficulties, unemployment, poor social support and a poor marital relationship are likely to be associated with caseness [7–9]. However, there are various other psychosocial circumstances which increase the emotional strain during pregnancy, thus constituting potential stressors triggering hidden areas of vulnerability in women who are apparently psychologically or medically healthy. These indicators are usually obtainable during a careful history-taking. Women may themselves request referral for psycho-therapeutic treatment or signs of distress might be observed by a perceptive health care professional during antenatal encounters.

7.3 CONFLICTED PREGNANCIES

This is a mixed category which can be broken down into 'Untimely', 'Unplanned', and 'Wrong' pregnancies.

a. An **untimely pregnancy** may be one where the mother is too young – adolescent girls torn between the wish to have a baby of her very own to love and the excitement of teenage sub-culture, or one feels herself to be emotionally too immature whatever her age. The pregnant body may have been used as a false means of resolving problems of feminine identity or to establish a differentiated sexual identity separate from her mother's, rather than representing a mature desire for a baby. A crisis may occur due to the superimposition of the emotional upheaval of pregnancy on the maturational turmoil of individuation during adolescence and early adulthood.

Conversely, a woman may feel too old – a mature woman who feels herself transgressing the generation gap with her own grown up children, who possibly have had babies themselves, or a 'last chance' conception in an 'elderly primagravida' (post-35) ambivalently torn between the dictates of the biological clock and her career (in a largely male world). The increased probability of birth defects and additional anxieties about physically coping with the stress of pregnancy and strain of infantile demands, broken nights and loss of high-powered identity, feature in later pregnancies, as do concern about possible emotional 'overload' and straddling the conflicting demands of the new baby, older children, her own, and elderly parents' needs.

A pregnancy might be too early within a relationship or emotionally too soon – a 'replacement baby' following an insufficiently mourned stillbirth or neonatal death [10], or else too late – a conflicted me following a guilt ridden recent abortion or an unresolved one of many years earlier.

b. An **unplanned pregnancy** foists new adjustments on the surprised parent/s-to-be. Although abortions comprised two-fifths of conceptions, fully one quarter of all births in 1984 were unintended pregnancies [11]. For a woman on her own it demands rethinking her single identity and whether she wishes to incorporate another unknown being into her life for the next two decades. Unplanned pregnancy may involve moral and emotional dilemmas, very real economic sacrifices and interference with career structure and work plans; it inevitably necessitates changes in life style. Unplanned conception may force a crisis in a fragile relationship, splitting a couple or bringing them closer. In a well-established marriage it may suddenly reveal bitter marital discord about whether to abort or start a family.

Needless to say, the fact of an ongoing pregnancy does not imply acceptance. It could mean any one or more of many things: it may represent the woman's breakaway or her rebellious overriding of her man's wish for an abortion or else could mean her resentful compliance with his wish for a baby or represent 'the lesser evil', a compromise solution to a no-win situation or be the result of their mutual indecisive procrastination or begrudging resignation to Fate. All these possibilities suggest open or covert antagonism between the partners and their future offspring, which augurs deteriorating emotional interplay among them unless harmonious communication can be restored. Resolution of such marital differences will affect not only the experience of this pregnancy for the woman, but is likely to determine the emotional quality of the child's future life. Couple therapy is often indicated.

For the western woman, coming to terms with an unexpected conception, above all means initially deciding whether to continue or abort her pregnancy. However, women who do not use their new-found prerogative of choice, constitute a particularly vulnerable group. Often, the pregnancy continues because of lack of conscious decision – or despite one. A woman may not be able to contemplate abortion for religious, ethical or health reasons. She may spend her pregnancy hoping that she will miscarry and not have to be judge and jury in doling out a life or death sentence to her unwanted baby. She may feel unable to face her partner's moral disagreement or parental disapproval and proceed to conceal the pregnancy for too long. More worrying are the cases who refuse consciously to acknowledge the pregnancy to themselves, and continue their lives seemingly oblivious to their own signs and symptoms, denying that a baby is expected. Since these women rarely attend antenatal clinics, they seldom come to the attention of professionals unless underage or under close scrutiny of people who care enough to get them to seek psychiatric or obstetric help. When these women lack a mate, unless emotional ownership of the pregnancy is accepted before the birth (either with a view to keeping the baby or relinquishing it for adoption), possible placement of the baby with a relative, temporary fostering or contested adoption must be considered as a postnatal alternative to the biological mother's care (Chapter 28). The woman herself needs psychotherapeutic intervention, if she will have it, and social work attention if not.

c. **'Wrong' pregnancies** could convey several meanings

(a) *Wrong mother*: the woman or her partner lack confidence in her ability to mother a baby, now or at all (see neurotic difficulties and historical sensitization below).

(b) *Wrong father*: tragic conception as a result of rape or incest raise particular problems (see below). However, in common with other 'wrong' impregnators like an unloved partner, an irresponsible man or 'substitute' for someone else, all of these mean that the woman feels she has growing inside her part of a hateful or distasteful Other. Unless this feeling can be resolved, the fetus who takes on these characteristic, is liable to remain an internal foreigner, barely tolerated or in constant danger of expulsion, and the baby will emerge part-stranger likely to be ostracized or punished.

(c) *Wrong baby*: this is an extension of these feelings, but might also be specifically related to the baby him/herself. A pregnant lesbian or rape victim might find the idea of carrying a male fetus within her repugnant and be determined to have an abortion should amniocentesis reveal a boy. A woman or couple eagerly awaiting a boy might be saddened to discover she's carrying a female fetus, or vice versa. More complex still, test results revealing a possibly abnormal baby, necessitate the agonizing decision of whether to keep this potentially 'wrong' baby or to abort it (see Chapter 29). Clearly, where these subjective emotions interfere with the ongoing prenatal 'bonding' process or if decisions must be taken, urgent psychotherapeutic intervention is indicated.

7.4 OVERVALUED PREGNANCIES

These include long-awaited conception following prolonged efforts to conceive; pregnancy following pseudocyesis; habitual miscarriages; ectopic pregnancy; previous still-birth, perinatal death or birth of a baby with congenital abnormalities. The hallmark of overvalued pregnancies is a heightened emotional investment in the process which takes on the quality of a Supreme Court trial. The woman feels that her ability to produce a live healthy 'special' baby is being tested from moment to moment, and the verdict will determine whether life-giving forces can triumph over destructive ones. A syndrome develops of oscillation between hope and distrust, elation and detachment, idealization and nihilism. Many such women experience the need to 'monitor' the pregnancy continuously as if their vigil keeps the baby in existence and even a fleeting loss of concentration will result in it vanishing. Untreated, these women become the disappointed mothers of ordinary babies who cannot possibly fulfil the grandiose expectations as maternal life-savers, or overanxious mothers who distrust the baby's ability to breathe through the night. For these women, unassisted waiting is intolerable and they will often present with hyperchondriacal anxieties which are a cry for psychological help.

7.5 MEDICALLY ASSISTED CONCEPTION

7.5.1 Artificial insemination with partner's sperm (AIH)

In some cases, conception following AIH due to male subfertility rather than female problems, can be accompanied by a residue of resentment that such medical intervention was necessary. The woman might irrationally feel slighted – as if she was not sufficiently 'attractive' for her partner to impregnate her without help. She may unconsciously feel derision towards her partner who was 'not man enough' or 'needed permission' and an intermediary in the person of the doctor to make contact with her ovum. He too, may feel unmanned by this operation and lacks the confident virility of his impregnating counterparts. Both or either might unconsciously attribute fatherhood to the doctor or regard the resultant embryo as less perfect than one originating in a night of passion. Marital disharmony and lowered self-esteem may necessitate counselling.

7.5.2 Gamete intra fallopian transfer (GIFT)

A GIFT pregnancy, where eggs and sperm are mixed and immediately replaced in the woman's fallopian tube, may arouse similar feelings, plus a sense of her vagina as destructive or his sperm too vulnerable to be viable without the doctor to 'neutralize' and help them by-pass their mucosoid and emotional incompatibilities. Nevertheless, relief at conception having finally terminated the period of unexplained infertility, usually overrides these initial preoccupations. When born, these babies are often still referred to as 'gifts', reflecting parental gratitude for this 'miracle' as well as the underlying sense of not having quite done it all themselves.

7.5.3 Artificial insemination by donor sperm (AID)

A pregnancy following AID may be accompanied by similar feelings to AIH with the added anxiety about genetic inheritance. Natural curiousity about the biological father's looks and characteristics may escalate into full worry anxiety or romantic fantasies about who the baby's father really is. (Some private sperm banks offer customers a (non-identifying) 'curriculum vitae' type profile of donors, including extended family background, personal shortcomings ('slight chin tick') and achievements.) These days AID may be accompanied by the dread of contracting the disease AIDS (both a phonetic association and a realistic one based on prevalence of the virus among homosexuals who were frequent sperm-donors). Such urgent fears may persist despite assurances of careful screening and semen-examination. A common initial experience among recipients of donor sperm, is the feeling of a foreign body embedded within her that is alien or 'adulterous' and makes her embryo feel unlovable. If she is in a relationship with a male partner, social secrecy about the means of conception may add to her burden. Unconscious resentment at his infertility, concern about whether her man and his parents could love a genetically unrelated baby and regret about his inability to share her biological predicament even vicariously, add to the complex emotions ordinarily associated with pregnancy. Further apprehension may focus on the future – whether or when to tell the child about his/her origins, whether the sperm register will be available to provide semen from the same donor next time to ensure that siblings may be full brothers and sisters; whether information about his/her genetic origins might be available in the future to allay the child's anxieties and prevent the most unlikely but still worrying possibility of an accidental incestuous relationship with a halfsib. The male partner, too, may require help to come to terms with his sense of failure and the issues of identity and attachment such impregnation arouses.

If the pregnant woman has a female partner, in addition to the above there may be uneasiness about the lesbian-mate's potential envy of her pregnant state and jealousy of her direct genetic relatedness to their baby as well as potential competitiveness for role of mother. Although many of these issues may have been tackled during the course of a mutual decision to pursue artificial insemination, nevertheless, during pregnancy, these feelings, like many others, are reactivated by the new situation and often require further working through, individually, in a special women's group or in couple-therapy.

7.5.4 *In vitro* fertilization (IVF)

IVF too, arouses many of the misgivings mentioned above and poses additional ethical issues, i.e. concern not only about the embryo(s) residing within her, but those fertilized eggs which have not been replaced. To some women, these eggs left in the laboratory, have the status of unborn babies whom she has abandoned to their fate [12]. There are women, to whom the risk of multiple pregnancy vies with trepidation about the implanted eggs not surviving. In some cases a pregnant woman might even have the additional embryos selectively aborted (a recent method injects the relevant cord of a particular fetus directly). While resolving the multiple birth problem, such intervention may give rise to subsequent worries about the physical and psychological effect of such a procedure on the remaining fetus [13]. The psychological traumata of prolonged infertility [14,15], consequent self-doubts and concern about the normality of a baby born of extra-uterine fertilization do not vanish with pregnancy and often persist for years after the birth.

4.5.5 Surrogacy

Although still relatively rare in Great Britain, surrogacy is a growing phenomena in the United States, and support groups for ex-surrogates suggest that feelings of grief, betrayal and guilt may be similar to those of women who have relinquished a baby to adoption, while the pregnancy is often fraught with additional stress of public curiosity and lack of support for the woman who has planned relinquishment prior to conception [16]. Furthermore, the act of surrogacy itself may constitute acting out of a neurotic disturbance which could benefit from therapy.

In all assisted conceptions, the ordinary course of pregnancy has begun differently, frequently following a period of prolonged emotional distress. Cases in which the woman appears overly anxious or when there is a fraught period of waiting to see whether the pregnancy will continue deserve special professional attention and offers of supportive help.

7.6 VICTIMS OF INCEST AND/OR RAPE

7.6.1 Incestuous pregnancy

Incestuous pregnancy is psychologically complex on many levels. Apart from the concerns about the baby's normality and family future, the woman herself is liable to have a mixture of feelings about her impregnator, and hence, the baby. Much depends on the degree of her own emotional engagement in the relationship. Many incestuous pregnancies are the result of an ongoing relationship with father or older brother that was foisted on the woman in her girlhood. She will have grown up with a sense of violation of sexual-security within the family and no entitlement to her own privacy and body ownership. Intimidation may have been used as a form of control and secrecy maintained under threats of expulsion or even murder. As incest victims testify, even when coerced into the intimate situation feelings of self-blame, internalized badness and humiliation are almost inevitable in an incestuous situation which she feels to be morally wrong even if she was coerced into it [17].

If her own father or step-father is involved, she will feel guilty towards the mother whose place she has usurped as well as a mixture of outrage, confusion and pain that her mother had not prevented this contact or even tacitly complied with its continuation. Pregnancy, in which she is harbouring her own sister or brother within her womb, brings about a further confusion of identity between her mother and the mother she is about to become. In brother–sister incest too, the real mother's failure to intervene will be held against her and affect the pregnant woman's relationship to her own 'internal mother' who has betrayed her, who is felt to be taking her revenge by inflicting this baby on her or by threatening to snatch it away. Maternal estrangement has been commonly reported in incest victims' families including maternal mental or physical dysfunction, or alcoholism: Mothers are also often victims of their husbands' abuse [18]. Transgression of generation boundaries, particularly with a child, not only involves violation, but constitutes a disillusionment – loss of trust in a father figure, loss of belief in unconditional parental love and protection, loss of the right to childhood innocence and a desperate yearning for a loving, forgiving, comforting mother who can never now be found. Pregnancy resulting from such a contact often forms a disclosure to the world of the secret incestuous relationship, possible imprisonment of the erring male, breakup of the family or ostracization of the now 'blackened' woman. She thus may not only be out on her own, emotionally and economically unsupported but also burdened by social stigma and rejection. Supportive health care is essential (Chapter 33).

Past victims of an incestuous assault or ongoing relationship, are also vulnerable during pregnancy even if conception occurred many years later. The fetus may be experienced as invasive, intruding into the one private place inside her which has been kept 'sacred' untouched by sexual violation. Conversely, she may have the fantasy that the fetus, being inside her, will discover her guilty secret or else will be badly affected by what she experiences as her 'polluted inner rottenness'. She may also feel that the incest had 'killed off all that was creative' inside her leaving nothing for this baby to feed off.

7.6.2 Rape

Rape victims who have become pregnant as a result and decided not to abort, have the most difficult task of differentiating between the baby and the experience of which he/she will forever be a reminder. This pertains not only to victims of rape by strangers but by husband, boyfriend, father or acquaintance. Women who have conceived by another man, years after the original violent incident, are also vulnerable during pregnancy to emotional revival of the sense of invasion as the fetus begins to move within them, a tangible male remnant now become an internal masculine presence. Research has shown that for many years after rape, victims are known to suffer from sexual difficulties even in a loving situation [19].

Inevitably, physical anxieties concerning internal examinations and genital damage during birth, especially episiotomies, may arise. Rape is not, as often regarded, a coerced form of intercourse. It is a violent and violating act which sometimes leaves the victim physically battered with her vagina torn and mutilated as well as emotionally battered, irrationally blaming herself for not escaping from an inescapable situation [20]. Being genitally manhandled during pregnancy and labour is very frightening to a rape-victim who is unlikely to make her plight known to obstetric staff. If a woman requests to be seen by a female doctor or is very anxious and tense during attempted examinations her reticence must be respected. Furthermore, a rape victim may still be harbouring her 'shameful' secret and fear that it will be revealed to professionals seeing her genitalia. Discretion and sensitivity are of utmost importance when rape is suspected. Finally, women who have lived with their own self-recriminations for not having successfully physically resisted their known or unknown rapist may feel further victimized by allowing medical intervention during birth. Birth itself may reactivate repressed memories of genital abuse, the effects of which can colour the woman's relationship to her baby, particularly if male (Chapter 33).

Clearly, the situation is one that requires great tact since unreported rape, like incest, is still surrounded by shame and secrecy. Calculations from classic survey data put probability of becoming a victim of rape or attempted rape in the USA at 46 women in any 100 [21]. All figures estimate that rape and interfamilial sexual abuse is much more common than official police reports suggest and possibly on the increase. Longitudinal follow-up studies of post-rape reactions reveal a 'rape trauma syndrome' [22] and long-term emotional and sexual sequelae many of which can be expected to be reactivated during obstetric procedures in women who do not necessarily confide their experience to attending staff.

7.8 HISTORICAL OBSTETRIC SENSITIZATION

Another particularly sensitive group are women with a history of unresolved abortions or miscarriages, obstetric pathology or morbidity, or primagravidae in whose immediate family things have gone wrong during pregnancy or delivery. Such women find it difficult to believe that they will be 'allowed' to have a new creative experience and often harbour irrational guilt and fear of retaliative predicaments. These include not only women who have themselves had miscarriages and still-births, but those with a history of obstetric tragedies in their families of origin or among close relatives, including sibling perinatal deaths or congenital abnormalities. These traumatic events may leave deep psychic 'scars' in a child's mind, sustaining guilt about childhood rivalries and severely inhibiting healthy aggression. The reality of obstetric problems in her immediate family also exacerbates the pregnant woman's common anxieties about the normality and viability of her own baby. Furthermore, a woman whose mother has died giving birth to her is particularly vulnerable. Not only does she carry deep guilt for having directly or inadvertently been the cause of her mother's death and the unconscious conviction of inevitable punishment by a similar fate, but she is acutely aware of what it means to be a motherless child. She may find it difficult to identify too closely with her doomed mother, fears she lacks the necessary experiential motherliness to tend her own baby while dreading what lies in store for her child should she herself die. To some degree, the latter is also true of women whose mothers died in childbirth of a subsequent sibling. In general, women who have lost their mothers during childhood have been found to be particularly vulnerable to depression in adulthood [23] and often lack access to many of the maternal resources mothered girls take for granted. When maternal loss occurs before adolescence, the young woman may have been deprived of the gradual experience of bodily similarity, mother–daughter exchange of feminine love and womanly interchangeability with her mother or a maternal substitute. Likewise, the daughter of a father who died within the period of her gestation or close on her birth will invariably be worried about a recurrence in her own partnership, partly as 'revenge' for having imagined she could 'get away with' having a family when her own mother didn't. Finally, a woman who was herself an adopted child, may find it hard to believe she will be allowed to keep her baby where her own 'birth-mother' was not. Difficulties also arise during pregnancy as she finds herself torn between identifying with the biological mother who rejected her, or the mother who kept her but was incapable of producing a child. Pregnancy may serve as a trigger to the adopted woman or her adopted spouse to initiate a search for the lost biological mother (see Chapter 28).

7.9 WOMEN ALONE

Between 1976 and 1986 the number of births outside marriage in the UK rose steeply from 9% to 21% (and almost 50% in Sweden and Denmark) [24]. In 1987, the proportion reached 23% in Great Britain, although approximately half of these were jointly registered by both mother and father residing at the same address. Similarly, the divorce rate has risen substantially, and rate of remarriage has fallen steadily for women [25], with UK holding the highest divorce rate in Europe in 1986. Hence, single and divorced mothers comprise 73% of all lone mothers in 1987 [26].

A single woman can no longer be ostracized on the grounds that she has 'fallen' pregnant since it is probable that she has consciously chosen to conceive or at least not to interrupt the pregnancy. Nevertheless, in a maternity world still geared to happy coupledom, when 'Ms X' is discovered to have no husband or stable partner the old stigma still emerges. In antenatal clinics and childbirth preparation class she is readily identified as 'the one without a man'. Invariably, she arouses curiosity. In some, she evokes pitying fantasies that she might be the casualty of a broken love affair, duped by a one night stand, a rape victim or widowed. Harsher critics imagine her finally paying the debt for her loose morals, or losing her gamble to use pregnancy to 'keep' a slippery man (who, nevertheless, slipped away) or naively finding herself 'with child' while the erring man got off scot free. Others might give her the credit of wanting the baby for itself, having chosen to become pregnant by a carefully selected 'genetic donor' or by artificial insemination, but this idea tends to provoke other negative reactions towards the woman who so 'cold-bloodedly' planned and executed her plan. Whatever the reality of her situation and motivations for conception, the point is that because she is on her own when many other women have a partner she tends to be regarded as 'different' and suspect; at best ignored, at worst treated in a manner which reflects the prejudiced assumptions and projected fantasies of her beholders. And if pregnancy and motherhood can be stressful in a cosy twosome, it is certainly taxing to meet the extra demands of single parenthood without adequate emotional, practical and financial support. Where these are lacking in the woman's close environment, a 'hierarchy of caring' which provides mothering for her so she has the resources to provide for her baby, may be implemented by counselling, social work or antenatal introduction to a local support-group network.

Women who find themselves alone following death, divorce or abandonment by the partner are particularly vulnerable, as in addition to the pregnancy they are coping with a highly distressing emotionally charged and, at times, unforeseen life-event (section 7.11). Unlike the single woman who has elected to become pregnant, these women are about to become single-mothers having neither chosen this status for themselves nor a fatherless state for the child. It is this lack of control over her own destiny and the unplanned dissolution of the couple at the very time when it was about to expand into a family, that a woman in this predicament finds so distressing. Furthermore, the inevitable emotions of grief, anger, fear, guilt, resentment, sadness and fragility conflict with the anticipation of a tranquil pregnancy and happy outcome. Unless such mixed feelings can be disentangled before the birth, the child may bear the brunt of unresolved 'baggage' which is not of his/her making – sometimes carrying into adulthood an irrational sense of having prenatally caused mother's unhappiness by 'killing off' or 'chasing away' the father, or by being so unlovable, that he couldn't bear to stay around to see his child born.

7.10 UNSUPPORTED WOMEN

The fact that a woman does have a partner, need not imply that she is supported. A husband may be present in the flesh but emotionally absent or, worse, abusive. It therefore may be equally invalid to assume that unlike 'Miss Z', 'Mrs Y' is getting what she needs from Mr Y even if he does accompany her to classes or clinics. He may be there not as a prop but to keep his untrusting eye on her. For all we know he may be pathologically jealous of her contact with male doctors, or envious of her capacity to carry a pregnancy, or distrustful of her ability to grow a healthy fetus or give birth 'properly' to his baby or he may be childishly worried about her attention being diverted away from himself. He may be seeking staff approval during ultrasound tests or antenatal examinations, or flaunting his virility ('isn't the baby large!'), or checking up on her 'credentials' as a baby-container ('should she be running so much?') or most likely, effectively preventing her from disclosing anything adverse about their relationship. Clearly, just because a husband exists does not mean he is a help and might mean he's a hindrance or an actual menace. This also applies to non-English-speaking women whose husbands are often used as interpreters by antenatal professionals.

Allowing each pregnant woman time on her own to talk about her feelings with a sympathetic counsellor or psychotherapist can allay unnecessary fears in women with adequate emotional support (and help them make the most of their existing resources) while also identifying women whose resources are insufficient. Offering the latter, group or individual support during pregnancy, or marital therapy where applicable, may help forestall postnatal maternal depression which has been found to be associated with poor marital communication [27] and possibly prevent future costly intervention. Furthermore, for many years I have been arguing that antenatal clinic waiting rooms are obvious spaces for educational programmes and videos as well as supportive discussion groups for all pregnant women either facilitated by a professional group leader, or self-help.

7.11 CONCURRENT LIFE EVENTS

Life events, such as moving house and changing jobs, cause some anxiety and confusion in everybody's lives. When occurring alongside the emotional upheaval of pregnancy, they increase the sense of disorientation and interrupt the psychological work of pregnancy by presenting intrusive or, at times, conflicting demands for readjustment. Thus, if for us all, on an unconscious level, refurnishing or renovating a house represents some degree of reparation of the maternal body, during pregnancy these emotional pressures in addition to the practical ones, may prove too great for a woman preoccupied with her own intrapsychic reparations and bodily creativity. Life events during pregnancy have been implicated in serious postnatal depression [28].

Painfully distressing and/or unexpected tragic events such as bereavement, eviction or dismissal, as well as pregnancy-related events such as negative results of fetal diagnostic tests, threatened miscarriage or death of a twin *in utero*, intrude into the natural emotional processes of pregnancy, invoking feelings of anxiety, grief, rejection, emptiness, limbo and loss at a time when the woman is psychically and physically geared to receptivity, incorporation hopefulness and fulfilment. It is not surprising that a pregnant woman might feel defeated by the critical overload of having to hold on to conflicting sets of feelings and integrate them despite their opposing connotations. She might resolve the conflict either by succumbing to her grief or by manically avoiding mourning. Both are partial solutions, the denied aspect of which cannot be ignored for long. Sensitive bereavement counselling or supportive therapy aims to enable the woman to experience her 'silent' feelings and work towards their resolution while sustaining the hopefulness of pregnancy.

7.12 SUBSTANCE ABUSE AND PHYSICAL VIOLENCE

7.12.1 Eating disorders

As noted in previous chapters most pregnant women are preoccupied with orality during this period. This may take the form of concern about providing 'proper' nourishment for the baby, 'eating for two' or trying to alleviate her suffering from morning sickness. Antenatal contact with professionals, too, to some extent tends to focus on this topic – weight gain, food intake and dietary instruction. A group of women who are particularly vulnerable during pregnancy are those suffering from eating disturbances such as compulsive eating, excessive nausea, self-induced vomiting and bulimia and those with a history of anorexia nervosa. Pregnancy increases their obsession with bodily intake, content, shape and symbolic meaning. For most women becoming a mother heightens the struggle with an archaic internal mother and the pregnant bulge forces a change of body-image, disclosing her sexual activity and physical maturity for all to see. The idea of a baby inside her feeding off her own resources, increases the panic-stricken sense of inner emptiness and need to binge. While true cases of ongoing anorexia are rare during pregnancy because of diminished fertility [29] active symptoms at the time of conception were found in nine women in a follow-up of 151 patients with a previous diagnoses of anorexia. This study also found twice the rate of prematurity and six times the expected perinatal lethality among the 50 mothers involved [30].

7.12.2 Alcohol

Excessive alcohol intake has been found to be associated with eating disorders, involving 50% of bulimics by age 35 [31] and estimates of incidence of fetal alcohol syndrome range from 0.4 per 1000 live births in the general population to 690 per 1000 among alcoholic women [32]. Drugs or cigarettes may serve similar gap-fillers or be used as a 'magic-wand' to create a sense of being given something, which sadly conflicts with the conscious knowledge of harming the real baby inside while cosseting the 'baby self'.

The flurry of unresolved emotions reactivated during pregnancy aggravate existing addictive conditions and professional assistance is often required to help women with these disorders to find a way of grappling with their conflicts in less concrete and bodily terms. In addition to the emotional vulnerability and physical risks for the fetus inherent in alcohol and substance abuse, with eating disorders there are the attendant dangers of maternal irrational diet, food refusal or obesity, as well as potential future feeding difficulties with the infant.

7.12.3 Physical assault

Fetal abuse by physical assault has featured with violent partners of pregnant women [33] (Chapter 33) and is also found in pregnant women themselves, hitting their bellies as impulsive expressions of rage towards the fetus [34], either under the influence of alcohol or in conjunction with other forms of ambivalence, such as chemical abuse. It is likely that fetal abuse precedes child abuse (low birth weight has been consistently found to be associated with child abuse). As will be shown, mothers' unconscious prenatal perceptions of their babies influence their postnatal maternal behaviour. Identifying babies at risk for maltreatment can set in motion corrective therapeutic and educational programmes to prevent future parenting disorders and child abuse. Early detection and intervention with prenatal psychotherapy or infant-centred maternal counselling during pregnancy can address disorders of attachment [35] and aims to alter maternal negative projections and attributions, thereby influencing the future mother–baby relationship.

7.13 AIDS-IMPERILLED BABIES

HIV threat to infants reflects a universal trend in which women of child-bearing age make up an ever-greater proportion of those infected with AIDS. World-wide, half of all the HIV-infected men and women are under the age of 25, most of whom were infected in their teens. Recent research suggests a transmission rate to infants of infected mothers of

25–50% (24% in European cities). The World Health Organization's Global Programme on AIDS believes that close to 80 000 HIV-infected infants may have been born in sub-Saharan Africa between 1980 and 1987. Projections are that a quarter of a million infants in Africa will have been infected with HIV from their mothers by 1992. In 1988, nearly 2000 babies in the US were infected and in the 1990s 75 000–85 000 uninfected children in New York City alone will be orphaned when their parents die of AIDS. Research has shown that infants born to seropositive mothers who had HIV-related illness during pregnancy were nine times more likely to develop AIDS or HIV-related illnesses very early, compared with infants whose infected mothers were clinically well. Contrary to earlier speculations, recent data indicate that pregnancy may not accelerate the rate of disease progression in HIV-positive women who are healthy. But a small study suggests that when a woman's immune system has been damaged, pregnancy may cause a more rapid acceleration of the disease. Exactly when HIV is transmitted across the placenta is still uncertain, but the virus has been detected in fetuses of 13–20 weeks. Studies show that the method of birth (vaginally or by caesarean) is not a predictor of HIV infection in infants. The WHO believes that the risk of HIV transmission from breastfeeding is slight and in developing countries, the benefits greatly outweigh the theoretical additional risk to the infant [36]. Women who have knowingly taken the risk of becoming pregnant while HIV-positive or ill with AIDS, have often agonized hard and long, weighing up the risks against the joys, pressured by their own precarious futures and uncertainties. These women must be distinguished from a second group who discover themselves to be HIV-positive during pregnancy, and have to face the fact of unwittingly exposing a baby to the dread disease while at the same time coming to terms with the personal implications of their own diagnoses. All pregnant women who are themselves ill, those who are potential 'carriers' or living with an AIDS sufferer should be offered the opportunity of discussions with a counsellor specializing in this area. In the US it was found that the majority of black pregnant women discovered to be HIV-positive while abortion is still an option, chose to continue their pregnancy [37]. For drug-addicted women pregnancy may be their first experience of special attention from partners and professionals and the baby offers a chance to 'reform'. Extensive support may be necessary after the birth, since anxiety and uncertainty are prolonged, and in the absence of a new test to detect the presence of HIV itself rather than antibodies to it, only negative HIV-antibody test results can confirm the child free of the virus, but up to 24 months, an infant born to an infected mother may show positive results due to maternal antibodies. Women who are themselves ill may be less able to nurture their children, and in addition to anxiety and guilt about infecting the baby they often suffer from social isolation, rejection by their families and worry over future care for the baby after her own death.

7.14 NEUROTIC DISORDERS

This group of women are difficult to categorize as deep-seated disturbance, often resulting from their own deficient mothering experiences might manifest in a variety of more or less apparent symptoms. While psychologists and trained therapists have the skill to detect pathological patterns, mental health professionals are not usually included in the antenatal care team. It is therefore up to the health care and educational personnel who do see many women during pregnancy, to learn to recognize warning signals in order to 'screen' the pregnant women in their care, make known the availability of psychotherapeutic services and facilitate referral for women in need.

a. There are gross signs of psychiatric abnormality which can be recognized easily by relatively unsophisticated workers, such as severe depression, phobias, delusions, depersonalization, derealization, and overt paranoia.
b. In addition, there are more subtle signs of long-standing psychological disturbances, psychosomatic disorders and symptoms specifically related to the pregnancy. A general umbrella description would identify women who have exaggerated reactions to the pregnancy, i.e. excessive anxiety (over and above the usual requests for information, reassurance and guidance); exaggerated and persistent worry about fetal abnormality or viability; panic reactions at routine testing, psychosomatic symptoms and undue dread of childbirth. Similarly total emotional detachment, denial of pregnancy or renunciation of future responsibility for the baby, are serious signs to be heeded. Psychotherapeutic treatment is effective. Hypnotherapy and biofeedback techniques have been used successfully to stem hyperemesis and premature labour [38].
c. Finally, a guideline for warning signals indicating disturbance which may not yet have developed into set pathology and therefore also more amenable to brief treatment. Difficulty in accomplishing the psychological undertaking appropriate to each stage of pregnancy. In other words, women who fall into the extreme categories of Facilitator and Regulator, described in Chapter 6.

The extreme Regulator syndrome would include a rigid defensive organization which prohibits adaptation to the emotional demands of pregnancy. This may manifest in an exacerbation of self-control; increased obsessionality; marked absence of emotions; a puritanical attitude towards enjoyment, self-indulgence or relaxation; or else frantic socializing, overworking and refusal to make any concessions to the physical demands of pregnancy, an expressed aversion to babies, feeling trapped by pregnancy or marked denigration of mothering. Conversely, extreme Facilitators may be recognized as women who become so overidentified with the fetus, so introspective and regressed during pregnancy, that they are unable to continue functioning effectively in an adult and responsible manner. This may become apparent in inability to concentrate, persistent forgetfulness, frequent missed appointments with vagueness about reasons; fantasies and imaginary conversations with fetus dominating and overriding social interaction; marked overidealization of the baby, pregnancy or motherhood; involvement in 'mystical' connectedness with the fetus to the point of voiced determination to go on being 'magically' fused or pregnant forever and denial of the imminent birth.

7.15 PREGNANT DISABLED WOMEN

The often grinding physical realities of carrying a pregnancy within a disabled body are difficult enough, particularly when the chronic disability involves pain and/or affects posture and physical functioning. However, a pregnant disabled woman also has to contend with additional psychosocial pressures while adjusting to ordinary demands of pregnancy. She also has to cope with these at a time when vulnerability is exacerbated by pregnant emotional sensitivity. Pregnancy suddenly makes her become more 'visible' to others and prone to receive thoughtless comments ('I never realized you had sex') idle curiosity and prejudice ('I wonder what her baby will make of her . . . '). Thus, cultural assumptions about asexual and childlike properties of the disabled (whether congenital, post-injury or illness) are violated by pregnancy, triggering alarm, ridicule or disgust [39]. In the antenatal clinic the visibly disabled pregnant woman becomes a focus for her able-bodied peers' fascinated repulsion since she visibly embodies their fears of a deformed baby. In the eyes of a disabled woman, the practice of fetal diagnosis is a eugenic insult to all handicapped people, differing from early abortion in the specificity of choosing to abort a particular fetus [40a]. Nevertheless, she herself may have to make this decision, if her disability is genetically inherited. Like all prospective parents receiving negative test results, therapy or crisis counselling may be indicated to tide them over the very difficult period of decision-making and its possibly long-term aftermath.

The disabled woman may also have to face parental and medical disapproval for having become pregnant at all, encountering dire warnings about its effect on her condition and, conversely, reminders of the limitations imposed by her handicap on her capacity to give birth and mother a baby. Being disabled, she may already have a back-log of painful or unpleasant encounters with the medical system, and while her experience might have made her 'hospital-wise', it also may have left her feeling powerless and fragile. She may need special dietary advice or coaching for labour, or in taking a physical risk, may appreciate counselling in this area, as well as welcoming the opportunity to discharge some of her accumulated frustration and discuss the physical and emotional effects of her disability on evolving mothering skills. Deaf and dumb women, or those who are blind, might benefit from special training before the birth in tactile and alternative communication with the infant. Most disabled women, who like all primagravidae cannot accurately foresee coping with the baby, may wish to be helped to envisage the practicalities of managing their new role, and find out about help they may be entitled to receive [40b]. As with all their clients, staff can facilitate possibilities for forming a support network with other pregnant women through antenatal acquaintance. Thus, in a caring clinic, pregnant disabled women may find the rare and satisfying experience of being accepted on equal terms by their able-bodied counterparts, all sharing the same miraculous female happening. Furthermore, pregnancy and birth can restore confidence and feminine pride to a handicapped woman and proof that her body can work and produce a healthy child.

7.16 PSYCHOTHERAPY WITH PREGNANT WOMEN

7.16.1 Pregnant women as psychotherapeutic clients

During pregnancy, women seek therapy to alleviate present and long-standing psychological discomfort and on behalf of their future selves as mothers. As such, therapy is both centred on intrapsychic dynamics within the woman herself and yet simultaneously it is relational and baby-centred. The pregnant womb, like the therapeutic session, serves as a receptacle for unconscious fantasies and actualization of feelings and wishes transferred from the past. There are other features that make pregnant women unique as psychotherapeutic clients:

a. Retention of almost intact ego resources despite the apparent disintegration of boundaries;
b. Accessibility of primitive fantasies coupled with an astute capacity for insight.
c. Influence of the physiological processes and fetal growth on the content of emotional preoccupations.
d. Representation of the 'baby self' often referred to in psychotherapy, in tangible form of the baby in the womb.
e. Psychic growth and rebirth metaphorically symbolized and concretely evident in growth of the pregnant belly and approaching built-in 'D-date', with pressure to achieve stability before the birth.

f. Rapid habituation, assimilation and absorption of psychological changes during pregnancy, and repression of most bizarre experiences within days or weeks of the birth.

(a) Features of individual psychotherapy during pregnancy

a. The sanctity of the dyadic treatment relationship is 'interrupted' by the presence of the fetus, and in it, the concrete representation of the sexual partner, or featuring as a competition to her attention, diverting her from listening to herself during therapy.
b. Focal preoccupation in the transference is on issues relating to maternal nurturance, fusion and autonomy, yet the fetus too is a transferential object, and a transference split may occur between the therapist and fetus.
c. Regression, passivity and dependence feature in heightened form, with oral preoccupations predominating in early pregnancy, differentiation from both fetus and mother (and therapist) in mid-pregnancy and mourning the loss of the internal fantasy baby (and ideal self) coupled with practical and emotional preparation in anticipation of the real baby and mothering.

7.16.3 Transference

Identification with the fetus heightens her transference to the therapist, who is experienced as an enveloping maternal womb carrying the client to her rebirth. In accordance with the specific feelings transferred, the therapist may be experienced as a nutrient-feeding placenta, both metabolizing material and transforming it for the patient's growth, and disposing of waste products, thus encouraging development or as a stingy or an abortive mother, resenting the presence and demands of her client, keeping or diverting good resources for herself while the patient suffers from 'placental insufficiency'. This focal preoccupation in the transference on issues relating to maternal nurturance, fusion and autonomy forms a complex theme as the woman links her fantasies about her own internal mother with those of the mother she is to become and the 'mothering' she receives from her therapist. Confusion may result from the triple identifications between self, mother and future baby and it is incumbent on the therapist to tease out the multiple levels:

('I'm afraid of not being able to carry on, getting fed up with being a mother, running out of energy – not having enough love to keep it going. When you're away, I just collapse now – what will I do when there's a baby around needing to be distracted and entertained and fed, washed, put to sleep? What will it do to my relationship – we're both so emotionally hungry and tired, barely enough time for each other now and we feel so inadequate and need to make up for so much deprivation. I dreamed my car stalled on a steep hill, couldn't go forward and started slipping dangerously back. I feel useless and hopeless, like my mother made me feel as a child, pathetic and with no power, just a great weight round her neck. What if the baby hates me, how will I stand it hating me and being furious with me like I was with my mother, making me feel the worthless mother she felt she was? What if it never grows up or just stays a great blob or is a greedy-guts manipulative little swine like my brother? I'd just want to smash it, get rid of it, kill it off like I lop off my own neediness).

7.16.4 Therapeutic themes

Although, as in all therapy, themes wax, wane and recur as they are worked through on different levels, during pregnancy, some issues are heightened by physical experiences and the timetable of fetal development. Regression, fusion and dependence feature in heightened form, with oral preoccupations predominating in early pregnancy.

('I'm afraid of being eaten by the baby, I'll just be devoured and vanish. But I'm also afraid of eating the baby – I would smother it, not let it live or breathe, just want to be controlling it, cuddling and smelling it or playing with it the whole time – I wouldn't be able to stop watching its every breath or else I'll forget to feed it').

In mid-pregnancy, differentiation from both fetus and mother (and therapist) occur. As another patient reports:

('I feel very chastened by realizing how remarkable these past few months with my parents have been: I've always been so quick to write him off and do what she said, to create a polarity with them as stuck and unchanging – a fixed point for me to define myself against. But now I see how much I'd have missed out on if I hadn't given them a chance to try again. I think its the baby whose taught me I can't have fixed ideas. Since it's begun to kick I'm so conscious of the unknown quality of the baby and myself. I had been quite angry about your refusal to tell me things, your saying "there are no right answers" – but find I can cope with unanswered questions and wait till I know. I'm exploring the whole world of babies from a stance of ignorance, all new or forgotten, just browsing. I dreamed my mother said: "I'm willing to help but don't know what you need; I'll just be available as a willing pair of hands or a blank cheque" but I realize I need to find out what I need').

During the last stage of pregnancy, mourning the loss of the internal fantasy baby features, coupled with practical and emotional preparation in anticipation of birth of the real baby. Women whose conflicts remain un-resolved may experience panic and apprehension (the same patient again):

('Now its so big, it might be born early. I feel my mother's changed – suddenly she's harrassing me like a witch, regimenting me with her time-scale, demanding I get things ready, talking to me in a loud voice like a fish-wife. I think she put the mockers on the baby, its turned and it wants to leave me. I don't want it to go – I don't know what shape I'll be in during the birth. How will I cope with all those contractions and the gratuitous back-pain coming at me from behind and the emptiness after, and everybody fussing over the baby and forgetting me'.)

Early referral gives the disturbed pregnant woman the space and time to make use of the full process of pregnancy within her therapy to attempt to resolve rearoused conflictual relationships with figures in her internal world, thereby freeing her to develop her capacity for 'reverie' and ability to relate to the real baby. Clearly, the deeper the problem and the more related it is to mothering, the less likely it is to be resolved during the course of pregnancy and the greater the need for continued treatment following the birth.

7.16.5 Features of group psychotherapy with expectant mothers

Where individual psychotherapy is not available, group therapy may be expedient in treating some of the issues enumerated above. However, this form of treatment differs from usual group therapy in various ways:

a. **All female group membership.** As noted in the literature, in general, same-sexed women's therapy groups have been found to facilitate more emotional self-disclosure and provide opportunities for role-modelling and empathy for sex-specific conflicts [41] by transcending sex-role stereotypes [42]. A pregnancy group has the additional features of a commonly shared ongoing quintessentially female experience, and heightened awareness of male-female divide.
b. **'Double' membership in the group,** which is comprised not only of participant pregnant women but includes the silent members, the fetuses 'listening in'.
c. **Two-fold (internal/external) foci of attention and communication:** As well as relating to group processes and interaction between group members, each woman is internally preoccupied, not only with her own feelings but those of the fetus. She is both distracted by movements and involved in monitoring and interpreting fetal 'responses' to communica-tions from group members. In addition, the tension between her experienced necessity for absolute honesty in deference to the fetus, yet her protectiveness, too ('not in front of the children') leads to

anxieties and a process of communication which at times takes place through the medium of verbal 'asides' to the fetus, or 'messages' from the active inmates ('my little one didn't like that comment') or oblique and deliberately obscure material ('if I use long words he won't understand').

d. **The 'two-tiered membership'** of primagravidae and multiparous pregnant women: sharing of mixed experience helps dispell unrealistic expectations about labour, birth, motherhood and babies, and these topics are central and take precedence over other personal preoccupations.

e. **'Triple time keeping':** The 'here and now' focus common to analytic-groups [43] is complicated by simultaneous preoccupation with futuristic anxieties about the birth and postnatal interaction, and powerfully revitalized infantile issues.

f. **'A multiple time-lapse view'** is possible in an ongoing pre/postnatal group, where the different pregnancy-stages offer some women a reminder of extinct previous stages, revived as newly pregnant members enter the group, and anticipation of future ones, in more advanced women and those, briefly absent during the puerparium now returning postnatally, as mothers with infants to the group.

g. **Transference:** As in many therapeutic groups, the leader represents a mothering figure [44,45] and the group itself represents a mother [46] or maternal 'breast' [47]. In a pregnancy-group, these metaphors are particularly salient as focal preoccupations revolve around the themes of containing, nurturing and merging. The group leader is invested with magical powers of preservation and the group itself symbolizes a containing, expelling and reuniting nurturing maternal body.

h. **Support:** The therapeutic group invariably serves as a potential pool for individual 'doula' [48] function during labour and takes on the function of a support group after the birth of the babies.

7.16.6 Therapist countertransference

The therapist working with individual pregnant women experiences a heightened awareness of time passing with the visible growth of the patient. She serves as 'historian' and 'recorder' of emotional processes which the client will forget. Time pressures and the physiological phases of pregnancy create their own momentum while awareness of the real dangers of childbirth, possible congenital problems and the momentous maternal task ahead necessitate a delicate balance of interpretation. This requires careful illumination and treatment of the pathological yet maintaining respect for harmless superstitions and necessary defences and preserving the modicum of idealization necessary for what Winnicott called 'Primary Maternal Preoccupation' [49]. However, the therapist's awareness of a dual-loyalty, and at times, contradictory responsibility towards both clients, creates a tension between speaking to the fetus, the child in the patient herself or the potential mother.

Further distinctions may be made between countertransference reactions in different categories of therapists:

a. The male or childless female therapist inevitably experiences disturbing twinges of envy and awesome appreciation of the powerhouse of live creativity. The sense of being in the presence of a mysterious, eternal and inexorable process may affect the humbled therapist's conviction of his/her own creative healing skills. The client's intuitive acuity and heightened emotionality may be disconcerting for therapists accustomed to working with non-pregnant patients.

b. The non-pregnant therapist: Access to primitive emotions, may re-evoke repressed elements from a female therapist's own previous pregnancies, arousing empathy, protectiveness, defensiveness, confusion or aversion. All therapists may experience particularly powerful transferential 'implants' from the pregnant client, with inducements to enact the parental figures, and a need to differentiate these projective-identifications from their own countertransferential feelings. A 'maternal' therapist may experience his/her own sense of being pregnant with, or anxious about and nurturing the expanding client, who is to be 'reborn'.

c. A pregnant therapist has in addition to her two clients, a third, her own fetus, who she might wish to protect from her work-stress or from the raw emotions expressed in sessions. Although her own heightened emotionality can serve as a refined intuitive tool, a fine differentiation must be achieved between her subjective arousal and that of the client. The pregnant therapist's vulnerability too, is increased, while her concentration may be decreased by a desire to introspect. Awareness of her own time pressures and impending maternity-break may create artificial acceleration of processes in her patients. Sexual curiosity, sibling rivalry, competitiveness and envy of her creativity and jealousy of the fetus have been found to occur in non-pregnant clients faced with a therapist's pregnancy [50–52]. In my own case I have found that in a pregnancy group led by a pregnant therapist, the nature of privileged communication changes, with the leader no longer entitled to special 'simultaneous translation' or neutral observer status [53].

7.17 CONCLUSIONS

To recapitulate, the reasons why it is advantageous to offer women psychotherapeutic help during their pregnancy rather than postnatally are as follows:

1. In practical terms they are more mobile, freer and available to look after themselves.

2. In psychological terms, the very accessibility of unconscious material during pregnancy makes these women more amenable to psychotherapy, more insightful at this time and better able to change.
3. In many women motivation to become 'good' mothers is high and although this means something different to each, to the psychotherapist it means releasing each woman's own strengths and resources so she is functioning to the best of her own ability.
4. In economic terms the 'built-in' termination date of the baby's birth invokes a sense of urgency to achieve growth and stability before becoming a mother, and is often reflected in a sense of personal 'rebirth' coinciding with that of the baby. Therapy reduces the likelihood of postnatal breakdown, suicide and child abuse.
5. Obstetric complications, too, have also been found to be associated with psychological stress and disturbance [54], which may be ameliorated during pregnancy.
6. From a cost-benefit point of view, where applicable, group psychotherapy made available to women attending for antenatal checkups or childbirth education is economical and has the added advantage of creating an ongoing self-help postnatal support group.

KEY POINTS

*Psychotherapeutic treatment during pregnancy can help a disturbed woman achieve better integration of internal resources and self-representations, thereby preventing postnatal maternal distress. Timely intervention can ameliorate negative prenatal bonding. Special features of psychotherapy with pregnant women include phase-related themes, unusual therapeutic structure, transference/countertransference issues for both individual and group work.

*Key therapeutic situations are indicated by delineating three somewhat overlapping subgroups of women, who may be particularly at risk during pregnancy due to emotional, social or physical factors in their current or past experience which constitute stressors when interacting with resensitized areas of intrapsychic vulnerability.

*Risk-indicators specified are:

– Conflicted pregnancies, including unplanned, untimely and 'wrong' (such as those resulting from incest or rape).

– Emotional sensitization: expectant mothers who for a variety of predisposing reasons (own or maternal obstetric history, previous still-birth or neonatal loss) or neurotic disorders are prone to emotional difficulties such as over or undervaluation of fetus/baby, pregnancy and/or birth.

– Complicated pregnancies: examining some of the possible concurrent physical conditions (maternal illness, substance abuse or eating disorders,

AIDS imperilled babies, threatened miscarriage or maternal disability, life events (bereavement, eviction, negative test results), socioeconomic difficulties (unemployment, housing problems, poor social support), emotionally impoverished marital relationship and unsupported women on their own.

*Prevention of future postnatal problems and alleviating existing suffering and pathology is partly a function of early detection of high-risk groups during pregnancy by the many professionals involved in antenatal care.

Chapter 8

The fetus – sociocultural beliefs, maternal fantasies and fetal abilities

'The things desired by the mother are often found carried at the time of desire. So it is concluded that one and the same soul governs the two bodies, and the same body nourishes both'. Leonardo da Vinci (cited by A. Macfarlane, 1977).

Until the invention of the fetoscope and ultrasound technology, the intrauterine world inhabited by the living fetus was dark and obscure. However, from the beginning of time fantasies and research have evolved to close the gaps in our understanding of fetal existence and growth.

8.1 HISTORICAL AND CROSS-CULTURAL BELIEFS

8.1 The fetus seen historically

Egyptian texts dating from 1500 BC reveal knowledge of embryonic formation, male and female contribution to conception, placental function and birthing techniques, such as podalic version [1].

Ancient Indian sources dating back to 1000 BC describe the complex processes and active principles which form the living entity of the embryo. Five primal elements constitute the material body of the zygote:

1. The 'thermal' principle from the mother's ovum
2. The 'placid' principle from the father's sperm
3. The three omnipresent cosmic fundamental reals – essence, energy and inertia
4. The five senses
5. The disembodied soul.

Fetal nourishment by the umbilical cord is described, with instructions for maternal variation of her diet in relation to fetal requirements at different phases of development [2].

The first recorded Greek embryological studies are recorded by Hippocrates in the fifth century BC likening embryonic development of man to that of inside a hen's egg. This misconception was followed by those of Aristotle in the fourth century BC, regarding the embryo as a formless mass developed from union of semen and menstrual blood, but also (like the ancient Indian conception) describing fundamental qualities contributing to embryonic growth: these humours – blood, black bile, yellow bile and phlegm – relate to the four primal elements of fire, earth, air and water, and qualities of hot/cold, wet/dry.

Roman embryologists followed the Greek and Alexandrine schools of medical and biological sciences. By the second century AD, Galen's book *Formation of the Foetus* described fairly accurately the placenta and amnion, ascribed conception to both female seed and male, and made an almost modern distinction in genesis as both alteration and shaping, i.e. growth and differentiation [3].

The Koran, holy book of the Muslims, believes the embryo to be formed by mixed male and female secretions, which settle, seed-like in the woman after 6 days (interestingly, the human blastocyst is now known to begin implantation 6 days after fertilization). The Koran depicts the developing embryo becoming human rather than leech like, after 40–42 days, developing within 'three veils of darkness' – maternal anterior abdominal wall, the uterine wall, and the amniochorionic membrane [4].

Ancient Jewish literature, restricted by prohibition on dissection, made allegorical references to cheese-making and potting. In allotting punishment for induced miscarriage, a talmudic distinction was made between an incompletely formed fetus and one who had assumed complete shape [5].

During the renaissance of the fifteenth century, Leonardo da Vinci introduced a quantitive approach by introducing measurements of embryonic growth into his famous drawings of the dissected pregnant uterus, also sketched by Michaelangelo, Raphael and others.

8.1.2 Crosscultural perceptions of conception and prenatal formation

Conception is not always seen to be inaugurated by intercourse. Trobriand islanders displace the human male progenitor, believing that pregnancy results from a 'baloma', the spirit of a dead person (usually female) inserting a spirit-child into the womb of the mother while she swims in the sea [6]. According to ancient Indian embryology (ca 1000 BC) conception occurs inside the womb by union of semen, ovum and a third essential force, the spirit, a male baby being conceived when sperm is stronger than ovum and vice versa for a girl [7]. The Walbiri Australian Aborigine women attribute pregnancy to a combination of copulation and 'guruwari' spirit entry into her body through vulva or crack in the sole of her foot. The spirit entity determines the child's sex, animating the opposite sex to that of the child's previous incarnation [8].

Concepts about development of the fertilized ovum into a human being by no means follow a linear pattern of growth. While many cultures recognize a continuum from conception to birth, some, like English common law, hold that life begins not at conception but at quickening. Muslim scriptures suggest life begins 150 days after conception. The Australian Anbarra talk of life beginning even before conception, when spirit children exist 'in the dreaming' [9].

Cultures differ in dating acquisition of human status, and its attribution to maternal or paternal sources. In some societies continuing fetal growth is partly attributed to the father 'feeding' the baby with his sperm during intercourse [10]. The Bambara of French Sudan believe in fetal development through spiritual forces received from the father in the first month of conception, the baby only acquiring maternal spirituality after birth. Jewish scholars regard the baby as an independent human being only after birth of the head. Before the onset of labour the fetus is considered an organic part of the mother. The Siamese hold the newborn breaks with the spirit world only three days after birth while Peruvian villagers continue to regard the neonate as 'embryonic' and the African Fang only name a child several months after birth [11].

8.1.3 Crosscultural beliefs about prenatal experiences and birth

The Eastern Ojibwa mother of Perry Island, Canada believes her child learns in the womb from the mother talking and teaching 'its soul and shadow such information as the habits of animals it would encounter as it grew up' [12].

The Arapesh of New Guinea believe the baby sleeps in the womb until ready for birth, then dives out. The Iatmul head-hunters of the Great Sepik river believe an unborn child can hurry or delay and chooses its own time of birth [13]. A Jewish folkloric belief holds that unborn babies know 'everything' but as the time of birth approaches, each is touched above the upper lip by the Angel Gabriel, whereupon s/he forgets all previous knowledge but retains forever the imprint of his finger.

8.1.4 Sex preferences

In many cultures, preference is expressed for male or female babies. In people of matrilineal descent, such as the Buka of the Solomon Islands, girls are desired to carry on the family line [14]. In many societies such as the Siriono of Bolivia, prenatal preference for boys is expressed; however, following birth both sexes are said to be given equal time and attention by parents [15]. In other cultures, such as some Muslim communities, boys are not only preferred but the birth of a girl is ignored or even mourned. Generally, in cultures where sociocultural patterns do not induce parents to discriminate strongly between the sexes and men are nurturant (such as the Arapesh described by anthropologist Margaret Mead [16]), prenatal sex preferences will reflect personal desires rather than social values. A mother might wish for a girl as a daughter helpmate; a baby minder; or a self-replica, companion, confidante or doll to be dressed prettily. However, in societies where boys and girls are allocated different work tasks reflecting gender differentiation and the relative status of men and women in that culture, conscious prenatal preferences are likely to follow prescribed patterns. A study conducted in Costa Rica found that the majority of pregnant women in that culture expressed a preference towards a specified gender which was oriented to the unborn child's future social role and status and based on sociocultural stereotypes. Thus, a peasant would wish for a male child as first offspring to help with agricultural tasks; whereas a middle class businessman might wish for a boy to perpetuate his name and company [17]. Reasons for preferring male children may pertain to privilege and protection bestowed on the mother of sons; to their physical hardiness and future work capacity; their supposed personality characteristics: more obedient, quieter, etc. In western societies we find a mixture of both social and personal conscious and unconscious preferences, which vary from woman to woman and in each woman, from pregnancy to pregnancy, often rooted in the constellation of her own family of origin.

KEY POINTS

*Crosscultural ideas about conception and the respective contribution of mother and father to prenatal formation reflect a variety of beliefs which affect the dating of fetus/baby's attainment of human status, and hence rulings about abortion, still-birth burial and infant rearing practices.
*Prenatal sex preferences differ according to sociocultural patterns of discrimination between the sexes.

8.2 PARENTAL BELIEFS

8.2.1 Mother's baby: maternal fantasies and projections

Unlike any other intimate relationship, the protagonists are invisible to each other. The pregnant woman cannot see her baby and usually does not know what sex s/he is. During pregnancy, the mother-to-be is provided with only minimal clues about this closest of relatives – the baby she is growing inside her. The mother–fetus relationship happens in the dark. Unlike most interactions, this one between the pregnant woman and her child is conducted for many months through an enigmatic veil obscuring sight, hearing, smell and direct contact. Therefore, what each mother makes of her fetus is largely of her own doing, assisted by spontaneous and reactive movements once the quickening is experienced. She can feel his/her movements thrusting against her insides but cannot get a grasp of the little limbs, or stroke the fetal skin. In fact she does not know who it is in there. In the absence of objective information, the baby she carries during pregnancy is the one she imagines. The baby, at this stage, is 'invented' by the mother, a focus for her desires, illusions and wishes. Elsewhere, I have suggested that the pregnant womb acts like a projective test, serving as a symbolic container into which each mother can confide her wishes, hopes, fears and fantasies and create the baby of her dreams or nightmares [18]. Into this inner receptacle she projects and transfers her current and archaic conscious and unconscious images and feelings about herself, her baby, her own parents and siblings, the baby's father, pregnancy and motherhood. From all these she constructs her imaginary baby. Researchers have found that prenatal perceptions of fetal personality remain stable in both mothers and fathers from late pregnancy to early infancy [19,20]. Also, since there is little objective relation between early neonatal behaviour and parental perception of it, these studies lend support to the belief that these attributions are based on fantasy [21] and on individual emotional differences in mothers (observable during pregnancy) rather than in differences of neonatal temperament [22]. Thus, already during pregnancy, each parent-to-be may be said to be guided by what Bowlby has called an 'internal working model' [23] a subjective body of expectations and symbolic representations based on their own significant experience and perceptions by which they construe their infant-to-be [24].

8.2.2 Mother's attachment to the unborn baby

Women differ in the degree of attachment to their fetuses. Most women have a complex mixture of feelings about the baby which vary at different stages of pregnancy and fluctuate at times in accordance with bodily experiences and external familial, social and even climatic conditions. Some women, as we have seen, have mainly negative feelings or tend to forego allowing themselves any fantasies about the forthcoming baby. Nevertheless, at an unconscious level, unless its existence is totally denied, every fetus assumes a meaning for the mother-to-be.

The nature of her attachment to the fetus she mentally conceives can be seen to be determined by many intrapsychic, psychosocial and cultural factors related to her motivation for becoming pregnant, readiness for conception and its timing, the place of this baby in the family and its relationship to mother's and father's own emotional and ordinal positions in their families of origin. Other factors include the woman's health and degree of physical discomfort during pregnancy, the quality of emotional support from her mate, family and nursing staff; the nature

of demands made upon her by other children, work, parents, her
mother's obstetric history as well as her own and her previous experience
with babies.

(a) Positive prenatal attachment

In my clinical experience, how much the expectant mother invests of
herself in the fetus will depend on her capacity for trust in a positive
outcome. Some women can afford to fall in love with the baby. A
prospective mother may have elaborate daydreams and conduct silent
imaginary interchanges and audible conversational chats with her internal
companion. She may imagine one particular infant, the child of her
dreams or herself in babyhood, or a baby she has felt close to or lost,
a faceless one or an infant with features she has made up out of fragments
of her own inner world. It may be the same baby in all her fantasies,
or differ from time to time as she 'practises' with a variety of infants
she may have.

(b) Neutral

Other prospective mothers hold their fantasies in abeyance. They feel
they cannot build a fantasy in case the reality doesn't live up to it. Some
pregnant women, particularly those with a history of loss (miscarriages,
still-birth, cot death) and/or older women, make a conscious effort to
have 'no feelings' and try to avoid investing their expectations in this
pregnancy for fear of something going wrong. Their dreams reflect these
fears – the images of a fetus thrown on top of rubbish in a dustbin,
wriggling but about to die; bathing a cooing, gurgling baby who suddenly
disappears down the drain or vanishes into thin air; labour ending not
in birth of a baby but of nothing or just a bloody mess of spongey tissue.

A cautious mother may feel the need to protect her other children
from too much emotional involvement with this fetus in case the baby
does not survive. By inhibiting her fantasies and minimizing her own
attachment, she feels she is safeguarding her future ability to continue
mothering her other children rather than collapsing with grief if
something tragic should happen. As we have seen, a Regulator may just
want the pregnancy to be over, counting the days until the actual baby
is safely delivered, like a parcel through the post. A woman who was
herself adopted may feel the conflict of becoming attached to her unborn
baby when her adoptive mother had not had this experience and her
biological mother could give her up following birth. A woman whose
history makes her feel that her pregnancy is always in danger of being
aborted cannot allow herself the luxury of being 'carried away' into
imagining herself with a baby for fear of prebirth loss. She cannot let

the baby be real to her. A candidate for amniocentesis may feel so dominated by the prospect of negative news that she cannot take the continuity of the pregnancy for granted. Only after this watershed can she begin to spin her daydreams although nightdreams, refusing to obey her, may have been erupting disturbingly, before this.

(c) Negative

Most mothers-to-be at times imagine their fetuses as incomplete, damaged or damaging to themselves. However, some women are constantly preoccupied with largely negative fantasies. Lacking an inner conviction of self-esteem, a woman may feel a sense of internal emptiness, fear destructive 'vibrations' emanating from the unseen baby or experience a wellspring of poisonous substances welling up deep within themselves. These may be sensations rather than verbalized thoughts, or may take the form of panic states and anxieties about the baby's normality or viability:

1. The 'monster' she will bring forth reflecting her own inner badness.
2. The baby harmed, lost or starved during pregnancy.
3. The internal damage she herself may suffer from the pregnancy or fetus and/or the birth process.
4. Bad 'substances' within her causing malignancies to the fetus or to her own internal body.

Such a woman might feel quite 'beleaguered' within herself, surrounded by people rejoicing and congratulating her on her pregnancy while she herself is possessed by thoughts of internal disasters and external inadequacies. ('Sometimes, when I'm exhausted, my baby seems so horrible, like a monster, vicious, greedy and bad. I end up like a monster myself, furious with my husband and with the pregnancy, just wanting to smash everything up, get rid of it all and force everyone out of my way. But I also feel desperate, like a screaming baby inside. What does all that do to the fetus? How will I bear its crying when it is born and I want looking after too? How will I cope without ever wanting to exterminate the baby the way I feel my mother would have liked to get rid of me?') She cannot imagine how women ever get through the long period of helpless waiting and may feel the need for almost continuous vigilance to ensure the survival of her pregnancy in spite of her internal turmoil. As noted in Chapter 7, psychotherapy during pregnancy ameliorates negative prenatal bonding.

8.2.3 Paradigm of placental exchange: a model of unconscious conceptualization of mother–fetus interaction

Because of human variability it is difficult to make any generalizations about the ways prospective mothers relate emotionally to their fetuses.

Nevertheless, it may be helpful to highlight an underlying unconscious paradigm or pattern for mother–fetus interaction which appears to serve as a basis for much maternal fantasy production – that of the umbilical exchange.

I have found that for many women, the placental processing of nutrients and waste during pregnancy serves as an unconscious model for her interaction with the baby postnatally [25]. During pregnancy, it can be assumed that the fetus remains unaware that with every heart-beat his mother pumps oxygen-loaded blood and nourishment into the placenta and removes carbon dioxide to be breathed out through her lungs and nitrogen compounds to be excreted by her kidneys in her urine Thus, already in the womb, the mother serves the function of container, metabolizer and waste disposer to that loved/hated parasite feeding off her tissue, directing nutrients from her blood to its own system and spewing out its deposits into her. We may say that during pregnancy she physically processes and transforms good nutrients and bad waste in the way that after the birth she will act as what Bion has called a 'container' [26] and transformer for her baby's complex experiences and feelings: cleaning his body of waste products, 'metabolizing' his unutter-able anxieties and feeding back a 'detoxified' processed version that can now be safely re-internalized by the infant.

I am proposing that interuterine processing and prenatal exchange can be seen to anticipate postnatal transformational interaction, when the nurturing mother is expected to contain her baby's emotions, filter noxious stimuli, remove unwanted aspects of the infant's reality and to replace them with growth-producing experiences.

8.2.4 Fantasies of placental interaction

In this sense, motherhood is foreshadowed by pregnancy, the maternal holding of the baby echoing the physical containment of the embryo within the womb. During pregnancy, these physical processes take place through the medium of the placenta. It is a commonly held belief that the generous mother grows this placenta for her baby. In actual fact, since it has evolved from the outer cells of the fertilized ovum, it may equally be said to be brought by the prudent fetus. Similarly, in viewing the placental exchange, one may choose to focus figuratively on the mother either as provider of nourishment or as passive container; an alternative view converges on the fetus either growing innocently unaware of the source of food or else, greedily devouring, stealing or polluting maternal resources. Indeed, some pregnant women imagine that their entire system is being drained or undermined by the ruthless parasite. How each woman conceptualizes this interaction affects her experience of pregnancy. Hence, one pregnant woman may attribute nausea to fetal excretions in her body; another might welcome morning sickness as a symptom that she is indeed pregnant in the early absence of other signs; while yet another might imagine the nausea to be the manifestation of her secret desire to get rid of the fetus by vomiting it out. Similarly, placental insufficiency could be unconsciously interpreted either as the 'stingy' mother withholding nourishment from her child or as the 'greedy' baby's needs outstripping what the placental mother can supply. A pseudocyesis ('pretend' pregnancy), or hydatidiform 'mole', rare in reality, are a common fantasy during pregnancy. Women dream of having the experiential appearance of a pregnancy which is all 'hot air' and imagination with no baby at the end. Nightmares consist of a belly full of nothing, or an imaginary mass of villi 'tentacles' multiplying inside her, swarming out of control, taking over her internal space from within, 'strangling' and killing her off.

8.2.5 Maternal unconscious value judgements

Moreover, the placenta not only conveys substances. It acts as a barrier; again, depending on one's focus, protecting either the mother or the fetus against harmful poisons produced or imbibed by the other. Conversely, the barrier must be permeable – good things need to cross: not only nutrients but antibodies to provide protection against diseases and placental hormones which help sustain the pregnancy. Thus, even women who have no detailed understanding of the physiological function of the placenta, imagine its activity as a filtered exchange between mother and baby, in which a transfer of substances occurs. Whether this exchange is deemed harmful or benign depends on the mother's self-image and unconscious concept of her fetus: she may imagine her own internal reservoir as good or bad and her fetus likewise, as good but vulnerable to her own badness or as bad and parasitically sapping her resources. The 'emotional barriers' between them operate according to her fantasy of their interaction as mutually beneficial or dangerous, with one or both of them needing to be hived off and kept safely separate.

Table 8.1

Mother	Baby	Placental activity
(a) SAFE/GOOD (processing/nourishing)	SAFE/GOOD (sustaining	common pool permeability
(b) SAFE/GOOD (bountiful)	DANGEROUS/BAD (parasite/polluter)	mother's defence barrier
(c) DANGEROUS/BAD (harmful)	DANGEROUS/BAD (harmful)	mutual barrier
(d) DANGEROUS/BAD (polluting)	SAFE/GOOD (innocent)	baby's defence barrier

The complex unconscious paradigm of imagined placental exchange between mother and fetus can be simply conceptualized as shown in Table 8.1.

(a) Good mother/good baby

A pregnant woman who views both herself and her fetus as benign and friendly to each other, can indulge in prenatal fantasies of reciprocal sharing. Identifying herself with the fetus, she feels both of them to be nourished by a common pool of good things which facilitates their exchange, and her permeability to introspection.

(b) Good mother/bad baby

Sometimes an expectant mother experiences her fetus as a potentially dangerous being, either greedily feeding off her resources or liable to pollute them with his/her excretions. She feels she must protect the good things inside her from this harmful influence, and erects an imaginary internal 'barrier' between herself and her fetus, to avoid her inner world being harmed by the baby or s/he taking over and sapping her emotional energies. Such a barrier may simply take the form of 'reserve', a refusal to allow her thoughts to become engaged by the fetus. She might feel the need for added precautions – 'eating for two' to avoid being deprived by the baby commandeering all the food; drinking lots of liquids, to 'flush out the baby's waste products'; resentfully attributing symptoms such as constipation, flatulence and palpitations directly to the baby's bad influence and a determination to continue to protect herself from its spoiling activities.

(c) Bad mother/bad baby

In a situation where the pregnant woman conceptualizes both herself and the baby as mutually dangerous, she tries to maintain an emotional boundary between them which is 'impermeable' as possible, and separate their existences. Thus a rigid barrier may take the form of the woman's refusal to think about the fetus or pregnancy at all. She may deny that her own alcohol consumption or smoking could have any effect on the 'insulated' baby or increase fortification of her own defences against regression, introspection or the dependence associated with pregnancy, indeed, to the point of manic stepping up of her own 'adult' activities without any concession to her 'condition'.

(d) Bad mother/good baby

Finally, where the mother experiences herself as potentially dangerous to her vulnerable, 'good' unborn baby, she may resort to magical superstitious activities to prevent anything untoward happening to her baby. Carefully monitoring her own thoughts to prevent 'seepage' of any negative emotions which might affect the fetus and subjecting her intake to rigorous screening, she might also compulsively feel the need to go out of her way to provide pleasant stimulation such as gastronomic delicacies, musical treats, soothing movement, a continuous 'feast' to mitigate her own bad internal influences which she fears may harm the baby growing inside her.

Most pregnant women's fantasies resonate with a particular set of attributes although some fluctuations between these various positions, according to their moods, daily or even momentary experiences, physical symptoms, external emotional 'reinforcements' or slights.

8.2.6 Facilitator/Regulator prenatal attachment

The Facilitator/Regulator model may now be seen within this framework always taking into account that there are few extreme types: many women vascillate in the mid area, or treat the fetus as a person.

The Facilitator tends to invest in the fetus an ideal baby part of herself. Based on an unconscious identification of her own imagined infant-self with the fetus, she attributes to it all the lovable and endearing qualities she feels her own, often unrecognized, baby-within-herself possesses. She communes with her fetus whom she feels to be responsive and communicative and in her identification often draws a mutual barrier around them both against harmful substances and external impingements. In fact, now that there is a tangible baby within her, the hidden baby aspect of herself can gain some recognition. She can allow these hidden fragments of herself their expression – she can regress, be dependent or demanding if she likes, she can have whims, cravings and capricious wishes which others will indulge or she can feel free to voice irrational fears or fanciful thoughts which others will not dismiss. All those childish facets of herself that she has kept at bay because she felt they might be unacceptable to other adults in her daily relationships, can now be indulged legitimately and find expression as features of her pregnancy, but, more so, as emotional parts of the baby that is there, inside her, visible for all to see. Depending on her own realistic integration of this baby-like part of herself, she will ascribe more or less glorified capacities to the fetus. In an idealized unconscious identification between the fetus and the extreme Facilitator's own imagined baby-self, they are both nourished from the common pool of mother–infant fusion and exchange ((a) in Table 8.1). Whereas, if she experiences herself as empty or full of harmful infantile residues from her own past she must separate their contact by erecting a barrier between them ((d) in Table 8.1).

Like the Facilitator, the Regulator also unconsciously identifies the fetus with her own baby-self, but in this case it is a denigrated, or repudiated baby-self, whose emotional demands she fears as potentially dangerous to her rational adult self. She may envisage the fetus as a greedy, savage little creature trying to grab all the resources for itself. A visit to the dentist for a filling, for instance, will reinforce her feeling of having been sapped by the parasitic fetus, who threatens to suck her back into toothless babyhood. She may feel at times that she is losing her grip as a competent adult person – distracted, clumsy, tearful – being dragged down by the fetus inside her, having the adult layers peeled off, until she is exposed as a great big baby. Putting up a final barrier to defend her external world from invasion by the baby, an extreme Regulator may resort to cutting off any identificatory resemblance between the two of them and refusing even to imagine herself as an infant or her bulge as a sentient baby. Alternatively, she may defend her hard-won autonomy by reminding herself that she is the adult and the fetus just happens to be residing inside her, two quite separate people. This solution is sought particularly when the fetus is felt to be so contaminating and greedy that she fears being taken over ((b) Table 8.1) or else, when she believes that she herself has poisonous residues from her own babyhood which might affect the fetus ((c) or (d) in Table 8.1).

In principle, the more the prospective mother has hived off and the less she has been in touch with her inner world before pregnancy, the greater the danger of being 'taken over' by identification with the fetus, for better or worse.

KEY POINTS

*During pregnancy, the mother-to-be is provided with only minimal clues about the baby she is carrying. Therefore, each mother 'invents' her baby as she invests the fetus with her own projected fantasies, wishes, hopes and fears and unconscious identifications.

*Prospective mothers vary in the degree of bonding to their fetuses and most women experience mixed feelings coloured by access to her own internal positive resources and to optimistic belief in fetal viability. Attachment is determined by factors in the woman's psychosocial and obstetric history as well as current physical and emotional experience.

*Fantasied interchange is likened to the placental exchange, with good and/or bad substances passing back and forth from the pregnant woman and her fetus, and internal 'barriers' are erected or dismantled according to perceived psychological dangers.

*One woman may idealize the fetus, her own capacity to grow the baby and the 'symbiotic' exchange, while another experiences pregnancy as an empoverishment, the fetus as an invasive parasite and/or herself as potentially harmful. The model is one of permutations of Good or Bad Baby in combination with Good or Bad Mother.

*In principle, the more the prospective mother has split off and the less she has been in touch with her inner world before pregnancy, the greater the danger of positive or negative by identification of her own 'baby' self with the fetus.

8.3 THE BABY TO BE: PRENATAL RESEARCH

We have come a long way since the belief that the sperm was a miniature complete little 'homunculus' who merely grew larger in the nourishing womb. Microscopic dissection techniques have revealed the pattern of embryonic growth, confirming rapid development from a single cell to formation of all the major organs and sense receptors by 11 weeks.

In recent years, our knowledge about fetal development has burgeoned due to more-refined ultrasound imaging, and recent technological advances have disclosed hitherto unknown capacities of the living fetus, either miraculously filmed through the introduction of fibreoptic intra-uterine film-photography or as observed by life-ensuring technology of ever-younger premature babies. While we have always been aware of fetal motor functions, we are now much more knowledgeable about sensory receptivity and possible integrative functions.

8.3.1 Fetal sensory abilities

(a) Hearing

Most pregnant women have known from experience that the moving fetus responds with a startle reflex to sudden loud sounds and differentially to classical or rock music. Studies conducted in the 1930s [27] with pregnant women whose hearing was obscured by headphones provided evidence that the fetus responds to sound and vibrations directly (i.e. bypassing the mother's reactions to what she has heard) and that s/he also responds to frequencies too low for the human ear to hear. Recent recordings made with microphones inserted into the womb have revealed that the internal pulsating noise of the mother's blood flow and digestive system obscure most ordinary external sounds that do pass through the amniotic fluid. The fetus spends the duration of its stay in the womb accompanied by the internal sounds of the mother's heartbeat and ongoing physiological processes as well as her voice, and external sounds loud enough to penetrate to the interior.

(b) Response to maternal emotions

An interesting development of this finding was Salk's study of infants' reactions to taped heartbeats. Not only were newborns soothed by exposure to regular (80 beats/s) heartbeats, and gained more weight than neonate controls, but their counterparts who were exposed to higher rates of heartbeats became distressed [28]. This postnatal finding suggests that chronic maternal emotional stress or physical strain which raises her heartbeat above a certain level might affect the fetus, as might increased hormonal activity that accompanies anxiety, stress or exertion. A study conducted as early as 1925 [29] demonstrated that fear and anxiety could be biochemically induced in animals and humans by injecting catecholamine chemicals from the blood of frightened individuals. Anxiety is the maternal factor most often studied and implicated in reproductive complications. A significant relationship has been found between maternal anxiety level and fetal activity [30]. In a recent study, when mothers who rated themselves as anxious were exposed to taped stimuli (of warbling sounds and babies crying) through earphones, fetal heart rate was markedly affected, although these pronounced responses were not found in the fetuses of women with self-rated high depression or hostility scores [31]. It has been also been demonstrated that not only does maternal smoking increase fetal heart rate, the pregnant woman just thinking about having a cigarette has a sudden effect on the fetus [32]. Further research suggests that changes in arterial pressure caused by maternal emotion or maternal hormones passing through the placenta barrier may similarly affect the fetus. Factors studied were both fetal reaction to maternal chronic personal stress (such as war-induced anxiety [33] and/or maternal attitudes towards the pregnancy [34].

Although findings of the many studies on birth complications must be interpreted cautiously because of complex methodological issues [35], a relationship has been demonstrated between maternal emotionality and reproductive outcome. Results suggest that babies born to rejecting or unhappy mothers may be more 'jumpy' and fearful and a correlation has been demonstrated between birthweight and the mother's prenatal psychological adjustment [36]. One carefully controlled study has demonstrated a significant relationship between chronic maternal anxiety level and fetal activity, with follow-up suggesting continuity between fetal and neonatal movement patterns and behaviour [37]. Ultrasound observation of fetal activity followed up by ongoing study of the same baby after birth, has shown marked consistency of behaviour before and after birth [38].

A complex interplay exists between maternal influences and inherent fetal characteristics, as other studies show that even young fetuses vary in the degree of their responsivity to stress. One study has found that prenatal 'low reactors' (judged by the steadiness of their heartbeat) differ when tested in their teenage years from those who were 'over-reactors' in the womb.

(c) Vision and dreaming

By nine weeks the eye is already formed and there is now evidence that during late pregnancy fetuses can distinguish between dark and light when a strong light is flashed through the mother's bulge and no doubt can do the same when she sunbathes. Some authors have tried to distinguish different states of quiescence, waking and sleep in the fetus [39]. Studies have revealed eye movements – both in response to his/her changing position and possibly due to dreaming as there is evidence of rapid eye movements (REM) accompanying sleep-type brain waves in fetuses. It is interesting to speculate about the content of fetal dreams since they have been exposed to so few visual stimuli. One suggestion has been the formation during sleep of 'internal representations' of the sensory stimuli experienced by the fetus, as filtered through the maternal container [40]. Babies monitored in the womb have exhibited similar brain waves to those of adults during REM (rapid eye movement) sleep when dreams are known to occur. Interestingly, although eye movements are difficult to detect in fetuses, it appears that mothers and their fetuses seem to exhibit dreaming brain patterns at the same time leading some researchers to speculate on a 'telepathic' link between the pregnant woman and her unborn child [41].

(d) Tactile sensitivity

Sensitivity to touch is revealed by responsive movements of the fetus either avoiding the source of touch or moving towards it, as well as by changes in facial expression. From six weeks, if the baby's budding hands touch his/her mouth area s/he turns his head away while opening the lips. Quite soon, the movement is reversed (similar to the postnatal 'rooting reflex') and the head is turned towards the hand and a finger inserted into the mouth.

(e) Discrimination and reactions

Sucking and swallowing are discriminatory; when sweet tasting saccharin is injected into the amniotic fluid, the swallowing rate doubles and drops dramatically accompanied by grimacing if unpleasant tastes are introduced. This capacity to produce varied facial expressions develops early (smiles have been noted in prems under 33 weeks), however at this stage we can only speculate about their emotional meaning.

There are researchers who attribute a great deal of sophistication to the fetus' ability to experience and discriminate emotions, both their own 'internally' experienced ones and maternal 'messages'. Although the autonomic nervous system develops early, it is only in the seventh month that development takes place in the 'higher' brain which later is known to control functions such as speech and abstract thought processes. Hence, making 'sense' of inchoate sensations seems unlikely to happen much earlier. Nevertheless, one school of experimenters report they can retrieve emotional memories from very early prenatal life [42]. Extending as far as beliefs about 'cellular memory' that can enable a person to recall being a sperm! [43].

Until we have further evidence it is enough to know that the fetus is a sensitive and reactive little being, aware of changes in maternal reactions, temperature, pressure, sound and light, affected by variations in her respiratory and vascular systems and her endocrine and circadian rhythms. In addition, the fetus is as much at the mercy of what passes through the uterine threshold as that which passes through the placental barrier. This places some responsibility on professionals in their dealings with the mother, both to facilitate her general sense of well-being and to protect the fetus from unnecessary impingements during investigations. Given the belief of many pregnant women that their unborn babies are cognisant to and influenced by much of what occurs to their mothers during pregnancy, common courtesy demands that professionals respect these beliefs and treat the women accordingly. Further, as will be shown in Chapter 9, antenatal caregivers are in a unique position as mediators to acquaint pregnant women with the remarkable capacities of their unknown babies, thus encouraging prenatal bonding and future sensitivity to neonatal needs.

8.3.2 Prenatal 'educational' psychology

In America, and to a much lesser degree in the UK, an alternative cult has arisen, capitalizing on the prospective parents' desire to be influential and involved rather than passive producers. Some experts in the private sector not only strive to make the woman a party to her own antenatal care but have taken to emphasizing the prospective mother's obligation to maximize the capacities of her unborn child. Thus, hypnotists will help the woman communicate her feelings to her fetus and 'speak out' fetal replies; guided fantasy and visualization techniques encourage prenatal bonding; physiotherapists will teach the woman to appreciate the baby's movements thus encouraging prenatal attachment; videos are available that teach fetal 'massage'; fetal-heart amplifiers are commercially available to enhance prenatal communication and a Californian 'Pre-Natal University' actually issues a diploma to fetuses, whose expectant mothers have optimized their potential by following a multi-sensory graded learning programme [44]. However, this concept is new only in its organized capacity: over the generations, numerous mothers have acted on their own belief in prenatal influence: conveyed ideas, words, music to their fetuses, stroked, danced, sung and each in their own way, communicated to their unborn baby the direction to fulfil their own fond wishes. (Thus a biography of Shirley Temple notes that her mother Gertrude played her dance records to stimulate the ambitions of her fetus [45].)

8.3.3 Fetal therapy

In medicine, the ever-increasingly refined techniques of prenatal diagnosis, aim not merely to identify severe non-correctable fetal disorders thereby presenting the mother with the stark alternatives of abortion or caring for a handicapped child. Development of techniques for effective fetal treatment have endeavoured to prevent manifestation of irreversible fetal damage *in utero*. Treatment, which until now was limited to manipulation of the mother and environment, has gravitated towards direct treatment of the fetus through drug therapy, surgery and interuterine transfusions [46]. Such interventions present ethical dilemmas recently debated in Parliament. They also raise our awareness of the fetus as a separate individual of controversial legal and moral status lodging within another person. We, therefore, find ourselves posing questions about 'fetal rights' and the 'ordinary expected quality of life' of fetuses. One such issue is whether, since the mother's state of mind constitutes part of the fetal environment, psychotherapeutic intervention might become a requirement for women suffering from anxiety and other emotional states which appear adversely to affect fetal well-being. Meanwhile, psychotherapy certainly should be made available to any pregnant woman who feels the need for it, on behalf of her own mental well-being and attachment to her baby.

KEY POINTS

*A review of research findings about fetal sensory capacities reveals the fine sensitivity of the unborn child with implications for health care professional responsibility to protect the fetus from unnecessary impingements during antenatal investigations and to acquaint the mother with fetal capacities.
*The recognition of the fetus as human before birth raises complex ethical issues relating to prenatal screening, 'education', therapy and preventive treatment.

Chapter 9

The professional as mediator between mother and fetus: antenatal care and assessment

'A woman about to become a mother, or with her newborn infant upon her bosom, should be the object of trembling care and sympathy. Wherever she bears her tender burden or stretches her aching limbs. God forbid that any member of the profession to which she trusts her life, doubly precious at this emotional period, should handle it negligently, inadvisedly or selfishly.' Oliver Wendell Holmes

9.1 ANTENATAL CARE

9.1 Antenatal services: expectations and reality

Antenatal care is an emotive topic. Babies represent the future of a nation and the production of healthy babies therefore becomes a political issue. As we have noted, each society defines the parameters of procreativity for women, and in Britain, these include provision of National Health Service antenatal care. From the perspective of the provider of maternity services, routine antenatal care is assumed to predict and prevent problems which might be avoided by appropriate prophylactic measures and to treat conditions which may have harmful effects on mother and/or baby [1]. The idea is promoted that attendance will ensure a normal pregnancy, labour and baby. However, the benefits of care have not been unequivocally demonstrated, and some interventions are of unproven value. The efficacy of routine antenatal care in respect of diagnosis of such conditions as pre-eclampsia, interuterine growth retardation and breech presentation is as low as 1%, suggesting that for the majority of women, four or five visits with more specific objectives at key points during the pregnancy might be as effective as the dozen or more visits currently advocated [2].

The conclusion is that heaith professionals, politicians and pregnant women might have unrealistic expectations about what may be achieved by routine antenatal care. Some women do not avail themselves of antenatal care and a historical review suggests that consumers who do, have voiced very similar dissatisfactions over the last 40 years [3].

These complaints usually focus on 'long waiting times, difficult access to clinics, lack of continuity of care, lack of opportunity to discuss things that women are worrying about, and the feeling that they are not getting as much out of it as they feel they should' [4]. Two competing ideologies of reproduction exist, and medical perspectives on good maternity care do not match up with those of pregnant women [5]. A conflict exists between two perspectives – that of the providers who feel women are remiss in not attending, and that of the users who cite defects in the service. This conflict is reflected in research which often fails to locate and question non-users (who tend to be the very young or very old, unmarried, low social classes and high-parity women), as well as consumers. One consequence of this non-complementary approach to the problem are gaps in our knowledge about the relationship between lack of satisfaction, reasons for non-attendance, and the mechanisms by which medical care and social factors of class and poverty influence perinatal outcome [6]. How can we bridge the gap between the providers and the users of a service, and between the expectations of all concerned and the disappointing reality they encounter?

Several attempts have been made to do just that. Increasingly, there is an attempt to implement the understanding that in order to be sensitive to all the needs of a pregnant woman, antenatal services should entail more than just medical screening and care and must involve agencies other than the health care authorities and would therefore benefit from being community based. Planning new antenatal care services have in some districts involved a partnership between various agencies such as District Health Services, Social Services, Department of Education and Adult Education Services, as well as voluntary bodies such as Family Unit Services, and consumer groups [7]. In my view, mental health needs of pregnant women must also be considered, as these are pertinent to her own general welfare, and that of her fetus and future relationship with her child. Integrated hospital and community-based obstetric services have been found to increase ease of attendance and communication by going out to the women (in larger group practices and community clinics) and providing continuity of care [8]. A study of the effect of such a scheme in Edinburgh found that the percentage of lower social class attenders rose dramatically as did that of very young women, with increased satisfaction for all participants and a steep fall in perinatal mortality of babies in the scheme [9]. This is an important finding as an earlier study had found working-class women less successful in obtaining the information and satisfaction they sought during antenatal care [10]. While evaluating further ways to improve antenatal care, the psychological and social expectations of pregnant women must be investigated to assess whether and how these may be realistically met. (In Sweden, a clinical psychologist is included in the antenatal care team).

9.1.2 Messages from the interior: the need for information

Motivation for attendance at antenatal clinics is not only determined by her belief in propaganda and health care but is also a function of the pregnant woman's need to find out more about her pregnant self and her unknown fetus. Given the inaccessibility of the fetus to the mother, the professional, who has the means of getting to 'know' what is happening inside her, becomes an important mediator between the pregnant woman and her inmate. In her eyes, people providing antenatal care have the capacity not only for measuring physiological processes and changes that she is aware of in her own pregnant body but of relating these to hidden fetal development. This is what the mother-to-be comes to hear: not how much weight she's gained or what her blood pressure is, but what this implies in terms of the tiny being growing inside her and how what she does can influence her baby's future for better or worse. To her, even routine blood and urine tests are 'messages from the interior' and she eagerly awaits the results: is the little fellow satisfied? Is she feeding her darling well? Is her blood 'rich' enough? What has the baby rejected? There are no poisons in her, are there? Is he bleaching her of essentials or are there enough for them both? Life and Death questions whose answers she needs to hear . . .

Similarly, although relieved to know that the symptomatic changes she has herself observed in her skin, eyes, nose, gums, breasts, breathing, heat sensitivity, etc., are 'quite normal', what she really wants to know is what they mean. Heartburn, runny nose, metallic taste, frequent micturation, will all be better tolerated if seen as consequences of other processes (increased blood flow, altered positioning of internal organs to provide more space, etc.) contributing to fetal growth and her baby's comfort rather than just as unpleasant side-effects of being pregnant. It is sometimes very difficult, when time and staffing resources are so scarce, for health professionals to be able to give more than a cursory explanation. However, in the interest of their own job satisfaction, relating to each individual client as a unique person whom he/she can get to know and observe growing month by month, can be infinitely more rewarding than the 'conveyor belt approach' which still operates in some antenatal clinics. Furthermore, in thus 'bonding' with her client, the professional can serve as a positive model and can help the expectant mother to increase her attachment and emotional dialogue with the unborn baby.

9.1.3 Access to the inmate

The professional can provide more direct access to the fetus. While uncomfortable, and sometimes felt to be sexually invasive, examinations and particularly internal ones are regarded by the woman as a secret pathway to her hidden baby. She tolerates them because she wants news: How is her baby doing? What is her baby doing? What has the doctor/ midwife found out? What can s/he feel? How big is her baby? and how happy – does s/he like it in there? The real unanswerable question asked in silence is: Who? 'Who is living in my womb?', 'Who will my baby be?'. She clutches at any scrap of information. The pregnant woman wants her excitement to be affirmed and to have someone share in the external reality of her internal world.

Dying to listen to her child's heartbeat on the stethoscope she may be too shy to ask for a go. She wants to hear from the busy midwife what it is like to watch a baby come out and how she thinks this baby is coming along but doesn't ask because time is short. She wants to talk and be recognized, to tell her version, to be asked to report her own internal experience of how each movement feels and tell them that she now can identify little limbs. Above all she wants to be treated as an adult person on a creative mission, an active, cognisant participant in a strange exciting experience not merely a dumb container come to the 'workshop' for a service checkup. This may be her first encounter with caring professionals. It may be her first experience ever of being treated as a woman with a 'treasure house' rather than emptiness inside. It may offer the only intimate opportunity she has to share some of her enjoyment or anxieties with anyone at all. To do so with an interested expert who has seen many other mother/fetus couples but treats her as special, takes her seriously and gives her time and space to explore her feelings, can be nourishing and healing.

9.1.4. The influence of professionals

During the course of her pregnancy each woman may encounter a whole host of different professionals (at times, she may be seen by as many as 28 doctors and midwives in the antenatal clinic alone [11]). Their potential influence on her is very great as they appear to have (and often make sure she knows they have) privileged information, vital procedures and immediate access to her fetus denied to her. They also know how she affects the baby. In traditional societies the initiated women who have themselves had babies mediate between the generations, offering ritualized guidance and reassurance. The western woman must find her own. She looks to health professionals to act as intermediary between herself and the fetus – giving her news from the hidden interior, formulating in words what she dimly experiences, telling her how to maximize growth conditions, enabling her to see pregnancy as benign and creative, reassuring her that she is not harming the fetus in any way, that she has what it takes to sustain this baby and that she is not herself being internally damaged in the process.

Professionals appear to hold the key. They present themselves as knowing the norms: they can judge how well her baby is growing, what riches might be missing in her blood supply, how the pregnancy is affecting her body, how her body is affecting the baby and when the birth is due to take place. They have the emotional power to induce her to change her eating, smoking, drinking and activity habits, and may prescribe tablets which she is to take on trust. They also have the controlling power over that most mysterious event, the birth: they claim to know what it will feel like and how it will happen; they can rule whether she has a caesarian or a vaginal birth; they possess secrets about procedure and process that she cannot even begin to discover until she is immersed in them; they might let her into the various choices or else, they can make decisions for her. But above all, during her antenatal care, their importance lies in their ability to gain and share with her, their understanding of the unknown – what and who is happening inside her.

At times, the antenatal professional may be so preoccupied with the well-being of his/her other client, the fetus, that the mother's thirst for knowledge is neglected. This is particularly the case where emphasis on the physiological overrides the psychological. Some women may comply, obediently attending antenatal clinic and classes yet feeling she has become merely a container – an 'incubator' – which must be maintained to provide optimal conditions for the growing fetus. Knowing what is happening seems superfluous. She needn't bother herself about it. Indeed, some professionals too, are convinced that mothers-to-be with a 'little bit of knowledge' are bound to 'meddle with the works'. Since she cannot know it all, better steer her away from questions and explanations. Not very long ago, the pregnant woman was told by the British Medical Association antenatal clinic handout manual: 'Never worry your head about any of these (examinations and chest X-rays) . . . they are necessary, they are in the interests of your baby and yourself and none of them will ever hurt you' [12].

However, we must recognize that the pregnant women's search for knowledge is not a form of idle curiosity but a sign of health. It is the beginning of responsibility as a mother and an attempt to reorientate herself by finding landmarks in an unfamiliar situation. It is a way of gaining access to an inpenetrable enigma that she lives with day in, day out, every instant of her pregnancy. Another person is growing underneath the skin of her body for whom she has life and death responsibility and she does not even know him or her! Little wonder that she turns to an outsider as a soothsayer, a bearer of news and imparter of information. The wonder is that we professionals could regard this information as belonging to anyone else other than the vital 'hostess'.

9.1.5 **The image of the professional as soothsayer**

Most cultures address the issue of Nature vs. Nurture – are we the malleable products of our environment or does basic personality exist from the start? These questions find purchase in the pregnant woman's mind – is she merely a hothouse for a preprogrammed baby or is she influential? Is she inadvertently liable, even prenatally, to change the course of his/her development and should she be deliberately acting in particular ways to ensure optimal achievement?

In traditional societies, women's anxieties are allayed by a predetermined range of ritual observances and avoidances, which are calculated by the elders to protect the baby from harmful influences and to procure a good outcome. As has been suggested, these shared beliefs, based on tacit cultural assumptions and an explanatory theory about the nature of their world, have evolved culturally to deal with the unforeseeable and politically, to maintain social control over childbearing. From the woman's own subjective point of view, such traditions acknowledge her anxieties as normal and assuage her fears about malevolent forces projected outside while reinforcing her internal benevolent desires to protect the baby. The pregnant woman may be regarded as reborn in a 'new bodiliness' – a progressive 'opening' of her body once shut by virginity. Gynaecological anomalies, whether the 'closed, bound, tied, entangled' states of barrenness or the complications of spontaneous abortion, premature birth, or still-birth, are subject to group diagnostic and therapeutic responsibility, including consulting a divinatory oracle and intervention which reintegrates the patient into 'the cycle of the continuation of the generations' [13].

In our own society, where these same basic psychosocial transitional needs have no overt traditional expression, a range of ritual activities have developed to fill the gap in proscribed behaviour and taboos. The pregnant woman clutches at any straw and uses what is available to her to meet her own needs for control over uncertainty. As with traditional witchdoctors, our western professional mystification and formalization of the split between 'scientific' understanding of physiological processes of pregnancy and the lay-woman's 'ignorance' of what is occurring within her, make the pregnant woman more susceptible to compliance. Indeed, her submissive obedience is often necessary to further political aims of centralizing childbirth. A major focus of professional activity has centred on institutionalized antenatal health care. The pregnant woman has been encouraged to attend clinics regularly, and follow a prescribed medicalized course of investigations. However, since their meaning has not been explained, to the prospective mother, weigh-ins, 'mid-stream' urine samples and blood pressure cuffs often have taken on ceremonial rather than medical importance during the long weeks when the expectant mother feels she has so little influence over the forces of pregnancy and so few rituals to mark the passing of time.

9.1.6 Ceremonies and taboos of pregnancy

These mysterious 'rites' are performed by professional 'high priests and priestesses' who often collude with the woman's transference and her suggestible need to believe in powerful authority figures, by patronizingly advocating blind obedience without informed understanding or feedback. Experts impart instructions to their pregnant clients who, in the absence of rational explanation, begin to feed off home-spun superstition and use expert advice as a magical means of alleviating anxieties about inadvertently harming or being harmed by the fetus. Another British Medical Association manual stressed the woman should 'keep herself regular' (bowels) adding paternalistically without specifying any reasons: 'Attention to your appearance and hygiene in pregnancy is very important, so make a special point of keeping yourself well-groomed, well-washed and sweet smelling' [14]. An influential consultant obstetrician warns 'suggestible' pregnant women readers of his book against 'Old Wives Tales' while simultaneously forbidding them to cross their legs during pregnancy, without ever explaining why [15]. Other experts specify activities to be avoided, such as hanging up washing or mountaineering, evoking fantasies based on folkloristic links with ideas about the cord becoming twisted as a result. Current 'remedies' for avoidance of stretchmarks similarly become ritualized, as do specialized diets, nipple treatment, the latest breathing exercises or high-tech routine investigations. Sadly, in their pregnant vulnerability and desire to do what they were told was best for their babies, many pregnant women tended in the past to trust blindly and follow their expert guides, who, in turn, did not always question the accepted practice. The appalling outcome of thalidomide and the long-term effects of diethylstilboestrol (DES) prescription to 3 million women during pregnancy shook the complacency of consumers and professionals alike. However, one recent study of a community antenatal clinic found that 93% of women had taken 'something' during pregnancy, the majority of which were iron and vitamin tablets, analgesics, antibiotics, antiemetics, antacids and laxatives [16]. Many drugs prescribed in Ireland still carry no pregnancy warning although they may have contraindications in the UK, and vice versa [17], and some of the latest technological advances, new inventions and current medical 'fashion', may, like ultrasound scanning, lack the necessary safety-clearing of randomized controlled clinical trials [18] or, like routine fetal monitoring, show no clear benefit and pose a higher likelihood of caesarian sections [19].

9.1.7 Increasing the expectant mother's involvement in her pregnancy care

The combination of the client's acquiescent unquestioning trust and the professional's empty reassurances or unexplained advice, results in activities becoming unconsciously rooted in sympathetic magic (nutritional instructions interpreted as taking iron or eating sweet and wholesome things to produce a 'good' or 'strong' baby); while other instructions may take on properties of contagious magic (recommendations to 'relax', 'read a good book' or 'take care of her appearance' seeming to indicate that such activities will enhance the baby's appreciation of beauty or culture).

We may dismiss these as laughable superstitions, or else, earnestly address ourselves to the power issue underlying some professional's need for activity and control. Pregnant women are more than the physiological containers of growing fetuses. Each woman is a potentially responsive and thoughtful person set on a course of being a mother to the baby (not 'fetus') inside her. Submissive obedience to expert advice may make her a 'good client' in a busy clinic but is not good practice for a woman about to become a responsible mother. Obtaining the woman's intelligent cooperation in her own antenatal preparation for the baby, increases the likelihood of her looking after herself post-partum. Similarly, listening attentively to a pregnant woman's reported problems and symptoms will encourage her to take her own observations seriously, to recognize signs of fetal distress, and to act promptly when danger signals. Recent experiments of women holding and reading their own notes (the total and sole obstetric chart of pregnancy) has resulted in one study of 250 women with only one woman arriving in labour without her records [20]. Finally, encouraging considered and well-informed choices by providing in-depth information and a variety of real alternatives also has an educational function in heightening the woman's awareness of health options and encouraging her own desire to meet the needs of her future baby in an individualized and thoughtful way.

9.1.8 Campaigners for reproductive rights

The 1960s saw the establishment of three major consumer groups, the National Childbirth Association (later 'Trust)') influenced by the findings of Grantly Dick Read, the Society for Prevention of Cruelty to Pregnant Women (later to become AIMS – the Association for Improvement of Maternity Services) and the National Association for Welfare of Children in Hospital influenced by work on maternal separation by Bowlby and the Robertsons at the Tavistock Institute, and more recently by Klaus and Kennell's work on neonatal bonding [21]. Their influence led to many advances involving both parents in pregnancy and birth. However, the ideological changes in all western countries of women regaining proprietorship of self and body have been far greater. Only 7 years have passed since thousands of people gathered on Hampstead Heath for a birth rights rally to protest about hospitals which denied women the right to participate in decisions and exercise choice about 'where and how to push their own babies out of their own bodies' [22]. A massive survey involving 6000 29-page completed questionnaires published the same year found that one in three of these respondents had not enjoyed her pregnancy, one in four did not enjoy the birth, 73% had never met the midwife who delivered the baby and nearly two-thirds felt they did not have reasonable freedom of choice about the position in which they gave birth [23]. *The Good Birth Guide* compiled a few years earlier had already made women more aware of the possibility of exerting choice to encourage hospitals to offer unavailable options by granting them 1–4 'star' status, like hotels [24]. Routine practices, epidural anaesthesia and drugs administered in childbirth and pregnancy have all begun to be questioned by consumers and a recent consumer organization, CERES, has been established to examine the ethical issues of medical research.

However, campaigners in this field have not merely been consumers and their partners. Midwives too, have rallied and queried the erosion of their role as upholders and mediators of women's reproductive rights. And this trend continues. Many changes are taking place not only in labour wards but within antenatal care, acknowledging the reciprocity of mothers and reproductive health-care workers. In a recent book on *'Sensitive Midwifery'* a central question revolves around how consumers could best benefit from antenatal visits and proposes innovative ways in which the care system can be run as a service that both meets the consumer's needs and increases the midwife's job satisfaction. This includes each midwife holding her own appointment diary, visiting her own clients in their homes or being a 'hostess' in her own clinic, inviting clients by friendly personalized letter for antenatal care (enclosing explanations about procedures), seeing her clients throughout the pregnancy, introducing women to each other, providing an educational function including discussions, films and talks and following each woman through the birth [25]. With this kind of concern for consumers, it is not surprising that women respond in their tens of thousands when a caring professional is suspended from her duties.

9.2 REACTIONS TO TESTS

9.2.1 The professional as interpreter of test results

In many western clinics, women routinely undergo ultrasound investigations at particular points in the pregnancy. Nevertheless, tests such as these which disclose detailed and potentially threatening information about the fetus, cannot be treated lightly however indiscriminately they are given. The woman herself faces them with trepidation: to her, scanning raises the possibility of discovering fetal defect, and however optimistically she approaches it, ultrasound becomes a 'Truth Test' which may determmine her baby's future. However, the 'oracle' is invariably obscured by the technician. It is still fairly rare for the screen to be placed at an angle where the woman can actually see her own fetus, for the scan operator to include her by pointing out what may be seen of her closest relative or offer her a photograph as a treasured momento. This extraordinary experience of being able to grasp visually what is hidden from sight, becomes a mundane task to the busy professional and a frustrating, tantalizing almost-event to the woman. Even if she can see the screen, she cannot make head or tail of the image and, often, no-one bothers to help her. What might have been a major 'bonding' session with her unborn child becomes a bladder-popping nightmare of endurance followed by an interminable wait for casually imparted results.

Conversely, where she and/or her partner are included in the experience, this event can become the turning point in prenatal bonding. Once the wriggling fetus is seen, there can be no doubt about its liveliness and humanity ('I swear he was waving to me!'). Maternal attachment to the fetus has been found to be enhanced by fetal movement perception [26]. Ultrasound enables both father and mother to become aware of fetal movement before it is actually experienced, hence, hastens the advent of second phase of pregnancy – awareness of the fetus as a separate, autonomous individual (Chapter 5). Indeed, studies have found a more positive response to pregnancy and the fetus following routine ultrasound screening for dates [27]. A study of the short-term psychological effects of ultrasound scanning during pregnancy found that its contribution is optimally informative and emotionally rewarding when women are given detailed feedback as a result of which they report feeling significantly 'more confident, more informed, involved, reassured and relieved' [28]. Women who have the test due to raised serum AFP (alpha fetoprotein) naturally find ultrasound more distressing than those having a routine test, but all respondents have expressed a wish to have sight of the screen, and to be given a running commentary, explanatory information and opportunity to ask questions [29].

In cases where the test does reveal abnormalities, radiographers are loathe to be the one to disclose bad news and are unauthorized to do so. Hence their predilection to obscure the screen and remain silent or non-communicatively cheerful throughout the ordeal. Nevertheless, we overlook the fact that very often bad news merely confirms what the pregnant woman has already steeled herself to meet after being offered the test (however routinely) and that attempts to normalize the situation with jolly chit-chat or conceal facts with awkward silence both alert the woman and leave her on emotional tenterhooks with her imagination running riot, often for some hours or even days until she is finally told the situation by the doctor in charge.

This problem has been the subject of much consumer discussion. A *British Medical Journal* editorial (1986) suggests explaining to mothers in advance that information on the fetus 'may best be witheld in confidence until management decisions have been made' [30]. However, advocates for improvements in the maternity services suggest streamlining the service by training specialized obstetric sonographers to be proficient in scan interpretation, evaluation and diagnosis combined with counselling skills and technical expertise [31]. In the meanwhile, professionals need to be aware that such 'routine' antenatal procedures are potentially emotionally disturbing rather than merely 'reassuring' to pregnant women, involving adverse psychological stress. In addition, tests such as these often arouse protracted worry about deleterious effects of the test itself on the fetus, and indeed, many experts argue that the long-term risks to living tissue of exposure to high-intensity ultrasound used in sophisticated diagnostic equipment are as yet unknown. Finally, many women hold unrealistic expectations about the potential of these tests for diagnosing abnormality, such that birth of a damaged baby may come as an unprecedented shock [32]. Conversely, with diagnostic refinements in prenatal screening an increasing number of lesser disorders can be detected, raising ethical, social and political issues which are only now being addressed [33].

9.2.2 Amniocentesis

Occurring as it does in the fourth month of pregnancy, this test looms large, as it will determine whether the woman can keep her baby or whether, as she half fears anyway, it will be snatched away from her. In a recent study, 78% of clients awaiting amniocentesis reported experiencing anxiety; 67% were anxious about a fetal injury and 53% worried about miscarriage [34]. Amniocentesis is a watershed – not a medical procedure but a life event. It is followed by a long wait for a verdict, during which the pregnancy feels as if 'suspended in limbo', neither cancelled nor affirmed. If the result is positive relief is great. Indeed, it may feel as if the pregnancy had been given a seal of approval and there is more assurance that there will be a baby at the end of it. If, in addition to a 'clean bill of health', the woman asks to be told the sex of the baby, part of the enigma melts away as she begins relating to a person of a particular gender who gradually acquires a name, clothes, a cot to reside in.

However in addition to their potentially fatalistic prophecy, fetoscopy and amniocentesis (un-like other tests such as post-rubella titre estimates and spina bifida blood sampling) also do pose a small possibility of inducing miscarriage in an otherwise healthy pregnancy. There are many women who do not relax into their pregnancy at all while awaiting these tests in their 17th week. They feel they are living on 'borrowed time', are reluctant to become attached to the moving fetus which might be snatched away or, worse, deliberately cut out ('everything has been dominated by the amniocentesis – it has been the biggest gamble of my life. I'm unable to deal with any of the alternatives it presents except a healthy baby. I can't allow the baby to become real and dreamt I was bathing a cooing, gurgling baby. Next thing I knew it had disappeared and I searched desperately but it had been washed down the drain as the plug came out, like a miscarriage or abortion'). Few women have these tests done lightly. In addition to the sense of endangering the fetus by allowing a needle to be jabbed into her abdomen, she knows full well that the results might expose her to a murderous dilemma: to kill or risk committing herself to a life sentence of endurance. During the 1–2 week waiting period for the 'Day of Judgement' following amniocentesis, although she tries to keep her emotions in abeyance, hope vies with grief, life-creating expectations conflict with death-dealing plans as the woman prepares herself for the worst: having to come to terms with the idea of terminating the pregnancy if gross abnormality or chromosomal deficiency is revealed or else contemplating a life of dedication to a handicapped child. Some women, unable to confront the enormity of personal responsibility, become fatalistic, flippant, blank or downright angry at having their pregnant serenity so disturbed by this hypothetical dilemma. Conversely, others feel that without the test they cannot relax until the birth.

9.2.3 Sexing the baby

Where results are satisfactory, a woman is naturally relieved. However, a spin-off of amniocentesis, 'sexing the baby', brings about its own dilemma. Does she really want to 'break the seal' before the birth and discover whether her baby is a girl or boy? Alternatively, can she bear not to know its gender, when strangers already do? Once again, this raises fantasies of 'tampering' with the mysteries of nature, requesting forbidden knowledge or foregoing it. With acquisition of gender the fetus is transformed from a mysterious unknown being into one with a definite identity. Clearly, the decision must be the mother's. However, at times a gap exists between her conscious desire to know the secret and her unconscious fears of knowing resulting in postknowledge-resentment at having had the choice at all and fear at having broken a taboo.

Furthermore, in communities which emphasize male primogeniture or superiority, amniocentesis tests may be abused as a means of sex detection. A study reported by *India Today* (31.1.88) showed that of 1000 abortions following amniocentesis, 97% were of female fetuses, leading to a possible change in legislation of these tests being used solely for detection of genetic disorders [35].

9.2.4 Infections, threatened miscarriage, missed abortion and ectopic pregnancy

Women who experience illness, spotting, bleeding or other symptoms during their pregnancy may be alarmed by these, alerting their GP or midwife immediately, or else may wait to 'allow nature to take its course' or seem unaware that anything unusual is happening. Sometimes the consultation may be made over the phone on the basis of description of symptoms or quality of bleeding. Some women may experience no symptoms but complain of no longer feeling pregnant even though bleeding has not occurred. While all these conditions will be discussed at length in Chapter 30, here we will briefly focus on the role of the professional as mediator between the woman and the meaning of her symptoms, helping her to understand the significance of what is happening in her body for herself, the fetus and the pregnancy, tiding her over the waiting period (which in the case of infections such as rubella or HIV may last beyond birth) and helping her to make the psychological transition from being pregnant to 'unpregnant' when loss is not preventable. In cases where a complication looms, a professional who has had ongoing contact with the woman during her pregnancy and perhaps, as in the case of a GP, before it, will be more aware of the nature of the emotional investment of this particular woman in her pregnancy and fetus, and how best to impart information to her. Unfortunately, in many cases the diagnosis is done in hospital by professionals who are strangers to the woman. Empathy is of prime importance, trying to experience what the woman must be feeling, gauging the amount of information she can take in, enabling her to express her anxieties, grief and vulnerability safely. She will need reassurance about her role in causing the problem, repeated explanations and follow-up, possibly including home visits. However as a female GP notes, women doctors may over-empathize with a problem they themselves have experienced to the point of clinical competence being hindered or be liable to aloofness when threatened by other women's maternity and its failure [36]. In many ways, all professionals are vulnerable when exposed to their own inability to prevent loss. Having to deal with the raw emotional suffering of another person without being able to do much to alleviate its cause, is a painful position to be in. When these emotions spillover into tears or angry accusations, it may feel easier for the professional to escape rather than comfort the woman in need. Embarrassment is partly due to lack of training in counselling skills and lack of opportunity to explore one's own deeper feelings. Staff support groups have been found helpful in relieving emotional stress.

9.25 'Positive' test results

Receiving 'positive' results of these tests constitutes a major blow to some women. When an abnormality has been discovered, extremely sensitive evaluation of the results and their subsequent transmission to the people involved is imperative, often requiring concurrent support and counselling in the face of the forthcoming decision-making and lifelong traumatic implications. Every attempt should be made to help the couple arrive at a joint decision. More importantly, particular efforts must be made to give the woman, who is to bear the brunt of the outcome, time and private space to verbalize her dilemma freely and express her own ambivalent feelings and the conflicts she may have with her partner and family, at this junction well into her pregnancy. Once the decision is made, whether to keep the baby or abort it, it is a binding one, the after-effects of which will remain with her for the rest of her life. Although the decision made may seem to be based on rational considerations it is most likely also to be influenced by unconscious emotional factors, relating not only to her present life conditions but to her past experience all the way back to her own infancy and feelings about babies in her family of origin.

Thus, it is not enough to impart the burden of bad news onto the woman/couple and abandon her/them to their lonely choice. The professional involved has a further informative role, to answer questions as they arise and repeat the answers in simple yet not simplistic terms, until the information is absorbed. Explanations will be needed about the possible causes of abnormality and implications of these findings. S/he will be required to provide a clear picture of the options, the quality of life expectancy for the abnormal baby as well as its duration, the availability of medical cure, amelioration or rectification of the condition, now and in the foreseeable future. Parents will also want an indication of the amount of professional help they will receive and the nature of daily conditions should they choose to have the child. They need to know the likelihood of diagnostic error and the probability of having a normal child should they choose to conceive again. In addition, the obstetric specialist must recognize his/her limitations and facilitate urgent provision of personal psychotherapeutic help if needed. Information can only serve as a guideline and framework within which the woman on her own or with her partner can envisage the future. A woman or couple who feel their internal resources ebbing away with their hopes will need bolstering up and access to deeper understanding during this crucial time of urgently making basic Life and Death decisions.

9.2.6 Decision-making and aftercare

Furthermore, once the decision is taken, follow-up care is needed. Support, help and guidance will be required during the rest of the pregnancy, and possibly the rest of their lives, for those who have decided to take their chances and have the child. Although some tests, such as CVS (chorionic villus sampling) may detect abnormalities during the first trimester, most others like fetoscopy and amniocentesis are performed between 16 and 18 weeks, meaning that by the time results are given, the women involved have experienced movement. Abortion counselling is hindered by time constrictions, which may determine the type of abortion she has, whether she can still have a suction abortion or a more complicated second trimester abortion. Nevertheless, although timing is crucial, most women need to spend precious time evaluating their motivation to keep or reject the fetus and to work through immediate conflicts.

A woman who has decided to abort will in effect go through childbirth with no prize at its end. She needs just as much, if not more, attention from nursing staff, as one having a live birth. With prostaglandin or saline induction, she needs to be verbally primed and taken through the various steps of the procedure, preparing her to anticipate the pain, onset of 'labour', the expulsion and its aftermath. She needs to foresee the immediate emotional toll of the experience: exacerbation of breast tenderness and possible lactation with no baby to suckle, followed by gradual loss of evidence that she has been pregnant at all, a hollow emptiness, sense of guilt and probable depression. Where possible, post-abortion counselling should be offered to work through the physical and emotional experiences of the actual abortion, her current reactions to the baby's father, family and pregnant friends, her own anger, guilt and grief at having been forced by the test results to undo the pregnancy she had already decided to keep. The woman is entitled to recognition of her state of bereavement. Although staff may feel she is better off rid of her burden, the unfortunate woman has lost her investment in the future. She is no longer a mother-to-be but 'un-pregnant', belonging neither to the world of pregnant anticipation nor yet able to return to her pre-pregnant state. She needs support during this period of slow recovery if she is to retain realistic faith in her creative capacity. (Further discussion of issues around abortion may be found in Chapter 29).

9.2.7 Moral, ethical and religious dilemmas

Finally, women in this state of emotional vulnerability are very sensitive to subtle signs of rejection or disrespect on the one hand, or condescending care on the other. This is an issue where professional awareness of the diversity of cultural attitudes is essential. Although nurses may have a straightforward expectation that the woman's problem is medically soluble by abortion, moral, religious and ethical dilemmas further complicate the issue. Thus, for instance, while Buddhist and Hindu theology do not prohibit abortion, an ethos of preserving life, however minute, counteracts it. Muslim scriptures suggest that life begins at 150 days after conception, Shinto religion believes life begins at birth, Judaism regards the fetus as part of the mother until its birth. However all these have a strict morality forbidding the taking of life. Abortion is prohibited in Talmudic law unless endangering the mother's life (or the result of an adulterous union), however, it is not seen to constitute murder. Nevertheless, in recent years prohibition on abortion is still upheld even in cases of mothers taking thalidomide or contracting rubella unless justified on grounds of the mother's health [37]. The Catholic Church prohibits abortion although tolerating it when underlying pathology demands it, and other churches maintain it is permissible when there is a strict medical necessity. Thus, the ethical issue of sin remains. Since abortion is tacitly disapproved of by many religious and social bodies, it is essential that professional staff are aware of their own possible ambivalence towards the issue and can be accepting and non-judgemental towards women who have had to make this difficult decision.

A woman who has had the experience of being given time and space to work through her distressing conflict under the guidance of compassionate and reliable people, can retain a sense of being cared for and having some control over her own fate at a time when Fate seems particularly cruel and uncaring towards her. Apart from the immediate benefits, such care inevitably helps foster a hopeful process of growing to believe that another pregnancy might have a positive outcome or coming to terms with genetic intervention, childlessness, or adoption. Genetic counselling must therefore be an integral part of follow-up care after an abortion due to fetal abnormality and even if she is not at risk, particular supportive attention must be given to the woman during any pregnancy that follows this traumatic termination.

Part Three

THE EXPECTANT PARTNER

Chapter 10

The father-to-be

Little one, lately/When you come to me,/
In the bed there seem/Not two, but three.
The third one, this stranger/On your side,
Has a burglar's eyes,/Where shall we hide?
He has cracked privacy/And flashes the sun
On us, like a torch,/Little one, little one.
. . . No, no, I love you./Do not cry. Please.
What I just said/Was merely to tease. (Taufiq Rafat, Pakistan. p. 33 in
I like that Stuff, Cambridge University Press, 1984.)

10.1 THE BURGEONING BELLY

10.1.1 Paternal experience and cultural variations

In many cultures, it is only at the point of conception that a marriage
is truly recognized by the extended family. As a woman's swelling begins
to disclose signs of a pregnancy creating blood-ties to her in-laws, she
is allocated a new position between the generations and between the
clans. It has been said that 'in the last analysis, a marriage is the
incorporation of a stranger into a group' [1]. Usually, the woman is the
stranger to her husband's family/clan/tribe and her incorporation into
her husband's group is via her child. Her man's acknowledgement of
the bond establishes him as father of the child to be. Of necessity, in
the absence of physical markers of pregnancy, he is dependent on social
tags and rituals declaring his expectant state. Thus, for all women but
adoptive mothers, pregnancy and motherhood is a biological fact.
Fatherhood is always a social construction. This basic difference has
pervaded the gendered experiences of pregnancy anywhere, anytime.
A man may have a child and not know it. He may have a child, of which
he is not the father. He is only a father if he acknowledges paternity and/
or engages in fathering behaviours. In western society, in recent years
'illegitimate' births have risen from 4% to 20% of all babies born. However, over half of these are registered by both parents, many of whom

continue to reside together although not married to each other [2]. On the other hand, as social mores regarding unmarried mothers change and single pregnant women elect to keep their babies while would-be-mothers among single women have easier access to artificial insemination, there are many truly 'single parent' families in which a father does not figure, even as a name. (Nevertheless, in these families too, as long as we retain a patriarchal bias, the awesome Father figure is present even in his absence, as an abstraction and as a representative of societal-law.) Finally, a new feature of our modern western world are many single parent households involving a father bringing up his child/ren on his own. In the USA, there are currently well over one million such families.

10.1.2 Acknowledgement of paternity

In some traditional societies paternal activity ritually begins only once the child is a certain age, when the child finally acquires the father's name. In others, conversely, it is the father who acquires a new name after the birth, and is now known as the father of his child ('Abu-X'). (In some cultures, this custom does not assert paternity but aims to protect the father's secret name from being divulged to others for fear of abuse.) In yet other societies, paternal recognition occurs even before birth. This may take the form of certain ceremonial rites or personal demonstrative gestures towards his wife or the woman pregnant with his child. Acknowledgement of paternity during pregnancy may involve protective activities which engage him directly, such as dietary restrictions, contact taboos, domestic avoidances or public rites to secure the child's safe delivery. In our own society, in the absence of a marital bond, or cohabitation, the partner's attendance at antenatal classes, clinics and/or the birth often constitutes a public acknowledgement of paternity.

10.1.3 Couvade

The ritual couvade has been practised throughout the world and was described by Diodorus Siculus in 60 BC [3]. Subject to local variations, it consists of simulation of pregnancy symptoms or childbirth, or abstinence from activities (hunting or dietary restrictions).

Much of the ethnographic literature has focused on couvade as a particular form of paternal acknowledgement – those ritualized practices, engaged in by the male mate of a parturient woman which mimic pregnancy, confinement and/or childbirth. These may involve the man retching with symptoms of 'morning sickness' during early pregnancy, or taking to his bed, writhing with 'labour pains' while she feeds and cossets him, or it may even take the form of him displacing her in the delivery-place immediately after the birth and 'nursing' the baby for 14 or 40 days. The last instance clearly encourages creation of a bond between father and baby, while, however, ousting the mother from the primary role. And indeed, paternal customs appear to serve many purposes on both intrapsychic and interpersonal levels – cathartic, integrative, political, ideological functions, to name but a few.

We may therefore treat couvade as a means of:

a.   Socially acknowledging the father of the child;
b.   Giving the man a protective role of diverting evil-spirits away from mother and baby;
c.   Deflecting his own ambivalence and sense of rejection by involving him in parallel creative activities while he is excluded from his wife's birth-chamber;
d.   Facilitating his empathic identification with her discomfort while mitigating destructive envy of her creative capacity to grow, contain, deliver and nourish life;
e.   Furthermore, not only does couvade encourage association with the maternal role, it also draws him into identification with the baby, being pampered and sharing in the infant's glory, rather than stewing in jealous resentment.

Couvade thus provides public recognition, social concern and an emotional outlet for the father in competition with mother and baby. We might say that whatever its form, couvade is designed to protect both mother and baby from the dangers of father's ambivalence and rivalry [4] while providing him with a focal role.

Many studies have revealed an increased incidence of psychological disturbance and psychosomatic pregnancy-related symptoms such as digestive problems, swellings, dental problems, backache, vomiting, weight gain, etc., in western fathers-to-be which may be considered as a non-formalized type of couvade [5–9] and although often related to anxiety about the birth, the relationship of the syndrome to this event may not be perceived by the sufferer [10].

10.1.4 Early identifications

Thus, for the man, pregnancy arouses not only male identification with the father, but the father-to-be identifies with his mother, too. This is not as bizarre as it sounds, since, as we have noted, in almost every human society, during their early years, boys as well as girls are brought up by a female primary caregiver, usually the mother. Therefore, when the father is less involved in early care, for both male and female children, earliest identification is with a maternal woman. Fathers serve many roles in babyhood, not least in offering alternative stimulation to the baby and replenishing the mother. The more exclusive the maternal care, the greater the need, with growing independence, to detach from their powerful mother and the fearful attraction of sinking back into fusion with her. The little boy breaks away from an engulfing early mother by emphasizing his difference from her. Like the girl, he is painfully disillusioned of 'unisex' fantasies about his unlimited potential, his omnipotent desire to be and have everything, a penis, breasts and capacity to give birth. When mother has been the primary caretaker he now has to 'dis-identify'[11] from the female who served as his sole original model in order to pursue masculine identification with his phallic father.

Interestingly, we find that in societies which emphasize prolonged suckling, there exist greatest envy, over-compensation and symbolic preoccupation with differentials between men and women [12]. Where boys are brought up mainly by women, male separateness develops into strong 'macho' institutions, with elaborate initiation rites and ceremonials to asset manhood, and to isolate themselves from women. Because motherhood is so much more easily grasped than fatherhood, the boy, exposed to maternal lactation and pregnancy, is forced from his early experience to realize himself as different from his mother, unable to make babies in his own body. Although some readers may feel I am overemphasizing this point, so central is this issue for mankind that anthropologist Margaret Mead has declared that 'the recurrent problem of civilization is to define the male role satisfactorily enough' to provide men with the sense of 'irreversible achievement granted women naturally in childbearing' [13].

Sociologists have stressed the irony of the absent western father who, in his elusiveness, presents a fallacious model for his children: his masculine reality is unknown; his work is elsewhere; its product is often intangible; he is largely unavailable to serve as a role-model and when he is at home, he is at leisure. The result is that many western boys have to construct his masculinity in negative terms, defined not by what it is but rather by all things feminine that it is not. In the past, boys have been taught that to be 'real' boys and later 'manly' men, they must repudiate any vestiges of their early feminine identification with their mothers. In societies of ideological male supremacy, unavailability of an early nurturing father means that the boy's negatively defined masculinity depricates female creativity or appropriates it, as we shall see below. Furthermore, since femaleness becomes associated with activity that excludes males, maleness has been largely underwritten and emphasized by practices and occupations which men deem forbidden to women.

10.1.5 The father and genesis – as conceived across cultures and generations

The genesis of offspring is not merely a bodily interaction but occurs within a complex social structure of complementary relationships which define the psychosocial origins of the baby, and the values placed upon the progenitive capacities of the father and of the mother.

In some cultures, not only does the father become the focus of social attention but he may actually supplant the centrality of the pregnant woman in procreativity. Social custom may declare that he has made the baby, she has merely 'grown' it. Such beliefs do not reflect ignorance of the facts of paternal contribution to procreation but an underlying ideology about the relative social importance of men and women. In some societies, there is a belief that the mother merely gives the child its body, while the father gives its soul [14]. Some practices of seclusion of baby and father after birth revolve around acquisition of the soul. Likewise, early protective rituals in many cultures restate the idea that it takes some time before the baby becomes fully 'human' and 'complete'. In some aetiological accounts of reproduction, the woman's contribution is minimized to merely functioning as container for the miniature 'homunculus' which the potent man has planted in her in seed form. Thus, although as we have noted, the egalitarian ancient Egyptians in 1400 BC recognized that both man's seed and woman's 'germ' contribute to conception, a thousand years later patriarchally minded Greek Aristotle assumed that 'the female does not contribute something to generation' [15] except the menstrual blood which was the material out of which the embryo was made, having been 'fixed' by the male semen. This attitude is not as far removed from our own 'modern' one as it appears. Many obstetric practices we encounter have been rooted in a paternalistic medical model based on the idea of woman as carrier of man's child, which is regarded as a foreign body lodged in her own whose needs are different from hers and necessitate her self-sacrificial attitude. Feminists have pointed out that according to this patriarchal model, drugs are evaluated on the grounds of medications harmful to the embryo rather than mother–fetus seen as an integral unit (i.e. nausea as a sign of protein deficiency). Likewise, labour may be regarded as a medical event to ensure quick and safe conduct for the (husband's) baby rather than a 'birthing' experience for mother and baby [16,18].

Paradoxically, the actual father may be overlooked. He may also be absent or minimized in conception. The Virgin Mother is a cherished myth that displaces the male progenitor, thereby both denying maternal sexuality and deflecting male rivalry between father and son ('*my* mother never did *that*'). Participation of a 'spirit' in conception occurs as we have seen in cultures as disparate as the Trobriand islanders, Australian aborigines and ancient Indians (Chapter 8). The latter imagined that a male child is conceived when the sperm is stronger than the ovum, and the reverse is true for a girl. This belief is not uncommon among modern 'macho' men who may unconsciously regard a baby boy to be special proof of their virility.

10.1.6 The dilemma of western expectant fathers

In western societies, fathers-to-be often feel themselves to be disadvantaged. Like their counterparts in traditional societies, despite having to achieve similar changes in self-image and identity as the expectant mother, the man has no visibly growing bulge or ongoing hormonal stimulation and physical experiences of change to punctuate his paternal development. In addition, there is usually little social recognition of his transitional state. Restricted by social conventions about masculine inexcitability, he is expected to pander to his pregnant woman's emotional disequilibrium, the expression of which is denied to him. In addition he lacks the support of built-in peer group identity, and those ritualized activities reinforcing the historical role of 'expectant father' about to move up the ladder towards the tribe-elders, which is provided to corresponding young men in traditional societies.

The dilemma of the western father-to-be is that he is confronted by the same transitional fears, anxieties and envy as his traditional counterpart, but has no transitional rites to express these. Each western man has to resort to his own individual means of finding social acknowledgement and achieving personal maturation during this period. This task is made more difficult by social restrictions on male expression of emotionality and a general tendency to focus on the pregnant woman's vulnerability and need for this protection. Constantly reminded of her susceptibility, he has to monitor ambivalent disclosures, and keep much of his own inner upheaval in check while forgiving her 'lapses' ('all her reactions are over the top these days – I try and keep my cool, but I also feel edgy – sometimes I wish I could just break down and cry and let it all out'). Driven underground, his feelings may erupt in strange and unconscious forms. Psychosomatic complaints may reveal his own unconscious need to experience the pregnancy physically. One multidisciplinary large-scale 4-year research project has found that up to 65% of prospective fathers developed symptoms resembling those of pregnancy, confirming that pregnancy is a critical period for fathers too [19]

Early 'uni-sex' wishes to be pregnant are revived, and while this period may be used by some fathers to work through reactivated envy of female creativity, nurturing their wives in identification with a nurturing mother, others deny the conflict through male competitiveness. The struggle to find affirmation and expression is reflected in the prevalence of expectant fathers' creative projects timed to coincide with pregnancy and reach their peak at the expected date of delivery. Some men try to share pregnancy: a growing number of fathers-to-be participate in preparatory classes on labour or prenatal courses on child care. Others also attend antenatal checkups with their wives or join in shopping expeditions for baby equipment. Nevertheless, despite the central upheaval in identity, it is rare that an expectant father has leisurely social opportunity to reflect upon the transformation of his relationship to his own father and mother as he becomes a father himself. Likewise, he is usually on his own with his awareness of the altered relationship to his wife and her changing figure, his worries and feelings about sexual contact and the revival or archaic fears of maternal powers of creation and destruction. It is here that discussion groups for expectant parents, both mixed and single sex, come into their own, by offering a means of exploring and working through some of the many feelings invariably aroused during this transitional life event. Similarly, prospective fathers who are in psychotherapy may relish this opportunity to allow feelings bubbling deep below the surface to rise and spill out in words.

KEY POINTS

*Fatherhood is a social construction. In the absence of physical markers, social or ritual acknowledgement of paternity establishes him as father of the child to be. The boy child, in turn, learns behavioural elements of 'masculinity' by secondary identification with his father, when the latter is absent or not involved in physical primary caregiving.

*Couvade provides public recognition and social concern for the father, enabling him to act in a protective capacity to protect both mother and baby from the dangers of father's ambivalence, rivalry and reactivated early envy of female creativity.

*In the West, attendance at antenatal classes, clinics and/or the birth often constitute such acknowledgement, while psychosomatic pregnancy-related symptoms may be seen as a form of couvade.

*The western father-to-be is doubly disadvantaged lacking both the physical experiences of change (of his partner), and the social recognition or ritual acknowledgement of his transitional state granted his traditional counterpart.

10.2 MATURATIONAL PHASES

Lacking a physiological component, the maturational phases in the father either roughly follow the trimesterial pattern of fetal growth as experienced via his pregnant partner or may evolve independently, focused on his own intrapsychic processes. Thus the initial response to being told of the pregnancy varies according to circumstances: whether conception was planned, mutually wanted, long awaited or surprisingly soon; its timing within the couple's emotional life together or apart; the manner of disclosure and the stage of pregnancy at which the man was told of his impending fatherhood.

10.2.1 Annunciation

In unplanned pregnacies the news may arouse shock, disbelief, guilt or a sense of being manipulated or entrapped in a relationship. Where the woman decides to continue her pregnancy against the wishes of her mate, their relationship may deteriorate into overt hostility, estrangement and eventual separation or covert antagonism. Where he prevails upon her to have the baby against her own better judgement, she may resent his symptom-free unpregnant exploitation of her as 'baby-machine' and vengefully expect him to carry full financial and/or practial responsibility for antenatal and child care. Conversely, sometimes a partner may seem obsolete once he has impregnated his woman, feeling rather like a spider about to be eaten by the mate he has fecundated. Ruminating that his only function in the relationship has been to provide her with the means of obtaining the child she craves to replace him in fulfilling her needs, his resentment may fester. Untreated, this state may result in a closed mother–baby dyad (twosome) based on mutual identification, excluding the colluding father. Given timely therapeutic help as a couple during pregnancy, a two-parent family may emerge. However, all too often, there is also professional collusion with this idea of the mother as solely responsible for her future infant, exemplified by a not uncommon practice of treating men attending prenatal parentcraft classes as 'invisible' or excluding them from antenatal clinics.

With planned pregnancies joyful tidings are not necessarily greeted with undiluted joy. Universally present preconceptual ambivalence stems from the unavoidable psychic fact, that on the level of unconscious narcissistic aspects of the parents, a child is always an intruder, a displacer, a rival, a threat. Thus even the most wished for, adored baby has had to overcome 'anti-reproductive trends' in his/her biological parents in order to be conceived and carried to term [20]. Realistically, conception heralds the end of exclusive dyadic intimacy for the couple. Two lovers are instantaneously transformed into a threesome, and awareness of the third 'sleeping' partner might affect sexual performance long before s/he becomes noticeably active. Nevertheless, where conception has been planned and awaited, and sex has become procreative rather than 'recreational', the news is greeted with pleasure, early pride, caution and, sometimes, unbridled excited elation.

10.2.2 Sexual intercourse

The father-to-be's preoccupation with the baby residing within the mother's womb may result in increased sexual activity – expressing both his tender affection for his pregnant mate and a means of caring for his growing baby, reaching out to the embryo inside the womb, nestling up close or even 'watering' or 'feeding' it in identification with the nurturing mother (penis = breast; semen = milk). A retrospective study of 103 expectant father's experiences of pregnancy found a substantial improvement in the men's sex lives following conception culminating at the end of the first trimester with new fantasies during lovemaking, of either an enriching or distracting and compulsive quality [21]. However, at other times, the expectant father may feel resentful towards the interloper, residing so peacefully in its father's 'place'.

In my clinical experience, in some men these ambivalent feelings may lead to decreased libido, fear of penetration or actual impotence reflecting concern about harming baby or mother during intercourse and a fear of being 'sucked back inside'. On an unconscious level, the father's close identification with the little interuterine fetus can lead to a sense of limp vulnerability. Impotence may signify that once he symbolically resides inside her in the form of his baby, he no longer feels the need vicariously to find his way back to the womb by means of his penetrating penis. Abstinence may also be the product of anxiety about the innocent, defenceless fetus being harmed by paternal intrusion or shocked by exposure to parental intercourse. Consciously, the expectant father may rationalize sexually abstaining as concern about dislodging the embryo through intercourse, a prevalent belief echoing traditional taboos on sex. Indeed, 30 years ago textbooks advised against coitus during the first three months and the last three months of pregnancy, although there is no evidence to suggest that these are related to adverse outcome [22]. Thus, already during the first trimester, even before the woman's bodily shape changes noticeably, and before fetal movements are experienced, the male partner is affected by the physical presence of his baby.

While during the second phase many men find their partner's pregnant bodies particularly attractive and sex unusually climatic, after the quickening, awareness of the fetus inside may be a 'turn off'. Although the baby now appears more robust and self-sufficient its very liveliness makes it more of a competitor for the woman's attention. Large enough to 'get between them' during intercourse, 'witnessing' private intimacies, s/he seems active enough to disrupt their love-making, to spy on the parents or even to 'grab' father's penis during intercourse! The woman's protuberant belly may also arouse old memories in the man of his own mother's pregnant body, reviving childhood jealousies of siblings whose birth disrupted his own intimate twosome with mother. This baby, too, may appear a rival, and the maternal pregnant woman, now equated with his mother, subject to incest taboos. Fantasies of a male fetus may arouse specific types of rivalry, a 'premonition' that a baby boy may take over, and overtake his father in his mother's affections (Freud claimed that a mother's relation to her son is 'altogether the most perfect, the most free from ambivalence of all human relationships' [23]). Such irrational ideas are by no means uncommon: we know that many fairy stories or legends, like the myth of Oedipus, begin with mountaintop exposure of a baby son by his threatened father. Among peoples such as the Eskimos and Spartans, where certain infants are abandoned to death as a threat to the race, it is the father who carries out the deed of exposure [24]. In recent years, a study of 51 first-time expectant fathers found rearoused oedipal feelings, sibling rivalry, reactivated infantile fantasies, feminine identifications as well as attempts to defend against ambivalent feelings through 'negation, denial, isolation, repression, intellectualization and reaction-formation' [25]. Another study describes expectant fathers' (of premature infants) preoccupation with gastro-intestinal symptoms during midpregnancy with a new focus on their 'insides', a wish to be both penetrated and penetrating and awareness of a sense of postcoital emptiness accompanied by prostatic contractions [26].

During the thrid trimester, the pregnant wife may loom so large and seem so strange as to be unrecognizable. Many men find this burgeoning fertile body quite magnificent, while others see it as endearingly overblown, 'flopping' about like a 'beached whale'. An expectant husband may find it rather exciting to have to evolve new sexual positions and techniques to accommodate his woman's altered anatomy. However, awareness of ambivalence towards both baby and wife create a 'dialectic between the notion of a nurturing and a punishing penis' [27]. Some men are so frightened of hurting the undeniably present fetus or their partner that they become unable to function sexually. Others find the ripening pregnant body repulsive or untouchable, disclosing their archaic anxieties, unresolved envy or deep-seated dread or maternal life-giving/death-dealing powers. However, their reduced sexual activity may also be the result of changes of libido in their partners. A study of female sexuality during pregnancy found marked reduction in frequency of intercourse in the third trimester and diminution of sexual enjoyment in 60% of women interviewed [28].

10.2.3 The father's father

On an intrapsychic level, the idea of becoming a father alters the father-to-be's relationship to his own parents as he ceases to be merely his father's son, and becomes a link within the continuous chain of genetic immortality ranging back to his great great grandparents and earlier, and forward to his own great grandchildren and onwards. Becoming a father thus inserts him into history. He is in the middle of the story, not the sole protagonist, no longer beginning and end of it. Orientation towards time alters with his changing sense of identity, and alongside identifica-tion with the fetus he once was inside his mother, a flurry of feelings come to the fore, related to the man who fathered him: love, fear, hatred, rejection towards the father he has had, tender yearning for the father he wishes he had had and poignant feelings about the father that he himself hopes/fears to become. As noted, sympathetic awareness of his own creative life-giving powers at a time when his father's are beginning to decline may increase the desire for a new reconciliation [29].

One study terms the midpregnancy turn towards father a 'fateful landmark in anticipatory fatherhood'. This work found that men who did not go through a 'refuelling' phase of sorting out in relationship to their own fathers seemed to become progressively less able to participate in the 'alliance of pregnancy', unable to turn away from vulnerability to feminine identification towards an internalized male mentor who could help them achieve a paternal role that was 'nurturant', involved and masculine'. In some men 'father hunger' due to his physical or emotional absence while growing up made them pursue 'males and maleness' through bisexual adventures or flagrant promiscuity in midpregnancy [30].

When a man's relationship with his own father has been particularly fraught, a further conflict may emerge as his wife becomes obviously more 'motherly' in appearance, related to resurfacing of unresolved oedipal dynamics. We now realize that all little children experience intense emotions towards their parents. As a little boy begins observing the differences between the sexes and acknowledging his own male gender, he has to relinquish his own desires to give birth like his mother and begin to experiment with becoming like his father, rivalrously wishing he, too, could have a baby with his beloved mother. Freud suggested that this desire was later repressed as the boy conceded the field to his stronger father under the threat of symbolic 'castration'. He extricates himself from the oedipal triangle, partially by repressing the conflict and by forming emotional attachments outside the family and partially by sublimation of his wishes through symbolic expression rather than behavioural enactment [31]. In adulthood, these early feelings are revived during pregnancy and making love to his expectant wife can become unconsciously equated with enactment of 'incest', and her pregnancy, evidence of his 'crime' of having usurped his own father. If he has not satisfactorily resolved these repressed primitive conflicts of love and hate, because of a too harsh or absent father, and/or if he did not have a satisfactory model of nurturant masculinity before the oedipal phase, current reactivation of old emotions will plunge him into regressive transactions with his 'internal' parents. In his inner psychic world, the image of 'Father' is occupied not by the real man, his father, now middle-aged, elderly or dead, but an abstraction of 'The Father', virile representative of an adult, authoritative world; the Father who is the Law-Giver, upholder of rank, establishment and male rule.

During pregnancy, confronted by a fertile, tender, motherly woman, oedipal anxieties are revived. Fears of impotence, passivity and/or a related dread of dying (being sucked back into the womb) may surface in him, expressing unconscious guilt and irrational fears of being castrated or killed as punishment for enacting his forbidden incestuous wishes. In sum, an anxious expectant father may feel the need to resort to extreme measures to relieve these archaic fears about retributive justice:

a. Denying that the child is his;
b. Becoming impotent, helpless and child-like in the marriage;
c. Distancing himself or developing an illness which prevents intimate contact;
d. Resorting to superstitious means of ensuring his safety;
e. Seeking out extramarital affairs or homosexual relationships;
f. Reverting to an unchallenging little-boy attitude towards his father and other men in authority;
g. Or, conversely, by a process of reaction-formation (doing the opposite) becoming belligerently possessive and challenging towards representatives of authority;
h. Counteracting fears of impotent passive waiting by promiscuity or reckless activity, such as dangerous driving and daredevil antics;
i. Developing psychosomatic symptoms which echo the process of pregnancy, thereby unconsciously 'choosing' to identify with the maternal love-object rather than copulate with her in rivalry to his father.

10.2.4 Maternal and paternal orientations

We have seen that masculinity and femininity are social constructs, determined by the culture in which they are defined. In western cultures, as in many others, masculinity has been associated with an 'instrumental' orientation of gettings things done, and problem solving whereas femininity, anchored in mothering, is seen to have an 'expressive' function, concerned with emotions, nurturance and welfare of others [32]. The latter feminine 'interconnected' orientation has been negatively contrasted by society with that of highly valued masculine independence and the male prerogative of concern for himself as an individual, and a free agent. Recent research has revealed this dual standard in the existence of two distinct moralities, a 'feminine' one that focuses more on complex interrelational aspects of issues such as abortion rather than a clear right/wrong division [33].

However, sex-role expectations appear to be gradually shifting with the double impact of Feminism and the cult of self-fulfilment. In line with Freud's belief in psychic 'bisexuality', recent research has focused on the concept of a single individual embodying within him/herself both 'masculine' and 'feminine' characteristics to varying degrees, although still defined and delimited by traditional sex-role identities and expectations of society. Whether and to what degree an individual is free to encompass traits associated with the other sex, is determined by a capacity to construe gender flexibly [34]. Both men and women are then freer of sex-typing and gender rules when definitive attributes of males and females pertain to recognition of anatomical genital differences important only for reproduction, defining gender in biological terms rather than restrictive cultural correlates [35]. These days, in the West, in addition to liberated women, we are seeing a new breed of young men who appear to cross the gender lines in their appearance, characteristics and interests. Nevertheless, they are not 'effeminate' in the old sense but rather seem 'feminine' and caring without losing their 'masculine' capacities. These 'all-rounders' become the nurturant fathers of a new generation of babies. Similarly, due to widespread influence of the Women's Movement, unlike their mothers, many young women no longer envisage themselves as appendages of men. Far from a future predicated on being 'feminine' to attract the right husband, and devoted caring for others, many a 21st century woman has a vision of self-realization, instrumental 'agent' of her own fate and creative enterprise, encompassing more than homemaking and having babies. Although our unconscious self-representations continue to harbour internalised cultural prescriptions, today many people embrace more fluid definitions of gender roles as Reciprocator parents attest, and they in turn, will raise children who can encompass a wider range of their own potentialities.

10.2.5 Gender and pregnancy

With pregnancy, gender is highlighted, as in few other situations. Following conception the biological bedrock is exposed as she grows their baby and he who sparked off the process, may not even know. Whereas in traditional societies paternal responses are governed by clearly defined social expectations, in westernized societies or those in transition, increasing liberalization of parental roles and childcare practices offer a variety of choices. Each man reacts to impending parenthood according to his current internal reality and personal construct of generative identity [see section 0.3.3]. His relationship with his father and degree of integration of his early identification with his mother, determines his adjustment to parenthood [see Chapter 24]. In recent years, this 'intermediate' group has swelled, reflecting these *Reciprocator* fathers' growing self-confidence and mature tolerance of role ambiguity and mixed feelings. Their hallmark is an intersubjectivity which allows greater spontaneity in both playfulness and nurturing than either the *'Participator'* who construes his parental identity on the basis of maternal identifications and the *'Renouncer'* father who having early on dis-identified from his mother, renounces 'femininity' remaining [36] strongly engaged with a concept of masculinity that is separate, and often the reverse of, feared or denigrated femininity. Clearly, since this is a model, there are in reality few 'pure' types who are exactly as described. However, as with their female counterparts, the Facilitator and Regulator, individuals gravitate towards one or other pole of the spectrum with an Intermediate group. During subsequent pregnancies and parenting of other children, men may change orientation in either direction, as a result of the experience of having fathered a baby and achieved a greater measure of inner integration or, conversely, having been hurt and retreated into a defensive position of rigid control. Chapter 11 discusses how they differ as prospective fathers, and what constitutes precipitating factors for psychological disturbance in fathers-to-be.

KEY POINTS

*Reactions to discovery of conception vary in planned and unplanned pregnancies, and are largely dependent on the nature of the relationship between the partners and unconscious meaning each attaches to the idea of having a baby.

*Preoccupation with the baby residing within the mother's womb invariably results in changes in their sexual relationship as does the man's fantasies and reaction to his partner's pregnant body, reflecting his early identifications.

*Relationship to his internalized parents is affected as he ceases to be merely his father's son and becomes a link within the continuous chain of genetic immortality. Early conflicts relating to his mother are revitalized as he is confronted by a wife turning into a mother before his very eyes. Archaic issues and unresolved oedipal dynamics rise to the surface, arousing fears of impotence and retaliatory punishments, to be reworked, avoided, or enacted.

*Male and female biological capacities and restrictions are physically emphasized by virtue of one partner being pregnant and the other not, raising queries about the social constructs of masculinity and femininity which now demand rephrasing.

Chapter 11

Participators and Renouncers and expectant fathers at risk

'The Child is father of the Man' Wordsworth.

11.1 PARTICIPATORS, RENOUNCERS AND RECIPROCATORS: A MODEL OF DIFFERENT MALE APPROACHES TO PREGNANCY AND PATERNITY

11.1.1 The 'pregnant' Participator

The Participator, as the name suggests, is eager to participate as fully as possible in pregnancy and later in primary childcare. He becomes actively involved in preparations for the labour and birth, reading baby-care books, attending antenatal examinations and birthing-classes, discussing pros and cons. Intrapsychically, he has free access to the 'feminine' 'maternal' aspects in himself, his tenderness, compassion, and gentleness. Enthralled by the 'miracle' of baby-making he craves to nurture and may desire to be the exclusive sole carer, with no restrictions on expressing his loving feelings; free to cuddle, to give warmth and understanding, and to protect the vulnerable infant of his making. If he can hold on to his own nurturant feelings without envying hers, these characteristics may find expression in cosseting the baby via his wife, cradling the bump, listening to the heartbeat, stroking and 'stoking' the growing fetus with good food and sperm, keeping it warm and safe while mothering her. Faith in the viability of his own contribution and trust in his partner's capacity to 'grow' the baby, determine whether he feels exuberant or anxious, or jealous of this arrangement in which the baby is nurtured by the woman and she by her man (and health care professionals too) while nobody looks after him! She seems privileged and he feels left out. Emotionally, a Participator may resent having to rely on his pregnant partner as an intermediary for information about *his* baby. Frustration includes the lack of social recognition of his impending fatherhood, the absence of obvious physical changes and no tangible reality of growing wriggling heaviness inside *his* body. Extreme Participators who cannot come to terms with sublimating rather than enacting powerful 'womb envy' covet the female partner's actual physical experience. This may take the form of constantly monitoring and admonishing his wife for her negligent eating or bad resting habits, proscribing and prescribing various antenatal activities, insisting on his choice of doctor, birth method and position, for all the world as if she were an extension of his own body or merely the container of his baby.

Alternatively, he may try to outdo her, actively taking over management of her pregnancy or enacting it himself. This may involve him practising all the relevant exercises, changing his own food intake, appropriating her antenatal classes and examinations, monopolizing conversations about pregnancy and intercepting her direct experience with his interpretation of it. As his frustration mounts with passive months of waiting, the extreme Participator may develop psychosomatic symptoms mirroring or competing with those of his wife, manifesting his deep-seated wish to be pregnant himself, or else he may lapse into a depression of hibernation, feeling by-passed and cheated of his 'birth right' to give birth to a baby like his mother.

In some men, preoccupation with the early mother is so enmeshed with the experience of being a baby to that mother, that his identification is not with the woman but mainly with the fetus. As infantile experience is stirred up during pregnancy, the male partner may feel helplessly dependent and needy himself or else constantly aware of his role as protector of and spokesman for the helpless, vulnerable and sensitive little person 'trapped' inside the mother. He may conduct a critical running commentary about the pregnant woman's activity, speaking as advocate for the 'imprisoned' inmate or acting as his verbal interpreter, which may coincide or conflict with the mother's own 'emotional listening' to the fetus.

11.1.2 The Participator and his Facilitator or Regulator partner

The degree to which the prospective father's behaviour will be tolerated and approved, depends largely on the dovetailing in their approach to the pregnancy of Participator and his mate. A Regulator may welcome her husband acting as intermediary between the fetus and herself, since she feels unable to form direct communication with 'it'. He can nurture optimism for them both, while she barricades herself against 'falling in love' with the fetus. However, if he goes 'over the top' in his intrusive bossiness or 'soppiness', she will resent his incessant preoccupation with the fetus, feeling she is being treated like a 'baby incubator' and ignored or devalued as a person.

Likewise, a Facilitator mother may eagerly lap up her husband's cosseting attention to herself and her fetus. However, if he crosses the boundary between his mothering of her (and indirectly mothering the baby) and begins to appropriate the function she regards as uniquely her own, she will withdraw inside herself to protect her 'mother-right' from his take-over bid.

Since both members of a couple respond to their own and the oscillating needs of the other, informed too, by the changing presence and significance of the interuterine baby, this situation will continually be in a state of stabilized flux, already a practice-field for parenthood.

KEY POINTS

*The Participator is the man who can be in touch with feminine and maternal aspects of his personality.
*How he resolves the early primary identification will determine whether he can sublimate it into protectively mothering his wife during pregnancy and postnatally, allowing her to mother the baby while he tenderly engages in 'fathering' it or whether his envy propels him into rivalrous 'out-mothering' or overidentification with the fetus.
*Similarly, postnatally, whether he competes with his partner over primary mothering or shares care-taking equally will be influenced not only by his own conscious and unconscious processes and needs but by those of his Facilitator or Regulator partner following the birth.

11.1.3 The Renouncer

The Renouncer poses a different set of questions. He is also acutely aware of male/female differences highlighted by pregnancy. As pregnancy progresses, and old repressed feelings are reactivated, he attempts to restore order into the inner chaos by re-imposing old solutions. Threatened with revival of archaic identification with his mother, he choses to reinforce his masculine attributes and identification with his own father and the paternal role. Although he may feel proud of his wife's pregnancy as external proof of his virility, he cannot empathize with her internal experiences, feeling ill-at-ease with 'feminine talk' or gynaecological symptoms. Unlike the Participator, he will treat antenatal clinics as a woman's domain, and if enticed by his wife to attend, feels disconcerted and out of place, asserting he is only there to support his wife. In some clinics, professionals share this attitude themselves, treating husbands as unnecessary appendages or chauffeurs, to be ignored, overlooked or talked down to. Nevertheless, being included in investigations and antenatal care makes the idea of an eventual baby more real and ultrasound imaging may serve as a watershed for all fathers, a major source of prenatal bonding. Actually seeing the shape and movement of their offspring provides an immediacy and a reality to the fetus, which many Renouncers lack. Many have fantasies about their offspring as fully grown children, or even college graduates. Sharing the sight of a somersaulting fetus arouses a glimmering of interaction of a new kind. Maternalistic behaviour in male mammals appears to relate to their presence at the birth or soon after. Although many Renouncers feel reluctant to stay in the delivery room (and this is to be respected), those who work through their anxieties long before labour commences, can experience early and intensive bonding, which may not alter their caretaking behaviour, but does increase compassion and tolerance.

11.1.4 The shift from hierarchical to flexible family structure

Whereas strict Renouncers were the norm during the 19th century and the beginning of the 20th, since the 1970's, distinctions between parents become less marked with each subsequent generation – and today many fathers are Reciprocators. As we saw in the previous chapter, the reciprocal of liberation of women's economic roles was freeing of men to engage in domestic pursuits. Nevertheless, despite the more egalitarian nature of western families today, some men still choose to follow the 'traditional' pattern of father as *pater familias* breadwinner laid down in their unconscious by identification with (or negation of) their own fathers and their image of the 'masculine role'. Yet fathers are as capable as mothers in looking after babies and reading their cues [1]. Microanalysis of split-screen neonatal video research suggest that men and women have inherently different interactional patterns with their babies (fathers' more exciting-vigorous-stimulating vs. mothers' more synchronous-soothing) [2,3]. These findings, claimed as true of both 'traditional' fathers and more 'maternal' ones [4,5] were interpreted as differences arising from mothers' physical experience of pregnancy and gradual bodily-attunement. Yet fathers differ from each other. We continue to be subject to subtle socially manipulated unconsciously held ideas of infants and mothers united by an invisible umbilicus, which may persist in affecting parental behaviours and maternal 'gatekeeping' even when they consciously chose to eliminate gender distinctions [6]. Interestingly, Reciprocators who choose to share primary baby-care are calming as well as arousing in their play suggesting that primary responsibility and intimate understanding of the baby's moods hold the key to attuned interaction rather than our sexed bodies. No doubt there are differences linked to the physical experience of pregnancy (that Participators try to attain indirectly), but I suggest this is conflated with unconscious social equation of mothering not only with 'the breast' but with *placental functioning* which prioritises females as nurturers. Be that as it may, differences between the artificially defined poles of 'Participators' and 'Renouncers' illustrate that these are psychosocially and culturally determined for each individual, as are all individual identities and interpersonal relationships, by their own current and past experiences with people and social institutions.

This brings us to a discussion of those men whose particular experience puts them at risk for developing symptoms of psychological disturbance during their woman's pregnancy.

KEY POINTS

*The Renouncer reinforces his masculine identity during pregnancy, when close contact with his wife increases his own vulnerability to and intolerance of his feminine identifications.

*Prenatal attachment to the fetus might be enhanced by ultrasound and participation in labour, if anxieties have abated, may increase paternal 'engrossment' in Renouncers, too.

*Loosening of social stereotypes has encouraged a less hierarchical male-dominated family structure; nevertheless, traditional patterns continue alongside new egalitarian attitudes. Research findings indicate that men and women have different interactional patterns with their infants, possibly based on the mother's physical attunement to her baby during pregnancy. We have yet to see whether these differences are minimized when the sons of Participators vs. Renouncers become fathers in their own right or whether the bodily gendered experience of carrying and bearing the baby will continue to override identifications where the quality of interaction is concerned.

11.2 EXPECTANT FATHERS AT RISK

11.2.1 Vulnerability in male partners

To recapitulate: in both men and women, pregnancy often constitutes a transitional crisis during which repressed conflicts are rearoused and require reworking and reintegration. It is thus a time of vulnerability to disintegration, while the old is obsolete and the new not yet established. The psychological pull towards regression, symbiotic merger and passivity is intensified by the proximity of the fetus within the womb, and this tendency towards dependence vies with the urge towards autonomy, independence and activity. For many men, the gradual transition from son-hood to fatherhood is a phase of maturation, an excursion into areas of fanciful elaboration, inner renewal and transfiguration of old wishes, postponement of immediate pleasures and modification of cherished boyhood aspirations and hopes into realistic plans. For others, the emotional experience is one of danger, of internal forces threatening to erupt beyond their control; of secret, incarcerated desires and ferocious conflicts bursting their age-old boundaries; of an outbreak of embarrassing childish anxieties preserved intact in repressed infantile form, now unleashed into subconscious awareness. There are many precipitating factors which can conspire to increase a man's susceptibility to psychological disturbance during the transitional crisis of pregnancy.

(a) Marked ambivalence

A man who has reason to be less than whole-heartedly pleased about the pregnancy is liable to express his mixed feelings in various ways. As in 'shot-gun' marriages, he may sense that this pregnancy is untimely, that he has been forced by circumstances into accepting fatherhood before he is ready for it. Whether the unaborted pregnancy has been foisted on him despite his objections or is the result of his reluctant agreement despite underlying, often unconscious, reservations, these usually relate to deep-seated feelings of unreadiness to test out his own ability to father a baby, at this time, and/or with this woman. Such resistance may have many sources, ranging from realistic considerations through to historical sensitizations.

(b) Life events

Even a planned and wanted pregnancy can constitute a threatening transitional crisis when unexpected happenings add to the natural stresses of this period. Events such as unforeseen redundancy or eviction create psychological tensions and economic strain, further exacerbated by the foreseeable increased expenditure of the baby's imminent arrival and probable loss of earnings of the housebound wife. Such financial considerations are not helped by the insufficiency of government maternity grants and hardship may be unwittingly increased by travelling expenses to antenatal clinics rather than local GP coverage. Illness or death of a close relative may interrupt joyous feelings surrounding the pregnancy, particularly death of a parent for whom birth of this grand-child would have been significant (as perceived by the expectant father). Bereavement, like job redundancy and loss of his own sources of creative activity, seems particularly poignant when his wife is flourishing with new life.

(c) Historical sensitization

1. **Paternal deprivation:** Men who have been deprived of close contact with their own fathers, either through their absence or death during childhood, or the emotional unavailability of a present but drunk or schizoid father, may find pregnancy a hazardous experience, lacking

the experience of an internalized paternal figure from whom to draw strength. Likewise, men whose fathers were brutally violent or emotionally abusive. Envy of this infant who will have two loving parents may increase his own hostility towards the unborn baby and a hardening determination that the child should learn early that 'life is not a picnic'. Conversely, wishing to envelop the baby in all that he himself did not have he may become painfully aware of his own lack of loving paternal models.

2. **Insecure masculinity:** A man whose masculinity feels built on shaky premises, may find his wife's inflating body grotesquely threatening. Since part of his own narcissistic masculine image revolves around possessing a wife with slim 'cover girl' looks, the thought that she may never recover her pre-pregnant figure mutilates his own identity. As one man put it: 'like buying a sports car which turns into a bus overnight' – a transformation that also converts the husband, i.e. glamorous racing driver demoted to being a public servant with a horde of passengers to look after!

3. **Insecure heterosexuality** may destabilize during pregnancy, both as a result of abstinence for fear of damaging/being damaged by the maternal body and as an enacted bid for his own feminine identification with his mother. The son of an overinvolved, idealized mother who has not resolved his dependency conflicts may be particularly fearful of the baby to come: jealous of the unborn child who will take his place in his wife's affections, while already awareness of her deficiencies as mother compared with his own, cause him anxiety and despair.

11.2.2 Symptoms of psychological distress

1. These may be identified first and foremost as extreme Participator or Renouncer stances: men who appear to be unable to continue functioning in their everyday lives, incapable of meeting the demands of their jobs and social lives without resorting to male 'pregnancy incapacitation' or morbid vicarious preoccupation with their wives' symptoms. Equally at risk are aloof men who show a determined lack of interest in the pregnancy, and distance themselves physically or psychologically from the expectant woman, appearing to deny that the birth will result in a baby or gratuitously planning activities that will remove them from home at the time the baby is due.

2. Incapacitating pregnancy-related **psychosomatic symptoms** and/or extreme 'couvade syndrome' type identifications (such as exhaustion, sleeplessness, stomach ulcers, breathlessness, etc. [7]) may well require brief focal psychotherapeutic intervention despite lack of insight into the source of the problem.

3. Men who display severe **psychosexual difficulties** could benefit from psycho or sexual therapy at this time [8]
4. Extreme **psychological defences** such as negation, denial, isolation, repression, intellectualization or massive anxiety are indications for psychotherapy if cooperation can be maintained. Lesser examples of these defences are within the bounds of normal crisis reactions but some sufferers would benefit from individual or group counselling offering a form of 'ventilation' and emotional support [9].

In need of immediate psychiatric treatment are men who show signs of:

1. **Clinical depression** (e.g. sadness, self-neglect, irrational guilt, feelings of worthlessness, obsessions, paranoid ideas, broken sleep and early waking coupled with lack of libido, various digestive complaints and appetite loss). All these indicate conflicting inner forces and a discrepancy between the wished for ideal and perceived reality. Threats of suicide must be taken seriously as the reality of imminent increased responsibility and decreased marital attention constitute major threats to a vulnerable husband.
2. **Paranoid delusions** and organized compulsive rituals and obsessions indicate a need to revive magical control to provide comfort and compensate for insecurity during a time of extreme stress and confusion.
3. Likewise, symptoms of **severe anxiety** and panic attacks (apprehension, hypochondria, irritability, insomnia, depersonalization and various somatic symptoms such as impotence, restlessness, sweating, diarrhoea without cause, palpitations, headaches and dizziness or unexplained pains), also benefit from immediate treatment.
4. Acts of sadism or **physical violence** towards the pregnant woman or substitutes for her are worrying signs that action is taking the place of understanding. This disturbance cannot be overlooked in the hope that it will not recur. Wife batterers very frequently become baby-batterers, particularly when violence begins during pregnancy [10]. This will be dealt with more fully in Chapter 33.

In conclusion, pregnancy can be a stressful time for the male partner. However, like his female counterpart, it can also be used as fruitful time of emotional maturation, resolution of conflicting inner tendencies and creative expansion. Psychotherapy, with its built-in (provisional and negotiable) deadline of the birth, if utilized fully, can lead to very substantial changes in the father-to-be. Untreated, these disturbances will continue to flourish in family relationships following the birth, in the form of absent, detached, violent or vulnerable fathers and emotionally deprived, disturbed or battered children. The following chapters explore the readjustments that pregnancy and anticipated parenthood impose on the couple's relationship.

KEY POINTS

*Fathers-to-be may experience their partners pregnancy as a time of increased vulnerability and crisis.

*Precipating factors which conspire to increase a man's susceptibility to psychological disturbance during pregnancy include internal conflicts, life events and historical sensitization.

*Some social, psychological, psychosomatic and psychosexual symptoms described constitute indications of a need for professional intervention.

Chapter 12

Lesbian partners

'When I kiss and stroke and enter my lover, I am also a child re-entering my mother. I want to return to the womb-state of harmony, and also to the ancient world. I enter my lover but it is she in her orgasm who returns. I see on her face for a long moment, the unconscious bliss that an infant carries the memory of behind its shut eyes. Then when it is she who makes love to me . . . the intensity is also a pushing out, a borning! . . . So I too return to the mystery of my mother, and of the world as it must have been when motherhood was exalted.

Now I am ready to go back and understand the one whose body actually carried me. Now I can begin to learn about her, forgive her for the rejection I felt, yearn for her, ache for her'. (poet Sue Silvermarie, quoted by Adrienne Rich, *Of Woman Born*)

12.1 DEFINITION OF THE NEW ROLE

The female lover of a pregnant woman faces complex psychosocial, legal and economic issues that lack precedents and role-models for people brought up in heterosexual families. In order to regard herself as a 'non-biological parent' to her partner's child, she may have had to negotiate an internal conflict of whether she wants children at all; whether to bear the child herself, of whether and how to facilitate her partner's wish for a baby, of how to explain to her family, friends, work colleagues and to the future child itself her connection to that baby (possibly having to 'come out' in the process of breaking the news), and finally, of whether to co-parent or co-mother, and what that distinction entails.

During her pregnancy, the pregnant lesbian will often be assumed to be heterosexual ('I didn't know you were married!'), and her partner is overlooked in a culture where traditionally a child has only one mother. Unlike the male partner of a cohabiting heterosexual couple, a lesbian partner has no legal claim over her lover's baby and cannot adopt the child unless the biological mother waives all parental rights. All she can do to protect her future relationship with this baby is to draw up an informal agreement with her pregnant partner that recognizes her parental role, affection and responsibility in the event that they dissolve their relationship after the birth [1]. The non-biological mother has to secure her right to be acknowledged as a parent by law. Unless she has donated her egg to be implanted by IVF, she has not contributed biologically to the making of the child, and furthermore, unlike AID (artificial insemination by donor) fathers, she herself has the potential capacity to bear a child. Having declined to use her prerogative, she may fear being regarded as secondary by the child who resided in her partner's womb, rather than her own. With unknown donors the 'fantasy father' who cannot be found in reality, may raise anxieties that paternal absence could lead to idealization and 'over-romanisation of men or to some gnawing sense of loss and mystery' [2]. Parenting is complicated by the ambiguity of this indeterminate role in the absence of social and legal definition within norm-setting lesbian communities and elsewhere. In feminist debates much discussion of personal life has centred around the politics of sexuality [3-6]. More recently sexuality, gender and reproductivity are demarcated as distinct systems of psychological constructs, social control and power. Increased awareness of diverse 'sexualities' and sociopolitical distinctions. Feminists have debated whether (heterosexual as well as homosexual) females who relate to other women but are non political 'give their allegiance to male myths, ideologies, styles, practices and professions' [7]) as opposed to women-identified lesbians, who through nurturant relations share 'the rich inner life, the bonding against male tyranny, the giving and receiving of practical and political support' [8]. New studies view lesbianism as a product of multiple influences rather than a traceable to a single cause, considering the 'total personal identity' informed by the wider social context rather than primarily a 'sexual condition'[9]. Research consistently finds lesbian non-biological mothers more involved than heterosexual fathers with their children. Prejudice still abounds despite studies confirming that children growing up in stable homosexual households do as well as others and do not develop disturbances of gender-identity. Much contemporary psychoanalysis is more accepting, believing that human psychic structure comprises homosexual and heterosexual components, since in its fullest form it is based on identification with both sexes, thereby enabling each individual to encompass both 'feminine' and 'masculine' aspects of themselves. According to Freud's view, the psychic 'bisexuality' resulting from these identifications means that 'every sexual act [is potentially] an event between four individuals' [10]. Clearly, for us all, choice of love-partner is determined by many factors at different phases of development, ranging from positive and negative qualities of very early relationships, through parental expectations and gratifications, social values and prejudiced restrictions, teenage delights and disappointments both with parents and non-relatives, and the search for emancipation from, transformation and resolution of, internal conflicts. There are various psychoanalytical viewpoints about lesbian choices. One believes that the homosexual component has two distinct aims: the desire for 'total possession of the mother in a world without men' and a wish to **be** the father through identification with masculine power so as to become the object of the mother's desires (while simultaneously proving that male sex organs are dispensable) [11]. Others regard gender role as distinct from erotic preferences, such that love of another woman does not necessarily reflect either masculinity or femininity, which in themselves have multiple determinants. Likewise, as in heterosexual relationships, psychic representations of the chosen partner are not necessarily congruent with their physical sex. Lesbian maternity comes under particular scrutiny, especially with egg-exchange. One (Kleinian) view regards same-sex parenting as an attack on the parental couple and 'creative sexuality'. Other psychoanalysts question the underpinning concept of an innate universal 'primal scene' phantasy, inviting reflection about the anxieties aroused by women having babies in the absence of men. In recent years, concern about legitimation of homophobic views has resulted in a critique of both theoretical conservatism and the 'fallacious' conflation of sexual orientation and gender identity [12,13], thereby encouraging fresh psychoanalytic debate.

12.3 REASSESSMENT OF HER OWN CONTRIBUTION

As in all close relationships, the dynamics of attachment/autonomy are also central to lesbian couples. However, as women, participants in a homosexual relationship have been found to value particularly equality of power, emotional expressiveness or intimate self-disclosure and similarity between partners [14]. When both partners' aim relates to possession of the mother through each other, the symmetry in their identification lends itself to the idea of mutual 'fusion', leading at times of stress to 'intense anxiety over any desire for separateness or autonomy within the relationship' due to female–female identification and blurring of boundaries [15]. I have found that pregnancy of one partner introduces subjective difference into their common mutual experience – one is 'full', the other 'empty'. The one who has conceived is clearly 'creative' and 'fertile', the other untested (unless they have taken 'turns'). One has been infiltrated by a male substance, the other is untouched. One is in direct communion with a third, the embryonic person, a potential invader into the close interchangeable lesbian 'mother–child' twosome. However, as in all couple relationships, such a difference, although rocking the emotional 'boat', can promote differentiation and growth towards personal individuation.

Like the expectant father, during the partner's pregnancy, a lesbian lover may feel disgruntled with all the attention lavished on the mother-to-be. However, unlike an opposite-sex relationship, she has a real option. At times she may regret that it is not she who is carrying the baby, and feel envious of the female experience that could have been hers. If she is menopausal herself or infertile, the bittersweet reality of having a child by proxy is nonetheless fraught with jealousy over the intimate 'closed system' connection between her expectant partner and the baby in her womb. When one partner has renounced her childbearing capacity, unconscious early longings might be stirred up in her during her partner's pregnancy. The pangs she experiences may be deflected in aggressive denial or sublimated in protectiveness. She may, however, also unconsciously feel deeply hurt that her partner has resorted to a search for something that could not be satisfied within the orbit of their relationship.

12.4 FEMALE AND MALE

Even if her woman was impregnated by insemination rather than intercourse, and even if the donor is homosexual, the non-biological mother may feel resentful at the intrusion of a male force into their female relationship, present both in the imagery of the male sperm making its way up the vagina to penetrate the female ovum, and in the fantasy of a male fetus residing within the female couple. In extremely female-centred male-repudiating atmospheres, even non-sexual insemination can be experienced as political betrayal. (In a study of a separatist lesbian community in New Zealand, one woman 'was said to have conceived parthenogenically' (eg. without a sperm) [16].)

Like all expectant mothers, the pregnant lesbian mother may have a sex-preference for a girl or a boy. However, the preferences of both partners may not coincide, and one or other may have strong negative feelings about boys. It has been indicated that some radical lesbian communities may seem ambivalent [17] or even rather hostile to male children ('my child is not a future rapist, which is how some lesbians like to think about boy children; the attitude in this community is oppressive and I feel antagonized by it' [18]). Other enclaves recognize the complex psychosocial problems and have evolved support groups to deal with some of the particularly volatile and difficult issues for lesbians raising boy children.

For the female lover of a pregnant partner, the issue of future bonding is complicated by feelings of alienation, superfluousness and exclusion not unlike those experienced by an expectant husband following his wife's donor-insemination. The non-biological mother also has to face the issues of bringing up a male child in a female household and/or one who belongs to a 'species' she may have politically repudiated and whom she might then feel to be inherently dangerous and/or oppressive. Alternatively, she may have to consider the right of the biological father to know and co-parent the child in the case of a known donor, and the child's possible future grief and anger at having no father but only two 'mothers' in a primarily heterosexual world.

12.5 REACTIVATED EARLY EXPERIENCES

Finally, like all expectant parents, the pregnant lesbian and her lover will find themselves reliving the emotional sequelae of being born of woman and brought up by one. However, in the case of the expectant lesbian and her female partner this process is further complicated by all the same-sexed identifications of being fetus and container, envious girl-child and pregnant mother, the one re-immersed in a childhood state of being displaced by the pregnancy of the other, feeling like an older sibling yearning for and excluded from the dyadic intimacy between fetus and beloved pregnant mother.

KEY POINTS

*A lesbian lover may experience her partners pregnancy as a time of increased vulnerability and identity crisis, necessitating reevaluation of her own contribution to the relationship.
*Both partners may experience doubts and conflicts about the biological father's input, the possibly male fetus and disturbance in their exclusive female dyad.

Part Four

PREGNANCY AS TRANSITION TO PARENTHOOD

Chapter 13

Anticipating parenthood: in the West and in other cultures

Situated as we are in the midst of the culture of our own upbringing, it is difficult to imagine the diversity of childrearing and childbearing methods and activities in other societies and in our own society in other generations. Crosscultural research, comparing different approaches to the same experience in different places, gives us an inkling of the wide range of human potentialities and widens perspective and insight into our own practices while enabling us to study the evolution of different cultural patterns in a variety of ethnic groups [1–5].

13.1 CROSSCULTURAL VARIATIONS

All known societies provide four kinds of help to childbearing women, the nature and extent of which varies culturally:

13.1.1

a. Help with fertilization (regulations determining acceptability of partner, timing of intercourse and rituals to ensure conception)
b. Protection from injury (physical protection from aggressors and inanimate dangers such as weather, water pollution or radiation, etc.
c. Economic aid while incapacitated (sharing, supplementing, concessions or grants)
d. Assistance with stresses of childbearing (help with other children and household chores before and after birth, and attendance during labour) [6].

13.1.2 Transition to parenthood

Most societies register a change in status when a person becomes a parent. In many cultures a marriage is only formalized during pregnancy or after a live birth. A barren wife may be stigmatized, returned to her family of origin or displaced by a fertile wife (for instance among the Yoruba, West Africa). Thus, depending on the culture, failure to bear children can be grounds for divorce, condoned extramarital sex or polygamy, or even lead to disgraced suicide, such as among the Lango of Nilotic Suda. Proclamation of pregnancy may involve rituals binding the two families closer together, with elaborate systems of gift exchange, as in Sumatra.

During pregnancy, in most societies it is customary for the social group to be solicitous towards the pregnant woman. Seclusion is often provided as she is regarded as physically vulnerable in her special 'marginal' state and endangered, as is her fetus, by various malign forces such as evil spirits in West Africa, the devil in Ukraine or ill-wishers in her own tribe. Among some people, like the Hottentots, or Guatemalan peasants, the woman herself is regarded as dangerous; among others, like the Lele of Central Africa or the Nyakyusa, her unborn baby is considered to be threatening, likely to affect sick people or the harvest. The pregnant woman is then secluded not for her own protection but to protect the group from her powers. Although accepted as a proud sign of male virility, in some societies, pregnancy is accompanied by shyness, reticence and feelings of sexual shame. Young brides who hide in seclusion, thereby delaying protective and health-care measures (e.g. Punjabi villagers, India, Bulgarian peasants or Nahane in Northern Canada).

In many cultures, dietary restrictions are enforced during pregnancy. These usually consist of avoidance of meat, fish and deformed plants and thus ironically may inadvertently reduce intake of protein and fresh vegetables. Other rules may serve to separate male and female principles now that in her pregnancy the woman is considered 'quintessentially feminine' [7] and dangerous. Yet other rituals keep categories of 'cold' and 'hot' apart while the pregnant woman's blood is seen to be in a heated state. Proscribed rites (of cleansing, eating, intercourse, geographical mobility, sacrifices or greetings) or avoidance taboos (omitting certain movements, foods, sights, thoughts, etc.) are seen to ensure a good outcome as the mother and/or father are deemed accountable for the baby's growth *in utero*. However, the degree of responsibility (and therefore guilt) ascribed varies in different societies from those in which parental negligence during pregnancy will be blamed for failed births or infant malformation to others operating varying degrees of acceptance of abnormality. Definitions of normality are culture-bound, such as the Siriono of Bolivia who nurture babies with club feet but regard twins as 'unnatural' [8]

13.1.3 Emotional commitment to the fetus

As has been noted, the point at which the baby acquires human status varies in different societies and determines timing and patterns of childcare, legal status and moral rights after birth. If the fetus is humanized during pregnancy, it follows that attitudes towards abortion, prenatal care, bonding and mourning practices following miscarriage or stillbirth will reflect this status. When the newborn has not yet acquired human status, procedures follow to humanize it if s/he survives infancy. Stillbirths and neonatal deaths may constitute a spiritual danger. The Yoruba of West Africa believe that 'Abiku', spirits of children 'born to die' haunt and torment parents and threaten a pregnant woman who goes outside at night [9]

The degree of emotional commitment to the baby is determined in any society by many factors such as prospects of viability and infant mortality rates, attitude to gender and sex preferences, birth order and patterns of inheritance, social class and circumstances of conception, and the degree of socio-economic stability enabling marriage to be conducted between individuals on an emotional basis rather than an expedient arrangement between families or clans. These forces also determine the degree of parental attachment which varies in different societies from proud devotion such as that of both father and mother, among the Siriono of Bolivia, who change their own name to suffix that of each new child irrespective of gender, to paternal indifference or hostility and even infanticide.

13.1.4 Paternal influence

Paternal influence over pregnancy may be central: for instance, the Ifugao of the Philippines do not permit a man to kill or cut anything during his wife's pregnancy; the Mundugumor must scrupulously avoid certain work activities and intercourse during pregnancy or his wife will have twins. In some West Indian islands, the pregnant woman, and among the Sea Dyaks, both parents are forbidden to bind, knot or braid anything for fear of creating a corresponding obstacle in the cord or woman's body. In the Toumbulauh tribe of North Celebes, after a ceremony in the fifth month, the husband is forbidden to tie knots or sit with his legs crossed [10]. Some fathers like the Arapesh of New Guinea, are required to 'build' the fetus with semen and blood or 'feed' the womb during intercourse; the Himalayan Lepcha have a ceremonial cleansing for both parents in the fifth month of pregnancy while others are involved during childbirth. A Pacific Ocean Easter Islander father has his wife recline against him during labour and delivery; and one study recorded 17 tribes from Asia, North America, Oceania and South America involving the father in couvade [11]. In yet other societies paternal recognition may only come after the birth or at some later date.

13.1.5 Social attitudes to pregnancy and labour

Female work roles during pregnancy vary widely across cultures, such that a Gujarati woman in India would be expected to do only light household duties throughout pregnancy; she is meant to enjoy pleasant thoughts as her ideas or actions are believed to affect the fetus. However, the most common single pattern of work activity across cultures involves some lightening of work in the majority of traditional societies, although in some, like the Ojibwa American Indians, a woman is expected to perform all her usual duties until the onset of labour. About one half of societies expect women to return to full duties within two weeks of delivery [12].

Similarly, the variation among societies in their attitudes towards childbirth as a natural event, a supernatural or sexual one or an illness in need of treatment, largely determines whether the birth is a private or social event, whether it is attended by midwife (as are the majority of births (60–80%) worldwide [13]), her own mother (in societies of matrilineal descent and matrilocal residence), in-laws or religious elders and whether men, including the husband, may attend the delivery.

KEY POINTS

*All known societies provide four kinds of help to childbearing women: (1) help with fertilization; (2) protection from injury; (3) economic aid; (4) assistance with stresses of childbearing.

*The nature and extent of these vary from culture to culture as do the change in status attributed to prospective parents; the type of solicitude demonstrated by the social group; the degree of accountability of mother and father to be for their offspring's normality; human status of embryo, fetus or baby; emotional involvement of father and ritual activity contributing to the well-being of the unborn baby; and the changing pattern of female work roles during pregnancy and the puerperium.

*All these taboos, rituals and duties serve as preparations for parenthood, affirming parental commitment to and responsibility for the baby-to-be.

13.2 HISTORIAL VARIATIONS IN THE WEST

Western society has seen far-ranging changes over the generations. A reduction of infant mortality rates, and recently, efficient contraception have meant fewer children per household, more 'wanted' babies with stronger overt bonding and emotional commitment to the physical and mental health of each child.

13.2.1 Changing attitudes to children

However, a look at the 'History of Childhood', shows how novel our current ideas about parenting are. Early European history sees parents engaged in an 'Infanticide Mode' of neglect rather than care, parents projecting their own devilishness into their repudiated children. From the fourth to the thirteenth centuries an 'Abandonment Mode' meant parents deposited their children on wet nurses, monasteries or foster families. Since 1250 an 'Ambivalent Mode' took over, with the child, still seen as wild and wicked, but being 'moulded' by parents, mutilated or 'beaten into shape' for their own good while also seen at times as miniature adults or even substitute parents to their own mother and father. Although infanticide was punishable with death, exposure of newborns was so common that a foundling hospital was founded in London by Coram in 1741 to save them. Nevertheless, this practice continued in England as late as 1890. In the eighteenth century the 'Intrusive Mode' predominated, with children treated by their parents more humanely, improvement of childcare and a decline in infant mortality. During the nineteenth and twentieth centuries the 'Socialization Mode' of training the child to meet society's regulations gradually gave way to the mid-twentieth century style of a 'Helping Mode' based on psychoanalytic insights [14].

13.2.2 Recent social trends

Thus, in our time, preparation for parenthood is affected by ideological changes on several interrelated fronts:

a. **Childcare.** The historical progression described above demonstrates an increasing awareness of children being in need of loving care rather than eradication of innate vices. Whereas medieval children shared the adult world of work almost from weaning, childhood has gradually emerged as a phase in its own right leading to prolonged adolescence and recently defined western expectations of exclusive and continuous mothering and such concepts as 'maternal deprivation'.

b. **Mothers.** In the West we have shifted from shared care in extended families to the mother as primary care-taker in an isolated nuclear family, equipped not with traditional knowhow but with fashionable books of expert advice on childrearing and up-to-date training in the latest innovations.

c. **Childbirth.** The historical pendulum has swung from female-based midwifery to male obstetric medicalization of childbirth; from traditional home births to early lying-in hospital deliveries, and then back to majority home births followed by the about-turn policy reversal of the late 1970s when 97% of babies in Britain were born in hospital.

d. **Fathers.** Victorian relegation of the cigar smoking husband to the waiting room during birth and children being 'seen but not heard', at least not by their fathers, have given way to the current trend for almost compulsory husband attendance at births, and expectation of paternal bonding and childcare participation.

e. Although still an innovation, classes in **parenting techniques** are now available, aimed both as promotion of babycare expertise and as discussion groups on the emotional needs and cognitive abilities of young infants. Studies of the effect of prenatal educational classes reveal that mothers who have attended have a lower incidence of postpartum disturbance and 'prepared' fathers feel a 'stronger attraction' to their newborns, change nappies more frequently and carry the baby more than non-instructed control counterparts [15].

KEY POINTS

*Western history has seen a gradual progression in childcare practices from an early mode of infanticide, through abandonment, ambivalence, intrusive-projection, to professed aims of socialization and, latterly, permissive care.

*An overview of recent times enables us to see fluctuations of ideologies from female based midwifery to male obstetric medicalization of childbirth, alternations of home and hospital births, changing beliefs about infant needs and the relative importance of parental care and, of late, classes in parenting techniques.

13.3 PROSPECTIVE PARENTS: CHOICES AND NEW VIEWS OF PARENTHOOD

In previous generations, parenting roles were fairly clearly prescribed along traditional lines of mothers fulfilling 'expressive', emotional and nutritive functions while fathers focused on 'instrumental' roles, economic responsibility and social authority [16]. Similarly, current beliefs about the state of the child's benign or 'devilish' nature determined prevalent parenting practices. In recent years, the post-war return of women to domesticity was accompanied by politically expedient idealization of exclusive, cloistered mothering by the biological mother. However, having had a taste of equality during the war years and proof of their own competent capabilities in hitherto 'masculine' enterprise, western women began to voice their dissatisfaction with secondary status and opportunities for growth. Concomitant with the revival of the Women's Movement and examination of sexual politics [17] and the 'Feminine Mystique' [18], a new trend began. This self-assertive trend which legitimized the questioning of established authority in all spheres (by students, women, blacks, soldiers, prisoners, etc.) has led to emphasis on personal fulfilment and individual choice. Parenthood too, has been affected.

With this new freedom, as never before in the West, parenting is at the locus of many options, no longer bound to follow the dictates of any one ideology. Personal beliefs, based on conscious knowledge and unconscious fantasies, now determine parental orientations and aspirations. Looking forward to motherhood, the pregnant woman, like her partner, now has a choice as to when, where, whether and how she is going to 'mother' her baby. In a circularity that recoils on itself, if she uses pregnancy to explore these possibilities in her mind and has insight into her own psychological processes, the choices she makes will not only influence her future interaction with the baby but will have immediate repercussions during the pregnancy on her prenatal bonding with the unborn baby which in turn affects her orientation towards mothering.

13.4 THE FACILITATOR/REGULATOR MODEL: TRANSITION TO MOTHERHOOD

The Facilitator spends her pregnancy rehearsing motherhood. She believes her baby is already alert and communicative in the womb, and will be born knowing what s/he wants. The Facilitator therefore believes that her future responsibility lies in spontaneously following the baby, listening attentively to his/her messages and protecting the infant against the impinging world. Since she feels her sensitivity is being biologically primed during pregnancy, she, the mother-to-be, will not need to learn how to mother 'artificially' through parent-craft classes but absorbs it through communion with the fetus within her. Mothering, to her, begins during pregnancy. She feels the need to be protectively alert to dangers and constantly receptive to communications from the fetus and assumes that postnatally, only she, the biological mother, will have this pregnancy-primed capacity really to understand and fend for her baby. Breastfeeding is seen as a direct continuation of pregnancy, and mothering is unconsciously equated with placental functioning. The Facilitator intends to function as an external nurturing placenta, intuitively gratifying her infant's needs, nourishing and containing, removing excretions and metabolizing bad feelings during the first month, if not years of her baby's life, while also monitoring any noxious infiltrations. Having been sensitized by maintaining close communication with her fetus throughout pregnancy, she feels she will continue to do so with the baby after birth. Her belief that only she can act as interpreter for the baby will necessitate her full-time presence, close proximity and exclusive devotion to deciphering her infant's cries and later verbal communications.

The pregnant Regulator regards full-time mothering as a trap engendered by society to keep women occupied at home. She believes that babies are born undifferentiated, asocial and understand very little about the world. Since adults know what is best they must regulate the babies' needs and train them to be socialized. Whereas the Facilitator plans to adapt to her baby the Regulator intend to teach her baby to adapt to the world which it will come to occupy. Mothering to her is an occupation, one role among many which she will play; maternal skills can (and must) be learned and, hence, are transferrable to others who can learn them too. Assuming that babies at first cannot differentiate between caretakers, she intends to institute shared care-giving at an early stage, either with her partner if willing, another mother with whom she can 'swap', a paid stand-in or doting relative. This will also necessitate shared feeding, so the Regulator plans ahead to introduce bottles and a schedule that can be followed by others.

13.5 PARTICIPATOR/RENOUNCER TRANSITION TO FATHERHOOD

Like the Facilitator, the male Participator believes the fetus is communicative and sentient. He makes great efforts to establish contact with his baby in the womb, loves attending ultrasound sessions or listening to the heart-beat on a stethoscope, 'playing' and chatting with the fetus and is very involved in preparatory classes for the birth and parenting. His own non-pregnant state heightens his awareness of the biological differences between himself and his burgeoning partner and, at times, he feels envious and dejected by the need for an intermediary between himself and his closest kin, the unborn baby. He is determined to 'learn' the baby's language and at times vies with the mother in interpreting messages from her interior. He intends to 'mother' the baby as much as possible, a welcomed proposal if he is married to a Regulator who wishes to share mothering in a non-sexist egalitarian way. However, if his partner is a Facilitator, she might feel he is already trying to steal into her special province as exclusive intuitive primary care-taker, and by withdrawal into herself curtails his 'access'. A compromise might lead to his mothering her now and postnatally so that she can mother the baby, or a negotiated modification of her own exclusive maternal role to allow joint mothering.

The expectant Renouncer finds himself quite fearful at the prospect of a new baby exposing him to raw emotions and crude messy infantile experiences. Many Renouncers spend the pregnancy planning their 'get-away': a walking tour, mountain climbing excursion or simple 'business trip' timed for the birth or as soon as decently permissible, serves the purpose of removing him from the threat of the newborn. Clearly, what the Renouncer cannot face is reawakening of old echoes within himself, residues from his own helplessly dependent and vulnerable babyhood. Like the Regulator, he prefers to regard the newborn as 'not all there', unable to differentiate or discern whether the father is around or not. If his partner is a Facilitator, he is happy for her to provide exclusive mothering care for the baby, although there may be a risk of being deprived of her ministrations to him. If his partner is a Regulator, he may approve her plans for shared care, provided he is not expected to look after the infant himself in the early stages. Needless to say, these paradigmatic people live in ideal worlds. In the real world of economic stresses and unforeseen events, plans do not always work out as they are made, and, in my view, postnatal distress in both women and men is caused by the *negative discrepancy* between these hopes, wishes and expectations of pregnancy and the reality of parenting experiences. This has now been statistically verified by several large scale studie s [see section 0.5 in the Update chapter].

KEY POINTS

*Pregnancy can be used to explore and formulate various options but choices are determined both by unconscious factors, conscious personal and subcultural beliefs about the baby's cognitive and social abilities before and after birth, and care required to meet infantile needs.

*A model was presented of maternal and paternal orientations and various permutations of partners - Facilitators with Renouncer or Participator partners, Regulators with Renouncer or Participator partners, and Reciprocators with any combination. Given their flexibility and tolerance of ambivalence, Reciprocators tend to fare well with either partner orientation).

* Increasing flexibility of parenting roles and new freedom of other choices mean that these orientations reflect personal predilections and unconscious representations rather than a social trend.

*Difficulties arise from mis-matches between the partners respective expectations about parenthood and when these fail to coincide with the realities of parenting. The greater and more unexpected the discrepancy between desire and reality, the more intense the postnatal distress.

* Distress pushes people towards the extremes and into the 'conflicted' area of parenting. Resolution of internal preoccupations and acceptance of ambivalence shifts orientations towards Reciprocation

Conflict/preoccupation

Facilitation   **Regulation**

Reciprocation

Chapter 14

Readjusting family relationships

'Thou art young and desirest child and marriage. But I ask thee: Art thou a man *entitled* to desire a child? Art thou the victorious one, the self-conqueror, the ruler of thy passions, the master of thy virtues? Or doth the animal speak in thy wish, and necessity? Or isolation? Or discord in thee? I would have thy victory and freedom long for a child . . . Not only onward shalt thou propagate thyself, but upward! For that purpose may the garden of marriage help thee! . . . *Marriage: so call I the will of the twain to create the one that is more than those who created it*!' Nietzsche, Thus Spake Zarathustra, 1885 (italics added).

14.1 IT TAKES TWO TO MAKE A THIRD: BUT HOW MANY TO MAKE A FAMILY?

Procreation is an act which requires two people to initiate it. We have each originated from two others, male and female. That vital combination of one sperm and one egg uniting lurks in the unconscious as an underlying prototype for one-male one-female heterosexual relationships. Like the gene-pool feeding the resultant fertilized ovum, a couple's relationship is the intergenerational sum total of all participants.

The couple may not be in evidence at all: a women may have been raped or become pregnant after promiscuous relationships or may approximate immaculate conception using a self-administered impregnation kit and anonymous donor sperm. Once the seed is sown a woman may try to destroy it or nurture it into life alone. Sometimes, it is the man who for various reasons may be left holding the baby on his own. Some expectant couples do not live together, or the father may not know he is one or the male partner may not be the father of the baby. They may not be a mixed couple at all but a lesbian pair or, infrequently two men and a baby. The ovum too may or may not be the woman's own. Sometimes the baby is not kept or does not survive. Nevertheless, once conception has taken place, the fetus forms the nucleus of a new family.

14.1.1 Contemporary changes in the family

As it provides an intermediary order between society and the individual, the family undergoes changes that parallel those of society as well as reflecting changes inherent in its individual members. Living as we do in a period of rapid social change, we find the nature of the family as we have known it in our own families of origin, greatly changed. Whereas only recently, while we were growing up, 'Adulthood' was synonymous with 'Marriage' and marriage with having children, many people are now refraining from making or sustaining relationships which would lead to marriage or establishment of a new family. In the United Kingdom, almost a fifth of women now in their thirties will remain childless; during the last decade the number of one-parent families has grown by one-third, and one in seven of all families with dependent children is single-parented. Nine of every ten one-parent families is headed by a lone mother [1]. These sexual and social changes seen at family level are the result of interactive repercussions of forces at societal, economic and political levels, such as the impact of the Women Movement, contraceptive trends, the advent of AIDS, increased unemployment, the energy crisis or metropolitan overcrowding. The necessity for living within old-style family confines has been further eroded by the gradual decline of the extended family structure, and transfer to the State of various social institutions, such as childcare, caring for the elderly, nursing sick family members, management of education, religion, work, security, childbirth . . .

Increasingly, young people find themselves uprooted from their places of origin, far from their families and separated from networks of childhood-friends who share common sources of understanding and familiar patterns of interaction. The challenge presented by the new confusing environment is to negotiate a tightrope between the conflicting demands of Social Acceptance and Personal Recognition. To belong, one must comply with the rules. To be noticed, one must be different. A contemporary emphasis in large centres of anonymity is one of 'Presentation' – creating a positive impression and packaging self and ideas in socially palatable form.

14.1.2 The family as a sanctuary

In western societies, the parents' task as advocates of society is to 'socialize' the child to meet the cultural demands of their community by establishing inner controls. What has been called 'a bargain' is struck [2]: In return for subordinating his/her desires to social expectations in the outside world, a sanctuary will be preserved in the home in which the child can revert to a less controlled and more expressive primitive form of interaction. To a degree within the confines of most accepting families, the child, and the adult too, can relax into being his or her spontaneous self.

In adult life, we all continue to crave this haven of an intimate relationship in which we can find the unconditional love, acceptance, freedom just to **be** without censure or fear of derision. Along with the loss of wider societal functions of the extended family, marriage has gained importance as a 'love-match' and a source of personal, sexual, emotional and even intellectual fulfilment. The current trend of almost one in two marriages ending in divorce reflects the heavy burden placed on marriages. Conversely, the idea of marriages ending in divorce raises fears of loss and abandonment which may induce some people to opt for a series of superficial relationships rather than a single stable one. Perfectionists may enter a succession of relationships with high hopes only to be disillusioned about marrying anyone. Nevertheless, however alienated from the idea of marriage, closeness and intimacy are sought. We each hope for someone on whom we can rely as upon the ideal parents of our childhood, to sustain and support us in times of confusion and sadness. We yearn to consummate childhood wishes and repair old wounds where parents and others failed us. We long for a partner with whom we can find, share and recapture happiness, in whose presence we can give expression to aspects of our inner worlds and real selves that have been denied expression; a true mate with whom we can have fun, make jokes, make love, promote growth, find healing and fulfilment and perhaps, even create a baby . . .

Thus, although the external aspects of marrige and our attitudes towards it have changed a great deal, by virtue of our human condition, many basic needs remain unchanged. An intimate sexual relationship potentially allows partners to come physically and emotionally closer than they have to any single person since being nurtured in infancy, the penetrating penis actually crossing boundaries between two separate bodies as nipple and milk did in infancy. In pregnancy, the woman comes closer still, with someone else actually growing inside her, initiated by a substance from inside another body. A third person will soon emerge – a mixture of them both.

The birth of that child will alter the relationship of a couple, from that of lovers to one between parents, a qualitative change without which the partnership cannot be resumed. Preparation for this transition to parenthood can occur during pregnancy, and, to be viable, necessitates changes in the couple's 'contracts' with each other. This chapter explores some of the conscious contracts and the less accessible components of a close relationship between man and woman, who have risked intimacy and are contemplating becoming parents or have actually initiated procreation. The next chapter focuses on the unconscious contracts underpinning their relationship. Our thesis is that parenthood will inevitably impose further changes and make extraordinary demands on the couple's emotional resources. Pregnancy itself activates psychological processes within the couple through which they can prepare themselves for parenthood before the birth by understanding weaknesses in their present relationship, identifying and strengthening internal resources and developing their potential for mutual satisfaction in the next phase of their family life-cycle.

KEY POINTS

*Partners and the family are influenced by the social forces which operate upon them from without as well as the individual forces from within.
*Despite changes in the structure of pair-relationships and the function of the family, the basic need of the individual for intimate gratification within a deep relationship remains unchanged.
*Understanding of their emotional and interactional needs by the couple before the birth of their child, will enable them to achieve mutual satisfaction during their transition to parenthood, thereby mitigating future complications.

14.2 PSYCHOLOGICAL CONTRIBUTIONS TO THE RELATIONSHIP

A marriage (used here to convey an emotional bond rather than legal status) is clearly more than the sum of the two participants. When two unique people come together to form an ongoing relationship, they enter it dragging their psychological histories behind them. Even if assertively independent, each still psychically belongs to his/her family of origin. When together they endeavour to create a new family, each releases into it, both intentionally and unknowingly, her/his individual personality, the psychic imprints, emotional deposits and ancestral pool of unresolved conflicts and attachments to their old family and those of their respective parents, siblings, at least four grandparents each and numerous predecessors ad infinitum.

14.2.1 More than a pair

Even an isolated single woman contains a male–female couple within her during pregnancy. Drawn not only from external reality but based on affiliation between internal parental figures. In an ongoing stable interchange, the 'relationship' which each couple creates, although abstract and unseen, has a definite identity. In essence, it is like a kaleidoscopic image constantly formed and reformed by interaction and reciprocity of both their contributions. Influenced by the nature of each of the parental couples in the partner's own childhoods, their own mutual relationship becomes a new prototype – the primary model which will determine all subsequent family interactions. Hence the parental couple's central place in this book, and the importance for professionals, who are transferentially ascribed parental characteristics, to recognize their own influence on the pregnant couple in their care, about to establish a new family of their own.

14.2.2 On giving and getting

People give in an intimate relationship and also get. What they get is not always what they want; similarly what they give is not always what they want to give or what is required by the other. Happiness depends on closeness of fit between the expectations of each participant and the generous fulfilment of these by the other. Clearly, since needs change and people differ, conflict is an inevitable part of all relationships, and if utilized constructively can promote growth. At no other time in life is progress as rapid and all-engulfing as in childhood. In the blink of a parental eye, babies elongate into teenagers while young mothers and fathers gradually mature into wiser middle-aged ones. While growing up, we have each looked on our parents as the stable adults, flexibly accommodating to our rapidly changing developmental needs, providing access to an increasingly wider, more diversified milieu and helping us to process its complexities. Our needs changed as we moved from the egotistic core of being a baby at the centre of the family, to becoming a special child in a nursery, to taking a place as one of many at school and then, out in the wide world. Parents meet or fail to meet specific needs according to their own capacities and human frailties, as each new phase of the child's development reactivates a flashback to a similar childhood phase in the parent and mobilizes the residue of their own cumulative developmental achievements and painful failures.

14.2.3 Making the transition to parenthood

In renaming what used to be called the 'crisis of parenthood', sociologist Rossi noted four social factors which impede the couple in their 'transition to parenthood' in western societies:

a. Paucity of preparation in an age-stratified society.
b. Lack of realistic training for parenthood during pregnancy.
c. Abruptness of transition to total responsibility.
d. Lack of guidelines to successful parenting, seen to involve a complex balance of individual autonomy and couple-mutuality, with each partner ideally fulfilling *both* instrumental and expressive roles [3].

Some of these shortcomings are now being rectified with our greater awareness of the problem. However, in western as in all societies, we find that in order to achieve an integrated (non-crisis) psychological transition to parenthood, the newly pregnant couple have to switch focus from being children of their own parents to a new mode of being a parent to their child(ren). On an emotional level, therefore, changes must occur on three fronts:

1. *Present*: on entering this new phase of childbearing in their life-cycle, the childless couple's 'relationship contract' with each other must be renegotiated.
2. *Future*: Homing in upon the baby they are about to produce, they now have to find nurturing capacities within themselves to play the role of those stable yet flexibly processing parents for their own rapidly growing child.
3. *Past*: Faced with parenthood, the relation to their own early parents is re-evoked in each for better or for worse. Old hurts and deprivations re-surface and to free parenting resources in themselves, need to be healed by internally forgiving the imperfect parents of the past.

14.3 A MARRIAGE OF FORCES

An adult marital-type relationship is a highly complex entity. No outsider can truly know what goes on between a couple. The fluctuating dynamic interaction, compulsive repetitions of the past, mutually destructive tendencies and reciprocal struggle to conserve, grow and promote healing, all differ in each relationship and also change over time. This inevitably means that generalizations always over-simplify. However, in a descriptive overview an adult intimate relationship can be envisaged as comprising three concentric layers, each of which is a tacit 'contract' between them, defined by a different set of forces – social, personal and unconscious [4]. When a 'marriage' fails, it is usually due to breach of contract, lack of fulfilment of expectations or infringement of rights on any one of these three levels.

14.3.1 The Social Contract: explicit and implicit cultural assumptions

The outer circle, or shell of the relationship, constitutes the Social Contract of the relationship: all the culturally determined expectations about 'marriage' that we have each acquired in the course of growing up in our society and our own particular ethnocentric niche within that. Some of these are explicit cultural assumptions that we have grasped by observation of other couples throughout the years, including our own parents (if they were in a couple) or their substitutes and other significant relationships. Other assumptions are reinforced by exposure of the media: novels, films and plays illustrating norms of interpersonal behaviour; TV and magazine stories featuring reciprocal roles; songs, jokes, games and shows all depicting or playing upon recognizable stereotypes of conjugal tasks and the marital 'rules' and standards advocated by society. Further expectations, based on implicit cultural premises, are woven from the intangible mesh of ideas, superstitions, symbols, legends and myths we have each accumulated in a lifetime. These cultural beliefs about marriage, like brides of old, are veiled in mystery; nevertheless, they silently operate on our special relationships, forming an undercurrent of expectations and aspirations.

Emotional reciprocity between partners in a long-term intimate relationship is an elusive entity which can only be fleetingly glimpsed by external observers. Even our long exposure from infancy onwards to the marriage of our parents does not make it clearer. On the contrary, the very specificity of their contact made us aware that parents have a private relationship of their own from which children and others are excluded. Hence, most of us retain a sense of mystery, a conviction of secrets withheld, clandestine intrigues jealously guarded behind the closed doors of the parental bedroom, hopefully to be disclosed, finally, with our own initiation into an adult parental relationship. In each society, much of the folk-lore seems to have sprung from an attempt to penetrate this marital mystery and dispell the parental enigma. In addition, Culture also expediently serves political ends, and myth-spinning about the nature and essence of marriage, in turn influences mythical expectations of our own relationships. As the Women's Movement discovered in western post-war societies, unquestioning reliance on these myths, hidden yet familiar since childhood has perpetuated a false social status quo through elaboration of a 'Feminine Mystique' [5]. It is my belief that the changes in marital patterns in recent years are an attempt to challenge several such underlying themes, now being exploded as we question the whole fabric of implicit political, social, medical and cultural pro-paganda. And each couple afresh, during transition to parenthood, re-questions these assumptions.

14.3.2 Once upon a time they all lived happily ever after

At the risk of exposing the obvious, I shall now try and spell out some of the evasive myths that I believe underlie many of our seemingly rational assumptions about love and marriage:

1. Marriage is an instant transformer and liberator: sleeping beauties awake and frog princes change with 'True Love's' first heterosexual

kiss, which rectifies their previous drab existence forever.

2. Marriage is an eternal fountain of bliss – all fairy tales introduce marriage as the end state following which only happiness flows.

3. Marriage 'Hollywood-style': mutual sexual attraction will ensure marital harmony between two glossy people. Conversely, sexual difficulties will magically vanish in a congenial marriage.

4. Love is an unchanging equilibrium: once achieved, marital bliss should remain constant and unchanging. (Such mythical 'stability' means fixed interactional patterns, needs and roles with no allowance for work towards changes, or place for maturation.)

5. 'Togetherness is all': marriage means never being alone. If happiness means being joined together in every activity, fusion and togetherness allow no place for personal growth and separateness.

6. Romantic love means selflessness, altruism and relinquished autonomy, hence personal strivings and self-realization seem incompatible with marriage.

7. 'Birds in their (marital) nest agree': conflict, friction, disagreements and anger are alien to this idealizing world of 'successful' marriages. (Ironically this is a self-fulfilling prophecy since once argument, the very corrective agent of change, is stigmatized and eliminated, few creative efforts to further or sustain the relationship are possible.)

8. Marriage is 'disposable': once (inevitable) disappointment occurs, new happiness can be found by discarding the now obsolete partner and taking on a replacement marriage.

9. Flagging marriages can be boosted by having a baby: even the most ill-suited couple will become compatible as parents (see Rumplestiltskin!) and the obliging baby will serve as super-glue or royal-jelly to rejuvenate the parent's love.

10. Do-it-yourself kits: Prince Charming/Cinderella made to measure! if you don't get what you want, do a remodelling job on your partner! Beauty did it on her Beast; Professor Higgins did it on Eliza. You too can do it . . . all it takes is fantasy living . . .

14.3.3 Outgrowing fairy tales

Such 'Love and marriage' myths are extremely persuasive and resistant to change even when reality proves them to be false. Often, mythical expectations still persist despite seemingly dramatic changes in the explicit expectations of a relationship, as evident recently in the re-allocation of male and female roles, dual career households, modified childrearing and egalitarian division of labour. Even after discontent has crept into a couple's home, it is often dismissed into the background or brushed under the family carpet and there left to moulder. Each disillusioned partner may experience a vague feeling of having been cheated out of a birthright yet is unable to share the poignant sense of yearning, of unfulfilled hopes and thwarted irrational expectations about their relationship.

The transitional period of pregnancy offers a unique opportunity for a shake-up of outgrown unrealistic misconceptions. Professionals who sense latent tensions or stagnant growth in the relationship of a couple in their care can introduce a breath of fresh air by offering opportunities in parenting classes or discussion groups for such vital issues to be freely discussed. Interracial or mixed marriages between members of different subcultural groups, although vastly enriching also pose a potential for unrecognized/unmet expectations. However, this danger is often averted by the very fact of these couples' awareness of their differences and their genuine desire to work at sharing their respective heritages with each other leading to readiness to clarify what is often mistakenly taken for granted as mutually agreed by other couples.

KEY POINTS

*An intimate relationship is formed by interaction and reciprocity of both partners' contributions, based on interactions with significant figures in their respectives pasts.
*To achieve emotionally the transition to parenthood, couples need to focus on present issues in renegotiating their relationship; cultivation of future resources for the parental role and resolution of past conflicts and deprivations by internally forgiving their own imperfect early parents.
*Marital expectations are derived from three sources: social, personal and unconscious and a 'contract' exists in each.
*The social contract between the couple is based on their explicit cultural assumptions about behaviour norms, tasks and socially defined reciprocity as well as on implicit premises such as those gleaned from cultural myths about love and marriage.
*Whereas the explicit areas can be consciously modified to suit changing times and the specific needs of each particular couple, implicit ones are more difficult to dislodge and often persist as undetected thorns in the body of the marriage.
*Conscious awareness of underlying mythical, irrational expectations as well as sharing realistically defined social assumptions can help eradicate mutual misunderstanding.

14.4 THE PERSONAL CONTRACT

The second layer of expectations in an intimate relationship resides in the personal contract between the couple. This is based on conscious goals and hopes each of the partners have when making a commitment to a long-term union and usually involves some arrangement of cohabitation.

14.4.1 Conscious goals and mutual adaptation

Living together demands complicated reciprocity. Adaptation will include:

a. Establishing an acceptable degree of mutuality in current shared and separate time, friends, activities, attitudes and interests.
b. Setting the rules for conjoint daily living, division of household tasks, financial resources and decision-making policies.
c. Negotiations about the degree of disengagement from or reliance upon their respective families of origin.
d. Developing new boundaries and patterns of couple 'identity' in sexual adjustment, individual gratification, social relationships and inter-personal communication [6].

Implicit in these exchanges is an attempt to arrive at a mutually satisfying viable relationship. The tenacity and ingenuity with which most pairs will attempt to iron out contradictions and continue to trust in the relationship despite emotional fluctuations, is a measure of their dedication to remaining together, although it may be fed by distorted as well as healthy forces. Compromises may be required to eradicate personal conflicts or resolve inconsistencies. However, if either member is too inflexible in bridging divergencies, a skewed relationship may emerge, stabilizing in their unequal contributions or resulting in the eventual break-up of the pair. As with all changes further adjustment is required in the couple's ongoing relationship when they begin to contemplate 'starting a family' or find pregnancy has begun.

14.4.2 Childbearing as a phase in the life-cycle of the family

When childbearing ends the 'couple phase' in the life-cycle of the family, pregnancy will usually be followed by a succession of new phases, such as the 'home-base'/toddler phase, those of school-children, teenagers, 'launching pad' and finally, 'empty nest'/retirement phases. Once they embark upon becoming a family, the nature of the couple's relationship must change to keep pace with altered roles and expectations.

A parallel has been drawn between the life-cycle of an individual and the history of a typical family, beginning with a period of dyadic closeness, growth with birth and development of the children, then a contracting stage after the mature children leave home and eventual decline of sexuality and death. Yet the family is not an organism and does not follow a rigid life-pattern or unfold in predetermined regular sequences. Nevertheless, it is useful to liken the family unit to a delicately balanced intermeshing 'system' [7] in which each shift of position in the family life-cycle imposes a need for acquisition of new skills, revision of old roles and attitudes and a general readjustment of all interacting family members to achieve a new equilibrium. During each transition between phases within the family, an emotional upheaval is experienced, as in first pregnancy. A series of interpersonal adjustments (which differ from couple to couple) need to be negotiated to enable growth and reallocation of resources in order to complete successfully the transition into the next phase. With each family, as with the individual, each developmental phase builds on the preceding one and underpins the following stage. Thus, effective mastery of one stage facilitates fulfilment of the next while incomplete consummation of the preceding phase may forestall or hinder smooth progress later on. At each point, earlier unresolved family issues are reactivated to be repeated unchanged or undergo further development and may then be reintegrated in a new form. We may say therefore, that the family is a product of interactive evolutionary processes – a flexible system that is formed by, adapts to and changes as the result of both internal and external forces.

14.4.3 Personal, couple and family boundaries

In the way an individual creates interpersonal boundaries to ensure the formation and preservation of his/her own identity, so an external boundary is drawn to delineate first the couple, then the family from the surrounding world. This boundary must be permeable to permit some exchanges to take place with other members and institutions of society. If the boundary is too tightly closed, the internal system of the family will become too isolated or insulated from the world and its realities. Conversely, if it is too loose and unselective, loss of difference between the outside and the inside will result, with loss of identity or cohesion between the couple or family members. Likewise, boundaries are drawn within the family around and between different members. Family therapists stress that these can be rigid or diffuse, creating disengaged-type transactional styles in the former and 'enmeshed' relationships where boundaries are too loose and members too close [8,9]. Within the family, in addition to a general mode of functioning, subsystems may arise, with the mother and child(ren) enmeshed and excluding the father, or the parental couple enmeshed but disengaged from the children. In principle, the more enmeshed and closely knit the family, the greater the reverberations of any one individual's stress or changes on all other members.

14.4.4 Division of roles within the family

As we have seen, pregnancy throws gender differences into relief. The woman carrying the child within her is to be a mother. Her male mate

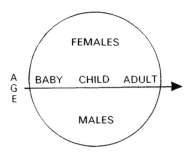

Figure 14.1 Determinants of structure in the family.

may or may not father the child. As the couple expands into a family, its structure and role expectations, once simply defined by their own genders, is now complicated by age factors (Figure 14.1). As children are incorporated into the male/female couple, they will have different rights and duties from adults within the family. Age differences determine a gradation of privileges and obligations within the child category as well, with increasingly complex expectations applied from toddlers to older children. In some societies babies are treated as asexual although expectations differ for boys and girls, and within the couple tasks differ, not only in conjugal roles as husband and wife, but in performance of parental roles as mother and father. Traditionally these roles have been regarded as inescapably rooted in the biological differentiation of the sexes. In many cultures, man was seen to be 'instrumental' in negotiating with the external world on behalf of his family. As such he was expected to be rational, efficient and an authority figure as opposed to his wife, who was seen to gain her status from her husband and children, centring on 'expressive' functions within the home – nurturing, giving affection and reducing family tensions [10]. Increasingly, this traditional dichotomy is being challenged as are all cultural stereotypes, while (as we have seen in the chapters on Facilitators/Regulators and Participators/Renouncers) 'feminine' and 'masculine' social roles (as opposed to male/female sex) can be seen to be undergoing reciprocal changes: as women demand more liberation and non-domestic involvement, men are increasingly less threatened in showing an interest in being expressive and empathic.

14.4.5 Dedifferentiation of masculine/feminine roles

One factor that appears to influence the degree of differentiation of 'masculine' and 'feminine' division of labour in marital roles is the couple's dependence on each other. A classic study revealed that when the family's social network was a highly connected one in which most of the friends know each other, the husband and wife tended to have more segregated and clearly differentiated masculine and feminine roles. Conversely, families with a dispersed network of friends who did not know each other were found to carry out many activities together with less gendered task differentiation or separation of interests [11]. While the social support network has been shown to have an important 'ecological' influence on parenting attitudes and behaviour [12], the marital relationship itself has been found to be a crucial determinant of competent parenting and subsequent child development, with marital dissatisfaction during parenthood following on marital dissatisfaction during pregnancy [13].

A study of 700 families conducted in the early 1960s in Nottingham found that patterns of marital cooperation were dependent both on personalities and on circumstances such as the man's work hours and his wife's earning capacity. In general, sex roles were seen to be more sharply defined and more rigidly typed as one descends the social scale [14]. A more recent study of 100 fathers also conducted in Nottingham reports an apparent contradiction between the egalitarianism expressed by the couple about their relationship (professing equality in terms of emotional reciprocity and the domestic work load) on the one hand and the realities of the differentiation between practical maternal and paternal roles [15]. Thus, professed changes in the renegotiated contract are not followed through in real practicalities. In fact, another study found a downward trend with a quarter of male partners sharing the burden of housework during early pregnancy yet only 6% doing so at 5 months postnatally. Participation in childcare falls from 20% in early weeks to 11% five months later [16]. (Achievement of the transition to parenthood and changes in roles postnatally will be discussed more fully in Chapters 24 and 25.) Suffice to say here that although marital satisfaction has been seen to decline for first time parents with household tasks divided in traditional gender-role allocation [17], changes in set perceptions of masculine and feminine parental roles may occur as a result of utilizing the readjustment momentum of pregnancy. One study of 511 couples found that active preparation for parenthood during pregnancy by attending classes, reading or caring for others' children enhanced men's sense of gratification after the birth [18]. Clearly, how the couple actually achieves a division of domestic and childcare tasks after the birth is a function of negotiations during pregnancy and often determined by the many factors influencing perception of their interlocking gender roles as spouses and parents – social, personal, and, as we shall see, unconscious influences from their own early years, too.

KEY POINTS

*Since the family is a primary group with a unity of its own, identity-defining boundaries and interrelating roles, any change in one member affects all others. External boundaries between the family and society and those inside the family between various members may be rigid or loose, and resultant relationships detached or enmeshed.

*Each shift of position in the family's life-cycle necessitates fulfilment of appropriate tasks entailing modification of previous roles, reallocation of family resources and acquisition of new skills.

*The emotional ripple accompanying each new transition may, if unresolved, trigger a crisis, as a new equilibrium is sought.

*The roles played by different family members are age specific and sometimes defined by gender.

*Segregation of male and female social roles has been found to be related to personality, socioeconomic factors and the degree of interconnectedness of the couple's social network: partners who due to mobility or choice have a dispersed set of friends, are more interchangeable in their household activities and spend more leisure time together.

*Changes in set perceptions of masculine and feminine expectations during pregnancy and early parenthood are influenced by social, personal and unconscious factors.

Chapter 15

Re-evaluation of unconscious contracts and therapeutic opportunities

'A thing which has not been understood inevitably reappears; like an unlaid ghost, it cannot rest until the mystery has been solved and the spell broken.' (Freud, 1909)

15.1 UNCONSCIOUS CONTRACTS

15.1.1 Choice of a mate

In addition to the external world which we share in common with others, we each also contain an inner world, peopled with significant figures from our past. If there is 'unfinished business' with these internal characters, a mystery or unbroken 'spell' as Freud suggests, compulsion to repeat the past may drive us to try and replicate these early relationships in our everyday transactions with others. Marriage, with its intimacy and special intensity of feeling, is the closest adult equivalent we have to the original emotional relationships with our parents. In strange ways, people select their potential mate with an intricate 'sixth sense' that makes subtle intuitive assessments, unconsciously picking up unintended cues while unknowingly sending out provocative signals. In the course of the couple's preliminary 'scanning' of each other, 'falling in love' means unconsciously recognizing interlocking communications from a concealed inner world. The Other becomes charged with special feeling as she or he rekindles hopes of satisfying passions, solving mysteries and gratifying cravings from a cherished past.

Sometimes marriages take place not between two real people, but between two figures inhabiting each other's fantasy worlds. A mate may be chosen to emulate an idealized parent figure or be selected by virtue of being very different to an ambivalently charged parent. He or she may be hand picked for similarities to overt or hidden aspects of oneself, or have imaginary qualities bestowed upon him or her. A marital therapist has defined several collusions which may occur in choice of partner:

a.   An attempt to break free from the past by finding a mate in contrast to negative aspects of the parents.

b. Choosing someone who will share a similar dichotomy: idealizing each other and projecting split-off bad and denied aspects of themselves outside their home.

c. Choice by complementarity: attraction to a partner who is unconsciously perceived as a symbol of 'lost' repressed aspects of the self and is chosen to enact them [1].

Building on (c) in this delineation we can see that when fantasies dovetail, each partner represents and acts out one half of a whole personality, liberated from a certain aspect which is then invested and secured in the other. Thus, a timid 'nice' person may admire and encourage their partner's outspokenness, cruelty or outrageous behaviour, or a neat and organized wife may scorn and rail against yet secretly relish her husband's 'dirty' habits, through which she can vicariously live out 'bad' and chaotic disowned aspects of her own.

Therefore, where the unconscious contract involves the mate as an embodiment of part of one's one personality, the spouse may be chosen:

1. To duplicate, validate or mirror one's own fragile self-image.
2. To represent one's ideal image and become the 'better half'.
3. To enact buried facets, achieving secret ambitions and restoring lost aspects one cannot afford to experience oneself
4. To complete one's own personality by personifying the hated or repudiated or dangerous parts one cannot claim.

15.1.2 Hazards of unconscious contracts

In partnerships where a spouse is chosen to contrast with disliked qualities of the original parent, a straight and narrow path is set from which he or she dare not stray. Any 'lapse' will evoke the original childish response, although secretly, the first partner may have actually engendered this failure to recreate a familiar and charged situation from childhood. ('As usual I trusted him, but I just knew he would let me down again'.)

Similarly, if s/he is chosen to represent idealized aspects of the parent, any 'fall from grace' is magnified out of proportion, as are autonomous exercising of parts of the personality unrelated to the chosen one ('Do you know, she painted her nails! I can't understand how she could do that to me!'.)

In situations where a couple projects badness beyond their nice clean good 'bubble', life becomes restricted as they live in barren beatitude off their meagre inner resources, unreplenished by external contacts or the vital life force of aggression. ('We can't believe the prejudice in people nowadays. There's simply no one you can talk to').

Conversely, in couples where dovetailing occurs, the partners each become two halves of one whole, 'seesawing' in their allocation of attributes ('She's changed from being a sweet loving person to a spoilt brat, wants it all but when she gets it, it's still not good enough. And I love her so much. I try so hard and ask so little and get bugger all from the bitch').

Or, a fixed allocation: one 'black' the other 'white' ('she's the happy-go-lucky one between us, and I do the worrying'). However when such splitting occurs neither partner is allowed autonomy or separate growth. Although hitherto hidden parts of the self may be vicariously expressed and find embodiment through the other in this externalized form they neither enrich the self nor become reintegrated by the rightful owner. ('My husband is such a baby, always whining or demanding sympathy. I can't understand how he can be so weak – It's pathetic! I've never allowed myself to make such a display'.)

While some or all of these collusions occur sporadically in most marriages, when they are the kingpin of the relationship, they endanger this couple, their children and their children's marriages and offspring in turn [2]. Likewise, relationships in which an interaction from the past is repeatedly enacted in an attempt to infuse it with new life, are doomed to failure: however close the partner's approximation to the original, s/he forever remains a stand-in for a past figure, never him/herself. However skilled the re-enactment, s/he will be blamed for being a mere replacement, while the yearned for gratification, like an elusive mirage remains always insubstantial and just beyond reach.

15.1.3 Three central clauses in unconscious contracts: fusion, power, inclusion/exclusion

(a) Fusion

In their relationship, many partners may retain an early childhood wish to be unconditionally loved and a secret yearning to recapture an illusion of fusion through the intimacy of sexual union or emotional merger. Most couples, like most babies, find renewed joy in their sense of individuality following ecstatic merging. However, some mates may use fantasy to deny their separateness, negating their adult differences. An unspoken clause of their unconscious contract might be that each collude with the other to sustain a 'Siamese Twin'-type marriage of conjoined inseparable identical two-who-are-one or male/female two halves of a whole. Another variation on this theme might be a silent agreement to repeat infant-adored-by-mother interaction, each partner alternating to meet the other's infantile needs or one regularly playing mother to the other's baby. A 'Hansel and Gretel' or what has been called a 'Babes in the Wood' type pattern involve the partners clinging to each other like motherless children in a harsh environment. Yet another variation is when one partner is a mirror to the other. ('I'm like a doll in a box, I don't exist unless he's looking at me. He's the person who makes me feel real, but he won't stay home')

Sometimes, as has been hinted at in the examples above, the scenario takes the form of one partner unconsciously setting up doomed situations which are bound to fail but which serve to prove and perpetuate the other's inadequacy as 'mother', as well as his/her own long-suffering deprivation and re-enactment of similarly disappointing interactions in early childhood. Again, it is as well to stress here, that most successful marriages grant the participants freedom to re-experience dependency and mothering in times of need and play. However, in a healthy union this is usually a fraction of the varied and complex interchange between them, not its mainstay.

(b) Power and control

A second type of unconscious contract is focused not on the issue of intimacy as above, but on a second critical dimension of relationships, power and control. This issue, too, has its roots embedded in early childhood conflicts, during what Freud termed the 'Anal phase' and Mahler has called the 'separation–individuation' stage of growing emotional independence and physical autonomy [3]. In marriage, which provides such a fertile ground for re-enactment of these early battlefields, the various 'you can't make me do it' and 'try and stop me' power games can be persistently put to the test, with partners varying their roles as manipulator and manipulated child or parent, often in an alternating 'see-saw' pattern of ascendancy and control. An example might be seen in Albee's play *Who's Afraid of Virginia Woolf?*. In some partnerships the power pattern is fixed. Ibsen's play *The Doll's House* illustrates a type of marriage which requires the wife's apparent helplessness to increase the man's sense of mastery and control. He can keep his own infantile longings and weakness at bay by projecting these into her.

In cases such as these, partners are 'substitute people' to each other forbidden to step out of role, unable to explore their own unique potentialities or those of the partner, or to create new transactions. The present real relationship becomes depleted, bound by obsolete roles in entrenched positions which reduce the capacity for change ('being with him is like nursing a terminally ill patient – he's brain dead'). Sado-masochistic relationships create another form of splitting in which each partner controls and is controlled by the tyranny of self-induced humiliation inflicted by the other partner who plays out in emotional or physical attacks, the repressed cruelty of the victim who sustains the attack. Similarly, use of external 'props' such as alcohol, excessive tidiness, suicide threats or agoraphobia, may be subtle variations on this theme of how one partner can control the other through power prohibitions or emotional blackmail.

(c) Inclusion/exclusion themes

The third type of unconscious contract originates in unresolved issues from a later stage of child development, designated a 'three-person' rather than the two-person psychology of mother–baby relationship [4]. Once the baby becomes focused on other people within the family, awareness of their relationships with one another come to the fore. Seeing mother in loving exchange with a sibling or the parents enjoying themselves together may arouse savage rivalry in the child, jealousy of their special intimacy, and awareness of one's own dependence on the source of goodies. As we shall see in the chapter on siblings, rivalry well handled can lead to constructive preoccupations with fairness, turn-taking and justice. Left unbridled, unexpressed or unguided it can develop into volcanic outbursts or deep rivers of poison. The manner in which parents deal with a child's rivalry is determined by the degree of resolution of their own internal conflicts about inclusion/exclusion.

The jealous little child's wishes for an exclusive relationship with his/her parent of the opposite sex vie with loving feelings and longings for the other parent too. How these 'oedipal' conflicts are resolved, depends largely on the specific family constellation and the parents' ability to handle their own oedipal feelings. For these issues are a three or more generational chain. The outcome hinges on whether parents can convey a sensitive appreciation of the child's budding feelings of sexuality without resorting to either seductive or punitive responses or scornful dismissal. If, on the basis of their own early experiences, the parents are secure in their own sexual relationship with each other and have a strong 'coalition' between them, the child will become reconciled to the futility of her/his wish to steal one parent from the other and at the same time will retain a fond hope of choosing a similarly loyal and loving mate in the future. In this case, in adulthood s/he will establish in turn a secure, intimate relationship with a partner who can share sexuality reciprocally and exclusively within the couple.

However, in families where parents lack sexual boundaries and intimate fulfilment in their own relationship, erotic sensuality is likely to be displaced by the parents onto interaction with a child, either in the form of overt incestuous assault or covert erotized contact, or else in a more generalized intensity of possessiveness, overinvolvement and deep emotional investment. Such near-realization of the child's fantasies endangers both the current family structure and future relationships, perhaps for generations to come. Likewise, parents who are insecure in their own sexuality or preoccupied with incestuous anxieties because their own childhood experiences, might inhibit their child's normal curiosity and sensual expression of affection within the family. This child could then grow up with unresolved forbidden passions and an inability to form new attachments outside the family. In most families, these issues are periodically reactivated, particularly in the 'oedipal' phase of the children or when these conflicts are revitalized during adolescence and the parental couple are called upon to respond. They are also present in new relationships where step-children are introduced into the lover-pair. However, in some partnerships the entire relationship is unconsciously exploited to enact unresolved scenes from childhood oedipal 'scripts', utilizing the partner to represent a loving or spurning parent, or to enact the excluded child, or sibling rivalries often involving a lover to complete the triangle. Once children are born, they too are sucked into the ongoing game either as unwitting actors or audience to a theatrical play from the distant past. Once again I stress that pregnancy forms a transitional junction at which, with help, a couple or family can review their hitherto pathological interaction and seek new patterns of growth.

15.1.4 Breaking out of the past

'Past continuous' is not merely a grammatical term but embodies a psychological truth. The past has a tendency to perpetuate itself. Begetting children in order to replace flagging actors or to rejuvenate a well- worn plot is as callous now as it was when the original scenario was set. Because of the 'layered' nature of intimate relationships, pathological interaction on an unconscious level is not necessarily detectable to others. The 'social' partnership they present to the world might conform to presentable cultural standards or even appear enviably perfect. Their personal behaviour at respective places of work or at dinner parties is quite ordinary; leisurely communications with friends or brief exchanges with professionals can be unremarkable. Only in the unconsciously motivated depths of their intimate relationship with one another as a pair or as a family, is the passion-play activated. Only the couple or their therapists may know of its existence. Ironically, some or all members of the family may not consciously recognize how deeply embroiled they are in a replay of former happenings, filling in the gaps in each other's 'emotional jigsaw puzzles'. Occasionally, one partner gains insightful perspective from a new growth-point in psychotherapy or both partners in a collusive relationship catch a glimpse of their deception in a revealing critical moment and find the motivation to eject out of the anachronistic spiral into present reality ('I've realized that this is a false life we're leading — a 'happy families' pantomime').

Time past directs present and future. Unless harnessed usefully it can be a brutal overseer. Couples enmeshed in the stronghold of the past may find release impossible to achieve without outside help. Untreated, the nexus of pathological interactions extend into future generations as mothers and fathers allow their pasts to intrude as 'ghosts in the nursery' [5], haunting the new family with shadows and projected resurrections. Old 'family myths' as they've been called [6], may take root in role-distortion and help the family avoid recognizing their pathology [7] while other types of shared unconscious fantasy may remain unresolved, denied and binding preventing the family from developing and its members from separating [8]. Exposure to parental distortion of the truth will result in the child's uncorrected defective adjustment to reality. As Skynner points out, 'if the parents preserve fantasies about themselves to hide painful deficiencies or perpetuate grandiose family myths to distract attention from skeletons in the closet, the child will learn to misperceive reality in similar fashion' [9]

Pregnancy with its attendant changes destabilizes the status quo and often provides a trigger for new insights and motivation for growth before the baby arrives. Professionals who are in touch with the couple during antenatal care can facilitate opportunities for exploration of their relationship.

KEY POINTS

*'Marriage' serves as a fruitful ground for repetition of old unresolved conflicts and challenges. In addition to couples' Social and Conscious Contracts, on a deeper level, Unconscious Contracts are made with a partner selected either by contrast to parental figures, as an idealized or caricature version, as part of an unfulfilled self or as an actor in a drama from the past.

*Unwritten 'clauses' of Intimacy; of Power and Control, and Inclusion/ Exclusion themes are central issues in the Unconscious Contract or marriage. The first is largely a two-person 'script', the second draws its salience from battles over autonomy, and the last originating in the oedipal phase of development centres on possessiveness, jealousy, rivalry, seduction, castration (and other retaliative punishments for intruders/transgressors).

*Featuring in the original triangular pattern of Father/Mother/Child, or a sibling variation on the theme, these family preoccupations are repeated in adulthood with a rotation of the triangle when the child becomes a parent. In childless couples, or during pregnancy the partner may be called upon to play the role of parent or excluded child while an extra-marital third is engaged to enact unresolved fantasies from the past.

*Unless resolved during pregnancy, children born into these unreal unions may be employed as marionettes and denied real identity outside the dramaturgical role imposed on them. The main hazard to the family is entrenchment in the past which restricts present spontaneity, authenticity and growth.

15.2 THERAPEUTIC OPPORTUNITIES

15.2.1 Self-help groups

Interaction with other couples undergoing a similar life-event enables partners to make comparisons and evaluation of their own exchanges. Such groups can take place within the context of preparation for parenthood or birth-education, accompanied by a professional who acts merely to encourage free-floating discussion and to contain the anxieties. Specific growth can be stimulated by a focus that is both interpersonal (between people) and intrapsychic (within the person) and based on increased reality testing, gradual disentanglement and separate individuation. These guidelines may help a group leader or couple.

(a) More realistic appraisal of self and partner

(1) *Working at it*
Recognition that all relationships require effort. Even a baby suckling at the mother's breast must work to get milk. Marriage, the most complex and closest interaction between adults, has to involve a great deal of subtle understanding to maintain a smoothly operating two-way process of give and take.

(2) *Improved communication and feedback*
We all retain a primitive wish to be magically understood without words. However, given the multiplicity of our mature needs, voiced expectations are more likely to be met than unspoken desires, and having to communicate verbally and clearly often brings unconscious feelings into conscious awareness and clarifies ambiguities for the speaker as well as the listener. Acknowledgement of grievances or gratification enhances the quality of the relationship and eliminates silent sulks or protective false jollity.

(3) *Developing the capacity to differ and quarrel creatively*
In contrast to self-righteous seething or martyred suffering which damage relationships while maintaining 'the peace', a flaming argument can do much to broaden the loving aspects of the relationship and confirm its viability. Struggle stretches the elasticity of the couple: developing a capacity to differ and engage in creative as opposed to destructive conflict engenders gradual disentanglement of collusively entrenched positions and increases self-knowledge and understanding of the other.

(4) *Encouraging authenticity and risk-taking*
Exposing underlying tensions, collusions and 'blind-spots' opens up the
field for new experiences. Partners discovering the safety of experimenting in each other's company can achieve a new freedom of being,
while hitherto inhibited aspects of the self can be given expression.

(5) *Increasing the range of feeling*
Where relationships have become 'land-locked' for fear of engulfing
tenderness or the passions of violence, verbally unbottling the anger often
serves to temper fury. Voicing the full range of feelings increases self-
knowledge and furthers tolerance of unexplored areas in oneself and
the other.

(6) *Cultivating physical tenderness*
The hall-mark of an intimate relationship is in the quality of touch. As
has been stressed, not since babyhood have such intimate physical
possibilities for demonstrative closeness existed. During pregnancy,
precisely because of the limitations of coital position and her new bodily
sensations, a couple may take new delight in love-making, their sexual
activity increasing in variation and inventiveness. Greater awareness of
the complexities of feeling between them may also increase the range
of affectionate exchanges, cradling, cuddling and hair-stroking, or warm
hugs which lead to laughter rather than passion.

(b) Gradual disentanglement and separate individuation

(1) *Increasing ownership of own motivations*
With confirmation that the relationship can withstand conflict, words can
begin replacing the festering antagonisms that previously found outlets
in action, aggressive sex, psychosomatic symptoms or disturbance in a
child. Conversely, recognition of the fact that words too can hurt increases
each partner's insight into their own motivation for sharing distressing
confidences or indulging in savage interrogations. Awareness that
honesty is abused to inflict pain rather than reveal the truth, may
eliminate those deadly 'games' in which 'telling all' is used as a deadly
weapon cunningly employed to gouge out counter-confessions or find
relief from inner tensions by dumping secret guilt on the other and gaining peace of mind at the expense of disturbing or punishing the partner.

(2) *Developing non-competitive cooperation and mutual interest*
Gradually, with a more realistic appraisal of partner and self, less role-
playing and more meaningful genuine interaction between them,
individual members of the marital couple become better able to disengage
their separate identities from the corporate identity of the marriage.
Newly developed respect for privacy and personal space allows for a

relaxing of boundaries which have had to be defensively rigidified for fear of take-over by the other. Reciprocity and mutual sharing now become a fruitful possibility.

(3) *Diversification and deepening of own interests*
Separate individuality also means self-fulfilment, as each discovers new skills and strengths, growing personally in areas hitherto dormant or building on previous interests and talents. Each may find freedom to encompass several roles within the marriage as well as outside it, and to cultivate unshared activities without detracting from the centrality of their relationship or the personal investment in it. In this way the diversity becomes a source of enrichment rather than a threat and the marriage can stimulate growth rather than the previous persecutory feelings of loss and deprivation.

(4) *Recognition of own parents as a couple*
During the course of achieving separateness from the spouse, issues of separation and individuation from one's own parents are revived. Utilizing the now warmly secure yet growth stimulating marriage, each partner can begin generating new solutions to old internal problems, no longer colluding in repeating the previous patterns. With development, in becoming parents, each may now find ways of liberating themselves from hidebound relationships with their own 'internal' parents, and in releasing these shady figures can begin to accept their real parents as people in their own right. In fact they may come to regard the parents as a sexual couple permitted to live their own separate lives and entitled to their own private idiosyncrasies. This in turn increases the young couple's ability to respond to each other sexually and emotionally as real, rounded and unique people in their own right, unhampered by shadows from the past.

Most of these psychological intra- and interpersonal tasks can be accomplished in the shelter of the marital relationship. Given stimulation and support from their peer-group and worked-through in the home, too, each partner within the couple can increase their 'degrees of freedom' and find their own thresholds commensurate with their courage, pain and capabilities.

However, certain types of problems, personal vulnerabilities and a high intensity of disturbances might tip the balance between the ability to benefit from self-help and the need for professional intervention. A guideline may be that outside help is needed when the stability of a marriage is threatened because too large a proportion of the marital resources are taken up with keeping the past alive or where precious resources are wasted in keeping too much of each partner out of the relationship, or too much work invested in trying to be what the other decrees to allow for mutual growth or self-realization.

15.2.2. Professional help

A couple seeking help or a health-care professional making a referral may find it difficult to choose among the confusing diversity of professional help available. Basically, professional psychotherapeutic assistance offered to couples experiencing emotional difficulties (or to individuals, for that matter) falls into one of two categories or a combination of both: A.Psychotherapeutic techniques which aim to increase awareness and 'insight. B.Structural and behavioural corrective approaches. In A. the therapist encourages free expression by the couple and uses verbal clarification, based on his/her assessment of the problem and observation of the couple's current emotional interaction with each other (and with the therapist), to interpret unconscious forces operating in each individual and/or in the relationship. In B, the second group of therapies, the therapist employs various strategies to manipulate and alter existing behaviour and promote alternative cognitive and behavioural patterns in one or both partners. To succeed, both types of therapy require the couple's commitment, cooperation and motivation to change, however, the former (group A) also requires a capacity for self-reflection.

(a) Group A: a variety of psychodynamically orientated techniques
1. Individual psychotherapy or psychoanalysis: a long-term intensive approach which is suitable when problems are experienced as intrinsically personal, of early complex and conflicted origin and where deep, far-reaching growth is sought by each partner to effect changes in themselves and the relationship as a whole, or when only one partner has the capacity or feels the need for change.

2. (a) **Conjoint couple psychotherapy:** addressing intra and inter-psychic dynamics and interpersonal aspects of chronic patterns and problems in the relationship. These are worked through in great depth over a long period, usually with two therapists of opposite sexes working simultaneously with both partners and providing a healthy interactive model for the relationship.

(b) Couple guidance or therapy: as above, with only one therapist.
(c) Couple counselling: short term active advice re specific problems.
(d) Couple casework: social work setting, supportive, long or short-term work, emphasising social/interpersonal rather than psychological aspects or unconscious contracts in the couple's dysfunctional relationship.
3. **Brief (focal) psychotherapy or counselling:** (individual or couple) to deal with specific distress and achieve predefined limited goals. Two to six sessions over an extended period or intensive and short term.

4. **Crisis intervention**: emergency treatment to restore personal or marital equilibrium following or during a crisis. May take place in the home setting by a specialist team.
5. (a) **Family therapy**: the whole family seen jointly as in marital therapy above, by one or usually two therapists, male and female.
   (b) **Extended family therapy**: as above but, at times, one or other of the partners is seen separately with all or some members of his or her respective family of origin with a view to tracing the root of the key-couple's present difficulties and working through these in the original context as well as the marital one.
6. **Couple's groups**: three to five couples seen simultaneously, usually by two (male and female) co-therapists. In some groups work is done separately with each couple, while others listen and learn by identification while awaiting their own turn. In other groups, individuals participate freely in group discussion, airing their own specific difficulties in the group situation, getting reinforcement and feedback from members of the group as well as elucidation from the leaders about the dynamics of their own particular pair-relationship as well as the dynamics of the group as a whole.

(b) Group B: behavioural techniques

1. *Contract making*: in the therapist's presence, the couple discuss particular difficulties between them, work out a detailed resolution and write a contractual agreement of behaviour to be encouraged or dropped. These resolutions are monitored at home on a chart or checklist and rewarded by agreed reciprocal behaviour of either spouse.
2. *Marital tasks*: the couple are instructed by the therapist to fulfil certain tasks jointly or singly, in order to alleviate the symptoms of marital stress of which they complain.
3. *Cognitive therapy*: a short-term structured therapy (about 20 sessions) which aims to identify the core pathogenic assumptions of the couple by using a diary of activities in addition to their reports and then trying to challenge their dysfunctional beliefs by helping them realize the illogicality of these ideas.
4. *Paradoxical prescriptions*: the therapist instructs the couple deliberately to reproduce the offending situation or symptom, thereby gaining control over its appearance by being able to produce it to order.
5. *Assertiveness training*: to enable one or both members of the couple to become more adept at asserting their needs, views, feelings as fully fledged partners in the relationship. In a group situation training is in the form of role play and personalized exercises.
6. *Sex therapy*: focuses on the physical aspects of the relationship,

encouraging improved communication between partners. Having identified the source of dissatisfaction, instructive techniques are employed to rectify these problems (such as impotence, frigidity, premature ejaculation). 'Homework' and behavioural tasks or very infrequently surrogates may be utilized.

(c) Therapeutic devices which may supplement or complement many techniques in either of the two approaches (A,B) (except A1.)

1. *Videotape feedback*: the couple are filmed interacting during the sessions; particular parts are played back in their presence to illustrate dysfunctional modes of interaction of behavioural patterns of which they are unaware. Interpretations of these sequences or corrective instructions are given by the therapist (type A or B respectively).
2. *Role play*: the partners are each instructed to play some role, and their improvisations are analysed with reference to their own difficulties; similarly, they might be asked to reverse roles and play each other, an exercise revealing much about their perception of each other and facilitating empathic understanding of what it feels like to be in the other's shoes.
3. *Psychodrama*: more complex scenes are improvised and enacted with a view to identifying unvoiced problems and unrecognized dynamics; their expression encourages exploration of new solutions.
4. *Family sculpture*: (particularly used in wider settings – group, family therapy, etc.). A three-dimensional 'living sculpture' is created utilizing the cooperative bodies of participants as building bricks, to illustrate family interactional patterns and myths, the 'postures' adopted signifying support systems, power structures, proximity or distances, and alliances between family members.
5. *Guided fantasy*: the couple are encouraged by the therapist to explore their own fantasies and 'led' into imaginary situations which they habitually avoid with a view to discovering, sharing and gradually neutralizing the fear and resistance. Other guided fantasy 'trips' may aim to explore levels of sensory awareness, hoping to recapture subliminal feeling experiences and reach universal symbols or themes or mystical (transpersonal) sensations.
6. *Gestalt*: a therapeutic framework that encourages partners each to take responsibility for their own behaviour, emphasizing present vs. past, the here and now. External props may be used, such as an empty chair which can be addressed in lieu of absent figures, or a cushion which may be pummelled instead of an exasperating other. Dreams and nightmares too are relived as if happening in the here and now, with dream elements acted out and extended. (Dream exploration is also extensively used in individual psycho-

therapy and psychoanalysis as a means of revealing a personal unconscious commentary.)

7. *Body work*: some therapies use body exercises to familiarize and sensitize people to their physical being. Others use 'body work' and shouting or screaming as a means of freeing what has become repressed, bypassing words where these are used defensively or regressing to a pre-verbal level of experience recaptured and expressed through bodily sensations. (Among the latter are various primal therapies who practise 'rebirthing', on the assumption that subsequent mental stress and disease result from bad experiences at birth. They do so by 'repeating' the original experience and/or living out a new one).

This overview is intended as a brief guideline for professionals intending to refer clients for therapy. It is by no means complete and both availability and practice may vary in different localities.

Chapter 16

Health-care professionals as guides in the transition to motherhood

'What choices do women have? They have precious few if midwives do not point them out to them. What choices do midwives have? They will only discover their choices when they really get to know a small group of women and follow them through their pregnancy, labour and puerperium. They will also discover their worth as midwives, how women need them and care about them, and the midwife's unique position and role in society . . . Mothers need midwives, but midwives need mothers even more'. (Caroline Flint, *Sensitive Midwifery*)

PARTURITION ACROSS CULTURES

16.1.1 Symbolic significance of female guides and midwives

Even in those many societies where reproduction is defined as a natural process, pregnancy and particularly childbirth are regarded as a time of increased vulnerability. A primagravida has a marginal social status while she occupies that transitional state when she is not yet a mother but no longer a maiden. Located between the past and the future, she is in temporal transition blurring social as well as spatial boundaries between inside and out and the corporeal entities of self and other. In many cultures, pregnancy also hangs between natural and supernatural. The woman, invaded by an alien being, possibly of spirit or ancestral origin, is regarded as being in contact with both the profane and sacred worlds; pregnancy may also be seen as a form of spirit possession, exposing the bearer to danger from malevolent demons or granting her extraordinary powers of sorcery or divination. In most societies, the marginal mother-to-be is provided with a female guide, who will act an intermediary between her and society.

16.1.2 Midwifery services

A World Health Organization cross-cultural survey estimated that the majority of women worldwide are attended by traditional birth attendants; in some parts of the world, where populations are sparse and dispersed, the role of indigenous midwife might be filled by female relatives, mother, mother-in-law or, rarely, a woman might be unattended. In some cultures, advice on fertility and birth assistance may come from spirit mediums and herbalists in addition to midwives; however, midwives, too, are often considered to have special powers. They may be granted religious legitimacy, seen as 'called' to the role by God or spirits, practising healing under ancestral mandate, ritually freeing pregnant women from sin and purifying them for a successful birth through confession and exorcism. Most midwives achieve their position by accomplishment rather than having it ascribed to them. Descriptions of traditional midwives from places as far apart as India, Pakistan, Bangladesh, Nigeria, Tanzania, Brazil, Mexico, Guatemala and Jamaica, emphasize the status of midwives who are mature women, and have themselves born children [1]. Their services extend well beyond the event of birth, ranging from diagnosis of pregnancy, estimated delivery date, advise on emesis, oedema, diet, physical work, coitus and abortion. Services may include massage prenatally and postpartum, herbal remedies, postnatal visits with practical domestic help, care of other children, and paediatric advice and companionship as well as assistance with supernatural powers and ceremonials. This range of activities is not inconsistent with the World Health Organization's definition of a midwife as: '. . . a person who is . . . trained to give the necessary care and advice to women during pregnancy, labour and the postnatal period, to conduct normal deliveries on her own responsibility, recognize the warning signs of abnormal or potentially abnormal conditions which necessitate referral to a doctor' [2].

16.1.3 The midwife's place in rites of pregnancy and childbirth

In many societies a sequence of ceremonial rituals during pregnancy serve to disconnect the prospective mother from her previous life, to shelter both her and the fetus while vulnerable, and to protect others from the danger or impurity the pregnant woman herself may represent. These rituals, during which she is often accompanied by her female 'mid-wife' (= 'with woman'), mark out her passage into parity. They follow the same structure of other transitional rites:

a. Separation from her previous life;
b. A transitional period with gradual removal of barriers;
c. Integration into ordinary life as mother [3].

In the case of the pregnant woman, separation might entail actual isolation from men and/or certain other women, restricted seclusion or prohibition from entering specified places or attending various rites. Or, as in our society, it may merely involve sexual or dietary injunctions, changes in work patterns, maternity wear and 'rituals' (such as antenatal checkups, hospital registration, shopping for baby equipment, filling out maternity grant and leave forms) to be executed at specified times. In many cultures, performance of ceremonies are located at nodal points (usually at the 3rd, 5th, 7th, 8th and 9th months) and may be accompanied by cessation or reduction of economic productivity.

The sequence culminates after childbirth with further seclusion, dietary and contact taboos for many days (usually counted in units of 10 – 10, 20, 30, 40 or even 100 days) and ritual purifications with gradual social acknowledgement of parenthood, return and re-introduction of the new mother and baby into ever-widening social contacts and finally, integration into her new status and peer group. In western societies, many of these processes are obscured by the isolated nuclear family structure coupled with the medicalization of birth and its institutionalization away from the couple's home. Often, in our own society, the social return from childbirth overlaps with the geographical return from hospital confinement, thus blurring the distinction between acquisition of social and physical parenthood. Nevertheless, looked at from an anthropological viewpoint, hospitals may be seen to induce segregation of the parturient away from her community, and to practise 'purification rituals' (enema, scrubbing, pubic shaving, separated baby-bathing, etc.). Although scattered among many professionals rather than a single midwife the health system implicitly recognizes the need for transitional care and re-integration: in Britain, nurses or midwives help the mother to establish breastfeeding, community midwives provide domiciliary continuity of care for 10 days following delivery at home or after discharge from hospital, the GP conducts a six-week checkup, and health visitors offer help, advice and practical assistance with the baby during the first year, while well-baby clinics provide mothers with opportunities to meet with their peers.

16.1.4 Ceremonies for the newborn child

Rituals performed after the birth of the child follow the same pattern of sequences:

a. **Separation** (cutting the umbilical cord, and, in societies where there is a belief in transmigration and reincarnation, rites of separation from the world of the dead);
b. **Transition period** of seclusion and protection (which may last well into childhood);
c. **Initiation** into human society, coinciding according to the mores of that society with baptism, circumcision, celebration of naming, first hair cut, appearance of first tooth, first outing, weaning, introduction of solid food, etc.

In each of these ceremonies, the female intermediary (often midwife) not only caters to the parturient's postnatal needs but also those of her infant by providing practical assistance and ensuring health and safety. Furthermore s/he serves a spiritual function to neutralize envy, banish impurity and/or attract sorcery to herself to protect mother and child. Above all she acts as a bridge [4] between the prospective mother and spiritual powers, between parturient and social milieu, and provides continuity between the woman's past life and future as nurturing mother.

KEY POINTS

*Pregnancy is regarded as a time of increased vulnerability during which the woman has a marginal social status between her old position and future one.

*In many societies a female guide is provided for the duration of her pregnancy, to act as an intermediary between the past and future, parturient and society, natural and supernatural sheltering both her and fetus while vulnerable, and protecting others from the danger or impurity she represents, and finally, acting as bridge back to her new status in society.

*The midwife-intermediary offers services far beyond the birth, ranging from diagnosis of pregnancy, estimated delivery date, advice, massage, herbal remedies, spiritual purification and practical help after the birth.

*She usually accompanies the pregnant woman through the various ceremonies which mark out her passage into parity through the means of: (1) separation from previous position; (2) a transitional period with gradual removal of barriers; (3) integration into ordinary life.

*Similar structures exist in western health-care patterns, albeit, usually with a succession of experts replacing the single guide.

16.2 EMOTIONAL EXPERIENCES OF PROFESSIONALS IN THE BIRTH CHAMBER

16.2.1 Psychological dangers in obstetric practice

Birth is a deeply arousing experience. The beholder cannot help but be confronted by fantasies of his or her own original journey from the female interior and archaic anxieties prevail, since, as Freud observed, birth is the prototype of all separations. In addition, the obstetrician or midwife assisting a labouring woman is informed too, by the physical dangers inherent in the situation and of their own godlike sense of responsibility for producing a live, undamaged child. Repeatedly these 'deliverers' are being tested: will their powers of creativity override darker forces? It is said that 'those who play God should not be surprised if they get blamed for natural disasters'. Sometimes there are conflicting loyalties towards their two clients, wishing to satisfy the woman's desire for a leisurely, natural childbirth, yet anxious about deleterious effects on the unborn child. While this conflict is no doubt resolved by experienced midwives, other unconscious anxieties continue to operate.

Birth-professionals have to contend with inevitable repeated exposure to pain, blood, mess, naked emotionality and urgency. The situation is further complicated by the fact that, unlike most patients, the woman in labour is not injured or ill; although there is one body in evidence, there are at least two people to be considered, one of whom is still unseen. Unlike most operations, the one 'patient' is usually fully conscious and often assertively insisting on managing the procedure herself. Her partner, and sometimes other relatives or friends are present, observing, commenting, supporting the woman, intervening, often advocating and championing her 'whims' against professional advice. Throughout the labour, physical intimacies may take place between the partners. The woman's nakedness is eroticized by the potent presence of her impregnator and his insistence on fondling, massaging and caressing her may embarrass the staff. Similarly, despite their neutral stance, professionals might feel stirred up by the woman's effusive emotionality. Her suffering, her ecstatic reactions or excessive screaming, her whimpering, crying out, beseeching or groping her helpers can provoke mixed reactions such as sympathy, distaste, empathic compassion or irritation. To remain untouched requires defensive manoeuvres that we all employ to some extent when confronted by repetitive stressful situations, chronic anxiety and prolonged trauma.

16.2.2 Defensive techniques of professionals and organizations

In institutions where the objective work situation is one which regularly threatens to evoke primitive responses in professionals, the organization itself evolves strategies to protect its members from the risk of being flooded with unmanageable anxieties. Menzies [5] has studied such socially structured defence mechanisms used within the general nursing service. She has enumerated strategies that have developed to minimize an anxiety-provoking person-to-person relationship between staff and patients. Many of these are also applicable to the obstetric situation.

(a) Splitting up nurse–patient relationship

The core of the anxiety situation is a close relationship with a dependent, often frightened, distressed and needy patient. Protection from anxiety is achieved by breaking down treatment into tasks, moving nurses around, minimizing nurse contact with patients as whole individuals, and reinforcing the myth that all patients are similar and all nurses are uniform and interchangeable. These features are applicable to the antenatal situation, where a woman may be seen by as many as 30 'interchangeable' hospital professionals in the course of one pregnancy and little attempt is made to acknowledge her as a special individual either before, during or after the birth. Furthermore, technological aids such as fetal monitors may also be used to replace direct contact with the woman during labour.

(b) Denial and detachment of feelings

Adequate professional detachment is a prerequisite of competence, necessitating control of personal feelings, refrain from excessive involvement and maintenance of a professional stance despite manipulation. However, in an anxiety-provoking situation, such detachment may be carried to extremes by denial of compassion or curiosity and standardization of treatment. In the nursing service this may be institutionalized as impersonal universality of staff functioning, ritualization of performance, and fragmentation of attachments among the nurses themselves by frequent mobility [6]. In the obstetric situation, there is often a 'production line' approach in antenatal checkups, with women literally laid out on 'slabs' dressed in identical robes, awaiting the detached probing fingers of doctor and impersonal blood-pressure-taking busy nurse. In many hospitals, physiotherapists giving birth-preparation classes rarely attend the birth of their clients, and nurses on the postnatal ward have rarely seen the new mother before her delivery. Even during the course of labour and birth, it is unlikely that the labouring woman will be handled exclusively by one individual as midwives frequently change shift, student doctors practise their skills and other personnel may casually come and go with little acknowledgement of the private nature of the birthing experience, its emotional significance and the disturbing feelings it arouses.

(c) Redistribution of responsibility

The burden of anxiety of having to make a final committing decision is dissipated among nurses by a system of checks and rechecks, delegation upwards, minimization of personal initiative and discretion, and a series of unconscious tactics enabling redistribution of internal conflict and uncertainty by splitting, projection, denial and avoidance of change [7]. In maternity nursing, there seem to be a situation which is further aggravated by hierarchical splits between obstetricians and midwives. Horizontal antagonism may arise between divergent styles of nurses and physiotherapists who also execute different tasks with the same patients [8].

The recent introduction of rapid change in obstetric practice due to technological advances and consumer pressures seems to have engendered new problems such as rigidification as some old methods are clung to, doubts as others are questioned and partially replaced, and confusion as yet other obsolete relics may be retained to 'calcify' alongside innovatory instruments. Because the social defence system has been constructed to help individual professionals avoid experiencing anxiety, guilt, doubt and uncertainty, any activities which threaten the status quo, are intensely resisted. However, the defensive techniques enumerated above not only protect staff members from emotional threats but also deprive them of job satisfaction by reducing them into task-orientated

Table 16.1 Emotional experience of birthing-care professionals

---

Professionals' exposure to emotional threats in the birth situation
  Chronic tension of uncertainty
  Acute stress of emergencies
  Maternal or neonatal death
  Birth complications
  Deformity of infant
  Maternal physical or mental illness

Exposure to primitive emotions – perceived and experienced
  Pain, eroticism; abandon; intimacy; passion; anxiety; rivalry; envy; fear;
  contagion; idealization; empathy; identification; reparation

Institutional defences employed as protection vs. above
  Staff denial of feelings
  Ritualization of treatment
  Depersonalization of encounter
  Interchangeability (of staff and of patients)
  Control of procedures
  Pain reduction
  Mystification

Emotional needs of paramedical professionals
  A staff support group enabling expression of feelings
  Opportunities to vent irritation, grievances and confidential
    complaints procedure
  Open channels of communication up and across hierarchy
  Continuity of caring for individual patients throughout pregnancy and birth
  Broad areas of responsibility, rather than task-orientated approach
  Space and time to form human attachments
  Individual and group counselling for staff encountering particular stress and
    opportunities to grieve for losses (i.e. as in neonatal intensive care units)

---

detached anonymous professionals and their patients into a succession of pregnant bodies. Both caring and gratitude are diminished in a system where people behave and are treated in a depersonalized way. Defensive strategies lessen personal investment in a job well-accomplished, together with inhibition of the many opportunities for personal growth, greater self-understanding and the gratification of expressing creative and compassionate aspects of oneself. As one experienced midwife puts it: 'The fragmented care we give most women at the moment might almost have been designed to stop us from learning about our role and to weaken us as a profession' [9].

KEY POINTS

*Researchers of social systems have described defensive techniques employed by staff members to lessen the experience of anxiety, persecution, guilt or doubt inherent in their work. These defences operate on both an institutional and a personal level and are highly resistant to change.

*In hospital settings, strategies employed to minimize concentrated anxiety-provoking person-to-person relationship between staff and patients include task-orientated rather than whole patient treatment; depersonalization and categorization of patients thereby reinforcing the myth that all patients are interchangeable and anonymous. Staff detachment and denial of feelings ensure standardization and impersonal universality of staff functioning; ritualization of treatment reduces uncertainty and the need for personal initiative and decision-making; and a series of conscious and unconscious tactics enable redistribution of conflict by splitting, projection and denial, and alleviation of potential worry and guilt by diffusion and delegation of responsibility.

*Such defensive techniques applicable to the nursing service in general, are pertinent to midwifery and obstetric care as it has been practised in recent years, a denial that limits effectiveness of care.

16.3 BIRTHCARE SEEN HISTORICALLY

Maternity care has been in the hands of women since the beginning of recorded history as Shifra and Puah, the midwives in the birth of Moses, verify. Midwives presided over pregnancy and birth in the ancient cultures of the Egyptians, Babylonians, Greeks, Romans, Chinese and Incas. Before industrialization, in western societies too, reproductive care was an indigenous female-controlled system, with a 'wise-woman' presiding over matters of fertility, contraception, abortion, pregnancy, birth and lactation. However, with medicalization of childbirth and suppression of female healers, specialized midwifery became a male province.

16.3.1 The history of midwifery in Europe and America

Medicalization of childbirth began with the establishment, in thirteenth-century England, of the Barber-Surgeons' Guild, whose right to use surgical instruments became a male prerogative. Embryotomies to dismember a fetus 'stuck' *in utero*, or caesarean sections to remove a live baby from a dead mother, could be performed only by specialized surgeons called in by midwives to attend a pathological delivery. With the professionalization of Medicine as a predominantly male discipline during the fourteenth to seventeenth centuries in Europe, practising wisewomen-healers/midwives, with their wide knowledge of anatomy, astronomy, psychotherapy and pharmacology, posed a threat to male doctors. In England in 1512, midwives were included in the Church licensing system which regulated medical practice; however, midwives were only licensed provided they swore not to practise witchcraft! Until the sixteenth century, a distinction had been maintained between 'good' and bad witchcraft, with the female 'good witch' healer defined by the 1548 English Witchcraft Act as an unlicensed practitioner of medicine, a distinction abolished by a later act in 1563. This was followed by several centuries of witch hunting. Persecution and execution of 'subversive' wisewomen healers were sanctified by Church authorities who regarded midwives as challenging established hierarchies. Midwives were considered to be in alliance with the Devil in their power to bring forth live babies. Also reputed to administer aphrodisiacs, they were deemed a threat to men's control over sexuality, and their potions and herbal remedies acquired supernatural magical properties [10].

Nevertheless, the 'pollution' associated with female bodies and sex was largely relegated to female practitioners until the invention of forceps in the seventeenth century, when male midwifery became elevated from surgical intervention to instrumental obstetrics dealing with abnormal and 'upper-class' deliveries. Restriction of female midwifery to 'normal' labour was officially recognized in the Midwifery Diploma first granted by the Obstetrical Society of London in 1872. However, with the redefinition of the role of midwife in the nineteenth and twentieth centuries, and her exclusion from medical and surgical training throughout Europe, midwifery became defined as a secondary status health profession practised among the working classes [11]. In 1902 in Britain, midwives organized and delineated an area of expertise over which they presided until as late as 1973, when the majority of all British babies – 70% of hospital births and 80% of home births – were still delivered by midwives. However, as male obstetricians monopolized 'pathological' births, the definition of labour underwent a change, emerging as an abnormal event requiring clinical intervention. With medicalization and hospitalization of childbirth, midwives were now to become mere 'handmaidens' to male obstetricians. Across the Atlantic doctors were at the forefront. In North America in 1964 only 1.5% of all births were delivered by midwives. For the first time in history, 'an entire society of women was attended in childbirth by men' [12].

During this era, hospital childbirth had become a high technology alienating event with the labouring women routinely immobilized in labour, absent in 'twilight sleep' or general anaesthetic in the USA – a supine body from which the baby was extruded by forceps delivery. With centralization of maternity services and mechanization of birth, not only did the mother lose control over her body and the experience of birth but the midwife too had become deskilled and a mere ancillary service to medicine. Previously a pivotal person in the community, engaged in teaching women to maximize their potential to grow, to give birth to and care for a healthy baby, her craft was now replaced by machines, and her emotional relationship with her charge broken into small units distributed among many practitioners and remodelled on a male medical basis of clinical neutrality.

16.3.2 The right to body ownership

Nevertheless, in the wake of the Women's Movement, women consumers have formed a childbirth reforming movement to restore parturient rights to female reproductive care. Their cause has been espoused and taken up by a sister movement geared towards restoring the independent status and skills of traditional midwifery. In America, by 1976, the Frontier Nursing Service set up in 1925 to emulate British midwifery, had trained 1800 certified nurse-midwives. Following the biting criticism of a courageous book exposing the 'Immaculate Deception' of childbirth as dangerous and requiring technological intervention [13], nurse-midwives in the USA bravely began questioning whether they had indeed, as accused, sold out to the medical establishment [14]. However, it was not only the midwives who were concerned. In 1976, an Interprofessional Task Force on Health Care of Women and Children was established by four professional organizations – American Academy of Paediatrics, the American College of Nurse-Midwives, the American College of Obstetricians and Gynaecologists, and the American Nurses Association. In 1978, this task force issued a statement on 'Development of Family Centered Maternity/Newborn Care in Hospitals' which clearly recommended reorganization of obstetric care to respond to needs on different levels – physical, social, economic and psychological. The psychological needs were defined as permitting women 'to achieve their own goals . . . within the context and cultural atmosphere of their choosing'. This interactional–ethical perception meant recognition of the necessity for 'team effort of the woman, and her family, health-care providers and the community', while changes on an organizational level suggested provision of a flexible system of obstetric alternatives necessitating regionalization of care through 'the cooperative interrelationships of hospitals, health care providers and the community so as to provide for the total spectrum of maternity/newborn care within a particular geographic region' [15]. With this reformulation a shift occurred from a medical 'expert'-orientated focus to a family-centred approach.

16.3.3 Changes in obstetric care in Britain

In Britain, a two-pronged movement of female consumers and midwives has brought about a similar shift in focus. Two nation-wide consumer organizations, the National Childbirth Trust and the Association for Improvements in the Maternity Services (AIMS) were founded over a quarter of a century ago to banish the 'dark-age attitude towards the psychology of childbirth' [16]. These were later followed by other organizations such as the Maternity Alliance. With increasing public awareness, the late 1970s saw the first gatherings and rallies celebrating a woman's right to be actively involved in decisions about the birth of her baby and her need to be treated as a 'whole' person rather than as a passive patient. Some corresponding changes of attitude occurred within the medical profession. However, the rise of routine interventions continued at such a rate that the General Medical Council queried the possibility that the Medical Defence Union were advising doctors to act unethically [17]. Petitions requesting Parliament to define and strengthen parents' maternity care rights by law (for instance, 22 March 1983 International Women's Council of Obstetric Practices' petition with 12 000 signatures) followed. Equally, midwives concerned with the erosion of their traditional role (due to obstetric takeover and abolition of home confinements) had begun to reexamine their dissatisfaction with the service they were offering. By 1983, three out of five midwives elected to the new English National Board were members of the Association of Radical Midwives. The latter repudiated the role of nurse-midwife which had become demoted to 'obedient female assistant of the doctor' [18] and have sought ways to reestablish confidence in midwifery skills both among professionals and in the community (see section 18.2.5)

16.4 REINSTATING THE CAREGIVER AS 'MID-WOMAN'

Vulnerable in her position as intermediary between the labouring woman and representatives of the State, i.e. the medical establishment, the consultant obstetrician who sets policies and her employer, the Health Authority, many a midwife has found that with increasingly advanced machinery her role has expanded to becoming a competent technician, and far from being the champion of her clients she find herself sometimes carrying out the very practices she decries, such as enemas, perineal shaving, episiotomies and acceleration of labour. A member of the English National Board of Midwives has stated; 'if midwives allow themselves to be participants in a system which dehumanizes care they must take some responsibility for perpetuating it' [19].

The call had sounded for democratic non-hierarchical staff groups to facilitate communication channels within the health service; for provision of continued education for qualified midwives in order to reinforce their unique expertise and for reorganization of the system to provide continuity of care throughout pregnancy and postnatally [20]. Throughout the western world, changes are occurring. A home birth movement has now begun even in Sweden, despite 95% of hospital births being conducted by midwives with much wider responsibilities than British midwives (to do inductions, intravenous drips, paracervical and pudendal blocks; perform vacuum extractions, do breech and multiple deliveries, perineal suturing and emergency manual removal of placenta) [21]. Although in 1984, 98% of births still took place within the NHS [22], in recent years an increasing number of midwives have been reluctantly leaving the Health Service to become independent (or doing home deliveries during their time off from hospital work). As general practitioner units are (sadly) contracting, private facilities offering a flexible variety of choices have begun to proliferate. Some American hospitals have responded to protest movements by remodelling their 'birthing rooms' while other, less cosmetic changes offer environments run entirely by midwives, with a single midwife attached to each childbearing family from the first antenatal visit through the birth, which takes place in a double-bedded motel-type room followed by a celebratory meal [23].

Many caregiving professionals are searching for new possibilities both within the existing mainstream and in innovatory experiments outside it to accept the modern-day challenge to redefine their role and the service they offer [24]. Obstetricians are looking to the future with a view to modifying current practice in antenatal, intrapartum and neonatal care [25]. General practitioners are questioning how GP training should be changed to accommodate future involvement in intranatal care [26]. Health visitors, too, are in a unique position to expand their service to a more comprehensive one spanning the antenatal to early parenthood period by initiating and running pre- and postnatal support groups as well as offering a highly personalized home-based support system for promoting health, early detection of abnormality and alleviation or containment of existing conditions [27]. Midwives, specifically, are seeking ways of regaining job satisfaction by reinstating their unique age-old position as female intermediary – 'she who sits with woman'. This may involve the need to reshape training [28], to expand and reinstate their position as health educator and parentcraft teacher [29], and above all 'friend' [30], confidante and personal guide throughout pregnancy, labour, birth and puerperium.

KEY POINTS

*Female control over reproductive care has been gradually eroded over the centuries in Europe and America. Defined as witches, public persecution and executions of 'subversive' wise-women healers were sanctified by Church authorities who regarded midwives as challenging established hierarchies.

*With the rise of exclusively male medical professionalism and redefinition of male technical and surgical intervention as obstetrics, female midwifery became restricted to an increasingly narrow field of 'normal' labour.

*As labour itself was recast as inherently pathological, and childbirth centralized and hospitalized, midwives have themselves become further deskilled as ancillaries to medicine rather than practitioners in their own right.

*Current consumer movements to reinstate women's right to female reproductive care is finding a corollary in the midwives' movement towards recovering their unique position as female guides in normal maternity.

Part Five

EXPERIENCES OF LABOUR AND BIRTH

Chapter 17

Anticipating Childbirth

'. . . elemental faith that life will conquer death. If this inner faith is lacking, the mother is in real danger; she may prove unequal to the possible difficulties of childbirth and its frequent physical surprises. In the polarity of life and death, the optimistic feelings are on the side of life, the anxious-pessimistic ones in the service of death' (H. Deutsch, 1945., *Psychology of Women*, vol. II.).

17.1 FEARS AND FANTASIES OF CHILDBIRTH

As the last weeks of waiting draw near, tedium mingles with suspense. The fantasy baby gradually gives way to anticipation of a real baby, however, excitement and curiosity are overshadowed by anxiety about its arrival. The pregnant woman feels she is caught up in an inexorable process. Carried along on a roller coaster hurtling in slow motion towards an unknown finish line; the timing and nature of the birth are beyond her control.

Birth anxieties may be categorized in various ways:

1. When/where will it happen?
2. How will she negotiate it?
3. Will her past catch up with her?
4. Who will emerge?
5. Out of where?
6. Who will be left?

17.1.1 Birth anxieties

To the outsider, birth is a life event, parturition of mother and baby. To the insider it is a primal event, thrusting life back to its origins. Anticipating childbirth, the pregnant woman richochets backwards and forewards, between the birth to come and her own birth out of a female body like her own, a dizzying zigzag of emotional confusion arousing primitive fears and passions. In her state of permeable psychic boundaries, seemingly rational worries reflect underlying unconscious fantasies and anxieties which in turn colour her conscious ideas about birth. Usually unvoiced, these strange fantasies find their way into words on the psychoanalytic couch, in close-support groups of pregnant women, and, more rarely, in women's writings during pregnancy. Faced with so many uncertainties, a particular anxiety may serve the purpose of anchoring her generalized sense of 'free floating' nebulous anxiety, giving a focus to her worry. Her mind is buzzing with unanswered questions, doubts, anxieties, enigmas and no-one can reassure her. She must live out these last weeks, tolerating these unknowns, bearing them as she bears her child, although at times it feels she can bear it no longer.

All she knows is that somebody else, living with her under her skin, is growing larger and expanding inside her body until it feels she will burst at the seams. Her body boundaries seem too tight to contain them both and clearly, one of them must go! However, in the deepest recesses of her mind lurks a primitive dread that the wrong one will be expelled. In her unspeakable fantasies she fears she will just vanish during the transition of childbirth and the baby will retain her body. Or else, that having sapped all her inner resources, the fetus will discard her desiccated body like an empty shell. A terrifying idea is that the baby will devour her own internal baby self, or having been inside her, emerge to show up all her inner badness. Or worse still, that nothing will happen and she will get stuck and remain pregnant forever.

These anxieties seep into her nightmares as she dreams of being pulled apart in two directions, of fading into oblivion or drowning; of being bludgeoned to death by an arm emerging from her tummy, or giving birth to a devouring monster or to nothing at all; or watches herself being drawn like jellified plasma out of her own vagina. She may dream of being entangled in seaweed or cobwebs or that her insides are all ripped to bloody bits by sharp hooks, or bitten by rats, or that she is locked out of a restaurant or has a baby and loses it. During pregnancy old mortifications are dredged up as she recalls feeling those times in her life when she has been made to feel 'not good enough', untrustworthy, and unable to care for things, useless, or chaotic and messy, with 'an interior full of junk'. Bitterly, she re-experiences the excruciating pain of being left out, excluded or doubted and devalued, and in her stirred up state is unable to believe that her baby will fare any better. She already feels envious of the care he/she is receiving inside her while simultaneously doubting her own capacity to give.

These fantasy and dream-images stay with her as a bizarre lining to her waking life, pricking her into emotional rawness as past hurts are rekindled despite being told that pregnancy is a joyful, carefree time. As she moves about her daily activities, she has a sense of indistinct but awesomely strange conceptions flickering just below consciousness, augmenting the science fiction weirdness of her reality – that a microscopic sperm has entered her body, joined up with something in her, taken over her interior and is growing perceptibly towards crowding her out. She herself has no knowledge of this thing that has taken possession of her – 'they' tell her it is a baby but it feels at times like an alien feeding off her lifeblood.

17.1.2 The moment of truth

The birth looms over her like a revelation, the moment of truth when the unknown internal being will emerge into the light and be seen.

- Will the real baby tally with her imaginary one?
- Will it be normal?
- Male or female?
- Will she be allowed to keep it?
- Or will it vanish into thin air or be snatched away from her by death or a vengeful, envious sorceress-woman, her archaic mother in the guise of an overzealous midwife?.

The moment of truth is also an exam: a fundamental test of her ability to give birth or fail.

- What will the birth be like?
- How will she behave?
- If she does give birth to a baby, will s/he live or die?
- Will it be perfect or deformed?
- On time, early or late?

The archaic clash between her imagined internal life-promoting and death-dealing forces is relocated in the arena of birth – the baby will be proof of whether she is creative or destructive, good or bad.

When birth unleashes the intensely potent forces she believes to be pent up in her womb, can they be constructively harnessed into labour or will they escape, flying about the labour ward wreaking havoc?.

And if she does endure this ordeal and survive it intact, what of the loss of pregnancy, loss of this unity she has felt with her unborn baby, the closeness as simple as breathing?.

Although eager for the birth she also dreads losing the baby from inside her, fearing the separation of being torn assunder and the sense of emptiness and impoverishment she suspects she will feel. She is also aware of the dangers to which she will be exposing her vulnerable child during birth, and the baby's poignant loss of the immediacy of contact with her, giving up the natural warmth and security of her cherishing womb.

17.1.3 Feminine mysteries of transformation

Self-doubt prevails:

– Can she trust that her ordinary body has access to primordial Feminine mysteries: those enigmas of formation, transformation, preservation and nutrition, which magically turn the tiny sperm and egg into a human being?

– Is she capable of forming perfect features and healthy limbs, preserving the fetus from internal danger, nourishing and sustaining it and, finally, transforming the growth inside her into a baby outside her?

– Can she, who has so far only expelled vomit, spit, urine, faeces and blood from inside her body, actually be capable of producing a good, viable real person?

17.1.4 Bodily fears

In this transitional phase awaiting labour, primitive anxieties are reactivated:

Where will the baby be born from: her vagina or her bottom as she imagined in childhood?

Will both she and the baby survive the age-old clashes between good and evil, inner and outer, life and death forces?

Will she be injured internally as the baby scratches, bumps and kicks its way down her vaginal passage or will she damage this fragile creature, who may get stuck on the way or bruised by her pelvic bones.

Suddenly what she knows of her body seems so incomplete. She has a limited acquaintance with its exterior, understands a bit about her inside and has experience of its everyday physical capacities. Yet the birth demands of her body extraordinary capacities of contortion, work and endurance of pain. Her little hole must become vastly enlarged or be slit to allow a head through; her uterus must contract and act as plunger to propel a body down a crooked canal or else she'll be split open to have the baby extracted. Despite rational knowledge to the contrary, at times she envisages her interior as a single large cavity, apprehensively imagining that once the 'plug' is removed everything inside her body could come gushing out. Lying awake in the dark she has the weird fantasy that the 'cord' might be connected to her vital organs and during its expulsion the placenta will yank them all out, her womb, stomach, lungs, perhaps even her brains.

Even if all her organs remain intact, will some essential essence of herself escape?

17.1.5 The ultimate test

Faced with the birth, she feels like a prisoner awaiting a torture session: – Will she survive it without irreversible damage? Will she scream? She fears disclosure and shame. If she does have a caesarian section, will the surgeons see all her innards? Will she reveal her innermost being? – Will her self-possession crumble under intolerable pain? – If she succumbs to overwhelming agony and loses control, will she disgrace herself? If she makes a fool of herself, will she ever regain her pride? Will all her innermost secrets be dragged out of her when the pain becomes too unbearable, like a confession drawn under interrogation, revealing her as a shameful coward or disclosing a hidden monster in the cold detached glare of the delivery room? Will she be isolated behind the barrier of pain, out of reach of husband or mother? Will she ever come back and be the same again?

Underlying all these is a primitive almost inaccessible fear of dying. Although modern science, surgery and hygiene have eliminated most of the lethal dangers faced by parturient women in previous generations and some other cultures, in the dead of night even in developed societies, a woman still experiences a chilling terror that she may not survive the birth. Vague trepidation is mixed with the dual dread of external and internal dangers of murderous retaliation by an angry witchlike mother and apprehension about the explosive release of internally confined destructive forces. This 'primal fear', the elemental awe of death continues to vie in the pregnant woman with the basic optimistic faith that 'life will conquer death'.

Finally, there are specific fears relating to the abrogation of body management: she fears the clinical atmosphere of the delivery room, the impersonal demands that will be made upon her to obey the rules when she is at her most vulnerable. She dreads the humiliation of becoming disorientated in the strange environment and situation, losing touch with her familiar body senses, unable to evaluate her own pain threshold or make sense of the strange sensations engulfing her, not really understanding what is happening to her and all this exacerbated by immobility, attachment to machines rather than people and being treated in a way that fosters her own depersonalization in the hospital.

The fears and fantasies of childbirth are schematized in Table 17.1.

17.1.6 Facilitators and Regulators: anticipation of birth

The Facilitator imagines birth as an exhilarating event, culmination of many months of waiting for this peak emotional experience. She believes that each baby decides when she or he is ready to emerge and activates the powerful process of labour, that will propel both baby and mother

Table 17.1 Fears and fantasies of childbirth schematized

1 Relating to feminine mysteries	**Predominant emotion: self-doubt**
Mysteries of formation	de-formation
Mysteries of preservation	inability to ⟨ contain / sustain / protect ⟩
Mysteries of nourishment	insufficiency of ⟨ 'inner breasts' (placenta) / male 'feeding' (semen) ⟩
Mysteries of transformation	failure to achieve transition from:

      seed (blood) into fetus
      pregnancy into baby
      bodily fluids into milk
      self into mother
      internal fantasy into external reality

II Transitional phase reactivation of infantile fantasies **Predominant emotion: conflict**
single internal cavity
cloacal birth
clash between ⟨ life/death / good/bad / inner/outer ⟩
birth ambivalence:
   (for baby) release into life (expulsion
      from interuterine paradise)
   (for self) separateness/loss of pregnancy

III Childbirth as a state of marginality **Predominant emotion: anxiety**
isolation behind barrier of pain
convergence of past/present/future
   ('Russian-doll' chain of mothers)
discontinuity of past/future
transmutation (own rebirth)
dangerous exchange between inner and outer
risk of depletion – loss of
   consciousness/selfhood/death

IV Fears of disclosure **Predominant emotion: shame**
loss of control – untamed regression
revealing viscera (caesarean section)
withdrawal of vital organs with baby or placenta
involuntary exposure of hidden badness and secret
   self
moment of truth – examination of own creativity
   and baby's normality

V Apprehension re abrogation of body management **Predominant emotion: humiliation**
trial of endurance
loss of dignity
desexualization (shaving; hosp. gown, no nudity)
depersonalization (anonymity, routine procedure)
immobilization (drips, epidural, monitors, supine)
ritual purification and mutilation (enema, shaving,
   ARM, episiotomy)
mechanizational (induction, monitoring, forceps)

From Raphael-Leff, J. (1985) Pre and Peri-natal Psychology Journal, USA Vol. 1. Spring.

towards an extra-uterine reunion. Labour is thus seen as a mutual activity, both the baby and herself reciprocally struggling towards each other, inexorably caught up in something greater than their individual capacities. Like the baby, she will have to surrender herself to the process, trust her body to retrieve age-old expertise to do this thing, which a primagravida, like the baby, has never done before.

If she is superstitious or believes in astrology or has a strong devotion to the 'natural', the significance of the baby's birth date and exact moment of birth will seem highly auspicious, not to be tampered with by inductions, or artificially speeded up during labour or hampered by physical restraints. Her main fear is that of being interfered with, bossed about or interrupted, thrown off course from intuitive dovetailing of the rhythms of her contracting uterus and those of the baby caterpillaring down the canal inside her. Ideally, the Facilitator wants to be free to get on with her own labour in her own way, 'letting nature take its course'. The less inhibited Facilitator hopes to engage in spontaneous activities and explore positions which assist the process, such as utilizing gravity and rhythmicity; visualizing the baby's journey; singing, swaying and practising self-adjustive breathing and panting or puffing. She trusts her body will 'know' when to alternate squatting, kneeling, lying, crouching and standing or sitting as contractions differ.

To the Facilitator, birth, like lovemaking, is an intensely private and intimate happening of an orgasmic nature, to be shared only with her baby, and possibly her partner, her mother, and/or her other children or a few well-chosen loved ones. She finds the idea that strangers should be present at such a highly charged emotional event embarrassing. Their proposed presence feels intrusive and unnecessary, since all she wants by way of obstetrics is a 'baby-catcher'. Her main aim is that the birth be as 'natural' as possible, and she fully intends to resist all pharmacological or technological intervention when offered.

The Facilitator hopes to find a midwife who can facilitate the birth experience she desires: someone patient, who can tolerate waiting, who will be willing to watch over her like a benign mother and sit it out with her rather than intervening. The mother-to-be knows what she craves: she imagines the final stage of birth, focusing all her energy into guiding the little head through, cupping it as it emerges and gently drawing the baby out onto her naked belly to suckle him or her even before the cord is severed. Many Facilitators are concerned that the cord should not be cut before it stops pulsating and worry about the fate of the placenta which they regard as a mysterious possession brought by the baby from its other existence.

The Regulator approaches birth differently. To her it is a medical event, an inescapable, painful crisis inflicted upon her which she intends to endure with minimal discomfort and maximum control. She wants the birth to be as *'civilized'* as possible, to make use of all the modern means available to shorten and anaesthetize the procedure. Although fit, she has no faith in her alienated body recapturing birth processes of her primordial ancestors and puts her faith instead in the wonders of scientific advancement and obstetric know-how, either submitting to the greater authority of physicians or surfing the internet to acquire information about analgesics and facilities so she can remain in control. This control may also include 'Active Birth' techniques, which a drug-spurning Regulator engages in differently from the Facilitator. *The Regulator's main fear is of loss control and dignity*: losing her emotional reserve during a protracted and painful labour and being excessively vulnerable and exposed on the delivery table. A marked discrepancy between her expectations and the reality of labour puts her at risk of postnatal depression. By contrast to the Facilitator, far from resenting 'strangers', she welcomes the idea of neutral carers whom she need never encounter again, professionally getting on with the business of delivering her. All she wants is for the birth to be over with as quickly, painlessly and properly as possible.

Table 17.2 Attitudes to labour

	Facilitator	*Regulator*	*Reciprocator*
Labour	'exhilarating' intimate event 'hard work'	'depleting' medical event inflicted pain	Unpredictable painful transition stressful&exciting
Ideal birth	'natural' birth no intervention	Civilized birth Analgesics Monitoring	best birth possible under circumstances

17.2 EMOTIONAL. PREPARATION

17.2.1 Emotional rehearsal for the birth As with all social and medical operations, inner preparation and mastery of the fears associated with an event contribute to successful outcome. Childbirth, too, benefits from previous emotional preparation. During the long months of pregnancy, each woman finds ways of accustoming herself to the inevitable.

Much of the emotional rehearsal takes place consciously, as the pregnant woman talks to 'initiated' mothers, comparing their experiences; as she attends classes, reads about labour and expresses some of her fears to friends, her mother or partner. On a less conscious level she works through her anxieties in repetitive dreams, in which identified with the baby, she too is immersed in later, swimming down a canal, traversing a wide river-bed or heaving herself, amphibian-like, onto land. Likewise, she may be emerging from a chrysalis, climbing a mountain, journeying through a tunnel or making some other transition from one state to another.

In her fantasies, the birth may be unconsciously equated with her own rebirth. She may imagine reliving her life as a male if she has a son, or as a different person, as a 'mummy' like or very unlike her own mother; she may simply be expecting herself to change dramatically under the intense impact of the birth experience or else hopes her world will be miraculously transformed by the arrival of a baby. Given time, by seeping into consciousness, these unrealistic fantasies are mellowed, affecting and affected by ongoing contact with her baby during pregnancy. Unmodified persistence of such fantasies undivulged even to herself, must inevitably result in postnatal disappointment.

Magical thinking abounds: in her waking life, she day-dreams both about her ideal birth and the very worst that can happen, and sometimes surprises herself engaging in superstitious beliefs – if the baby is born on a Wednesday it will be X; if she goes into labour on a particular date, the birth-announcement will have a special ring to it (i.e. 1.9.91, Valentine's day, February 29th in a leap year, an anniversary or family member's birthday, etc.). If she sneezes three times in succession when thinking about the birth, everything will be alright on the day, touch wood! Or even just if her partner is there with her, or a particular mid-wife, or if she has her talisman necklace on or a purple pair of socks . . . Whatever the magical belief which the woman finds herself shamefacedly clinging to against her rational knowledge, its function is to lessen the intolerable uncertainty.

A further unconscious device employed to ensure safety during birth is the attribution of magical powers to the professionals she encounters. The idealized male obstetrician may be granted the authoritative omniscience of a childhood father, while a female doctor or midwife, like the archaic mother, is ascribed life-giving and healing capacities of a good mother or the witch-like attributes of a bad vindictive one. Other women feel that it is only by virtue of their own efforts that they will survive the birth intact, or achieve the experience they crave. Before the advent of birth plans and protocols, these women had to prepare emotionally for the paradoxical effort of assertiveness at a time of supreme vulnerability, having to steep themselves in foreknowledge to prevent circumvention of their heart-felt desires by some well-meaning but dogmatic profes-sional 'helper'. For each woman, this once-in-a-lifetime event is a day she will remember for the rest of her life which she is therefore trying to safeguard as special and unique and her own.

17.2.2 Finding emotional allies

For many women, emotional preparation for the birth may be enriched by participation in a discussion group for pregnant women. First timers are assisted by multips; women with later due-dates benefit from seeing the live offspring of their counterparts and to all there is the advantage of expressing fears and fantasies which otherwise fester untold, and the discovery that these are normal and not harbingers of disasters to come. As I have advocated such groups may be led by a counsellor or group-conductor or run as self-help groups brought together by simple stipulation of meeting-date, time and venue in doctors' surgeries, hospital antenatal departments, community centres or, better still, in well-baby clinics so that mothers-to-be become acquainted with these future havens of good advice. Alternatively, a community midwife or GP may facilitate introduction of pregnant women in the same geographical area, so that they can establish a type of informal support group long before the birth of their babies. Needless to say, women who are showing signs of extreme anxiety about the birth, panic reactions, insomnia and birth-related phobias should be offered psychotherapeutic help long before due date (see Chapter 7).

17.3 PHYSICAL PREPARATION

17.3.1 Physical preparation for labour and birth

The pregnant woman's body inaugurates its own preparation for the birth, softening of ligaments, Braxton–Hicks contractions and engagement of the head. However, given the stationary lives many lead, some pregnant women wish to become 'fit' for the hard physical work of labour and attend antenatal exercise classes to help limber up. Many also wish to learn techniques of breathing and relaxation which they hope will be beneficial to them during labour. To some relaxation offers a means of restoring physical energy and a sense of well-being after contractions. To others, these techniques provide a sense of control or an activity to divert attention from the pain. With hindsight, participants in antenatal classes report that these are most beneficial when run by or attended by women who have actually experienced childbirth themselves and allow exchange or realistic information as opposed to the 'birth is like passing a watermelon' variety. Furthermore, women welcome candid yet non-sadistic descriptions which help them anticipate labour realistically and break the 'conspiracy of silence' about pain, unexpected interventions and postnatal discomfort. Childbirth education varies from limbering exercises to spiritual preparation and a birth 'philosophy' [1].

Two basic approaches are represented by (a) the psychoprophylactic (distraction) techniques and (b) the body-harmony range.

The former, once fashionable in the United States, was introduced to the West by Dr Ferdinand LaMaze who saw the Pavlovian method in operation in Russia. It aims at a 'painless delivery' by distracting the woman's attention from pain with a learned drill of patterned breathing during contractions and conscious control during second stage labour. Other psychoprophylactic techniques might encourage her to engage in singing a song in her head or aloud, envisage a relaxing pastoral scene or occupy her mind away from the bodily sensations.

The second approach, that of 'ecstatic childbirth', was first developed in England in the 1940s by Dr Grantly Dick-Read, often called the father of 'natural childbirth' and later introduced to the USA by Dr Robert Bradley as 'husband-coached' childbirth [2]. Dick-Read identified a self-perpetuating syndrome in birthing women, that of the 'fear-tension-pain' cycle. According to this syndrome, fear and apprehension produce a muscular tension which attempts to stop the opening of the cervix until the 'danger' has passed, thereby working against the normal functions of the labouring uterus. He believed that women could overcome not only their fear but the self-induced pain by knowing in detail what happens inside the body during labour and by using deep breathing to calm the woman, relax her body, dispel fear and hence pain [3]. Interestingly enough, experiments with environmentally disrupted labours of mice [4] as well as rabbits and red deer [5] illustrate muscular tension as a result of fear, labour discontinuance and prolonged or abnormal labours, akin to human uterine inertia due to anxiety. Shorter labours and fewer complications have been recorded for women who had attended childbirth preparation classes [6,7].

A variation on prepared childbirth also influenced by Jacobson's 'progressive relaxation' [8] as was Dick-Read's, is the 'psychosexual' method evolved by Sheila Kitzinger, advocating physical and psychic education to foster a woman's 'delight in the rhythmic harmony of her body's functioning' [9] and training to maintain her conscious participation, 'power of self-direction . . . and active cooperation with doctor and nurse' [10].

Other methods of childbirth training such as 'Active Birth' techniques focus not only on relaxation, but actively controlling labour through understanding, free determination in changes in posture, use of gravity, breathing and 'natural expulsive positions' such as kneeling, squatting or sitting [11].

17.3.2 Match and mismatch

Clearly, all these different classes which often encourage partner participation as well, serve not only as 'training camps' for physical labour but prepare the couple for a shared experience of birth and parenthood, from which single women might feel excluded (see also section 7.9). However, they also offer a chance to meet like-minded companions, to compare notes and find support in the transition to parenthood.

As we have seen, instruction in methods of preparation for labour varies in different antenatal classes and some obstetric teams not only prefer their 'patients' to be taught in classes run on their own premises but may be somewhat dismissive of what women have learned elsewhere. Although appreciated by many midwives and doctors, some professionals hold the view that childbirth educators whether attached to private clinics, or the 125 or so NCT (National Childbirth Trust) branches (as well as 'crankpot' antenatal classes) collude with women by encouraging unrealistic expectations of an ideal birth which can only be attained under optimal conditions, and is unlikely to be available in the less-than-perfect state of the National Health Service today. Yoga practices or preparation for 'Natural' or 'Active' birth are deemed particularly threatening to members of a hospital department geared to high technology. Staff might feel that such women are primed unrealistically to expect an 'ecstatic' birth experience. They regard these women as arriving in hospital inflexibly armed with preconceived ideas about mobility during labour, the evils of ARM (artificial rupturing of membranes), episiotomy, fetal monitoring and pain relief, and an insistence on upright or all-fours position during birth. Although the obstetric staff at such a hospital may argue that women wishing something different from what is on offer should go elsewhere, it is equally arguable that many women do not know their local hospital's labour policy. A report by AIMS finds that some hospitals refuse to release their statistics of labour induction and intervention to the consumer [12]. Although the Community Health Council has a statutory right to obtain these if requested by consumers of the local services, few pregnant women follow up this procedure. As a result of this lack of knowledge, or in some instances, lack of choice, a mismatch may arise between hospital obstetric policies and the customer's desires. Such a situation can be avoided when, in addition to the focus on physical preparation for the birth, hospital antenatal education gives participants accurate information and video-film illustrations of the degree of active management of labour by staff, labour intervention and expected practices, thereby enabling pregnant women to prepare for labour in a realistic manner and to make a truly informed choice about the prospective birthplace.

17.4 PRACTICAL PREPARATION

17.4.1 The place of birth

The choice of venue for the birth is therefore a crucial decision which must be made well in advance. Although in the late 1970s 97% of women had their babies in hospitals [13], increasingly, home birth remains the choice of many women even though not all those who choose it secure this option. The majority of government reports have recommended hospital births as safer; however, a review of the issue by the National Perinatal Epidemiology Unit in Oxford concludes that there is no evidence to support this claim [14] and there are statistical data to suggest that for low-risk healthy women, home birth may be safest [15]. By Law, any woman may decide to have a home birth and her decision must be respected by her doctor and the health authorities who are obliged to provide a domiciliary confinement service [16]. The woman might choose to have a midwife only, or accept GP cover as well. However, the midwife, as an independent practitioner in her own right, does not require the service of a GP for patient referrals for special tests or emergency admission to hospital, wherein a medical clinician is obliged to treat the woman on her own terms or find a suitable replacement for his/her care. The midwife may also be obliged by the Health Authority to accept a high-risk case and would then be expected to take reasonable precautions to deal with a crisis, such as taking a second midwife, bringing with her IV infusion, plasma and resuscitation equipment for the baby, and ensuring a qualified medical practitioner also attends the home birth. Unless the midwife was negligent in her duties, should disaster occur, neither midwife nor mother can be held responsible even if they have signed consent forms [17].

A woman/couple choosing to have the baby in a hospital setting have a variety of options, although not all may be available in the local area:

1. Hospital
(a) Teaching hospital
(b) Consultant unit
(c) private hospital.
2. GP unit
(a) separate unit
(b) GP unit within a consultant unit
(c) GP beds within a consultant unit

Sadly GP units are being phased out along with small maternity units and midwifery clinics. Choices amount to a hospital birth under various schemes:

1. Consultant care
2. Shared antenatal care between GP/community midwife and hospital
3. Domino birth: the woman attended by her local midwife antenatally, at the hospital birth and for ten days postnatally, thus providing continuity of care.

4. 6 or 48 hour discharge after delivery by hospital midwife
5. Private care

Practical preparation means each woman/couple researching all these various options through talking to her doctor, community health visitor or midwife; reading, chatting to acquaintances and mass-media exposure. Having chosen, choice may be secured by booking or writing to the appropriate authorities.

17.4.2 Birth plans and protocols

However, merely booking in still only secures the venue, not the preferred procedures. This is where the idea of birth plans has evolved to fill a gap between parental desires and hospital procedures. A woman/couple's desires relating to their birth are as special and individualized as love-making. Research has shown that the quality of birth has long-lasting effects on the relationship of the mother and father to their baby and to each other for years to come [18,19]. Although emergency intervention is necessary in some cases and unexpected occurrences necessitate a change of policy, nevertheless, most couples have a clear idea of the kind of birth they would wish to have under normal foreseeable conditions.

To facilitate meeting these needs, some hospitals have introduced forms in which during pregnancy the mother or couple can formulate their requests and requirements from staff regarding labour and birth. Birth plans give the woman peace of mind. She feels she has stated her desires and need not spend precious energy during the labour reiterating these and arguing out discrepancies. Birth plans enable the woman/couple to list any special practices they wish to avoid under normal conditions (enema, episiotomy, monitoring, pain relief, etc.) while specifying emotional requests they feel may get overrun by medical practices in the excitement of the birth (partner's presence throughout all examinations, birth on hands and knees, immediate suckling, no separation from the baby, etc.). They may have wishes which are contrary to current hospital practices, such as a desire to be ambulatory during the first stage or a request that the cord is not cut until pulsation ceases. Ideally, in such cases, a practitioner might meet with the prospective parents to discuss their divergent ideas.

However, birth plans are likely to back-fire if couched in negative terms, instructing care-givers to abstain from intervention. They can also be counter-productive, leaving little room for manoeuvre, actually bringing about more of the intervention the woman has sought to avoid [20]. Some hospital-generated birth plans have been criticized on the grounds that far from offering women a real choice, they seek to assert the power of the institution by defining and limiting the parameters of choice by presenting a restrictive 'menu' [21]. Paradoxically, units where birth plans are most welcome are also those in which the underlying approach makes them least necessary. In all events, the woman/couple should be notified if there are items on their birth plan which are unlikely to be respected, so that they can make a decision whether to pursue the birth of their choice elsewhere or compromise some of their requests. It is unfair to leave the consumer under an illusion that the birth plan is being taken seriously when there is no intention of fulfilling its requirements. This emotive issue very clearly brings out discrepancies between a stark medical focus on safety or staff convenience and the customer's concern with emotional quality of birth, as well.

The introduction of protocols, which are a set of guidelines for obstetric staff, aimed to 'encourage consistency in practice and a yardstick against which future developments can be assessed' have been accompanied (in a unit in which they were assessed) by a fall in induction rate (from 23% in 1980 to 6.1% in 1985). The number of normal deliveries increased (from 63.2% to 70%), while the number of forceps deliveries declined (from 19.1% to 14.4%). Of the women delivering in this unit 50% had epidurals and 12% caesarean sections [22]. Nevertheless, there is some debate as to whether these protocols are appropriate for normal parturients.

Practical recommendations for improving the system have been formulated by consensus of professional participants of a meeting of the Forum for Maternity and the Newborn at the Royal Society of Medicine:

1. Use professional journals to encourage discussion of birth plans and protocols.
2. Encourage Health Districts to make existing protocols available to women in antenatal clinics.
3. Provide time for discussion of these with a view to drawing up a personalized birth plan.
4. Encourage all units to publish annual figures of intervention rates.
5. Encourage professionals to place more emphasis on promoting health and normal physiology rather than detecting and correcting abnormality.
6. In line with the Griffith report, establish an effective system of feedback from consumers.
7. Commend to all districts the appointment of full-time obstetricians for the labour wards, as under the present system abnormalities are sent by midwifes to junior doctors who are inadequately backed by their seniors.
8. Attempt to equalize the 'power struggle' between consumers and caregivers by providing continuity of care by independent midwives [23].

17.5 PREPARING FOR DISAPPOINTMENT

17.5.1 Consumer/carer negotiations

Once women/couples are assured that their wishes are being taken into account and that the professional staff are willing to accommodate these if possible, most prospective parents will readily acknowledge that safety must take precedence. Despite heart-rending disappointment a Facilitator will agree to an induction or caesarean section, if she trusts that her caregivers have her best interests at heart, that a natural vaginal delivery is truly out of the question, that it is necessary for the baby's health and that today's action does not rule out the possibility of a future vaginal birth. Similarly, a Regulator might accept that despite her pain in the transitional stage she cannot have any more analgesics because it will affect the baby. She is concerned to do the right thing by her baby, not merely to rid herself of short-term discomfort.

It is useful therefore for the professional to be able to distinguish between Facilitator/Regulator type orientations: realization of what constitutes failure and violation for each woman will help the practitioner to ease the situation accordingly. Thus a Facilitator having to have a caesarean section would appreciate an epidural and early contact with her newborn; similarly, a Facilitator mother of a baby in intensive care would want to be maximally involved in caring for that baby and would wish skin-to-skin contact with her incubated prem should that be possible. Many Regulators would accept an induction that allowed for planning rather than the unpredictability of spontaneous labour. She might wish to have electronic monitoring, pain relief and constant checkups rather than being left to get on with it naturally. Similarly, when she phones up in the very early stages of labour, she prefers to be asked to come into the hospital rather than having to wait it out unsupervised at home until the correct interval between contractions. What she is most afraid of is getting out of control, and she needs people in authority to ensure that all is under control. Nevertheless, both types of women are sometimes caught in systems which disregard the deep importance to them of their respective aims, and leave them feeling not merely bullied or let down but with a deep sense of personal failure which may persist for years, clouding the early relationship with this baby and their partner who allowed the violation to take place. For it is a violation. Even in an emergency, respect for the patient comes across, as does high-handed disregard. In obstetrics as in any other professional contact, trust is the essence of client confidence in the practitioner. Unfortunately in some hospitals, trust has been eroded by medical mystification, routine practices and authoritarian non-explanatory control.

In recent years, patients throughout the western world are increasingly concerned to be actively involved in making informed choices about their health. Many consumers have become disaffected with a medical system that has indiscriminately and without forewarning fobbed them off for years with addictive tranquillizers and sleeping pills, antinausea drugs that cause malformations and contraceptive means with side-effects of infertility [24]. Pregnant women have been at the spearhead of the patient-rights' movement, presenting a particularly vocal and active group since they are not ill although often treated as such, and have a 'client' of their own to protect, namely, the baby. Clearly, professionals, too, can fall into the categories of Facilitators who adapt to their client's needs and try to promote gratification of their wishes, or Regulators, who believe there is a 'right way' to which they expect the client to adjust.

KEY POINTS

*Emotional preparation for the birth takes place during the long months of pregnancy, through conscious learning activity and gleaning of information and unconsciously, in dream-work and confronting her fantasies and fears, although some of these may be deflected by attribution of magical powers to antenatal and birth attendants. Discussion groups for pregnant women can support and enable anxious women to express their fears and fantasies, and work through them before the birth.

*Physical preparation is aided by antenatal classes offering either psychoprophylactic or relaxation techniques of various kinds. It is good practice to ensure a match between antenatal preparation and hospital obstetric policies.

*Practical preparation includes finding out as much as possible about local resources, making an informed choice of birth venue; filling out birth plans (and ensuring these tally with hospital protocol). Professionals have recommended a variety of practical ways in which communication with consumers can be improved.

*Preparation for disappointment enables the woman to accept that her birthgiving may not be the ideal she envisaged. Nevertheless, professionals can mediate on behalf of the consumer to help her achieve her aims insofar as these are feasible. To this end they may find it useful to distinguish between the labour/birth expectations of Facilitator/Regulator clients.

Chapter 18

The birthplace and birth process

'The first objective of those caring for pregnant and childbearing women is the removal of anxiety and dread'. (Ballantyne)

18.1 CROSSCULTURAL VARIATIONS

18.1.1 The Eternal Mother in the birth-chamber

Childbirth is the bedrock of difference between the sexes. Only women give birth. Each and every one of us anywhere in the world throughout the ages has slithered out or been retrieved from a woman's body. Our flesh was contained within her flesh; life began within her fertile womb; we too, were propelled along a birth canal by a contracting uterus or lifted out, unpummelled, from a slashed belly. Since human time began, in most known societies, birth has been regarded as a significant awesome event, a moment in which one becomes two or more and a hidden tethered being comes into separate being, and begins its solitary course towards mortality. Left alone, the infant would surely die, for human infants are all born prematurely, unable to fend for themselves. We who have survived infancy have all, therefore, been dependent on the generosity of a nurturing Other, almost invariably a lactating, caring female, who fed, cleaned, soothed, smiled, wiped, played, scolded and cajoled, to whom we each surrendered and against whose authority we each gradually revolted, humiliated by her power over our bodily weaknesses. In the deep recesses of the unconscious, therefore, Woman has become the receptacle of all our hungry angry feelings of corporeal rage, disgust, wonder and sensuous yearning. The shadow of this primordial care-taking mother hangs over the birth-chamber of every woman in labour affecting both the birthing mother and her attendants. In the grips of her own contraction, the parturient grapples with her mother's experience of these pangs when giving birth to her. Onlookers unconsciously connect the pain-wracked body of every labouring woman with the tormented flesh of their archaic mother. A pregnant body is the home we each once knew before exile into the world, and witnessing the act of birth, we rediscover our own origins in the body of a woman. Tables turned, we may be tempted to revenge all the dependent humiliations of infancy in our power over her physical vulnerability.

Birth is thus a numinous event which arouses unconscious fears and fantasies relating to the inherent emotional attraction and repulsion of maternal flesh. Birth assistants who, being female themselves, carry the 'burden of shame and sacredness' [1a] consigned to women, can draw on identification with the nurturing mother, offering comfort and succour to the labouring woman. However, in order to maintain a 'mid'-position the birth attendant requires freedom not only from external constraints and pressure from above but also from internal compulsion and overidentification with her client. To be effective she needs to be free to think her own thoughts, free to operate within a calm space so that she acknowledges and responds to the woman's suffering but is not sucked into it. On the other hand men, or women who have repudiated this early identification with their mothers, may abuse access to childbirth as a means of reinforcing their punitive contempt for the maternal body through intervention in and control over the birth process.

18.1.2 Cultural beliefs about the birthplace

The manner in which birth is conducted, and its venue in any given society serves as an index of cultural values and reflects community beliefs about women, men, bodies and babies. In the light of practices from around the world we can re-evaluate our own methods of dealing with labour and childbirth.

(a) The meaning of birth

In many societies, birth takes place in seclusion. The labouring woman is isolated in a special hut from which all men and most women are excluded. In some other cultures, a woman gives birth in the privacy of her own bed at home, with a midwife or a few chosen birth attendants [1b]. Yet other people, such as the Navaho Indians of south western United States deem birth as a social event openly accepted, accessible and celebrated by the community [2]. The place of birth is determined by fantasies about the birth process: it may be seen as an auspicious occasion, or as a dangerous physical crisis. As a secret or sacred mysterious happening, or one which is potentially polluting. Our own changing attitudes over the last century have transferred birth from the context of a homely, private event to one conducted in a place reserved for illness and death, in need of specialized, mechanized attention among strangers. From being a personal issue of emotional intimacy, we have medicalized it, centralized its venue, stressing danger and pathology over normality, and state ownership over individual right.

(b) The dirty female

Among various peoples, such as the Arapesh of New Guinea birth takes place at the edge of the village in the 'bad' place 'reserved for excretion, menstrual huts and foraging pigs' [3]. Similarly, we find postpartum purification ceremonies in diverse cultures right across the world, such as the South African Hottentots, the Jordan village people of the Middle East, Caucasia region of Russia, women in India and Vietnam, are evidence that birth is regarded as dirty and defiling [4]. Laws governing ritual purification of women following childbirth in Judaism, Islam and Catholicism illustrate male horror of contagion. The newly delivered woman is generally regarded as particularly dangerous to men, as is the menstruating woman. Both are debarred from ceremonial activities, and in some societies their male partners are also disqualified, polluted by association. Not only menstrual blood and vaginal discharges, but all body products of the new mother, such as nail parings, hair clippings, excrement and other bodily secretions are taboo to men. It is believed that exposure to these, eating her cooking, or even contact with her possessions could result in men's debilitation, illness or death. Postnatal rituals of purification are necessary before women can be safely reincorporated into society. Cleansing rites, like purging, play a similar role. It has been suggested that enemas or suppositories given to labouring women in our own society, and the effort invested in regulation of parturient bowel movements in hospital may serve a comparable function [5].

(c) The dark female

In most societies, as we have seen, women are the primary care-takers, and so embody all the wonderous/terrible powers invested in the mother by the helpless dependent infant. Being ascribed these seemingly omnipotent capacities, women have always been regarded as closer to the darker forces of nature, in touch with elementary passions and magical powers. Furthermore, the body of a woman is symbolized in art, dreams and the poetic language of primary thinking, as a vessel with a dark interior where transformational mysteries happen. During menstruation, birth and lactation when internal corporeal conversions come out of the body, a woman is considered to be particularly enigmatic and powerful. Both 'open' and potentially polluting with all that oozes out of her and yet also vulnerable and receptive. She is unguardedly open to spirit entry from the outside and, in her contact with the fetus who comes from the 'other world', close to supernatural forces dangerous to the uninitiated. In some societies the woman in the throes of labour is regarded as 'possessed' by spirits or susceptible to demoniacal forces beyond her control. Christian midwives in Zaire, Zimbabwe and Zambia ritually purify women through confession and exorcism to free them from sin which is believed to obstruct childbirth [6]. During childbirth, with its altered state of consciousness, the parturient is seen by the Navajo to be entering the magical dimension of 'dreamtime', embarking on a mysterious journey which her shamanic midwife shares [7].

Other cultures ascribe special powers to the birthing woman herself while in her liminal state between this world and the twilight one. She may be seen to possess telepathic powers of thought-reading, clair-voyance or contact with dead ancestors or be deemed capable of malignant influence. In these cases, seclusion safeguards the community and postnatal purification rituals are necessary to 'decontaminate' her before her return to society, while also preserving mother and child from the threat of the unknown and the powers of darkness through which they have passed.

18.1.3 Fantasies about the process of birth

(a) Woman's curse: birth as a painful process

From biblical times, childbirth has been associated with punishment for the transgression of that first pollutor/temptress Eve. So ingrained was the belief that woman was cursed to bring forth children in sorrow and pain, that there was a public outcry by church ministers, scientists and politicians against the use of chloroform to ease the pain of childbirth until it was accepted by Queen Victoria in 1853 for her own labour. The martyred *mater dolorosa* forms a pivotal concept in patriarchal western civilization. The colloquial name for menstruation testifies that her monthly bleeding is regarded as an evil 'curse', proof of women's degraded position, as is childbirth. When an entire culture deem pain and suffering to be the due destiny of women, women too must approach childbirth with foreboding and an unconscious expectation of punish-ment, atonement and payment for the baby with passive endurance of female agony and masochism. Only when the ancient curse of being female is lifted socio-ideologically and in the mind of the pregnant woman and her birth attendants can childbirth constitute a celebration rather than a trial.

(b) The erotic female and libidinized birth

Pregnancy begins with sex, and many cultures recognize sexual and erotic connotations in birth. In most cultures, modesty prohibits men, other than healers from entering the birth-chamber, and in some African tribes, when a 'marabout' (Mohammedan hermit or saint) is called in for consultation in abnormal labour, he must stand outside the tent and not come near the parturient woman [8]. Until recently, in American hospitals, where male physicians have been the principal attendants, drapes discretely concealed much of the labouring woman's vagina. Female modesty dictated that doctor-attended deliveries in the eighteenth and nineteenth centuries were entirely conducted under a sheet tied round the mother's neck on one end and the physician's on the other.

In societies where the sexual partner is allowed in the birth-chamber during labour, his physical presence and ministrations underwrite their original coitus. Uninhibited by social restrictions, the Easter Islander of the Pacific Ocean has his wife recline sensually against him during labour and the delivery [9], a method that is beginning to be introduced in some western delivery rooms [10]. Indeed, the recent inclusion of husbands has heightened the libidinized atmosphere of birth, as the couple bare emotional and physical intimacies to which birth attendants are exposed. As we have seen, many conventional practices such as dressing the woman in a hospital nightie and the man in a white gown, placing him at the head of the bed, etc., have sought to restrict erotic overtones. However, with increasingly 'sensitive' obstetrics in home births and more liberal hospitals, the partner may actually be encouraged to massage, kiss or caress his labouring partner's body to encourage labour [11]. Women who are capable of unselfconscious abandonment to the sensual experiences of their labouring bodies, report orgasmic-type pleasurable sensations rather than pain [12]. It has been noted that in societies where the 'male participates in his wife's delivery as a husband, not a magician or a priest, there is an extremely uncomplicated attitude towards birth; women do not scream, but instead work, and men need no self-imposed expiatory activities afterwards' [13]; in other words, when birth may be seen as a natural outcome of the initial loving intercourse, it can be registered by both partners as a sensuous happening.

(c) The bodily product of birth

All societies appreciate the physical difference between male and female bodies in terms of the woman's creative interior which men lack. To compensate for the intangibility of male reproductivity, culture itself is largely man-made and inherently male in its social conceptions. Anthropologist Margaret Mead has suggested that male imagination, uninformed by immediate bodily experience of birth may have contributed disproportionately to the (man-made) cultural superstructure of belief and practice regarding childbearing [14]. Folk models of body functioning and specific imagery of the human body may be seen to underlie cultural management of the birth process itself. For example, in societies where male envy of female procreativity must be denied and negated, giving birth may be construed as equivalent to defaecation, i.e. demoted and common to both sexes. The birth canal is then equated with the alimentary canal, as a tube with an opening at either end, the same for males and females. This may in turn lead to the fantasy of the baby rising up during birth into the mother's chest to choke her, necessitating massage or binders to ensure its descent. Ideas about labour are, therefore, affected by analogies with other processes, and obstetric traditions arise to meet these fantasies. Commenting on the western woman's alienation from her own body during the birth process, Mead remarked that if in industrial societies the imagery of the human body is analogous to a factory that manufactures human beings, the products of the body become non-personal and 'the orientation of the individual to the outside world is made more prominent as the relationship to her own body shrinks' [15]. This view anchors western woman's estrangement from her bodily processes in a mechanized world which assumes that the process must be monitored, birth can be 'streamlined' and babies 'improved'.

(d) Birth as a dangerous process

In some societies, male envy of women's capacity to give birth has resulted in punishing taboos and protective rituals, seemingly intended both to control his dangerous projections and confirm the male view of her body as inferior and handicapped by her natural physiological functions. These societies attribute great danger to the act of birth. The Aztecs saw the heavens red with the blood of men killed in battle and that of women who died in childbirth [16].

Such cultural impositions have served to complicate normal birth process and prolong recovery. However, in subsistence societies fraught with other dangers and hardships, the parturient takes birth in her stride. Thus, in some food-gathering cultures, such as the Bushmen of South Africa and Australian aborigines, women resume their normal way of life immediately after the birth [17] and even in the South Pole the Yahgans have been said to do so [18]. In migrating tribes a woman might fall out, give birth, catch up and continue the march.

In the West, from the seventeenth century, with the advent of male-controlled labour, physicians, somewhat prejudiced and handicapped by ignorance of female anatomy and false assumptions biased by their own very different experience of procreation, evolved corresponding strategies of intervention and, later, hospitalization. These unfortunately actually introduced morbidity into childbirth in the form of uterine infection, puerperal fever and asepsis, paradoxically confirming the belief in it being a dangerous process. Anaesthesia, forceps, lithotomy and caesarian interventions followed, turning a normal active female experience into a technologically controlled confirmation of the idea that women's inferior bodies cannot cope unaided with the painful and dangerous situation of birth.

KEY POINTS

*In most known societies women are the primary care-takers, and so embody all the wonderous/terrible powers invested in the mother by the helpless dependent infant.

*The manner in which birth is conducted in any given culture serves as an index of social values and reflects community beliefs about women, men, bodies and babies.

*The place and status of birth is determined by fantasies about the birth process: it may be seen as an auspicious occasion, a dangerous crisis, a secret mysterious or magical event, or one which is dangerous, dirty and potentially polluting.

*Attitudes towards the experience of birth as a painful, sexual, intimate or dangerous event vary according to local beliefs which are often generated by men in that culture.

*Male envy of women's capacity to give birth and lack of immediate access to the physiological experience of birth have in some societies resulted in false assumptions, taboos, protective rituals and cultural superimpositions which complicate the normal birth process.

18.1.4 Labour and birth patterns around the world

As we have seen, cultural values and beliefs about women and their bodies determine the procedures of labour which surround, shape and influence the universal biological process. Thus, although partially an instinctual process which we share with other primates, human childbirth is culturally determined and varies across societies. In a rapidly changing civilization such as our own, procedures not only vary in different birthplaces but even in the same hospital over short periods of time or in different departments. Once again, a glimpse of labour and birth practices in different cultures might serve to throw our own ideas into perspective.

(a) Sensory stimulation

In many societies, birth is accompanied by enactments of the dramatic forces which are believed to be operating within the woman's labouring body. A shaman might intervene in a difficult labour to sing the baby out of the mother's body with a song-saga as that of the Cuna Indians of Panama, describing the search for the god who resides in the uterus [19], whereas in other birth-chambers the midwife or village elders might perform a dramatized myth relating this birth to the universal forces of good and evil, life and death. A recent revival of American Indian shamanic birthing ceremonies, such as the Navajo 'Blessing Way' and 'Monster Way', provide a ritualized means of 'confronting unseen forces and fears which might obstruct childbirth' by means of chanting, song, visualization and touch [20]. Music, incense or perfume, visually attractive or provocative decorations and (often lewd) verbal banter accompany labour in various places. Other sensory stimulation of the parturient woman may take the form of abdominal massage lubricated with saliva (Kurtachi) or pollen (Navajo) or melted butter (Punjab) and manipulation, manual or knee pressure to her back or perineum. Heat application to vulva or abdomen, fumigation and steam baths are used in different cultures to enhance or facilitate the experience of birth [21].

(b) Biochemical supplements

Midwives throughout the world have used various herbal potions and poultices to relax the birthing woman, to ease her discomfort, or to speed up a flagging labour and increase the efficiency of contractions. In medieval Europe these prescriptions contributed to the prosecution of midwives as witches. Where traditional remedies have been subjected to pharmacological research, many have been proven to have oxytoxic, analgesic or therapeutic properties, and some have been adopted by western drug manufacturers.

(c) Nourishment during labour

Hospitalized western parturients are usually prohibited any food or beverage intake and dehydration/low blood sugar in prolonged labours are combatted by intravenous drips. In many traditional societies labouring women are fed honey, soups, herbal or spice teas, various foods rich in vitamin B_1 and other beverages which are believed to have magical properties to 'open' the body, unblock the pasages and free it for childbirth.

(d) Posture during labour and childbirth

In most societies women are active and upright during labour, sitting, standing or walking about, using gravity to assist the baby's descent. Mexican sand-pictures and ancient Egyptian stelae depict women squatting to give birth with the head emerging from the bulging perineum.

Dr G.J. Englemann wrote a book in 1883 entitled *Birth Among Primitive Peoples* which investigated birth positions. He found the three principal positions were squatting, kneeling (including all-fours and knee-chest) and standing. A more recent cross-cultural survey of 76 non-European societies found that in 62 places women used upright positions during delivery. In 21 of these the woman gave birth kneeling; in 19 cultures she sat, in 15 she squatted and stood in the other 5 [22].

Some cultures offer a choice of several patterns of delivery depending on the circumstances of birth, as defined by midwife or chosen by the mother. Thus the Siriono woman will lie in a hammock for the delivery of the baby grasping a rope above her head; she then kneels beside the infant to expel the afterbirth. During childbirth, the Goajiro woman chooses between four different positions [23]. The forward 'curved back' seems typical of most birth positions, whether sitting, kneeling or squatting although in some societies, the woman is supported from behind or leans backward. Sitting may involve spread or folded legs or drawn up knees, often with the midwife 'heeling' the pelvic outlet with the heels of her feet, or supporting the perineum with her toe to prevent tearing [24].

Supine immobility in western societies appears to have been intro-duced to accommodate the heavily sedated parturient and for the convenience of pelvic examinations. The fashion for horizontal labour is attributed to Louis XIV's desire for an unimpeded view of his mistresses giving birth, and later to the invention of forceps. Dr Caldeyro-Barcia, then president of the International Federation of Gynaecologists and Obstetricians, commented wryly on the harmfulness of the lithotomy position: 'Except for being hanged by the feet, the supine position is the worst conceivable position for labour and delivery' [25]. Recent research findings show shorter duration of labours in women mobile and upright during labour, enhanced dilatation, maximized inter-pelvic pressure and optimal fetal oxygenation.

(e) Aids to birth

Bracing, pulling or pushing devices are used in many traditional societies: ropes are used by groups in Asia, North Africa, North and South America; poles and stakes may be used for grasping during labour or feet may be braced against them [26] while birthing stools, neck rests and human support are used elsewhere. In West Africa a woman may swing from the rafters or crouch between two house-posts pulling herself up and down, then squatting for delivery supported and massaged by four midwives [27]. In societies in transition, where trained midwives are taught to deliver in the lithotomy position, village women may opt for 'untrained' traditional midwives who allow them to move about freely [28].

Until recently, western women were usually supine during delivery. Although a 1964 American text book discussed the possibility of delivery in the lateral position on her side, in the United States until the 1970s most births were treated as a surgical procedure with parturient women heavily drugged or anaesthetized. Unconscious, or in a state of 'twilight', women were therefore immobilized on their backs on delivery tables by means of stirrups, straps and cuffs. British hospitals conceded a wedge to raise women slightly from the lithotomy position during birth, which however, remained almost supine (and its angle often causes slippage). More recently, some western hospitals have introduced birth chairs or elaborate birthing beds into delivery rooms, which ironically, may have the disadvantage of preventing choice of position and spontaneous mobility [29]. Following the Active Birth movement, many western women give birth squatting or kneeling. Given free choice of position, only two women out of over 1000 giving birth in an extraordinary clinic in Pithiviers in 1981, chose to have the baby lying down, and some immersed themselves in warm water [30]. A radical Russian innovation by Dr Igor Charkovsky introduced underwater delivery by (female) obstetricians wearing snorkel and goggles and the baby floating underwater for some minutes. A less aquatic version involves home-birth midwives delivering women in their own bathtubs or in larger mobile fibre-glass tubs which may include the partner while the professional leans over the edge.

(f) Assistance or intervention

In many parts of the world, 'sluggish' labour may be tolerated patiently or accelerated by herbal remedies, sensual stimulation or verbal means (encouraging or disparaging comments). Vaginal lubrication with sap or oil may be used in some cultures to facilitate birth, while expulsion of the placenta is sometimes hastened by tickling the nose to induce sneezing; in other places, manual extraction is performed. In some cases, vigorous physical measures are used to speed delivery. In parts of East Africa a woman having a long arduous labour may have her vagina packed with cow dung 'meant to encourage the birth by letting the child smell how rich its father is' [31]. The Hottentots stretch the vagina manually and pull the baby out by the chin once the head is delivered [32]. And the Chagga have developed a kind of episiotomy for use in difficult labours.

Downward pressure on the abdomen of a woman supported from behind, accompanied by verbal encouragement has been described among the Aranda and the Navaho, while extreme measures such as strong pressure on the abdomen, a tight belt or binder, or even kneading or treading on the abdomen occur in Burma and some parts of Africa.

Oxytoxic medications are used to speed labour in Mexico and North America, and breast stimulation is used in labour by the Lepcha of Asia and Siriono of Bolivia to this end. The Bahaya of Africa administer a drug of powdered bark and dried leaves which is so strong as frequently to cause rupture of the uterus. Although some societies practise long delays in cutting the cord until the arrival home of the father from hunting, or to 'strengthen' the infant, other peoples sever the cord immediately after or even before delivery of the placenta, depending on their methods of staunching the bleeding [33].

18.1.5 'Natural' childbirth?

Thus, from this review of the range of intricately different labour and birth patterns practised in both developed and developing countries across the world, it is clear that we cannot speak of a 'natural' childbirth. Births vary as to the amount and type of intervention, whether social, verbal, manual, instrumental or technological, and the degree of personal choice and active participation granted the woman by her attendants. These are considered 'natural' for that society at that time. Given our own range of choices, when a western woman expresses a desire for 'natural' childbirth, what does she have in mind? She probably means she wants a place and a helper who will respect her right to experience labour and birth physically and emotionally in her own way, the way that she feels is natural for her. This entails provision of a cherishing atmosphere of acceptance and care in which she can relax sufficiently to savour her own feelings. It may involve the midwife as nothing more than a 'baby-catcher' or might necessitate various forms of active help and intervention – the important thing is that she experiences herself being supported in her wishes rather than interfered with.

KEY POINTS

*Procedures of labour in any society is determined not only by the specific conditions of each individual woman's needs, but by the cultural values and beliefs about birth, women and their bodies.
*Various sensory stimulants may be employed to encourage the progress of labour, such as music, drama, decorations, massage, aromas, baths and distractions. Biochemical supplements, herbal remedies and nutriments may be used to revitalize flagging labour. Birth may be aided by implements such as ropes, poles, birth stools, etc., or human assistance such as tickling, massage, pressure, manual extractions, surgical procedures and oxytoxic medications.
*Given the range of variation, 'natural' childbirth must be defined as that which each society and each woman within that culture deems natural to her.

18.2 CHILDBIRTH IN THE WEST

18.2.1 Hospital births: facts and figures

In many western countries today, hospitalized childbirth is still the medical ideal. In England and Wales, at the turn of the century, when the Midwives Act of 1902 was passed, virtually all deliveries occurred at home. In parallel with the gradual establishment of a maternity hospital service and the founding in 1929 of the Royal College of Obstetricians and Gynaecologists, the proportion of births occurring in hospital rose steadily from 15% in 1927 to 98% in 1984 [34]. During those years, maternal and perinatal morbidity rates fell equally steadily. However, we cannot draw conclusions of direct causality since this decline must be seen as partly attributable to epidemiological considerations, such as altered patterns of childbearing age, number of children and improved health, nutrition, hygiene, education and living standards of the general population rather than merely reflecting improved treatment, such as blood transfusions, antibiotics, anaesthesia and early detection of problems [35]. In Holland, where hospital confinement rates are only about two-thirds of those in England, overall perinatal mortality is one of the lowest in the world. Futhermore, for births occurring in Dutch hospitals, perinatal mortality rate is six times higher than that of Dutch home births, confirming that with careful selection and proper care, home births are safe for the majority of women. The fact that these Dutch figures are in striking contrast to data from other industrialized countries, suggest that in other European countries, home confinements may often be 'neglected confinements' [36] or that the published rate of morbidity is increased by statistical inclusion of pre-term unattended home births [37].

Despite these mediating factors, the association between increased hospitalization and decline in perinatal morbidity has been interpreted as unequivocally causal, by such authoritative bodies as the Peel Report in 1970, culminating in pressures to decrease the practice of home delivery, proclaiming hospital births to be safer while producing no evidence from randomized control trials about outcomes for low- risk women. When the 1975–79 data were analysed in detail, perinatal mortality rates for non-high-risk women in their late 20s were found to compare favourably with the corresponding rates for births in hospitals with consultant units [38]. This question of safety, effectiveness and appropriateness of birthplace remains a controversy, as influenced by politics as it is by statistics. Meanwhile, in recent years, Britain has had the highest rate of technological intervention in the whole of Western Europe. Nearly one in three deliveries in 1985 were induced or accelerated and one in ten babies were born by caesarean section [39].

The prevailing view of hospital safety might be challenged by stating that even taking into account the difficulty in extrapolating across countries where statistics are based on different definitions [40], the British figures for infant morbidity remain high despite only 1.2% of women having their babies at home!

18.2.2 A sociological view of hospital procedures

In recent years many hospitals have undergone a shift towards lower intervention rates and more lenient procedures. Aware of the pitfalls for both staff and inmates, of institutionalization, many hospitals are also trying to provide a homely atmosphere with attractive wallpaper, curtains and rocking chairs. Nevertheless, these changes could become merely cosmetic ones if in time there is an inadvertent reversion to the old practices under new guises within the revised environment. A 'bird's eye' perspective of hospital procedure might be useful in mapping out danger zones of potential backsliding and pin-pointing areas which require further change.

(a) Reception

Hospital staff who spend many hours each day or night in their particular institution may not realize quite how frightening an experience it is for a woman in labour entering a hospital, perhaps for the first time in her life. To begin with, hospitals are places usually associated with injury, illness and death not joyous creative experiences. Second, even if she has become familiar with the hospital through antenatal visits and tours, on admission the woman herself is in a state of emotional vulnerbility, stress and uncertainty about outcome. She may be experiencing fear in addition to physical discomfort and her body is labouring in the throes of unfamiliar activity. On arrival she is often confronted by strangers and unsympathetic bureaucracy: Where are her notes?. Who is her doctor? Is she registered? What is her number? – a host of questions to be answered during contractions, often in the reception area. In sociological parlance, she is undergoing 'admission procedures' which are a feature of all residential institutions.

First analysed in 1960 by Goffman [41] for 'total' institutions in general, these procedures are still prevalent in many institutions and his analysis may be applicable to maternity wards in some hospitals despite the enormous changes that have occurred in others. The introductory procedures may be seen to contribute to a process of 'curtailment of self' practised on inmates in such institutions, as a means of ensuring a temporary break with the external world, role dispossession and compliance with house rules. The labouring woman is then 'relieved' of her clothes and personal belongings, issued a hospital gown and subjected to a series of routine checks to establish her condition.

(b) Treatment

Unlike a garage or workshop where the faulty machine is left for repair, the process of observation, diagnosis, prescription and treatment must be conducted on her body 'while she waits'. Nevertheless, the medical model preserves a workshop system since the body has been established as a 'serviceable possession'. In obstetrics, one solution to the problem has been anaesthesia, another is staff-segregation and mystification with specialized instruments, hi-tech equipment and 'non-person treatment' whereby the patient is not acknowledged as a social person or even as owner of the 'inanimate object', her body or entitled to know what is being found or done to 'it'. Furthermore, rules of procedure are an established feature of each institution, such as routine artificial rupture of membranes in some, drip, fetal monitor and policies regarding restricted duration of labour, defined by cervical effacement and measured dilatation or in other hospitals, taken from the time of the woman's arrival. Once she enters hospital a 'cascade of interventions' [42] may follow in predictable fashion to ensure safe delivery. Inevitably, the so-called 'patient' (for she is not ill) usually has to abide by the rules for the duration of her stay in the 'workshop' particularly in the 'active treatment phase of the repair cycle' although she may be opposed to what is happening there. To facilitate her assimilation she may have to be deceived about certain procedures, since, as Goffman pointed out, some of the hospital routine will be dictated 'not by medical considerations but by other factors, notably rules for patient management that have emerged in the institution for the convenience and comfort of the staff' [43], for instance, the lithotomy position. Furthermore, in such institutions, 'the management of inmates is typically rationalized in terms of the ideal aims or functions of the establishment, which entail humane technical services' [44]. However, a conflict may arise 'between humane standards . . . and institutional efficiency' [45].

(c) Procedure

In obstetrics, we have also heard similar rationalization of what are clearly mortification procedures on medical, sanitary or safety grounds:

1. Personal defacement (stripping of personal possessions and appearance);
2. Physical indignities (enemas, pubic shaving);
3. Forced deference patterns ('Please nurse, could I have just one tiny

sip of water?' 'May I see my baby now?');
4. Permanent mutilations of the body (episiotomy);
5. Lack of physical privacy (non-fastening gowns, orderlies trotting in and out of labour and delivery room, collective sleeping arrangements, public breast feeding);
6. Violation of informational reserve (history taking of marital status, previous pregnancies, abortions and other demographic facts recorded in the patient dossier available to staff, not patient);
7. Verbal exposure (intimate questions about stitches, nipples, bowel movements in earshot of others);
8. Infantilization ('Are we feeling better now?' 'Have you done a big job?');
9. Lack of autonomy ('There is no choice! you eat what you're given or don't eat at all'. 'No, you can't go to the toilet now – the doctor is coming!')
10. Loss of bodily comforts (high narrow hard bed; noisy ward; nocturnal lighting; early wakening).

While many of these procedures have become obsolete in most hospitals, others remain either because they have not been questioned or are defensively ingrained in the hierarchical system (section 16.2). As consumers become more vocal, midwifery status and training increases, and wards change to accommodate new ideas, far from being a miserable time spent in a drab atmosphere, the days in hospital can be a joyous and enhancing experience for the parturient.

18.2.3 Hospital sanctions

In many old-style hospitals, there has been a subtle and not always conscious system of rewards and privileges which have been held out in exchange for obedience to staff and house rules, while punitive measures, restrictions or verbal threats often meet the 'rebellious' or 'stroppy' woman. In the maternity unit these may range from simple busy disregard – leaving her alone for much of labour, neglecting to give her a bedpan after delivery, citing rules of no first breakfast unless ordered before the hour of her entry to hospital, restricted access to her baby while it is whisked away 'to be weighed/bathed/observed' – to officiousness, such as unsolicited bottle feeding with dextrose or curtailing of visitor access 'so she gets some rest'. Although not consciously intentional, obstetric staff are also in a prime position to administer physical chastisement: rough handling during an internal examination, withholding of pain relief, or an unnecessarily long episiotomy. Even though most birthing facilitators are caring and helpful, verbal intimidation is not uncommon. AIMS (Association for the Improvement of Maternity Services) has received hundreds of letters from consumers describing incidents which they term alarmist 'shroud waving'. Many a woman in labour has been informed by staff that there will be dire consequences for the baby if she refuses to have a drip or that they will not help her is she insists on an upright birth although they may fail to inform that she herself has a right to dismiss her attendant and have him/her replaced.

Women are particularly sensitive and vulnerable at this juncture, and often remember every word their carers utter. It is not unknown for a woman discharging herself early from hospital to be cautioned that her baby will die and 'on her head be it'. Comments casually dropped by nurses during these critical hours of birth or early days postpartum, reverberate in the mother's ears and are still carried many years later.

We are all fallible and prone to human frailty, particularly when working long hours under stressful conditions. While most professionals do their duty out of a strong sense of righteous procedure, nevertheless, if they stop to question their own behaviour, each may find that she or he too has inadvertently fallen into treating people as patients and process as fixed. There are many institutional and emotional factors that contribute towards this (Chapters 9 and 17) and each individual member of staff is under professional pressure to carry out their job within the context of official doctrines of the institution. However, each is also personally exposed daily to raw feelings and crude demands in their encounters with vulnerable women who arrive in hospital in pain, fearful of strangers, often defensively spiky and expecting highly individualized care and attention. Finally, in the situation where each professional encounters a stranger, s/he is at the mercy of their own reactivated unconscious experiences of primal envy, awe, revulsion and a host of mixed feelings which cloud the encounter, and, as in the case of all authority-hardened practitioners, engenders internal splitting off of human empathy and guilt. Human relationships are built on acquaintance ripening into compassion and caring. We have placed an impossible demand on birth-care professionals by expecting them to 'bond' instantaneously, to care deeply, and attentively mother a stranger. However, since that is the expectation, we must anticipate this crucial junction, for the sake of both professional and client. Ways must be sought of fostering an early and continuous involvement which facilitates gradual 'bonding', not at the end point of labour but throughout the continuum from conception to birth.

18.2.4 Alternative institutions

Throughout the western world, alternative birth centres are springing up in an attempt to combine a cosy home-like atmosphere with centralized modern emergency facilities for use in the event of complications.

While architectural arrangements vary from double-bedded carpeted rooms with private bathrooms en-suite to ordinary labour rooms with chintz curtains, the main difference from old-style hospitals is one of philosophy. The underlying attitude is that birth belongs to the mother or parents and the baby. The professionals are there as assistants, invited to participate in the experience without spoiling or artificially attempting to enhance it. Nevertheless, we often find that what starts out as an open-minded facilitating place may become somewhat evangelical in its adherence to a particular ideology.

An example might be practice of the Leboyer technique which pledges to minimize impact on the newborn of the abrupt transition between pre-natal state and post-birth experience. Dr Fredrick Leboyer's own sensitively phrased pleas are for birth which extends rather than severes the intra-uterine connection – a muted environment with no loud sounds and dimmed lights in the birth-chamber, cutting the cord only when pulsation stops, followed by symbolic rebirth in a warm bath and massage. However, in some centres these recommendations have been elevated to rigid formulae of absolute silence inhibiting the labouring woman's vocalization and parents' spontaneous joyous greeting of the newborn, and bathing which precedes cuddling or suckling. Strict adherence to the 'rules' of cord-cutting may result in possible prolongation of non-breathing and, as apparent in Leboyer's own films, professionals playing the role of 'rebirthers' may in effect be denying the mother immediate physical access to her baby while it is bathed or stroked by the specialist. Furthermore, since the fetus is exposed to vocalization and noise *in utero*, silence might be quite unnatural. And it is conceivable that skin-to-skin contact with the breast may be more in keeping with the tactile birth process itself than immersion in warm water.

Other birth places offer various 'extras', and in North America these have begun to proliferate. For instance, the Berkeley Health Centre in California provides indirect hypnosis and hypnotic suggestion, meditation and visualization techniques assumed to 'change the brain's sensoriat from an augmenting mode into a reducing one' [46]. Hygieia College in southern Utah offers perinatal professionals training in shamanic midwifery skills to inspire 'purebirth' [47], other centres offer 'transformational fantasy', 'guided imagery', under-water births, or partner-assisted childbirth and many other variations of ideologies.

The point is that even the most tolerant institutions have a way of fostering a climate of professionalism. Without randomized double-blind or matched-controlled trials we cannot know that any one 'method' of 'enhancing' birth is intrinsically better than another. The parents' guess is as good if not better than the professionals' where their own experiential quality of birth is concerned and, what's more, they are the ones who have to live with the emotional consequences for years to come.

If the duty of freedom is to preserve respect for individual differences, what becomes essential in childbirth, as in any other sphere, is provision of a variety of choices that encompass and facilitate expression of each individual's preferences rather than a single method which soft-talks parents into blind belief in the professed Truth or capitalizes on the charisma of carers within an institution, however well-meaning and humane.

18.2.5 Home births: facts and figures

The Government-set target of 100% births in hospital has almost been achieved, but the trend appears to be reversing as women exercise their right to choose where to have their babies.

In previous generations many people were born and died in the same bed in the same house. The home was the core of their experience, for better or worse. Contemporary hospitalization of birth and death, national centralization of education, health care, monetary activities, safety provisions and entertainment, ensures a basic standard of provision of all, but means that few of the salient activities remain in the control of the family. Privatization, the current palliative, appears simply to change the paymaster instead of providing a wider range of individual choices within the health service.

Whereas many women choose to have their babies in hospital or birthing centres, many others would wish to have them at home. Although hospital births are claimed to be safer, careful analysis of statistics relating to perinatal mortality and place of birth in England and Wales, provide a consistent picture of excess mortality rates for both higher and lower-risk groups compared with non-obstetric GP units or home births, lack of advantage in hospital delivery regarding the incidence of abnormality or outcome, higher mortality rates in GP units attached to obstetric hospitals than in those not so attached; and finally, it seems that the increase in hospitalization, far from hastening the decline of the national perinatal mortality rate has retarded it [48]. Nevertheless, it has been noted that without a truly randomized trial the difficulties in matching risk factors and other methodological problems cloud the evidence of whether hospital or home is actually safer for delivery [49]. However, the Dutch experience of domiciliary confinements indicates that careful selection and good transportation and back-up facilities can result in a perinatal mortality rate that is six times lower in home births than hospital ones (3.0 per thousand vs. 17.2 per thousand in 1979) [50]. In addition to continuity of antenatal care, these home confinements also provide a specially trained home-helper or maternity-aid nurse to assist the mother in her home (with childcare, budgeting, shopping, cleaning and cooking) before, during and for 8–10 days after delivery (which is conducted by a midwife). In the United Kingdom, help with cleaning is available after home births or early discharge, but this is not widely publicized and the Health Education Council 'Pregnancy Book' makes no reference to it at all [51].

It is the legal right of any woman to have a home birth; however many are intimidated by incorrect implications by some Health Authorities that responsibility and liability for tragedy rest entirely with the mother [52]. Home births with a private midwife are costly, and some GPs (in breech of contract) have been known to strike a woman off their list rather than deliver her at home. Furthermore, when provision for hospital births was increased the domiciliary midwifery service was allowed to decline. As a consequence, fewer NHS midwives are experienced at home deliveries. A study conducted for the Royal College of Midwives found that 50% of qualified community midwives interviewed had done no home deliveries at all in 1978. The number of community midwives dropped from over 4000 in 1972 to 3000 in 1979, and they were responsible for only 5.4% of the total births [53]. Unfortunately, GP units are being curtailed and some Area Health Authorities withdrew the flying squad service, thereby threatening emergency provision for home birth as well as for premature labour and postnatal haemorrhage of women booked into hospitals. Clearly, as one report states, 'a divergence exists between central policy which maintains that choice must be there and local policy which often makes this choice difficult, if not impossible' [54].

It has been pointed out that disillusionment with current obstetric care has resulted in significant numbers of women in the United States resorting to having their babies without recourse to medical care [55]. In England, where midwives have always been a stronger presence, the Association of Radical Midwives (ARM) was formed to 'restore the role of midwife for the benefit of the child-bearing woman and her baby'. The Association of Radical Midwives are campaigning for responsibility for all normal deliveries both in hospital and at home, to be handed back to midwives, and emphasize that the latter have a much longer training in their subject than do obstetricians [56]. In 1980 they stated their aims as follows:

a. To re-establish the confidence of the midwife in her own skills
b. To share ideas, skills and information
c. To encourage midwives in their support of a woman's active participation in childbirth
d. To reaffirm the need for midwives to provide continuity of care
e. To explore alternative patterns of care
f. To encourage evaluation of development in this field [57].

These aims agree with an NCT study of reasons given by women for choosing home births:

a. Objections to hospital routines and impersonal atmosphere;
b. Wanting a spontaneous birth without drugs or other interference;
c. Concern about emotional bonding, in a situation where mother and child are frequently separated;
d. Wanting the birth to be seen as a normal part of life by other children in the family;
e. Continuity of care by a familiar and trusted midwife;
f. Wanting the baby's father to share as fully as possible in the birth;
g. Wanting the delivery to be as gentle as possible and postnatal care to be sympathetic [58].

It seems that when consumers and birth practitioners can overcome unconscious prejudices, anxieties and dread within themselves and practical deterrents to meeting each other's needs, a creative partnership may be formed.

KEY POINTS

*The coincidence of increased hospitalization and decline in perinatal morbidity must be interpreted with caution as many questions of safety, effectiveness and appropriateness remain a political as well as medical and statistical controversy.

*Many hospital procedures have been found unconducive to the consumer's mental or physical well-being at a time when they are particularly vulnerable and dependent.

*Many institutions place an impossible demand on birth care professionals, expecting them to 'bond' with and care for a strange client.

*Alternative birthing centres advocate client-centred policies. However, they too may fall into a form of institutionalism if they fail to provide consumers with choice.

*Consumers and midwives alike have been campaigning to reinstate home births as a practical and safe choice for normal deliveries, with continuity of care a central issue, as it should be in all deliveries.

Chapter 19

Uncomplicated spontaneous labour

'The lesson of history . . . to accept that the great and admirable improvement in obstetric care is only important in the handling of pathology; in no way can we improve a normal pregnancy and labour in a healthy woman – we can only change it, but not for the better'. GJ Kloosterman (*J. Psychosom. Obstet. Gynaecol.*, 1, 1982)

19.1 FIRST STAGE: DILATATION

The point at which labour commences may be defined physiologically if an obstetric professional is present. However, in most cases, it is the woman herself who, on the basis of a psychosocial interpretation of her own physical condition, subjectively determines whether or not labour has begun. Conversely, her psychological approach influences the course of labour, as her conscious behaviour and unconscious emotional conflicts acts upon her sympathetic and parasympathetic nervous systems responsible for innervation of the uterine muscles.

Thus, different evaluations of the same physical processes influence the outcome. One woman may present herself in hospital too early and be rejected as a case of 'false labour' which leaves her doubting her capacity to judge her body. Another woman continues with her daily activities during the very early contractions until these are fairly frequent, but when she enters hospital and is put to bed, the supine position depresses labour, and leads to an eventual definition of sluggishness requiring intervention to speed it up. A third may recognize labour but delays entering hospital, enduring much of the initial discomfort at home. Her labour, defined by the staff, dates from her admission, and therefore when compared with her early-admission counterpart, even if both women are equally dilated, the late arrival will not necessarily encounter the same interventions. A fourth woman may deny her labour is 'real' until well advanced, and arrive in hospital during transition while a fifth may find her frequent contractions stop once she is strapped to a monitor. In each of these women, their specific psychosocial past, maternal obstetric history, current emotional support, readiness for this child and crucial events during this pregnancy all combine to determine the moment at which she will identify labour as such and what she does with this information influences the process.

When labour begins with a 'show', some women panic, expressing the irrational feeling that now the 'plug' has been removed, the baby is about to 'fall out'. If labour is heralded by leakage of amniotic fluid or gushing as 'the waters break', the experience paradoxically revives old childish sensations of bed-wetting and incontinence while simultaneously catapulting her into a new and uncharted womanly happening, arousing apprehensive doubts about her ability to cope. Her lived subjective experience of labour will be influenced by the degree to which she can listen to her body from within or define its activities from without. The very process of hospitalization partially dictates the quality of her response: as the familiar Braxton–Hicks 'practice' contractions and 'period-cramp'-type sensations gradually escalate into active labour, the necessity to define a cut-off point at which she will transfer herself to a strange place reserved for illness, promotes anxiety and establishes labour as a crisis situation given current emphasis on the need for professional assistance, institutionalization and medicalization. Women having a home birth will have to determine when to call in the midwife, but the process of labour progresses within the same environment. (Home confinements will be discussed at the end of this chapter.)

In addition, our stratified society and nuclear family structure isolates many a parturient from her mother and other, older, initiated women who could reassure her during this fraught time. Their absence may induce her to take flight into the desired 'haven', in the hope of finding a place of female experts who can help her and keep her baby safe. It is difficult to convey to health professionals who work in hospitals and see women in established labour on a daily basis, just how confusing the onset of labour can be for an uninitiated woman and how bewildering the formal admission to hospital, with all its morbid connotations and strangeness, at a time of pain, apprehension and anxiety.

The reception a woman receives on her arrival may affect the course of her labour: haughtiness about her 'false labour' may shock her into disappearance of her fragile contractions; whereas, a warm greeting that conveys understanding of her turmoil, reassurance that Braxton–Hicks do serve some preparatory function for actual labour, and guidance about the signs to expect, help her to go home and return to hospital when in labour, in good time, sure of a welcome, with less trepidation and more trust that she will be helped there. Similarly, if admission to hospital during labour is greeted with form-filling and history-taking by non-clinical staff who will not assist in the birth, they may be unaware of her inability to answer during contractions, or her need for cossetting at this tense time. Conversely, when intake is conducted by the midwife on duty, base-line measures of physiological parameters and labour status can be accompanied by assessment of the woman's coping skills, her emotional preparedness for and responses to labour, the relationship between parturient and her companion (if she has one) and their need for support and explanations. There will also be a further opportunity for them to reiterate their special requests and feelings about use or non-use of medication, episiotomy, partner's presence or absence during the birth, infant contact and breast feeding after delivery, etc. [1].

19.2 THE FACILITATOR/REGULATOR MODEL OF LABOUR

The Regulator, who presents herself in hospital very early on in her labour to counteract her anxiety, is a familiar figure to staff. Her labour, too, tends to follow a predictable course of more interventions [2] which have been found to follow early hospital admission [3]. However, where the Facilitator is concerned, much of the first stage is never seen by professionals but takes place at home. This timing is partly determined by her anxiety about institutions and semiconscious decision to keep away from hospital and delay going in as long as possible for fear of interventions, such as ARM (artificial rupturing of membranes) which might take place routinely. However, staying home during the early part of the first stage also reflects her intuitive need for familiar privacy and is a manifestation of 'nesting' behaviour: following close of the flurry of physical activity immediately preceding labour (such as oven cleaning, floor polishing and reorganizing of cupboards), the Facilitator spends early labour putting the final touches into 'feathering' the baby's cradle/room/home to resemble the safe warm womb and preparing the first homecoming for her cherished, long-awaited soul-mate.

Unlike the Regulator who responds to the first contractions or show as a trigger to seek medical help, the Facilitator treats these as a fetal announcement of his/her readiness to emerge. Excited at the prospect of their imminent meeting, she experiences each contraction as bringing them closer. She submerges her natural anxieties in joyful anticipation and her elation is enhanced if she has a supportive partner or friend who will 'do the worrying for her', enabling her to give up all practicalities and concerns while she 'goes inside herself' surrendering to the rhythmic waves of contractions, listening to the heartbeat or to carefully chosen music in a darkened room, relaxing into her breathing patterns and experimenting with different reclining or crouching positions while her back or hair is stroked by her adult friend or her other children. Once the crucial interval is reached (according to her own understanding of the process), she agrees to enter hospital, reluctantly trading the secure intimacy of her own cosy comfort for what she fears will be the anonymity and cold glare of the institution.

If, despite her trepidation, she finds a homely space in hospital, she is overjoyed, and, in the exhilaration of her labour, endows her helpers with special qualities. She is sorely disappointed, therefore, if they prick her bubble of specialness by treating her as 'just another delivery'. To her, this is the ultimate experience – the triumphant event she has been working towards for so long. In this spirit, internal examinations may be seen as milestones along the way or else as unnecessary brutal interferences in the natural rhythm of labour, depending less on what is said than on how it is conveyed, reflecting her sensitivity to subtleties in the manner of relating by birth attendants. A woman in labour has a heightened awareness of non-verbal cues, listening to the tone rather than the words, sensing brusque roughness of touch or a disparaging glance, picking up unspoken 'vibrations' of anxiety, acceptance or disapproval, all of which speak to unresolved conflicts within her at this sensitive time, when she is in a state of emotional transference to her 'deliverers' as to her earliest carers at a time before she understood the meaning of words.

19.3 MEN AND BIRTH: PARTICIPATOR/RENOUNCER MODEL

As has been shown in earlier chapters, the private relationship between two intimate people is so complex that only those engaged in it have access to some of the many layers and facets. Whether the male partner accompanies the labouring woman or not is partly a function of her current psychosocial situation and historically determined emotional needs, and partly to do with the man's own orientation. The woman who arrives in hospital may not have a male partner. She may be a lesbian whose female partner attends the birth, or stays at home of her own volition or at the parturient's request. She may have a male partner but refuse him access to the birth of her/their baby, or may wish to include someone who is not the baby's father in the birth process. The baby's father may have not even been informed of the pregnancy or birth, or in the case of a single woman having had artificial insemination or many lovers or a post-rape pregnancy, may not even be known. On the other hand, the parturient may choose not to have him present at this highly emotional and vulnerable time despite a continuing relationship. She may love him dearly but feel that his presence would inhibit her or affect their relationship adversely. He too, may have his own reasons for not attending.

A Renouncer may feel his masculinity will be endangered by exposure to the 'ultimate female experience'. He may imagine himself being 'unmanned' by the feelings aroused in him as he watches his woman in the grip of a powerful solitary experience from which he is excluded or he may fear standing by helplessly, watching her surrendering to

'sword thrusts' of pain or feeling guilty about her suffering so much with
the emergence of the baby he has 'lodged' in her. Unconsciously fantasizing a scene of internal female 'stuff' pouring out of her body and
primaeval emotions saturating the atmosphere, if he does attend labour,
a caring husband may sense a reproach in his wife's beseeching eyes,
blaming him for her agony. He may be quite claustrophobically threatened by exposure to such primitive passions, dread the spilling out of
'gore and guts', and feel this would have long-lasting implications for
their sexual relationship. A Renouncer may feel so overcome by the subjectively perceived dangers of the experience that he has to resort to
fainting or bolting as a means of escape. However, a 'sensitive' midwife can provide 'help, guidance and support' by making him feel part
of the whole process, which however long and gruelling, for him too
can be a peak experience [4]. Gentle introduction by his Facilitator mate
from early labour onwards to a sense of purposive activity, such as
massage, occupying other children, producing beverages for assistants,
helps to encourage a Renouncer to participate, however minimally, and
induce a sense of belonging without endangering his masculinity. Those
who make it through the birth and have early visual access to the newborn
are usually thrilled to have done so. Clearly, only the two people involved
can assess their own intricate dynamics and sensitivities under stress,
and all members of the obstetric staff can do is estimate what might be
disturbing, convey this tactfully, and allow the woman to choose. This
may apply to his presence during internal examinations, spinal epidural,
episiotomy, forceps delivery, caesarian section or simply prolonged
exposure to female suffering. It is probable that increased participation
of Renouncer partners in recent years is due not only to encouragement
from peers but the use of epidurals providing effective pain relief to
Regulators, which in turn enables their men to tolerate the experience.

Equally complex is the relationship between a Facilitator or Regulator
and their Participator partner. The latter might be so eager to participate
in labour and birth that he virtually steals the show. He might take over
'coaching' and management of breathing regulation to such a point that
the Facilitator feels stripped of her own capacity to engage in her internal
experience. Conversely, he may confidently guide a panic-stricken wife
through labour or stimulate her during a flagging labour. On the other
hand, he may restrict her autonomy, for instance, by refusing his
Regulator spouse permission to have pain relief for the birth of 'his' baby
or insisting on her trying longer for a vaginal delivery when a caesarean
section is indicated. He may become so engrossed in the process of labour
that he forgets the centrality of the woman immediately involved in it,
or may feel so envious of her capacity to do what he is physiologically
denied that he spares her no suffering, withholding his tender words
or tactile support. Similarly, a Participator can become so appalled at his

partner's ingratitude for his presence and lack of staff appreciation of what he is going through that he sets up a competing demand for attention and recognition. He may subtly take control or overtly and at times, aggressively, set himself up as 'patient advocate', even at variance with her own expressed desires.

Alternatively, and more often the case, the labour partner, whether Renouncer or Participator, may simply be lovingly there, doing the very best he can in an extremely arousing, stressful and potentially overwhelming situation, and as such deserves staff recognition and encouragement.

19.4 SUBJECTIVE MEANINGS OF PAIN

19.4.1 Facilitator/Regulator interpretations of pain

A little-researched area is that of the subjective meaning of pain for various sufferers. Clearly influenced by cultural norms and expectations, responses to pain are not only expressed in different ways, but pain itself is perceived and interpreted uniquely by each individual. Experience of it at any one time is determined by concurrent emotional factors such as anxiety, uncertainty, fatigue, depression or panic.

Pain presents a threat and a challenge to the Regulator. To those engaged in controlled childbirth, self esteem is rested either in a capacity to endure the 'torture' stoically or a determined effort to deflect what she perceives as an inflicted agonizing ordeal of suffering. Whereas the Regulator tries to assert her dominion over contractions by actively controlling the level of pain rather than passively suffering its distressing imposition on her, the Facilitator refuses pain relief. She believes herself to be as caught up in the inexorable trajectory of her contracting uterus as is the baby. Her entire body is suffused with sensations which she defines not as pain but as sensual excitement. The Facilitator therefore rejects any attempts to tamper with the finely tuned process which she senses exquisitely building up towards its crescendo. Nevertheless, discomfort is experienced and can be reduced by sensitive nursing care such as support, reassurance, massage, encouragement and information about naturally occurring endomorphins which build up with increasing contractions, help the woman to cope better with her pain. Ironically, women in whom this natural process of escalation has been by-passed by the pain relief of epidurals may find pain overwhelming at the end of the labour if they allow analgesic effects to wear off so that they can push.

19.4.2 Professional's interpretations of pain

Health professionals vary in their attitudes towards pain. To some, pain is a symptom to be managed; a side-effect to be monitored, regulated, restrained. To others, pain resonates with punitive implications, retribution for immorality or insolence, warranting pain relief for worthy sufferers and prolonged birth-right 'sorrow' for the rest. To yet others it is part and parcel of morbidity, and as such demands medication, local or epidural anaesthesia. While yet other birth practitioners regard it as a function of a normal physical process to be tolerated while it lasts. Thus Facilitators may be considered 'brave girls' or foolhardy masochists and martyrs depending on the outlook of the tending professional, whereas Regulators may equally be seen as 'sensible', 'spoilt', 'selfish', 'cowardly' or 'compliant' in their demand for or acquiescence to pain relief. These attitudes reflect the helper's own ideas about pain: while many professionals have healthy compassion and a rational respect for their client's solitary experience, others may use the repeated drama of labour and birth as a theatre in which their own emotional preoccupations find enactment. Such birth attendants may proffer drugs to mitigate labour-pain because of personal difficulties in facing their own helplessness or an inability to tolerate exposure to suffering or, even worse, they may allow their internal conflicts to endow the labour-scene with morbid fascination, promoting intrusive overinvolvement or detached intellectual observation of how others cope with torment or even, in rare cases, sado-masochistic pleasure in withholding requested pain relief.

Needless to say, given the range of different thresholds for pain and the variety of individual interpretations of experienced contractions – from 'twinge' to 'excruciating agony' – the decision about whether she has pain relief or not must rely on the woman's own informed choice, although, clearly, what is administered and how much is determined by clinical expertise. To make decisions, the woman must be forewarned about the possible duration of labour, the intensity of present contractions compared with later ones, the effects of the drugs on her baby, the efficacy of her own means of lessening the pain. Caregivers must consider not only the physical advantages but also emotional disadvantages and after effects of certain treatments, such as a long-lasting sense of deprivation caused by epidural block in a woman who wishes to experience the accomplishment of pushing her baby out herself, or the frightening aspect of drugs which induce clouding of consciousness in a woman who wishes to retain control over herself during labour, or the consequences of a splitting headache on bonding with a neonate.

Furthermore, staff may inadvertently compound disagreements arising within a couple about the use of drug relief. A Participator husband married to a Regulator may try to encourage his wife to do without drugs, inducing a sense of failure and betrayal if she 'succumbs' while a Renouncer may encourage his Facilitator wife to partake of pain relief because of his own inability to confront her prolonged agony. Each partner and also the birth attendant may each have a different appreciation of pain. How pain is perceived depends on its personally restructured meaning for that individual. Professionals administering pain relief, whether of the pharmacological variety or in the form of reassuring explanations, must learn to recognize the subtle variations in non-verbal expression of pain and ask themselves and their client, in each case what the subjective meaning of pain might be and how it is best approached for the particular woman experiencing it at that time.

19.5 SOME DIMENSIONS OF THE EMOTIONAL PROCESS OF LABOUR

19.5.1   Activity
/   \
Resistance Acquiescence triangle

In addition to pain tolerance thresholds, a kinetic dimension of responses to labour may range from resistance through to activity.

As the hours slowly tick by, a Facilitator may attempt to keep mobile, by pacing the room or corridor or adjusting her position on the floor to suit or resist the contraction. (Up to fairly recently, in some labour wards this behaviour was regarded as unseemly and a woman might have been told to 'get back into bed'). She may have brought a tape-recorder with carefully selected music to tide over the wait, but this sound, like emitting groans, moans, shrieks or even singing, has been frowned upon in many hospitals where it was deemed to disturb other women but rather seemed to threaten the staff's sense of decorum. Today, most maternity units are much more flexible in their approach, recognizing the importance for the woman of freedom from inhibition during labour, and the need to recreate a little corner of her home in the strange room. (Some hospitals even provide bean-bags, low beds and curtains and encourage women to bring in their own pillows, photographs, clocks, nightgowns, etc.). A more passive Facilitator may forego mobility and, yielding to the process of labour, may spend time between contractions dozing or even experiencing hypnogogic dreams.

The Regulator too, may passively give way, however not to the process but to the physician or midwife, expecting him or her to take over and provide her with a 'civilized' (rather than 'natural') birth. Alternatively, an assertive Regulator may feel the need to be active or resist pain. Resenting this process that has taken control of her, she feels the need to do or take something in order to feel less helpless and to regain her composure.

19.5.2 Introspection–Extraversion continuum

Women vary in the degree of their preoccupation with the internal sensations of their labouring bodies. Some focus all their attention inwards, either going inside themselves, 'going with' the pain and experiencing each contraction in its full intensity, or controlling pain-perception by self absorption, muscular relaxation or breathing techniques. Yet other women or the same woman at different times seek external diversions, concentrate on extrinsic input or hope for relief to be bestowed from outside in the form of encouragement, hypnosis or sedation.

Fortunately, nowadays, in most hospitals, the labouring woman is no longer left virtually alone for much of the first stage. Even when accompanied by a friend, many parturients can feel isolated, fragile and bewildered by the unfamiliar contractions. A Regulator particularly if accompanied by a Renouncer labour-partner, may feel she has to keep up her social manner, even, and especially now. Her partner may feel guilty about not sharing her pains and responsible for having made her pregnant. Immobilized by drip and belt from early on in labour with her internal bodily-feedback partially obscured by numbing pain relief, the Regulator and her companion become reliant on the graph-producing monitor to chart her labour, trying to control their mounting tension and anxiety in a barren room dominated by the bleeping machine. Desperately in need of human contact and caring acknowledgement of her helpless dependence, yet equally needing to preserve her demeanour, if left alone, the labouring Regulator may resort to calling the staff in the only way she feels is legitimate – by requesting physical ministrations, further pain relief or permission to be heaved into a change of position or examined for progress when what she needs is feedback.

Conversely, the introspective Facilitator may regard all social contact as an intrusion and diversion away from the central task, resenting small talk and cheery encouragement as demeaning. At times she may seem far removed and unresponsive, because she is so involved in her labouring. Her need is for a warm, physically caring, calm, quiet environment with dimmed lights and few distractions or unnecessary interruptions to her internal reverie.

19.6 TRANSITION FROM DAUGHTERHOOD TO MOTHERHOOD

The craving for warm mothering is one of woman's central preoccupations during labour. Her physical vulnerability, emotional fragility and regressive sense of being little and helpless in the grips of a process larger than herself intensify her need for motherly support and soothing. Furthermore, as she makes the transition into motherhood herself, a primapara in particular needs maternal reassurance that she is permitted to enter the realm of mothers and of her own mother and that she will be allowed to have and keep her live baby. Unless she feels free to experience her own labour in her own right as a new potential mother, the parturient may feel unconsciously compelled to re-enact her mother's labour (what she has been told or imagines of it), especially where this has had unresolved disastrous effects. Therefore, during her labour, the woman has a heightened awareness of her female attendants' responses including those conveyed in subtle gestures of tender approval or withheld in dutiful bustling or silent disapproval.

Warm cherishing acceptance, permission to 'be herself' and settle into a gradual process of escalating labour gives the parturient time to absorb the transition from being a daughter to becoming a mother and to feel she is earning the right to possess and enjoy her own baby. However, oxytocin augmentation and introduction of new standards accompanying 'active management of labour' have reduced the definition of prolonged labour from 36 to 12 hours. This evidence of the efficiency of artificial speeding-up of labour, like jet travel as opposed to ocean liners, overrides the Facilitator's desire for unhampered leisurely progression towards motherhood; it also places the Regulator in a stringent test situation of achievement before the 'deadline', and no doubt contributes to the jet-lagged bewilderment of early motherhood.

19.7 THE EMOTIONAL ROLE OF THE PROFESSIONAL BIRTH ATTENDANT

Professionals, too, harbour unconscious ideas about labour and birth. Indeed, in a questionnaire filled in by several series of student midwives in a London teaching hospital, to the question about the ideal birth they would wish for themselves were they in labour, the majority replied 'spontaneous, natural childbirth'. When asked what their ideal birth would be as a baby, the same young women replied 'Caesarean section' [5]. These responses suggest an unconsciously perceived conflict of interests experienced by some student midwives regarding the stresses undergone by their two clients. More experienced professionals may have resolved their unconscious dissonance by conceiving of the process as a dovetailing whole. A healthy acceptance of each client as different and labour as a multi-optional experience enables the professional to provide space and support for the parturient to experience her own labour in her own way. However, all too often, with accumulation of experience, birth attendants, like all professionals, may become static in their approach, evaluating each labour on a 'success–failure polarity' [6] in the light of their perception of the 'right' routine procedure. Dilatation during this first stage, thus may be regarded as a complex physiological transition to be naturally awaited or one to be pharmacologically promoted. The midwife may patiently await natural rupture of the membranes or feel impelled to perform an amniotomy. In a 'slow' labour, she may be content to sit and bear with the woman or feel the need to intervene actively, impelled to 'do something' which may range from an extra internal examination to officiously straightening the bed covers, or even introducing an augmenting drip. The woman herself may be overlooked. Unconsciously dehumanized, she may be regarded either as a labouring body going through its paces at more or less satisfactory rates, or as a series of tasks to be ticked off, a collection of physiological parameters to be monitored, areas to be palpated, responses to be written down or registered. Detachment and fragmentation control her anxiety.

Her own capacity for empathy will determine the degree to which a birth assistant can recognize the influential role of psychological processes in labour in maintaining the steady activity of dilatation and productive contractions. Ethological research has found that labour is delayed or comes to a standstill in animals as different as sheep, deer and rabbits, who are interrupted, intruded upon or threatened during contractions or between them [7,8] It is not surprising then that the mere presence of a medical student or other outsiders can inhibit a self-conscious labouring woman, while muscular tension induced by fear of pain or anxiety about unnecessary interventions may result in uterine inertia [9,10]. Conversely, a quiet, relaxed atmosphere respectful of the process and supportive of the labouring woman are conducive for steady progress. Indeed, the continuous presence of a caring but unobtrusive companion (female 'doula' = 'woman's servant') has been shown to reduce duration of labour and perinatal complications [11] compared with unassisted labours. By staying with her for the duration of the shift, keeping out intruders, providing creature comforts and close contact, the midwife can protect her client's basic rights to privacy, dignity, security and personal care, while implicitly 'allowing' her permission to have her baby. It is within the power of the caring birth attendant to negate or create a warm, calm atmosphere with few distractions from this primal experience.

19.8 TRANSFERENCE TO BIRTH ATTENDANTS

During labour the woman unconsciously transfers many feelings from past key-relationships onto those caring for her at the moment. These may be loving feelings for a helpful figure or paranoid anxieties about being diverted or attacked; she may experience one of her attendants as a callous and unfeeling parent, passively standing by while she herself is in agony or else as a sad but resigned parent unable to offer help. A split may be maintained between the all-powerful midwife 'mother' and the ineffective obstetrician 'father' or between any other two attendants, thus splitting, locating and controlling good and bad sources of power. The professional may be used as a 'savour', a repository for hope and confidence or as a container for fears, anxieties or weaknesses to be repudiated by projection. Above all, s/he is invested with the power to withhold or give permission for birth. S/he may be seen as the parent whom the woman can never please, or a disinterested parental couple involved in their own relationship, or a wheedling mother intent on her own glory. 'Deals' may be made with the ancient powers-that-be via the faceless birth attendant – 'if I survive this I'll give up X' – or a mute plea to keep her safe during the interminable experience that she believes will never end. ('Just hold me together through this terrible ordeal while I'm in danger of breaking into scattered bits'.) A central question (that often cannot be answered) for the professional attending a birth is who (what qualities) the midwife, doctor, orderly, nurse, medical student represents to the patient and what role is s/he playing for the labouring woman? Simply posing the question affords the professional some realization that not all that is directed at him/her is personal. This is where community midwives who have seen her during pregnancy and have some personal knowledge of the woman and her family background are at an advantage. They know more about her, but also she knows more about them. All a birth attendant can do is be themselves, as naturally and unaffectedly as their defences allow, and in knowing themselves can measure the discrepancy between what is projected onto them and what is a response to their own personality and devoted less than loving care.

In addition to these 'counter-transference' feelings by which the professional gauges what the labouring woman is projecting into them, there are other feelings which the birth attendant may project into the stranger who seeks his or her help. Omnipotence, omniscience and power over life and death are heady attributes to encounter daily and may intoxicate the professionals who are placed or mount themselves on a pedestal reserved for gods. Birth attendants who have unresolved conflicts about their own early life might exploit deliveries to master disturbing fantasies about their own birth or repeatedly to compensate for the labouring experience of their archaic mothers. Awareness of his/her own complex feelings about women, babies and birth may help each professional to alleviate an intrusive spillover of their own personal needs, thereby helping to contain such feelings as rivalry, envy and controlling bossiness, and to increase their empathic ability to tolerate exposure to suffering and intense emotions. Only self-knowledge can provide insight into one's own motivation for being a birth attendant, and self-knowledge can transform a crippling unconscious compulsion into liberating self-confidence.

19.9 TRANSITION

The transition stage when pain peaks and contractions are longest, most intense and very close together, is often accompanied by a sudden change of mood. In the grips of the powerful contractions with no time to rest between them, the parturient may feel that her pain is unending and the birth will never happen. Her temperature control goes awry as she feels hot yet shivers, squirms and twitches uncontrollably or develops cold feet. Often she loses her cool control over her emotions too, whimpering, screaming, begging for relief or crossly blaming those around her. The hitherto content and placid Facilitator erupts into irritable tetchiness towards 'frustrating' helpers who insist that she delays pushing despite her increasingly overwhelming urge to do so, while the restrained Regulator may become angry, abusive or resentful towards her unaffected attendants or the unimpaired man who put her through all this. They may respond to complaints by topping up her epidural or administering drug relief where explanations about the escalating pain and proximity of birth may suffice to encourage the woman to ride the acute discomfort of this short phase, knowing she is so close to her goal. Promotion of pain relief at this point may also reflect a media-promoted common misconception of birth as the painful pinnacle of a prolonged process rather than a subjective transition in which, once purposive activity takes over, pain recedes and in which, unlike labour, the woman can achieve a vigorus concentrated sense of self-affirming accomplishment and long-lasting enhanced self-esteem.

A Facilitator who gratefully acquiesces and accepts drug relief at this point may feel this 'failure of nerve' clouds her relationship with the baby right from the start – both in the emotional sense of a shattered ideal and in the realistic sense of a baby born unresponsively drowsy or herself being artificially 'high'. A Regulator may beg to alleviate her suffering when it seems never-ending, but retrospectively might feel she has missed-out on a gratifying experience of energetically putting her body to the ultimate test. Professionals have a difficult task trying to be tolerant in the face of undeserved abuse and having to find the patience to reassure the woman/couple that bad temper and loss of control are normal reactions. It is often tempting to be punitive and difficult not to be insulting or to abandon the ungrateful woman to her own rude resources. So much maturity is required to continue to be helpful, to empty her bedpan, clean up her mess and not to be rough while conducting a vaginal examination to confirm full dilatation. The situation is helped if the frustrated attendant bears in mind that it is a panic reaction rather than true hostility motivating the patient's response to transition. Such reactions appear more likely to occur in a noisy and confusing atmosphere or one where tension exists between the woman and her partner or health professionals caring for her. A difficult situation may temporarily be eased by designating another helper to provide primary support thus relieving the member of staff who has been targeted for abuse by the parturient. S/he may then take a break to express their feelings away from the patient, find support for themselves and restore his/her own objectivity before returning to the labouring woman refreshed. Women entering hospital at an advanced stage of their labour pose extra difficulties since trusting relationships with staff members have not yet been established before the tense phase of transition.

19.10 THE SECOND STAGE OF LABOUR

In hospitals where there are restricted facilities, transfer to the delivery room unfortunately may take place in the midst of the crisis of transition, with the uncomfortable 'journey', new place and strange equipment adding to the woman's confusion and anxiety. Increasingly, women are transferred to the labour ward when they know labour is established and when they feel they need privacy, determining this for themselves. With her contractions coming fast and long, the woman often needs physical help climbing onto the delivery table, and wants to be braced with good back support for the second stage. If her partner is with her, a stool positioned near her head will provide him with some comfort while he supports and caresses her and serves as 'mouth to ear mediator' between the midwife and her preoccupied client. However, he may wish to position himself at the foot of the bed so as to watch the actual birth. As she is scrubbed for delivery, the patient needs to be forewarned of the unexpected sensation as cleansing solutions are cold and may burn. Finally, the panting–puffing parturient is given permission to push. All her pent up energy is released in massive bearing down as she tries to push effectively (despite being stranded in the lithotomy position in some cases). In many hospitals, awareness of the positive force of gravity and women's differing needs has brought about a change in midwifery training and an ability to accommodate a variety of delivery positions. As Flint points out, granting women the opportunity to choose increases the excitement of midwifery as then 'each labour is an adventure and a tremendous learning experience' [12].

An air of tense urgency in the room stresses unknown dangers lurking in these last minutes, which resonate with the woman's own inherent fear of damaging her emerging baby or of herself being damaged in the process of birth. If her bearing down is to be effective, she needs active encouragement and praise, truthful feedback and reassurance that her actions are not harmful to the emerging baby. More and more, as normal birth becomes the province of experienced, caring female midwives, the experience of birth can be a mutually joyous powerful occasion, gratefully remembered in years to come. However, less-sensitive professionals can turn an enchanted moment into a nightmare. To the parturient focusing on her internal sensations of tightness and the gradual heavy rotating sensation of the head crowning, unannounced invasive prodding, tugging fingers of the midwife, feel more hurtful than helpful, violating her inner impressions. Then, often, without warning she suddenly experiences a last ditch betrayal and humiliation: the chewing sound and uncanny feel of apparently blunt scissors casually sawing through layers of her most private female flesh turns the seemingly innocuous episiotomy into the mutilation it is for the parturient, confirming unconscious fantasies of punitive retaliation against her dangerously restricting 'vagina dentata'. If present, her partner, quite unprepared for the shock of seeing his wife's vagina sliced and blood pouring out, may find himself too overwhelmed to take in the momentous moment of birth.

Nevertheless, the Facilitator's own urge to push takes precedence as she struggles to 'listen' to her own sensations above the insistent call of midwifery instructions to 'PUSH' or 'PANT'. However, the Regulator is druggedly unsure of when she is contracting, her eyes closed in breath-held effort and a desire to escape this nightmare. She feels like a child on a potty urged to do her stuff despite her lack of sensation. She is naturally relieved when it is done for her, baby-evacuation assisted by episiotomy, forceps or vacuum extraction. The Facilitator cranes to watch her bulging perineum release the baby's head, her episiotomy numbing the stretching and retraction that helped her gauge her achievement by internal sensation. (Once again, to prevent the reader forming an inflexible view of these Facilitator/Regulator orientations, it must be remembered that the descriptions are intended as a model to illustrate two poles of a continuum).

With a final mighty bearing down the head pops out, several further quick pushes produce the slippery shoulders and torso and she has a first glimpse of the screwed up little face as it relaxes momentarily before being manually lifted by feet or head. Once again, hospital professionals, increasingly aware of the importance of these first moments, sometimes allow the woman to draw her own baby out, or gently deposit the newborn, still attached to the cord onto the mother's abdomen. GP units and birthing centres tend to differ from hospitals in their approach to this second phase, using birthing chairs or stools or enabling the mother to take up a supported kneeling or all-fours position on the floor, and in some places, adhering to 'Leboyer' type instructions of dimmed lights and muted sounds, skin-to-skin contact possibly followed by bathing the baby with a view to minimizing the birth trauma.

19.11 FIRST CONTACT

Struggling to cradle the baby on her still swollen abdomen, the Facilitator reaches down, and gently touches her infant with her fingertips, as the cord is clamped and she feels an unexpected injection in her thigh. Yearning to smell, cuddle, be close to this little scrap who has just emerged from within her, she finds it unbearable if the baby is whisked off to be weighed, 'cleaned up' and Apgar-scored while the midwife tugs on the placenta and the crying–laughing mother seeks out her detatched baby with her eyes and ears, desperately aware that her sensitive newborn is ingesting smell, sound and touch of people other than herself. Deprived of cutting the cord himself, the Participator father is torn between sharing his elation with his excited wife and following the nurse to retrieve his newborn daughter or son. A Renouncer who has stayed for the second stage may find himself fearful if handed the baby, yet feels superfluous wiping his wife's forehead as womanly things still go on at her other end; and the Regulator, feeling battered and exhausted as well as excited, may desperately wish for peace and solitude.

19.12 THE THIRD STAGE: MYSTICAL PROPERTIES OF THE PLACENTA AND MEMBRANES

As she finally suckles her infant, her expanded senses heightened by the exhilarating activity of birth, the Facilitator experiences her contracting uterus expelling the placenta, marvelling as it slithers out liver-like accompanied by the opalesque blue umbilical cord. As the cutting of the cord forms the symbolic prototype of separations, so birth of the placenta conjures up unconscious imagery of a magic powerhouse, conceptually preceding the idea of the bountiful breast. In many cultures, the placenta is deemed magical, fed to the new mother to nourish her or in powdered form, given to barren women to increase their fertility. The cord and/or placenta may be regarded as highly personal attributes of the newborn, and hence require ritual burial to sanctify them and protect the baby from evil-wishers who could misuse these vital possessions for spell casting. Both in Africa and the West Indies the placenta is buried near the baby's home. In rural England too, until recently, the placenta was buried, often under a tree planted in the family garden, or near the threshold of the house. According to seventeenth-century English custom, apparently still prevalent, midwives would burn the placenta to find out by the number of 'pops' how many children the woman was destined to have [13].

By association with that other universal womb, the sea, amniotic fluid too is held to have special properties, offering protection from drowning. In many ports amulets containing amnion are sold to sailors to keep them safe at sea. Likewise, a baby born with a caul is seen to be destined to become great (as was Freud), and doting parents may wish the caul to be preserved, sometimes for fear the child would pine away or be a 'wanderer' if it wasn't cared for. Other superstitions hold that the state of a person's health could be determined by his caul, it protected him/her from drowning and if carried aboard ship could prevent shipwreck. Midwifes were also known (according to the Treatise of Witchcraft, 1616, to sell cauls to 'credulous advocates and lawyers, as an especial means to furnish them with eloquence and persuasive speech' [14].

19.13 EPISIOTOMY AND REPARATIVE 'EMBROIDERY'

The long-term emotional effect of the episiotomy cannot be underestimated. In some birth situations, the Facilitator who has laboured bravely towards a natural childbirth, often struggling against a temptation to give in and accept offered pain relief such as 'gas and air', finds herself caught unawares by a needle-prick of local anaesthetic and the surgical cut just a few contractions from the end. The Regulator too, who has managed to keep her dignity in the face of threatening experiences, finds herself exhausted and battered, trapped like a butterfly on a pin, trying to make polite conversation from her top end while her slit perineum is laboriously and slowly sewn up. The most frequently given reason for performing an episiotomy is to pre-empt a tear which would be more difficult to sew up. However, even in the early 1970s, a careful trial showed that in births conducted by experienced midwives, only 6.6% of women tore [15]. Unfortunately, the enthusiasm for routine episiotomies has only recently abated and in the interim resulted in loss of the art of delivering babies over an intact perineum [16]. Letters to childbirth consumer organizations, and surveys conducted years after the birth find many women still complaining about the ongoing discomfort of their episiotomies – tenderness, stress incontinence due to cut muscles, hypersensitivity, loss of sphincter flexibility, pain on intercourse and other complaints which tend to be dismissed by their doctors as fictional or trivial [17]. Furthermore, psychoanalytic clinical experience reveals that an episiotomy is often felt by women as a deliberate attack, a violation, the scarring of which serves as a constant reminder, not of the birth, but of the cavalier male whose hand casually made the cut. Due to successful campaigning by maternity organizations representing consumers, routine episiotomies are no longer the norm in most British hospitals. However, they nevertheless continue to be widely practised in some centres, often justified on dubious medical grounds such as prevention of prolapse, and conducted without any long-term follow-up. Today, with perineum massage, hot pads and squatting, episiotomies can be avoided in many cases and, where inevitable, can be sutured by midwives who are now trained to suture small and medium size tears [18].

19.14 THE FOURTH STAGE

Once the flurry of activity around the birth and its aftermath has subsided, all most couples want is to be left alone, to reorientate themselves and/or to become acquainted with the baby. Institutional needs differ, and paradoxically, in the past, it was just at this point of heightened need for closeness and privacy that nurses chose to send the husband out, insisting on washing the woman or removing the baby to the nursery (at times, politely proceeded by the question : 'Have you bonded yet?'). Such lack of consideration for the intimate needs of the new family are grounded in hospital routines and attention to procedure (albeit thoughtlessness towards the consumer) but also reflect unconscious underlying feelings of exclusion which are inevitably aroused in the staff confronted by a happy couple's radiant happiness. When a midwife has shared the exciting adventure of birth with a couple whom she has come to know intimately, having partaken of their joy, she will sense their need for privacy as she has gauged their need for her presence during labour, and will find ways of enabling them to be alone in comfort. Naturally, it can be very distressing to the couple when the intimate time they are allowed together is limited, inhibited and interrupted by a stream of strangers popping in and out of the delivery or recovery room (in some cases without even knocking on the door).

Creature comforts become very important as both partners (and the midwife, too) become aware of the physical and psychic strain they have all been through together. Provision of tea is traditional in British hospitals, but usually no food is offered even though both are tired, have been awake, active and deprived of intake for many hours and the woman has been engaged in the hardest work of her life. Nursing care is focused on assessing the woman's bodily symptoms. However, equal thought must be given to the emotional needs of the couple who may require reassurance about her physical state and discomforts (afterpains, nausea, leg cramps, chills, etc.) or retrospective explanations about the birth. They may need calming down if overexcited and the comforting presence of someone maternally competent if they feel emotionally insecure.

19.15 ALTERNATIVES TO HOSPITAL BIRTH

Birthing centres differ from hospitals in their approach to this phase, often supplying the couple with a private suite and double bed in which the partner and other children are welcome to spend the night rather than tear themselves away from their loved ones at the height of emotional climax.

GP units have all the advantages of hospital coupled with some of those of home birth, too. In addition to the familiar presence of her own GP during the last stages of labour, the community midwife, who has cared for the parturient during her pregnancy, not only accompanies her to the delivery unit, but is likely to provide reassurance while attending to her during the first stage at home, thus prolonging comfortable occupancy of her own home, and reducing the number of hours spent in labour in hospital. This simple fact has been found to reduce the likelihood of intervention in this low-risk group (and raise the Apgar score of their babies) compared with those who have shared care with their GPs and are delivered in consultant units in hospital [19]. A further advantage for some women of this and the 'Domino' scheme is the early discharge (after as little as 6 hours) into the care of their community midwife. However, there are women who prefer to have a longer hospital stay, needing time away from household and family demands to recuperate and bond with the baby, benefiting from the 24 hour presence of nurses during this bewildering time and enjoying the continuous support of other parturients. To some, the care they receive during labour and their stay in hospital is the only form of tender mothering care and emotional support they have had in adult life, and as such it is a healing and strengthening time.

19.16 DELIVERY AT HOME

Once the automatic birthright of everyone, home birth is now one alternative among several. It is not usually available to primaparae or where complications are foreseen, and is not sought by all women, some of whom prefer to be secure in the knowledge that high obstetric technology and neonatal intensive care expertise are available. In some areas, lack of resources has reduced this option to a privilege sought out by the few women who are prepared to fight their case, at times against guilt-provoking pressures from alarmist authorities. However, backed by the safety net of sophisticated modern obstetrics and a (sadly dwindling) 'flying squad' service for emergencies, home birth can offer some healthy women a secure and protected environment coupled with continuity of care.

During the first phase, the midwife, by now well known to the labouring woman from ongoing antenatal care, is an inspiring female presence, available in the background, not in competition with but as complementary to other key figures in the woman's home, infusing life into her age-old internal mother. The midwife spends much of the time during this early phase creating a peaceful, calm atmosphere by reassuring the woman's supporters, looking after the emotional needs of other children, preserving morale, nourishing the woman physically and emotionally and instructing helpers in preparing utensils and an area for the birth. Success may be gauged in the unselfconscious activity of her trusting client as she relaxes or walks about between contractions, and during them, uninhibitedly breathes, hums, moans, cries out, rocks and sways as she kneels, squats, or leans against her intimates.

As the day or night progresses in the familiar security of her own home, the labouring woman can partake of tea, juices, light meals and clear broths in homely contrast to the parturient in hospital who is often forbidden any intake by mouth in anticipation of possible anaesthesia (necessitating an immobilizing intravenous drip in lengthy labours). As contractions increase in infrequency and duration, the midwife offers more bodily contact, keeps check on physical changes and teaches the husband, mother, children or friends to massage and stroke the labouring woman, rubbing her back or applying pressure, washing her down or sponging her forehead, offering her sips of juice and helping her breathe calmly and fully. The parturient may feel like taking a shower or warm bath, finding the sense of weightlessness and buoyancy of the water help her to remain relaxed. In some home births, the second stage of expulsion may actually take place in the bath and the baby is born under water, moving imperceptibly from the watery medium of the amniotic fluid to the warmth of the bath water.

Throughout the labour in a home birth, the midwife will be making the same kind of clinical evaluations as she would in hospital about progress of the labour and fetal well-being. However, here she is on her own [20]. (Although in some cases a domiciliary confinement might be conducted by a General Practitioner [21].) The main function of the carer is that of a 'mid-wife', a 'with woman' who can sit it out with the parturient, patiently waiting, reassuring her of the normality of her condition. Being a guest invited into the women's home to partake in a birth celebration differs from catering to the needs of a visitor to her place of work. In the home setting the carer may feel her main function is that of a midwife. Like all midwives, she has the capacity to 'hearten' her client and emotionally tide her over the difficult contractions, holding her anxieties for her, giving her 'permission' to give birth and physically cradling her. Her own confidence is naturally increased when she herself can be secure in the knowledge of a reliable emergency backup, in terms of a transfer to hospital when labour deviates from normal.

In the home setting, the parturient can feel less inhibited as the midwife tolerantly enables her to surrender herself over to the process, to trust her body and yield unselfconsciously to doing and saying anything she desires. If there is a partner present, tact will dictate when the professional leaves the couple together during this arousing emotional happening and when she intervenes. As the birth approaches the parturient herself finds her own position, and the midwife follows suit – sitting on the floor in front of a squatting woman, on the bed below a standing woman whose one leg may be propped on the bed, kneeling behind a woman on all fours. The father may be supporting the birthing woman physically or emotionally, or poised ready to catch the infant. As there is no sharp artificial distinction or interruption of the natural rhythm of the phases due to external change of scene or staff, so in these final stages, the transition eases itself into the birth. If she has succeeded in creating a relaxed atmosphere, the solitary midwife has a chance to utilize her professional skills of preventing the upright or crouching woman from tearing, as she helps the mother ease out the baby's head, and lift the son or daughter out of her own body. In the absence of small talk, bright lights, extraneous distractions and multiple attendants, a calm prevails unlike the urgent bustling activity and excitement of the birth in some hospitals, while the father and other children or intimates watch quietly engrossed as the wide-eyed undrugged infant snuggles into the external 'womb' of the mother's arms and bed, and looks around. Ethological and human research indicates that exposure to the newborn at birth heightens emotional bonding especially when primed by first-hand active involvement in the labour and birth [22]. The presence of those closest to the baby during or immediately after birth, in their own safe familiar milieu, offers an opportunity to get to know each other closely and celebrate uninhibitedly. (The baby also acquires the bacterial flora of those closest to him/her rather than foreign ones of hospital personnel.)

Ideally, if midwives straddle both services, and have ongoing contact with the parturient antenatally, hospital births can become more home-like in their continuity of care, and home births can benefit from the knowledge that in the event of difficulties, the client can be transferred with her hospital-experienced midwife to a high-technology institution where she will be welcomed and offered the benefits of high technology and obstetric expertise.

KEY POINTS

*The course labour takes is influenced by a woman's psychological approach; the real and perceived reception she receives in hospital and individual threshold and interpretation of pain for both herself and her birth attendants. Throughout parturition, she is hypersensitive to non-verbal communications, intended or unconscious.

*The woman's response to labour depends on her personal under-standing of the process and significance of birth and where she places the locus of its control. In 'kinetic' terms, we may chart her coping-style as oscillations on a **Resistance–Activity–Acquiescence** triangle. In addition, the parturient's locus of concentration and centre of 'gravity' can be defined by an **Introspection–Extroversion** continuum.

*Facilitators and Regulators respond differently during the early stages of labour: they regard it as a mutual–labouring of self and baby towards reunion, or an inflicted painful event respectively, and have a divergent wish for birth to be more 'Natural' or 'Civilized'. Participators and Renouncers experience of labour is determined by their subjective conceptualization of threats.

*The process of labour will be affected by the atmosphere created by the midwife, her recognition of the importance of psychological factors and awareness of the complex feelings transferred onto her by the labouring woman. During transition and birth, archaic emotions (such as rage, terror, elation, defencelessness, disgust and confusion) may be intensified, bewildering both the woman and her birth attendants.

*The professional's handling of delivery procedures, whether in hospital, GP Unit or at home, including episiotomy, birth, placental expulsion, and introduction of the parents to their newborn, have long lasting effects on the emotional life of the family.

Chapter 20

Managed childbirth

'Birth is both the first of all dangers to life and the prototype of all the later ones that cause us to feel anxiety, and the experience of birth has probably left behind in us the expression of affect which we call anxiety. Macduff of the Scottish legend, who was not born of his mother but ripped from her womb, was for that reason unacquainted with anxiety' Sigmund Freud (*A special type of object-choice*)

20.1 VARIATIONS IN INTERVENTION RATE

As we have seen, there are variations in the degree of obstetric intervention in normal births cross culturally, and birth complications are dealt with differently, both within and between more and less technologically sophisticated societies. In the West, variations are found between countries with differing obstetric policies (such as Holland with a high proportion of home births and low caesarean rate, to the obverse in the USA) and also within the same country, over time.

Figures illustrating UK trends in induction, episiotomies, caesarean sections and instrumental deliveries between 1955 and 1978, show steep rising graphs (45 degrees) for the first two, and a more gentle gradient for the latter two. Evidence of relatively high levels of intervention in private deliveries compared with the NHS, and day of the week variation in hospitals with consultant obstetric units [1], all suggest some degree of flexibility in obstetrics and elective intervention in addition to that which is inevitable. A paediatrician cites induction figures for 1977, stating that in some English hospitals 6–7 out of every 10 women are induced compared with others where only 1–2 out of every 10 women are induced [2].

Caesarean section rates fluctuate considerably over the years and although the rise in the United Kingdom has been gradual, from about 5% to 10% during the years from 1974 to 1982 [3], in the United States, the rate for caesarean sections between 1970 and 1984 quadrupled. Data from the National Centre for Health Statistics show that the American rate has risen by a steady 1% per year, from 5.5% to 25%, and that 40%

of these operations have been done 'simply because of a history of a previous caesarean section' [4]. Rate variations are thus clearly dependent on non-medical factors in addition to fetal or maternal health, and correspond to various technological advances such as fetal monitoring (the period specified above coincides with introduction of ultrasound into established practice), sociopolitical trends such as insurance considerations, increased malpractice litigation, almost universal hospitalization, or changes in medical practice like rate reduction due to vaginal deliveries following caesarean in multiparae, or policy reversal about breech presentations. Caesarean section statistics also vary regionally in the same country, between hospitals, and, at times, even among consultants within the same hospital.

In addition, research findings suggest that the woman's mental state and particularly her anxiety level during pregnancy and labour may contribute to complications of labour and the degree of intervention. Similarly, obstetric interventions and outcome are likely to have postnatal psychological repercussions for both mother and baby. These findings will be examined in detail in section 20.8, but first the relationship between obstetric outcome and psychological functioning during pregnancy and labour will be examined, followed by psychological reactions to induction and various types of instrumental deliveries.

20.2 PSYCHOSOCIAL FACTORS IN BIRTH COMPLICATIONS

Although many studies exist which relate psychosocial variables to obstetric outcome, the field is riddled with methodological problems due to small samples, lack of matching controls, retrospective designs and diversity of procedures making comparison of results across studies very difficult as research reviews demonstrate [5,6]. Nevertheless, over 100 studies have related problems in pregnancy to anxiety [7] and higher levels of general maternal anxiety feature as a predictor of birth complications. Obstetric difficulties have also been predicted by maternal age, educational level, menstrual history and an unrealistic attitude towards pregnancy [8]. A significant relationship has been shown between neuroticism scores in pregnancy and both assisted delivery and length of labour [9] and although another study failed to duplicate these findings a non-significant trend towards higher ratings of pain in labour in women who had higher ratings on depression, tension and anxiety in pregnancy [10]. Uterine dysfunction has also been shown to correlate with the woman's attitudes towards labour pain [11], with 'character disordered coping styles' actively avoiding pain and pain-provoking situations.

A prospective multivariate study found that 38% of medically low-risk women became high-risk during labour, strengthening the view of birth as a psychophysiological process. This study found more severe psychiatric diagnoses among women having complicated deliveries; character disorders were more commonly linked to caesarean section and uterine dysfunction, to greater use of defences of denial and repression of emotion, projection and somatization, by working out stress through the body. Anxiety measured during the first trimester of pregnancy was found to be highest among the women who later had caesarean sections, followed by the uterine dysfunction group [12]. It is as well to stress that in all these studies a moderate measure of anxiety was found to be normal, and many researchers emphasize that pregnancy is accompanied by 'behaviours and mental states of psychiatric significance', reminding us that even in a medically uncomplicated population, emotional states 'rooted in the woman's background' may have an 'impact on perinatal events and infant functioning' [13].

Clearly, psychological factors can be useful predictors of complications during birth. Ongoing access to a psychotherapist or counsellor during pregnancy can help to alleviate some of the longer-term psychological disturbances which possibly contribute to complications during labour, and good childbirth education can reduce anxiety about labour. The continuous presence of a mental-health professional as part of the obstetric labour team may be a further asset, both in direct contact with his/her clients and in training obstetric staff to help reduce the stresses provoking the woman's anxiety and defensive reactions, and to circumvent distress-causing mismanagement. S/he may also support staff members and alleviate the need to intervene as a response to the patient's anxiety. A surprising finding in recent research is the degree of influence a parturient's psychological bearing has on her attendants' obstetric decisions. One study has found a significant relationship between higher educational attainment and fewer inductions [14]. Regulators have been found to have had significantly more instrumental deliveries and caesarean births than Facilitators defined by independent measures, albeit retrospectively [15]. Another study has also shown that caesarean sections performed for ambiguous reasons appeared to have been brought about by the staff's inability to tolerate their patient's excessive anxiety [16].

Findings confirm that women are not passive recipients of treatment but influence management reactions in a variety of ways. These may relate to medical considerations of psychologically induced phenomena (such as dystocia due to tension and fear or an excess of pain relief drugs); they may constitute a professional response to overt requests for instrumental intervention; or else, they may be due to inadvertent or unconscious collusion of staff with patient pressures or the woman's overbearing manner which subtly sets off a cascade of managerial responses to her anxieties in her birth attendants, culminating in her passive delivery. How the woman copes with labour is clearly a function of many interacting, past and present psychosocial variables: emotional, cognitive and behavioural factors which affect not only her perception of pain and capacity to labour but also influences and are influenced by her birth attendants' responses.

20.3 INDUCTIONS

In some cases inductions clearly save lives and prevent morbidity. Other advantages cited are unrushed admission, maternal stamina (and empty stomach), and predictability of dates. Disadvantages to the mother are speed of labour, more painfully accelerating contractions, with resultant panic, often leading to less-efficient breathing, more need for pain-relieving drugs, which in turn have been found to affect the neonate's behaviour [17]. Studies also show a slightly higher occurrence of jaundice and a very high rate of admission to special care for both medically and 'socially' induced babies (34.4% vs. 17.4% non-induced babies) [18].

Women react to inductions in a variety of ways. Regulators may be relieved to know in advance when they will be delivered as this affords them a measure of control and the ability to plan ahead. Some Regulators have been known to arrange to be induced so as to procure the presence of a particular obstetrician who is due to go on holiday or to coordinate the birth with other activities. Although medical necessity for an induction invariably increases anxiety, particularly when it is due to maternal ill-health or placental insufficiency, the Regulator nevertheless feels comforted by the fact that events are predictable, that she is safe in the hands of her physician and being looked after in hospital rather than sitting at home worrying, and that the pregnancy will be shorter rather than drag on until an indefinite 'D-day'.

Nevertheless, to the Regulator, the doctor's pronouncement that she is to be induced also feels like a confirmation of her own unconscious beliefs that she and the fetus inside her are incompatible. She has often imagined that her placenta is 'insufficient', that her interior is harmful, that the baby can stand her no longer and 'wants out' or that she is unable to continue containing the child without damaging it or being poisoned by it. This fantasy takes on a poignant reality when their rhesus blood groups are different or if she has pre-eclampsia. However, these ideas may occur in any of the conditions necessitating inductions, and reassurance to the contrary will greatly assist the woman in future positive bonding.

By contrast, the Facilitator is appalled by the idea that her baby should be removed before it is ready to emerge. She tries to delay the induction in the hope that she will go into premature labour of her own accord, which indeed is known to happen. Failing this she desperately tries to weigh up the risks to the baby or herself if the pregnancy continues and the risks she feels the baby faces if born before it is due. Underlying these seemingly rational calculations lurks desperate guilt that she is failing to provide the perfect prenatal environment, despair that she cannot protect her baby from this impingement, sometimes, superstitions about meddling with 'destiny' and the baby's 'intended' birth date and invariably a sense that their relationship is being spoilt even before the baby emerges.

A Facilitator who has been confined to hospital for observation or bed rest preceding the induction will alternate between gratitude to the staff for helping her keep her baby well and resentful ruminations about their interference with the course of nature. Entering the hospital for the induction she feels cheated of a home birth, if planned, or at least a spontaneous early labour in the calm atmosphere of her own home. During labour she is torn between the induced need to expel the baby and her innate desire to retain him/her inside for a while longer. If the professionals caring for her can help her by verbalizing this conflict, it may alleviate the ambivalence, which unresolved can influence the progress of her contractions.

Given a choice, the Facilitator will usually prefer to be induced by surgical method such as ARM rather than hormonally, feeling that this offers a better chance of 'natural' childbirth since she still hopes to avoid any pharmacological intervention which she believes will affect the newborn. Given her aversion to artificial pain relief, the induced Facilitator finds herself in the throes of rapidly escalating labour, often unable to employ her breathing techniques, immobilized by monitor and drips, in a 'nighmarish rollercoaster of pain' where all her dearest wishes about this birth are being negated and she feels she has lost touch with her baby too.

The presence of a confidante – husband or intimate friend – throughout her labour is even more essential for women during labour following induction, particularly for a Facilitator who is not reconciled to the prematurely induced birth. She desperately needs the presence of a good mother figure who can reassure her that she is not a bad mother by failing to allow her baby to go to natural term. Many of these feelings also apply to spontaneous pre-term labour, where guilt is exacerbated by a sense of rejection as the woman feels her baby has chosen to abandon her.

20.4 INSTRUMENTAL DELIVERIES

In this decade, nearly one in four babies in the West will have had an instrumental or caesarean delivery. Some of these are avoidable. A study on the effects of continuous support during labour found fewer perinatal complications (34 vs. 74%), less medication (4 vs. 19%), and shorter labours (8 vs. 14 hours) in women who had a continuous caregiver present. The rate of caesarean section was significantly greater in the control group who did not have a 'doula' present (17 vs. 7%) [19].

The emotional effects of an instrumental delivery may remain with the mother long after the event, and have been found to be a determinant of postnatal depression [20]. In recent years, there have been many studies examining psychological effects of instrumental deliveries on the babies involved [21]; researchers claiming to uncover birth memories stress the profound long-term effects of such births on relationships [22] and resultant psychological pathology [23]; therapists engaging in 'rebirthing' equally stress the importance of the quality of birth, and use their method to try and 'undo' these births and rectify the damage [24]. People born by caesarean section or having had an instrumental birth have expressed their sense of betrayal or convictions about the influence of the delivery on their personality [25]. Although such claims are difficult to establish scientifically, the mother's immediate emotional response during instrumental deliveries is readily available to scrutiny and is the clear domain of every birth-attendant. As such it justifies exploration.

20.4.1 Forceps delivery

To the Facilitator, being unable to push her baby out of her body leaves her with a sense of an incomplete cycle from the creative intercourse through pregnancy to expulsion. It feels as if her trusted body has let her down, and she is letting her baby down. Delivery of her baby's head by forceps assumes the frightening dimensions of a torture instrument which she has permitted to be applied to her baby's tender head. She is alarmed by the artificiality of the process, the sense of being emptied while the baby is 'dragged out' and the resultant moulding, swelling or bruising of her baby's head. Despairingly she feels that not only has she failed to propel her baby out herself, but she has had to succumb to pain relief for the operation, whether epidural or local pelvic block which prevent her feeling the baby emerge, and which she believes will affect the baby. Even when forceps have been applied because the head is large or the baby lying awkwardly, she feels responsible and guilt-ridden.

For many months if not years to come, an anxious mother will watch her child to determine the long-term effects of the delivery, whether in terms of minimal brain damage or emotional trauma. During the birth she needs to be held securely and lovingly by midwife or partner to decrease her sense of rape or personal guilt and lonely abandonment. After a forceps birth, the mother is in need of reassurance from the birth attendants that far from causing damage, the forceps have protected the baby's head in a precipitious premature or breech birth, and have been specially designed for the purpose. Also, that given its diameter the baby's head would have most likely have looked misshapen after a spontaneous delivery. However, if she does feel violated, such technical reassurance on its own will not suffice to eradicate her anxieties and she may continue to harbour resentment against the staff whom she feels did not give her the chance to push. Conversely, some women may be afraid to push too hard for fear of harming the baby. A Regulator mother may be glad to have this responsibility taken away from her by the instrumental delivery but nevertheless may experience it as an attack. Where feasible, it is important to give the mother as much encouragement as possible to bear down while natural expulsion is still an option, and as full (and repeated) an explanation as time and the situation allows if forceps are to be applied, plus instruction to push during contractions, whether she feels them or not, to give her some sense of active participation and control in an otherwise gruelling process. Flint suggests telling the woman 'it will feel horrid for you as if your whole insides are coming out but I will hold you in my arms and together we will count up to 85 . . . ' [26a]. Indeed, women undergoing unexpected instrumental deliveries report feeling very frightened and distressed ['I was trying to be really grown-up and helpful, but when they broke the waters I just lost my mind. The contractions suddenly came non-stop and I had no chance to catch up and adjust to the excruciating waves of pain. I panicked and just couldn't stop screaming, and then when the baby got stuck and I heard them say: 'Get the forceps, cut her!' it felt like an attack. Afterwards, there was blood everywhere as if a murder had taken place . . .'].

22.4.2 Vacuum extraction

To many Facilitators this slower procedure seems more humane than that of forceps or caesarean section. However, with this method too, the mother feels that her baby, rather than being wrenched is sucked out from inside, yet still prevented from popping out through reciprocal labour. She fantasizes that his/her tardiness is a sure sign of not being ready to leave her secure womb and that they, the doctors, will not respect the delay. Needing to lash out in her disappointment and guilty sense of being at fault and 'too feeble' to push vigorously enough, she may blame her husband for having 'put in the breech baby upside down', or the professionals for not having turned the baby or the midwife who should have prevented fetal distress, or the childbirth educators for having led her to believe she could give birth naturally.

Depressed, furious and resentful about her brutal introduction to her baby and the baby's to the world, she may suffer from tearfulness and self-recrimination during the first days after delivery, or may develop a longer-lasting postpartum depression. In the long run, it may emerge that the technological delivery has sorely influenced a Facilitator's relationship with her baby, to whom she may unconsciously become a 'therapist' trying to repair the psychological damage she imagines was caused by the instrumental birth, rather than just being a devoted mother. Although the Regulator does not feel the same sense of personal inadequacy or failure relating to her baby, she may resent having been out of control with the unexpected instrumental delivery for which she was unprepared, railing that 'they' the doctors or midwives have 'botched the job'. Conversely, a Regulator who has a venthous or forceps delivery as a result of an elected epidural will not feel as dissatisfied with the experience she has anticipated and chosen in full knowledge of the consequences, and indeed, will be grateful for the technology that has enabled her to minimize the pain of labour. As noted in Chapter 7, women who have been sexually or physical abused may struggle and respond agitatedly to an unexpected instrumental birth, which revives the concrete experience of violation and its inevitable emotional repercussion.

20.4.3 Caesarean section

A distinction must be made between the emotional effects of a planned caesarean when the woman or prospective parents can anticipate the operation and decide how it shall be conducted, and between an emergency caesarean with no preparation. In the former case of elective caesars, as in all surgery, the patient benefits from getting used to the idea, being gradually introduced to the procedures, having time to absorb information and being able to ask for explanations. She/they can assess pros and cons of various choices, such as whether to have an epidural or a general anaesthetic, whether the partner will be present or not, whether the baby will 'room-in' or be in the nursery and whether she will try to breastfeed despite the postoperative pain. In some cases, a Regulator may actually choose to have a caesar hoping to avoid the pain of labour, feeling it offers her more control, decreases the risk of her 'doing the wrong thing' and seems to entail a lesser degree of emotional involvement. It may also tally with childhood fantasies about birth, and by-passes anxieties about her sexuality being affected by a vaginal birth. Other Regulators appear to bring about a caesarean section through demands, anxiety and subtle manipulation of the health professionals attending them. As noted a significantly higher proportion of Regulators than Facilitators were found to undergo surgery [26a] and studies of 'ambiguous' caesarean sections suggest that anxiety induces action in professionals [27].

Although most childbirth education classes mention the possibility of a caesarean birth, few actually prepare mothers either emotionally or factually for the unanticipated eventuality, by telling them what to expect, teaching specific pre- and postnatal exercises and breastfeeding/childcare techniques for the postoperative period. As a result, an emergency caesarean comes not only as a shock but often finds the woman in a state of ignorance. She will be alarmed by the strange surroundings and hi-tech equipment, the masked doctors and unintelligible noises, unknown sensations and unfamiliar smells. If she has a general anaesthetic she may fear dying on the operating table or never waking up. It is important therefore, for the familiar midwife to accompany her into the operating theatre and keep physical contact and a 'running commentary' going in her comfortingly familiar voice in this 'nearest brush with death that most of us experience in our lives' [28]. The sense of failure and disappointment at not having experienced a vaginal birth is greater following childbirth education classes which take this often greatly idealized birth for granted. Where feasible, it helps to give the Facilitator, in particular, the sense of having tried other options. An American study found that for the vast majority of women 'allowing a trial of labour is a safe alternative to automatic elective repeat caesarean sections' [29]. With primaparae, a trial of labour and forceps in the operating theatre will have provided time to warn both patient and staff of the possible caesarean and may be beneficial in facilitating vaginal delivery with a subsequent baby [30].

Women who have had a very prolonged painful labour may feel relieved that the caesarean means it is finally all over. Similarly, retrospectively, they may feel pleased at having at least had the experience of labour, unlike their set-caesarean sisters. When the caesarean is a direct consequence of fetal distress, the mother will be grateful and relieved that her baby has been saved, even at the expense of a 'natural' birth. However, when it is a consequence of genital herpes, the mother may feel especially downcast at her 'sexual past' catching up with her in this way. In addition to the required formal consent of the woman, where feasible, it seems wise to obtain joint agreement of the couple to the operation. Tension about the vaginal birth having been 'sacrificed' by the husband's compliance to doctor's 'enthusiasm' or his accusation that she succumed to a 'knife-happy' surgeon's charm, can taint the relationship with grievances of betrayal for years to come.

Whether the caesarean section is performed under general or epidural anaesthetic is inevitably determined by medical considerations. However, where there is a choice, parental decision will rest on emotional factors. A Regulator might wish to abdicate responsibility for the birth, feeling that it is preferable to 'put herself out' and let the specialists take over. Alternatively, she may be fearful of losing control to that degree and prefer to maintain consciousness despite the discomfort and fear, or else hopes to be anaesthetized when the incision is sutured. A squeamish Renouncer may prefer not to be present at all even if his Facilitator wife wishes him to remain with her. She would wish to have an epidural so as to be fully present at the birth, hoping to be given the baby to cuddle on her chest while being sewn up. A Facilitator/Participator couple may try to avoid any separation from the baby (and each other). A Participator may wish to take over the holding, caring and feeding of the newborn while his wife Regulator recuperates, staying with them all day and in an ideal set up, rooming in with his family. In some cases of caesarean birth, paternal bonding with the newborn is enhanced by his early contact and greater involvement in childcare, due to maternal anaesthesia and post-operation recovery (21.1.7). A Facilitator may need special help establishing breastfeeding to counteract her sense of having failed her infant and a Regulator too might need her self-esteem boosted after her failure to give birth 'properly'. Both need to be reassured that the difficulties in breastfeeding are temporary and due to recovering from an operation, exacerbated with a drip in her arm, a sore abdomen, inability to lift the baby and a bloated stomach. Some women might feel so 'knocked out' after the operation that they prefer to bottle feed their babies and to have them sleep in the nursery. Other mothers may object to a full-term healthy baby being removed 'for observation'. Yet others might feel that postoperative recovery requires quiet conditions which a postnatal ward cannot supply. Clearly, the emotional needs of each individual/couple must be respected where possible, and awareness maintained of the emotional trauma which a caesarean section constitutes for many women.

20.5 POSTPARTUM REACTIONS TO INSTRUMENTAL BIRTH

Reactions of disappointment, disorientation, depression, inadequacy and detachment have been commonly found among women following an unplanned caesarean, as they grieve over loss of the birth they had desired [31]. Similarly negative feelings about an instrumental birth may stem from reactions to the actual bodily process or relate to its implications for bonding. The former are rooted in the woman's relationship to her body. Because our very first self-awareness in infancy is somatic, the first ego is a body-ego, and our sense of reality is filtered through bodily experience. Therefore, enforced alteration of the body-image threatens both our sense of self and perception of reality. A woman whose idealized body image is disturbed by the traumatizing experience of mechanized labour and forceps delivery may suffer severe disappointment at her body's failure to function normally. She may feel abused by professionals who artificially intervened in the natural process; she may feel judged as inadequate by her partner, the baby or staff; she may feel humiliated by having needed help with bodily functions or having succumbed to distress or 'submitted' to the doctors' orders for caesarean section. Postnatally, she may find that her body-image has been so changed by pregnancy and the birth that she is compelled to reverse the effects of change by punitive slimming or exercise regimens. If her anxiety focuses on the belief that her genitals have been stretched or mutilated by the birth experience she may suspend intercourse for many months (also see section 25.5). When this feeling includes a more generalized distortion of her mental representation of her sexuality, she may abstain from intimacy with her husband, averse not only to sexual stimulation but all close contact. Where pre-genital disturbances are evoked, the woman may feel unable to bear being touched (physically or emotionally) and resorts to defensive avoidance of arousing sensations. Ordinary responsive fondling of a snuggling baby will be jeopardized, as will breastfeeding and loving physical care. Psychoanalysis or psychotherapy are indicated. This 'postnatal anticlimax' may thus be accompanied by bonding difficulties. The alienation reaction of doubting that the baby is hers is a well-documented phenomenon, particularly in women who have had a general anaesthetic and were not 'present' at the birth. Some are reassured of the baby's identity by their husband's attendance at the delivery or outside the window, however, the doubt about the baby's identity is not rationally based but is an expression of having 'woken up to motherhood' rather than actively accomplished the transition. She has not given birth to the baby – the baby has been 'taken' from her. She may feel violated or robbed, of the baby inside and of her fantasy baby as well as of the experience of giving birth 'normally'. Her sense of feminine pride may be hurt as she feels inferior and inadequate, unable to do what every woman around her seems to have done so easily. Emotional preparation for the anticipated operation and the opportunity to talk to other women who have had caesarean sections can alleviate much of the postnatal anticlimax.

Long separation after birth, due to maternal post-surgical recovery or infant isolation and special care, increase the likelihood of estrangement. A woman who had planned to breastfeed may resentfully feel cheated of this possibility too, and opt for milk suppression. Timely encouragement by an understanding midwife may make all the difference, enabling her to persevere with expression or difficult feeding conditions. Furthermore, postoperative pain and complications render the woman vulnerable and in need of cossetting herself, rather than feeling receptive to meeting the demands of a needy infant. Just the effort of turning over in bed or trying to cough may reduce a woman recovering from a caesarean section to helpless tears of frustration and disappointment. Several studies have found a significant relationship between postnatal depression and complications of delivery [32–34].

20.5.1 Long-term effects

The long-term effects of an instrumental birth on the relationship between parents and child are as yet unclear. Several studies have found ongoing disturbances in family interaction. A study of socially advantaged women who had emergency caesarean sections for 'ambiguous reasons' cited earlier found that when compared with a matched control group, these women were shown to be more depressed, more anxious, lacking in confidence in mothering abilities, took longer to identify their babies as 'personalities', had less eye contact and showed less appropriate mothering behaviour when interviewed when the children were three years old [35]. Others report an alarming tenfold higher incidence of child abuse in children born by caesarean section rather than vaginally [36], due to factors preceding childbirth or interacting with it. In the latter case, protracted physical or emotional illness of the mother during pregnancy, or loss of key family members have been seen to cause stress leading to dysfunctional labour; complications of parturition or acute illness of baby or mother all contribute to bonding difficulties [37].

Some researchers assume the difficulties lie not in the mother's incapacity for positive bonding, but in the effects of a less than optimal birth experience on the neonate's responsiveness and the child's developmental progress. Thus following complicated deliveries some newborn babies have been found to sleep more during the early days and suck more sluggishly due to excessive narcotics given to the mother during labour [38], and persistent motor and cognitive deficits have been found in children of women who received large doses of drugs during birth, when studied at 4 and 7 years [39]. Again, interaction of such factors as prematurity and congenital defects with both the necessity for instrument deliveries and the possibility of later developmental deficits, make it difficult to tease out cause and effect. One researcher proposes that obstetric complications lead to 'irritable new-born behaviour' which may pose difficulties for parents, who then exacerbate the irritable behaviour by their responses, thus leading to a 'maladaptive developmental pathway' [40].

Retrospective research have linked birth procedure and mental ill-health. One such study found adolescent suicide to be correlated with respiratory distress at birth [41]. Others have attributed hyperactivity, dyslexia and other disturbances to birth complications while various schools of therapy advocating 'rebirthing' attribute virtually all psychological pathology to birth trauma. Some mothers, too, attribute the child's subsequent pathology to events at birth, either indirectly as a result of her own inadequate mothering (instrumental birth is often reported as a factor in postnatal depression [42]) or due to its direct effect on the child's personality. It is not uncommon for a Facilitator to feel so guilt-ridden at having deprived her baby of the experience of birth-canal stimulation and spontaneous birth that she may believe that she has predetermined his/her personality to by-pass conflict, avoid work processes and/or seek premature gratification.

Given the interaction of many complex physiological and psychological variables of the mother during pregnancy, birth and postnatally with circumstances of birth, personality factors and developmental history of the child, it is difficult to isolate any one agent as a primary determinant. A more useful clinical approach may be for professionals simply to recognize the additional stress imposed on a new mother's relationship with her baby by recovery from a complicated delivery and, particularly, the caesarean experience. Additional stress includes the psychological shock of unexpected intervention, and a trauma for which she was insufficiently prepared; possible imposed separation and anxiety about a high-risk infant; post-operative pain or episiotomy discomfort while breastfeeding, lifting, sitting or walking; sleep disturbance and fears of splitting her stitches while tending to the baby; anger, grief, guilt and shame about her 'failure'; envy of vaginally delivered women or those without episiotomies in the postnatal ward and resentment towards their menfolk who have literally left them 'holding the baby' and got off scar-free.

Such feelings heightened in many women who have had a caesarean section can be greatly ameliorated by exchanges among them. These may be facilitated when possible by members of staff tactfully introducing mothers on the postnatal wards to others who have had similar experiences, or arranging for them to room together, and putting them in touch with the caesarean society or a local branch of the NCT Caesarean Support Group. In addition, visits to the recovery room and postnatal ward by staff who were on duty during the parturient's labour can help her work through her disappointment and confusion regarding her instrumental delivery or emergency caesarean section and the necessity for its occurrence.

KEY POINTS

*While many instrumental births are the result of a purely medical reason, others are triggered by psychological factors in the woman, such as anxiety, both during pregnancy and in labour. These may operate directly on complicating the progress of labour, or indirectly by inducing the caregivers to offer her instrumental help.
*In some women (mainly of Facilitator orientation), an instrumental birth may have immediate psychological repercussions, such as postnatal depression.

*Long-term effects of birth complications are difficult to separate from personality factors in the woman, which might have induced her to have the instrumental delivery in the first place.

*Effects on the newborn's responsiveness have been well documented; some researchers have found associations between behavioural maladjustment or psychosocial difficulties and caesarean births or obstetric complications. It is suggested that these long-term effects are not necessarily the result of neurological damage, but may be psychological disturbances as a direct consequence of the birth or due to impaired family interaction.

Part Six

COPING WITH
THE OUTCOME

Chapter 21

The newborn: parental responses and neonatal sensory and cognitive abilities

21.1. PARENTAL RESPONSES

'Into the flowing stream of love-oriented feeling chance drops a variety of crystallizing agents – words, events, other people's examples, private phantasies and memories, all the innumerable devices used by the Fates to mould an individual human destiny' (Aldous Huxley, *The Genius and the Goddess*).

21.1.1 Reality vs. fantasy baby: immediate maternal reactions

As the baby is drawn out of her, the mother begins a further transition, back to external reality from her intense inner preoccupation during the stage of expulsion. Matching up the real baby who has come out of her with the imaginary baby who has been inside her for so long demands an effort of integration by no means spontaneous. Many mothers peer at the infant unbelievingly – where is the little girl she anticipated? . . . who is this 'bony frog-like baby'? . . . is it really all over? . . . Far from 'instant bonding' a study of women giving birth in a London Teaching Hospital revealed that up to 40% of 120 new mothers reported that their predominant emotional reaction when first holding their babies was indifference. Although by the end of the first week most mothers in this and other studies report feeling some positive emotions, onset of maternal affection is found to be delayed by artificial rupturing of membranes, painful labour or high pain relief dosage [1]. We cannot underestimate the importance of psychosocial factors in this most delicate of emotional transactions.

With the phasing out of home births, wide geographical mobility and insularity of nuclear families, relatively few adults in western societies have ever encountered newborn babies. Their moulded appearance differs considerably from romanticized media pictures. Indeed, some women feel revulsion for this messy, squashed-faced squalling creature who is so dissimilar to the pink, chubby baby envisaged. His or her features are unfamiliar and disappointingly unlike those of her fantasy baby the mother has nourished for so long. Far from being joyful she may feel cheated. When responses immediately after the birth are recorded, feelings of strangeness and unfamiliarity abound [2]. Studies of mothers' responses immediately following the birth, have found that after 'greeting' the baby, laughing, smiling, and looking, a detailed (sometimes verbalized) examination follows, as mothers show some preoccupation with getting the baby to open his/her eyes, and make an adjustment to the sex of the newborn [3]. In culture where the child's gender determines the mother's status, a parturient has rapidly to become reconciled to the birth of the wrong sexed child, to find the strength to console her husband and relatives or resign herself to his cold disapproval or the active resentment of her in-laws.

In a classic study of women allowed to have their naked babies with them under a radiant heater, the mother's first tactile contact (between 30 minutes and 13 hours after birth) was found to follow such an 'orderly and predictable pattern' that it was felt to be species specific. The tactile progression began with hesitant touching of hands and feet with her fingertips, intense interest in getting the baby to open his/her eyes, and bolder full-hand caresses amid mounting excitement, which diminished with dozing as the 'examination' ended [4].

21.1.2 Psychological bonding: myths and facts

Although varying in the duration of alertness, undrugged newborns have been found to be particularly alert in the first hour after birth [5], their open-eyed intentness thus dovetailing with the alert state of the excited parents. It has been postulated that this responsiveness is geared to maximize attachment between those present at and immediately following the birth. Following this early 45–90 minutes phase of alertness immediately following birth, the newborn tends to sleep and it may be days or even weeks before s/he returns to a state of similar degree of prolonged alertness. It is, therefore, essential that where health allows, this prime time with the baby is allocated to the parents to use as they wish and not be taken up by delayable nursing, cleansing or practical procedures. Nevertheless, it must be recognized that, for many women, the baby is a stranger. The mother might feel embarrassed or even harassed by having the baby publicly foisted on her by well-meaning nurses eager that she 'bond' before it is 'too late'. She needs time to become acquainted, perhaps in private, in her own way, at her own pace. The original Klaus and Kennell [6] studies on the beneficial effects of early parent–infant bonding have often been misinterpreted to mean that there is a critical sensitive period during which close contact magically produces 'bonding'. These researchers have repeatedly stressed the multiple individual differences of mothers and fathers and the need for respect of parental variations [7]. Bonding is not to be confused with 'imprinting'. It is a two-way process of great complexity which transpires and is reinforced by many subtle exchanges. While an enraptured mother might fervently refuse separation from her precious newborn who is still part of her, a chilled, aching parturient may feel so exhausted and deeply drained that having checked the infant for blemishes all she wants is to hand it over to the father or a nurse before she drops it. Other mothers may want to be held themselves. A parturient may be in a state of shock or too excited and aroused to settle. A tired woman may find herself crying uncontrollably in the aftermath of birth, both to relieve the tension of long hours of effort and stress, and from joy and disbelief. Inevitably, each mother experiences some mixed feelings after a birth: a sense of loss of the baby moving within, deflated anticipatory excitement, possible disappointment with the birth itself, a bruised perineum, ambivalence about becoming the careworn carer rather than the pregnant focus of attention. The setting in which these intense emotions are experienced, whether in public or private, in a caring context or left to her own resources whether in a hospital delivery room, birthing centre or her own bedroom, all clearly affect the ease with which initial responses to the newborn are registered and expressed overtly, overcome or harboured to fester inside her.

21.1.3 Physiological bonding in mammals

It has been pointed out that while the baby's need for the mother is absolute, the mother's need for the baby is relative [8]. It is in the neonate's interest to 'activate' his/her mother into close and attentive contact. Whereas among lower primates the young is able to cling to the mother, gorilla and human babies are reliant on being held, which necessitates attachment by the caregiver. In most mammals although transient hormones of parturition prime the female to nurse, these soon dissipate and unless followed through with external exposure to the newborn, no maternal behaviour will follow. Conversely, exposure of newborn rat pups to virgin female rats or adult males, creates maternalistic caretaking behaviour without hormonal priming [9] and the same has been shown with rhesus male monkeys. Evidence points to the premise that caretaking behaviour in adults is induced by the offspring, cued by features such as odour recognition which activate attachment. A review of ethological studies has shown that in mammals, mother–newborn separation affects maternal behaviour, such that the mother will treat as alien a pup, cub or member of the litter that she has not licked, smelled and nursed at birth [10]. Human attachment theory has been founded on the belief that maintenance of proximity to caretaker and their mutual bonding has survival value to humans, protecting, as it does, young mammals from danger and predators [11]. Adult human behaviour is rooted both in highly complex and sophisticated feelings which are 'overdetermined' by historical, emotional and intellectual factors yet also influenced on a non-rational primitive level by sensory factors such as smell. Neonates have been found to show preference for their own mother's smell [12]. Less recognized is the observation that mothers, too, unknowingly relate to the smell of their own babies, can differentiate their own from others and even later into childhood, can distinguish the smell of each of their children from each other. Similarly, many mothers learn to distinguish the cry of their own baby on a busy hospital ward as their discriminating 'let down' reflex verifies. It is well known that women in dormitories unwittingly tend to synchronize their menstrual cycles, so it should not come as a surprise that two people who have spent nine months, one within the other, should learn to contemporize. Indeed, microfilm analysis reveals that mother–infant couples in close contact achieve an 'entrainment' of almost imperceptible movements [13], coordination of circadian bodily rhythms and interactional synchrony [14]. The neonate's licking of the nipple triggers oxytocin release in the mother, hastening uterine contractions and reducing bleeding, and also increasing her prolactin level inducing milk secretion. A recent finding that the neonate acquires bacterial flora and yeasts from those in close physical contact immediately after birth, suggests that if handled by doctor and midwife rather than parents, they will colonize these 'foreign' strains rather than the familial ones [15]. Some mothers feel that a similarly contaminated experience of stranger-'imprinting' occurs with the newborn's exposure to nurses' touch, smell and voice rather than their own.

21.1.4 The context of early caregiver responses

Clearly, as with 'falling in love', bonding is a highly personal affect. Postnatal attachment to the 'real' baby builds on the positive or negative bonds forged with the imaginary baby prenatally. Some mothers experience 'love at first sight' with their infants; to others love grows slowly. All need to progress at their own pace. The fact that generations of parents have established loving relationships with their babies despite enforced separations during the early days, is evidence that humans are adaptable and that the early prime time is not crucial for bonding [16].

The setting in which the birth takes place influences the bonding process. Following a home birth, attachment may be furthered for the mother by seeing the baby at a slight distance, held physically or emotionally by a loving father or adoring relatives who appreciate her baby, applaud her achievement and also pamper her. Unfortunately, the hospital experience imposes a dysjunction from her usual framework, separating her from caring relatives and familiar tasks at which she has established her competence. Learning new skills in a strange situation deskills her. Similarly, exposure to rows of babies lined up in a nursery or ward is counterproductive to forming a realistic intense relationship with one unique individual: idealization becomes exaggerated in the competitive situation, where the mother has to reify her imaginary baby in order to differentiate hers from all these other ordinary ones. Conversely, mothers whose fantasy babies unconsciously reflect their own weakness, may try to maintain their adult separateness from the baby by over-emphasizing negative qualities exemplified by the horde of crying infants.

Over the past decade consumer concern has been aroused by professionals assuming responsibility for decisions which are felt to lie in the parent's domain such as how much contact they have with their own newborn. Attempts to force 'bonding' in parents who are not yet ready for close contact, may do more harm than good and certainly reveal arrogant presumption and interference on the part of some professionals. Such meddlesome behaviour can only engender self-doubt in new mothers who feel guilty at their lack of 'maternal instinct' and who resent the needy baby. Luckily, most professionals are very sensitive to the issues and provide motherly care for the woman who is recovering from her own ordeal of birth. Their concern for her and unfawning appreciation of her infant plus approving assistance with babycare are far more likely to endear the baby to the mother than disapproval about her lack of maternal feelings. By providing a strong model of motherliness to be internalized, the carer can affectionately convey in her helpful behaviour what some mothers may have lacked in their own mothering. Her presence during early feeding sessions, her patient demonstration of caretaking tasks, her tacit acceptance of the baby's soiling, regurgitation and burping, benignly guide the mother through this perturbing time. By pointing out communicative signs and responses in the infant, and encouraging the mother's own intuitive responses, the sensitive midwife/nurse on the postnatal ward can help the mother overcome her fear of the fragile-looking infant, introducing her to maternal strengths within herself and teaching her to recognize robust and vital aspects of the little being for whom she is soon to be totally responsible on her own.

21.1.5 Objective measures and unconscious preconceptions

It has long been observed that infants reveal individual differences in their characteristics, modes of response and arousal levels from birth [17,18]. Babies can be studied by observers, and/or be 'asked' to respond to environmental challenges. In this sense, even newborns can act as 'informants', 'reporting' on their own psychological processes of habituation, discrimination, conditioning and many sensory and motor functions (section 21.2.3). The study of these diverse capacities can help to identify babies whose early behaviour and development may have been compromised by perinatal hazards and to gain better understanding of fetal and neonatal aberrations [19].

Babies' reactions have shown to be affected by drugs administered to their mothers in labour [20]. Obstetric complications have been found to predict child developmental problems, due not only to neurological deficits but to social interactions with caregivers. As Rutter says, 'differences in nature lead to differences in nurture' [21], with excitable infants provoking a different set of interactions with their caregivers than placid babies. However, in addition to the neonate's objective characteristics, are those perceived or ascribed by the parents. Recent research has been conducted on the effect of obstetric factors on maternal perception of their newborns. Although professionals observing the babies found full-term newborns with poor obstetric histories to be less alert and more fretful than comparisons, mothers' diaries, ratings and impressions did not reveal awareness of these differences [22]. This does not seem surprising since 'rooming-in' mothers, particularly first-timers are each only relating to their own baby, and even if comparisons are made with others, these are clouded by unconsciously determined subjective perceptions of their own babies.

During pregnancy a woman often forms a prenatal 'model' of the infant based on desired or feared facets of significant others, or on the internal image of a baby part of herself, either idealized and perfect or a split-off weak, vulnerable, greedy or demanding aspect she cannot tolerate in herself. For the mother to relinquish her unconscious fantasy and begin to see the baby as a unique person in his/her own right, she must be able to re-possess her projections, which is no mean achievement. Reconciling the real baby who has slithered out of her body with the internal image she has cultivated for so long is a subtle process of adjustment which continues for some weeks (in some ways is never completed), enhanced by close reciprocal interaction with the alert and responsive infant. These preconcepts of the baby, or 'working models' constructed during pregnancy have been shown to influence maternal perceptions of their infants (anxious mothers find their babies more 'difficult') and postnatal responses to them [23]. In the study cited earlier, the researchers state that the new mothers' 'perceptual disposition' and expectations have been shown to influence their views of their offspring, which comprise 'a significant attributional . . . component' in addition to the baby's actual characteristics. This maternal perceptual process has also been shown to affect their behaviour towards the infants, and to override the subtle effects of obstetric adversities [24]. Clearly, mothers assign meaning to their own perception of the infant's behaviour. The model of Facilitators and Regulators can be used to illustrate how this mechanism operates with positive and negative attributional orientations.

21.1.6 Differing experiences of very early contact: Facilitators and Regulators

A Facilitator unconsciously identifies the newborn baby with her own ideal baby-self, reborn in tangible form in this little scrap of life. In the hours following the birth, the woman with this orientation ascribes familiar features to her baby, whom she feels she has known almost since conception. Her elated state of heightened maternal sensitivity has been termed 'Primary Maternal Preoccupation', and likened to a 'normal illness' of preoccupation with the baby to the exclusion of other interests [25]. She often spends the first hours oblivious to the world, just staring at the newborn, crooning, cooing and talking to her infant in a high-pitched voice. Many Facilitators find they are so exuberant that they cannot sleep for the entire night following birth. Some would prefer to have the partner there too, to share in the wonderous excitement and to talk over the extraordinary experience of producing a baby from within her. Another may feel quite content with the mother–baby dyad. The baby seems the manifestation of all that is good inside her. Cherishing the perfect infant, she lavishes all the motherly love and care she herself has been craving, merging their identities in a symbiotic fusion, as in her fantasy she becomes her own mother adoring her reborn baby self. She attributes to the infant, sensations she believes she has had and by gratifying the imputed needs, she feels her own infantile needs to be vicariously satisfied. As during pregnancy, she immerses herself in this new experience, striving to maintain an ideal psychic atmosphere free from impingements from within or without.

The Regulator by contrast, during pregnancy, has invested the fantasy child with repudiated baby aspects of herself – dependence, weakness, helplessness, neediness, greed and rage. Following the birth, as during pregnancy, she tries to maintain her own familiar identity, to keep separate from this emotional infant who seems to reflect the worst qualities she has striven to overcome in herself. In her detachment, she feels little spontaneous affection at first, holding the baby slightly away from her and reluctant to come too close. The real crying baby seems to accuse her of being a bad mother, a feeling that is reinforced if a disapproving nurse criticizes her equivocal handling of the newborn. Also, since this baby has been inside her, she unconsciously feels that not only does he/she know her 'inside out' and can pass judgement on all that is buried within her, but the baby can parade her own 'badness' for all to see. Her early experience with the newborn is thus one of 'Primary Maternal Persecution', as I have termed it [26], in which she feels threatened by loss of control due to rearousal of unmet infantile needs within herself. The baby thus poses a threat, as she is caught in a situation of fundamental competitiveness with her own mother and the insatiable baby. On the postnatal ward, a caring nurse can become a buffer between the Regulator and her persecutory baby, by introducing the new mother to her infant's good features. By helping her to identify the baby's needs and to recognize that these are not wanton or excessive she can also help to meet them generously and to find ways of replenishing her own resources when she feels drained by the baby.

Although influenced by the quality of the birth experience and the personality of the real baby, the mother's prenatal perceptions and orientation continue to operate. However, under certain conditions a would-be Facilitator might become a Regulator and vice versa. In unusual circumstances, for instance, following an unexpectedly ecstatic birth for a Regulator which sets the scene for a benign interaction, or a particular gruelling nightmare for a Facilitator which makes her feel all is now spoilt, the mother may be jolted out of her pregnancy orientation into a mixed or intermediary approach towards her baby and motherhood. In the course of the early months, a switch may gradually occur, as an infant who is extremely assertive, unsoothable or exceptionally winsome may win (or force) the mother over to his/her mode of operation, be it a need for structured regulation or spontaneous facilitation. (This is explained more fully in Chapter 24.)

21.1.7 Fathers' early interaction

The inclusion of fathers in the birth process is a relatively new concession. Many mammals and most Old World primates exclude the male from birth and childrearing. Over 70% of human societies ban men from observing or assisting their wives in birth [27]. In the West, fathers excluded from labour and delivery rooms, were usually informed of the mother's progress, told after the birth the sex of the child, and possibly allowed to see or hold the baby briefly. Undoubtedly, as well as reflecting cultural stereotypes of aloof 'tough' men disinterested in 'womanly' matters and tender infants, this policy of excluding them has also reinforced such ideas. Indeed, human research indicates that fathers who are present at the birth of their babies become more involved with childrearing in the early months, although this is possibly a tautological argument since one could assume a prior emotional difference between fathers who choose to attend the birth and those who don't (i.e. Participators and Renouncers). A father watching his baby emerge from the mother's body has to find an emotional location for his nonphysical paternal connection to the child. Exposure to an alert newborn and observation of the way in which the infant responds to sound and touch and seeks eye contact, encourages emotional engagement with this little person, involving a strong attraction. A term has been coined for such paternal bonding – 'engrossment' – meaning both involvement and 'enlargement', the baby seeming larger than life, and the fathers growing in the process [28]. It has been noted that exposed fathers are just as responsive as mothers to infant cues such as vocalizations, although fathers respond by rapid talking and mothers by increased touching [29].

In situations where fathers were offered longer early contact with their babies following a caesarean birth, three months later they were found to show significantly more touching behaviour with their babies than fathers given the regular amount of contact [30]. In an uncomplicated birth fathers may find themselves holding the newborn while the mother is being stitched, washed or fed following the birth. In the original studies on paternal 'engrossment' the researchers singled out seven different experiences in the initial peak feelings of engrossment: intense visual and tactile awareness of the baby; uniqueness and perfection of this infant; the father's attraction to the newborn, his elation and increased sense of self-esteem [31]. An orderly progression of paternal contact with the infant has been charted from films immediately after caesarean birth. Each father began by gently touching the infant's extremities, then gradually proceeded using fingertips, then palms and finally the dorsal side of his fingers to touch the rest of the body and face. Interestingly, unrelated adults (medical students) also demonstrate a touching sequence similar to fathers [32]. Although mothers giving birth in hospital follow a similar touching sequence when handed their nude infants, home-birth mothers have been observed stroking the baby's face with fingertips, rather than extremities before breastfeeding or birth of the placenta [33]. These differences possibly reflect institutionally induced inhibition and the mother's sense that her hospital-delivered baby does not entirely belong to her. Similarly, a father's engrossment in the newborn can be helped or hindered by hospital procedure or attitudes.

21.1.8 Participators and Renouncers: fathers' early contact

The Participator is eager to greet the son or daughter who for so long has been veiled and withheld. Finally, he can touch and caress the little limbs directly, search for resemblance in the baby's features and interact directly with the newborn without the mediating woman. Feeling 'high on the miraculous experience' of seeing the baby born, the new father's attention is 'rivetted' by the neonate, and a would-be Renouncer might unexpectedly be so captivated by a pleasurable birth experience and alert newborn, that he begins Participator-like bonding. Marvelling at the relative size of their respective hands, gleeful about the baby's cleverness in yawning, blinking or peeing, the elated Participator father cannot get enough of his offspring. He is content to prattle and coo long into the night, while his Regulator partner is being washed or rests, or his Facilitator wife tries to get a look in. This 'reunion' might be exhilarating or fraught, depending on whether the husband feels himself to be a rival to his wife or complementary to her, and whether she needs mothering herself, wants to share her postnatal elation, yearns for privacy and rest or craves exclusive contact with her baby. Given the complexity of these permutations and the intensity of post-birth feelings, professionals can only try to respond sensitively and non-judgementally to parental requirements.

The Renouncer may feel somewhat threatened in the moments immediately following the highly arousing birth experience. The disturbing arrival of the bloodied baby from between his wife's legs in the tense atmosphere of the second phase, may leave a husband feeling slightly stunned and awed by this extraordinary happening. If a well-meaning professional then suddenly hands him the strange creature that has come into being under these mysterious female circumstances, he may feel overwhelmed by a sense of his own male inadequacy and fearful of 'dropping' the fragile baby or being 'contaminated' by this alien, newly emerged from the mother's womb.

The Renouncers who have spent a lifetime cultivating a cool-headed competent masculine manner will feel threatened by the emotions which well up inside, culminating in a sense of insecure vulnerability and the defensive need to repudiate any identification with the helpless volatile newborn engulfed by an omnipotent mother. Again, each Renouncer's experience and perception of the newborn partially depends on his own psycho-history and current circumstances but is also influenced by whether his partner is a Facilitator merged with her idealized infant, or a Regulator who herself feels threatened by the new arrival. Watching the former he may be relieved at not having to be involved or feel jealous of the infant's joyous reception. With a Regulator partner he may have the intimidating baby given to him to relieve her or he may wish to spend time on his own with her to restore their adult relationship, the baby having been safely removed by accommodating nurses.

KEY POINTS

*Following birth, in order to see the baby as a unique person in his/her own right, each mother has to reconcile the real baby with the imaginary baby of her pregnancy. The ensuing attachment is a function of each parents' historical, emotional, intellectual and sensory factors interacting with the specific constitution and personality of the baby.
*Her view of the baby is influenced by maternal unconscious prenatal representations (invested with a baby part of herself, either idealized or a

split-off aspect she cannot tolerate in herself). For the mother to relinquish her unconscious fantasy she must be able to re-possess her own projections and identification with the baby, a task only gradually and often partially achieved.

*Most newborns are highly alert and responsive in the first 45–90 minutes, postulated to maximize attachment between those present at and immediately following the birth. 'Bonding' may ensue.

*However, given the complexity of their unconscious processes at this transitional stage, many mothers feel indifferent towards their babies initially, and need time to become acquainted.

*Rather than force the issue, nurses may benefit the bonding by looking after the woman and recognizing her individual needs, thereby providing a strong example of caring motherliness to be internalized.

*A model is presented, illustrating differing experiences of very early contact of Facilitators and Regulators as determined by prenatal expectations.

*Paternal interactions with neonates differ from those of mothers, and a variety of responses are noted among fathers, as illustrated by the Participator/Renouncer model.

21.2 NEONATAL SENSORY AND COGNITIVE ABILITIES

'People say and believe – that a newborn baby feels nothing. He feels everything. Everything – utterly, without choice or filter or discrimination. Birth is a tidal wave of sensation' . . . (Leboyer, *Birth Without Violence*)

21.2.1 Consciousness at birth

Recent neonatal research has scientifically confirmed what many nurses and mothers have realized for generations, that from the moment of birth, babies are far more sophisticated and discriminating in their behaviour than they have been given credit for. The newborn has the capacity to see, hear, smell, suck, taste, feel and to seek out sensory stimulation [34] and signal for help [35]. Findings from a wide range of empirical studies provide conclusive evidence of consciousness at birth. From the moment they first open their eyes postnatally, babies employ routines of active visual pursuit and rhythmic scanning as well as visual preferences and 'listening' behaviours. Neonates are 'curious, attentive and exploratory' [36]. Experiments have illustrated that newborn babies have distinct preferences. They differentiate between various shapes, sensations and sounds, recognizing and showing preference for their own mother's smell [37] and voice [38] after less than 12 hours of contact. But above all, recent findings based on refined experimental techniques and technological advances demonstrate that the newborn infant not only experiences sensory stimulation but coordinates information from different sensory systems.

On the basis of continuous observation, Wolff [39] delineated six different states of consciousness in newborns, ranging from deep sleep, through light sleep and drowsiness to screaming, with two different states of alertness – active (occupied) and inactive (responsive). Following the short phase of alertness immediately after birth, newborns tend to sleep as much as 16 hours a day or more during the first week, with disruptions peaking on the third day. Between the second and fourth day, babies often have 'jittery, disorganized periods' when they are hard to rouse or over-react with startles and excessive crying [40]. These disruptions may be attributed to the neonate's need for reorganization of natural biorhythms after the disequilibrium of birth. Various researchers have noted indications that dreaming takes place during this period, possibly to assist organization.

Impaired habituation in newborns appears to be related to the amount of anaesthesia administered to mothers at birth, as are low Apgar scores and brain damage. Long-term deleterious effects of inhalant anaesthetics have been illustrated even after one year and later [41]. Needless to say, drugged or impaired babies do not respond well to parental efforts at interacting and may result in serious delay and difficulty in bonding. Furthermore, sleepy or damaged babies may develop feeding difficulties if the mother perceives the baby to be uninterested in sucking at her breast.

21.2.2 Active engagement

Above all, recent neonatal research has confirmed that babies are clearly social beings who seek out and actively relate to humans, and are able, even at two to three days, to discriminate and imitate smiles, frowns and surprise expressions [42]. Newborns display a special predilection for humans, preferring face-type shapes and human voices to other shapes and sounds, and displaying preferential responsiveness for their primary caretakers with whom they have most contact. In addition to these pre-adapted innate behaviours which are activated within the context of the caregiving relationship, newborns differ strikingly from each other, not only in responsiveness and capacities but in temperament. Some infants are more tolerant of frustration, others are more volatile. Research has illustrated a tendency towards 'behavioural synchrony', suggesting a biological predisposition of infants to 'mesh' behaviour with their primary caretakers, with gradual internalization by the infant of the mutual relationship pattern [43].

Thus, in terms of the Facilitator/Regulator, Participator/Renouncer model, we may suggest that the nature of the relationship will largely be determined by the degree to which there exists a 'good fit' between baby and parents and by the specific infant's flexible capacity to adapt to that particular maternal/paternal couple's orientation or to influence it to change.

Their reciprocal exchange involves dynamic alteration. Fine-grained analysis of split-screen videos reveals that ongoing interaction between the infant and parent involves complicated transformations, with each partner in turn engaging in communication while the other attends. So subtle is the coordination of this interactive process that it is only when disruptions occur in these exchanges that the infant's own complementary adaptations and regulatory function can be seen [44].

21.2.3 Cognitive abilities

Babies form and test out hypotheses [45] about the experiences they encounter, and show an interest in problem solving [46]. Careful empirical observations suggest that babies evolve abstract cross-modal representations of 'invariant' (unchanging) properties of the world about them. They are not only able to recognize patterns in one modality (i.e. visual, auditory, sensual) but to coordinate information and transpose perceptual experience across sensory modalities. This allows the baby to develop an experience of perceptual unity as the meaningful separate unrelated happenings gradually and progressively become integrated around an emergent sense of a core-self [47]. However, it seems that newborns are unable to conceive of objects and people as integrated wholes with independent existence, differentiated from their own action. This is only gradually achieved by progressive discrimination [48]. There are indications that dreaming takes place during which the baby might be mentally 'digesting' the many complex novelties which they encounter in their environment.

21.2.4 Affective reciprocity

During this REM (rapid eye movement) 'dreaming' sleep, newborns express a full range of facial expressions including smiling. Their crying is purposeful and spectographic analysis reveals distinctions between birth, umbilical clamp, pain, hunger and pleasure cries [49] while further studies match 'cryprints' of baby to mother's speech rhythms [50]. Newborns of only one hour old can imitate adult gestures such as sticking out a tongue [51] thus displaying interactive attentiveness, and social responsiveness. By two weeks they clearly discriminate between the mother's and a stranger's face, and can associate her face with her voice [52], and respond quite differently towards people and objects [53].

As we have seen, parents too, appear to display intuitive responsiveness to their newborns, a species-specific sequence of touching behaviour, exaggerated greeting responses, imitation of the baby's facial and vocal expressions, 'mirroring' and simple repetitiveness in interactions, pitching their speaking-voices high and maintaining eye-contact. However, these may differ in the case of home births and hospital deliveries, where clearly, in the latter, the parents are more self-conscious. A 'cascade of interactions' of interlocking behavioural, immunological, endocrinal and physiological systems has been postulated gradually to establish 'locking' of parents and baby together and 'ensuring further development of the attachment' [54]. This sociobiological predisposition of parents and infant to mesh in reciprocal interchange is clearly a delicately balanced complex mechanism which can all too easily be upset by ordinary factors occurring in every hospital delivery room and postnatal ward, e.g. stranger-scrutiny, lack of privacy, sedation, glaring lights, constant mechanical and artificial noise, unsafe, uncomfortable furniture in ugly surroundings and thoughtless intervention on behalf of well-meaning professionals. Since policy has dictated that the majority of births take place in a foreign and daunting institutional atmosphere, special provisions must be made to protect parents' and baby's right to become acquainted in privacy, intimacy and comfort.

21.2.5 Emotional needs of infants

We must be cautious in speculating about the internal states of infancy, which we can only infer from observed behaviour and childhood recollections or adult reconstructions. Nevertheless, there are generalizations we may now make with some confidence. Neonatal research has shown that even very small infants have the capacity to relate to other humans, a selective alertness which appears to consist of a built-in orientation and readiness to interact, rather than specific anticipation of care. The neonate's sensitivity to speech patterning and preference for certain human stimuli (taste of human milk, maternal smell, voice, heart beat, visual images of human faces) and ability to discriminate and organize information cross-modally, seems to indicate, over and above the need for proximity and physical gratification, a desire for reciprocity, recognition and response.

Despite theoretical variations and different approaches, most psychoanalysts and neonatal researchers alike appear to agree that 'good enough' maternal care is rooted in the caregiver's capacity for sensitive responsiveness and 'attunement' to the baby's emotional cues and signals through which the parent can fathom the preverbal child's needs. 'Paternal'-type interaction appears to involve a greater degree of playfulness and provocative stimulation than mothers, possibly due to lack of intimate familiarity with the baby's own biorhythms. Equally, there appears to be general agreement among most professionals whatever their theoretical leanings, that it is in this early context of intense emotional experiences with primary caregivers that basic levels of security and trust are established, distortions of which can influence later vulnerability through increased sensitivity to stresses.

One view, that of the psychoanalyst and pediatrician Winnicott, is that the mother's 'holding' function consists of 'mirroring' back her baby's feeling and her own enjoyment of mothering so that the child, searching the mother's face can come to see and value him/herself (if she is an 'accurate' mirror). By 'feeding' the world to the infant in appropriate little 'doses' and by warding off 'impingements' and the unpredictable, the mother maintains for the child an illusion of his/her own omnipotence. Ideally, as the baby grows and is no longer absolutely dependent, so the mother resumes her own independence, and through her gradual failure to adapt to the child s/he becomes aware of dependence, and differentiates 'me' from 'not me' in an emotionally significant way [55]. Dovetailing with this theory is that of another psychoanalyst, Bion, who regards the mother's capacity for 'reverie' as the essential containing function, the 'well-balanced' mother accepting the baby's fears and managing them until the infant evolves his/her own capacity for holding onto thoughts, and thinking realistically, which coincides with recognition of and toleration of frustration [56]. Thus, there is agreement that to be effective, caregiving must progressively change to meet the developing needs of the child, and that parents vary in their capacities to accommodate different developmental phases in the growing child.

Disturbances in close early relationships affect later parenting capacities. These are dependent on realistic self-appraisal and assessments of the baby's needs. Good caregiving is rooted in the adult's capacity for positive unconscious identification with the infant, having successfully worked through similar developmental stages in her/his own childhood. When the parent retains 'unfinished business' from their own early experiences they will be driven to exploit the baby to their own ends. However, in addition to the past, the present is a potent stimulus in its own right and the intricate mechanisms of exchange between primary caregiver and infant occur in a series of reciprocally affective interactions, in which the parent, too, is continuously influenced by his/her own subjective interpretation of this particular baby's response.

The picture that emerges, therefore, is an intergenerational one: the caregivers' receptivity to the infant and capacity to observe accurately and respond sensitively depend on their own sense of psychological well-being, in addition to the specific infant's capacity to 'signal', initiate and respond. As we shall see in later chapters, unless counterbalanced by the child's resilience and utilization of other nurturing experiences, disturbances in early parenting may create and perpetuate emotional disturbances in relating to self and other, which uncorrected, may be transmitted during their own parenthood, to future generations.

Chapter 22

Early days: getting acquainted – unconscious identifications and gender differences

'If we look at the attitude of affectionate parents towards their children, we have to recognize that it is a revival and reproduction of their own narcissism, which they have long since abandoned' . . . (Freud, *On Narcissism*).

22.1 'THERE IS NO SUCH THING AS A BABY'

A British psychoanalyst who was also a paediatrician once shocked his colleagues by remarking excitedly: 'there is no such thing as a baby'! [1]. What he meant, of course, is that without the attentive care of the (m)other the baby would not survive. This 'other', in most societies has been designated as the woman who gave birth to that baby, although in many a preindustrial society any lactating woman could act as wet-nurse caretaker, and in bottlefeeding societies, theoretically, anyone, male or female, young or old, can nurture. However, the desire to provide loving maternal care for an infant is by no means universal, and although it may be activated by exposure to the baby during birth or immediately after, it is not uncommon for a sense of mother-liness to be tardy, triggered slowly on acquaintance with the infant or, in some cases, not at all. 'Becoming' a mother is not an overnight happening or one that automatically coincides with the birth. The biological mother undergoes a psychological 'gestation' before she feels herself to be a mother. Her emotional attachment to the baby is a function of her own receptivity to this particular infant and the baby's capacity to evoke her responsiveness [2]. Early responsibility for care of the newborn appears to foster nurturing. Fathers of premature or caesarean-section born babies have been found to be more deeply involved in their infants than other fathers or, sometimes, than the incapacitated mothers in the early days [3,4]. However, in the usual course of events paternal attachment reactions may be delayed due to lack of close contact and opportunities for emotional exchange in the early days (fathers are therefore dealt with in more detail in Chapter 24).

22.2 EARLY POSTNATAL AFFILIATION

We have all been babies. Exposure to a dependent newborn uncannily touches us. Often arousing a mixture of protectiveness and pity, as we are each reminded, not only of our own origins, but of the poignant aspects of that dependent state. Each mother unconsciously responds to her new baby with the full force of her real and imagined history of having been mothered, reawakening fantasies and memory traces of bliss or painful frustrations from her own subjective infantile experience of helplessness. Since early pregnancy, the nature of her relationship to her 'internal' parents and her emotional relationship with her partner have constituted the matrix for her orientation towards mothering her fantasy baby. Now, the encounter with this tangible fragile newborn adds the crucial element – the real baby she is to mother. Gazing at her baby, she imbues the infant with the home-spun emotional aura of her unconscious ideas, coloured by her own unmet infantile needs.

Clearly, each mother differs in the degree to which she has come to terms with the imperfections of early experience and the mother she carries within herself. More emotionally mature women, content to be 'good-enough mothers' [5], have found ways of resolving unrealistic idealization or resentful denigration of their mothers while others still maintain old resentments and skewed expectations about motherhood, and are determined to be different or better than their own mothers. Young mothers oscillating between insecurity and overcompensatory self-confidence may be categorized as 'overindulgent, oversolicitous, over-protective and/or perfectionistic' [6].

Who the baby represents in her own mind is a further strand in the fantasy relationship that is transferred onto the infant. She may attribute various features to the newborn, seeing a family resemblance or similarity of temperament, ascribing meaning to little gestures or sounds. Conception may have occurred following a loss, with the baby serving as an unconscious replacement for an adored lost relative or lover. The early encounter with her newborn simultaneously weaves together myriad connections ranging from realization of the imaginary child she has dreamed of since childhood; repayment of a debt to her mother now transmitted to the infant; tangible resurrection of the unmourned dead or, depending on the constellation of her family of origin, this baby may be unconsciously equated with a loved or hated baby brother or sister. All this, in addition to emotional tallying with unconscious aspects of the woman's own self. Needless to say, during these first days, the father too is involved in coming to terms with the birth of a real baby, whether he is in touch with it or engaged in a 'flight' from fatherhood. The process of reconciling the external baby with the fantasy one of his imagination is a different experience for men, who, unlike their pregnant partners, have not had the benefit of the reality of direct prenatal interaction with the fetus, and are excluded from close ongoing early contact while wives and babies are in hospital.

22.3 NAMING THE BABY

Some parents now bring out the secret name that has been stored up during pregnancy, superstitiously awaiting the birth before it is shared. In some places such as Scotland and Shropshire, it is regarded as unlucky to divulge the name of an infant before s/he is christened [7]. Others drop the nickname of pregnancy for the 'real' name. Yet others spend these first days 'playing' with different possible names, or searching the child's features for the name that will 'emerge' and declare itself. Although choice of the name is often accompanied by much conscious deliberation, like the date of birth, it is often shadowed by unconscious determination. The name is a live myth to be bestowed upon the child. On a deep and primitive level it is not a label but an attribution. In discussing the magical properties and importance of names, Freud states the early belief that a man's name is 'a principal component of his personality, perhaps even a portion of his soul' [8]. In many cultures a person's name is regarded as a concrete part of themselves, so that s/he may be harmed by its misuse by people or demons. Personal names may be duplicated or kept secret for this reason as among some Australian aborigines or a special sacred or unmentionable name will be kept for solemn occasions only, as with the ancient Egyptians and Brahmins. Many diaspora Jews still give their infants a Hebrew name for religious purposes, in addition to their locally determined name in daily use. Customs also dictate who the baby may be called after – whether an infant may be named after a live relative as in many Christian societies; the degree of predetermination of calling a new baby after a dead ancestor as in Judaism or its taboo as in some South Indian, Japanese and Philippine cultures, for fear of ghosts. Similarly in Ireland naming a baby after a dead sibling is said to be a 'certain way of bringing early death' [9]. One text reports that among the Lapps there is a belief that a deceased relation will inform the woman in a dream who is to be born again in the infant [10]. In some countries a baby is named after the saint on whose day s/he was born or after an animal or hero in the hope of being empowered with its attributes.

However, in most cases in the West, lacking all but the broadest of traditional guidelines, the parents are personally faced with the arduous responsibility of saddling their child with the name that will accompany him or her for the rest of life. And in so doing, they often unwittingly assign unconscious legendary or personal meanings and messages in either overt or disguised form. Many years later, a parent may be surprised to realize the obscure origins in his/her unconscious of the name chosen. In larger families, children's names, jigsaw-puzzle like, may interlace, each having some attributes of one or both of the parent's or some other significant person's name, or else their cumulative initials may form an acronym, or their full names form a historical progression or chain of associations which can only be completed with the birth of the last unconsciously planned baby or may include miscarried or lost babies.

22.4 REACTIONS TO THE SEX OF THE BABY

Anbara aborigines traditionally classify the newborn with the fetus, a fetus outside instead of inside, lacking gender distinction until, with the smile it gains humanity at 6 weeks by showing a capacity for social interaction, and becomes a male or female 'small one' [11]. Westerners tend to emphasize the newborn's gender and there is research evidence that from birth, parents interact differently with their newborn male and female infants. One study of mothers' delivery room reactions to newborns found a correlation between satisfaction with the baby's gender and having a name for the baby, a sense of accomplishment and general happiness; mixed feelings about the baby's sex were associated with maternal distraction, whereas displeasure with sex of her child significantly correlated with a report at the 6 months' follow-up of colic [12]. My own psychoanalytic observations [13] suggest that, 'whichever sex she anticipated in fantasy, there is a vast difference for the parturient mother in relating to her son as opposed to a daughter, who Russian-doll fashion, already contains within her ovaries the eggs of her own future fetus and the womb in which her baby will reside. On an unconscious level, the woman imagines the daisy-chain of successive 'navel-strings' connecting her baby girl backwards to her mother and through her to maternal grand- and great grandmother, and forwards (if she is to have a daughter), to her female descendants. The female infant denotes for the mother an interiority and an umbilical lineage which stops short at the male. Her body is a miniature copy of the female body in which the mother lives, whereas a newborn son thrusts his male differentness at his mother'. How each mother reacts to son or daughter is also embedded deep in her own affirming or negating relationship with her own early mother and father and other significant figures. The parturient's relationship to her male baby is greatly affected by her close relationships with other males; her own father, brother(s), impregnator, partner. These will determine whether this baby must become a substitute for an impoverished love-life or compensation for an unsatisfying erotic relationship; whether he is identified with his loved or disappointing father or invested with qualities of a yearned-for past lover; whether he represents an envied brother or a wished for penis, or the reincarnation of a loving relationship, or the projection of her cumulative negative past experiences with members of his sex.

Similarly, a woman's relationship with her girl baby is from the start coloured by her own experience of being a daughter to her mother, being feminine in a patriarchal world and what it has meant to her to occupy a female body.

22.5 GENDER DIFFERENCES AND ASCRIPTION

Gender stereotyping begins at birth, with parents differentially attributing 'feminine' or 'masculine' qualities to their female and male babies. Although each baby's experience of male or female genitality is formed by living in a male or female body, social evaluation of that experience is subtly determined by parental definitions and expectations which are conveyed to the infant from the moment of birth, in the robust or tender way he/she is held, fed, cleaned and caressed; in the teasing, seductive, serious or attentive tone of voice in which people talk and coo at him or her and fine-grained differences in the way she or he is exuberantly encouraged to be assertive or tacitly devalued. Some studies have found that fathers more than mothers tend to encourage sexually stereotyped behaviour [14]; flirting and treating their baby daughters as little 'glamour pusses' while attributing greater strength and valour to their sons. Fathers have also been found to diverge from mothers' soothing approach in their handling of babies of both sexes in a more playful, 'rough and tumble' and stimulating way [15,16]. Nevertheless, a research experiment demonstrated that when parents' autonomic arousal was measured in response to watching videotapes of a smiling/crying infant, psychophysiological responses of mothers and fathers were indistinguishable [17], suggesting that women do not have innate superior responsiveness to babies as ethologists had proposed but that both sexes are potentially equally sensitive in responding to infant needs.

Furthermore, parent/baby interaction is affected by more than corporeal gender of the baby and parental fantasies or male and female type social interaction of parent. Recent research suggests that neonatal differences between the sexes are not only anatomical but possibly mental as well, due to the organizing influences on the brain exerted by hormones determining structural variation [18]. Indeed, studies of expressive actions of neonates suggests that innate characteristic differences may exist between the sexes, with male babies being 'more vigorous and assertive' and females 'more observant of the mother and making more prespeech and more delicate gestures' [19]. However, it is difficult to determine the extent to which these differences are innate or arise within the context of a predominantly female primary care set-up, and maternal ascriptions. Furthermore, we also must assume gradual accretion in each baby of distinctive male or female genital experiences which develop into different mental representation of body-image, as receptive enclosed inner space vs. external erectable penis [20,21]. Nevetheless, careful research into hermaphrodites has disclosed that parental ascription of 'social' gender from birth onwards usually over-rules the genetic determination [22]. In other words, a chromosomally male child brought up by the parents as a girl will usually regard himself as one. Such is the psychosocial power of the primary care-taker.

22.6 CIRCUMCISION

The debate about the efficacy of circumcision as a preventive measure still rages in the United States where for many years it was a routine procedure. About 58% of newborn males are still circumcised in the USA, and the Californian Medical Association passed a resolution in 1988 declaring that circumcision is an effective public health measure. On the other hand, the Canadian Paediatric Society reaffirmed its own stand against routine circumcision in 1988, and the American Academy of Pediatrics still maintains its 1971 finding of 'no valid medical indications' for routine circumcision [23]. An interesting twist to the debate involves Swedish researchers who have suggested that the prepuce, or foreskin, presents a problem in societies where childbirth is attended by good hygiene. In 'biologically natural settings' mothers, who give birth squat-ting or kneeling often defaecate during childbirth, thereby colonizing the baby with their own aerobic and anaerobic intestinal flora. In sanitary hospital maternity units, the baby's gastrointestinal tract and genitals may be colonized by strains of non-maternal origin to which the baby has no passive immunity. The Swedish paediatricians' conclusion is that urinary tract infections should be prevented not by circumcision but by encouraging more natural colonization of the baby with his mother's gut flora [24].

In the United Kingdom circumcision is usually practised only for religious reasons by both Muslims and Jews. Freud suggested that on a deeply unconscious symbolic level, circumcision is equated with castration, a fantasy which fuels antisemitism among non-practising people [25]. Although surgeons sometimes oblige and the 'plastibell' method is available in some hospitals, Jewish circumcision is ritually performed on the eighth day of life by a special religious official, the Mohel, who usually conducts the ceremony at home. Sometimes, a doctor may also be authorized as a mohel. Although conducted without anaesthetic, the baby is given some sweet kiddish wine before the procedure which is performed on the lap of his godfather (with the father standing by), and special prayers are said entering the baby boy into the covenant of Abraham, who circumcised his son Isaac at this early age, blessing him with entry 'into the Law, the nuptial canopy and into good deeds' [26]. In Islam male circumcision is also the rule but may be carried out at any time before puberty. Following birth a specific faith-affirming ceremony for the newborn male in which the *adhan*, the call to prayer of the faithful, usually declaimed from the minaret of the mosque, is immediately recited, in the delivery room if necessary, by the father or a senior member of the Muslim community [27]. In some immigrant communities, especially from Somalia, female circumcision or infibulation of prepubertal girls is still practiced. Invariably, even a routine circumcision causes both baby and parents some distress and despite cultural dictates, many parents now choose to forgo it. Previously, before the current trend of questioning authoritative injunctions virtually all Jews and Muslims, whether practising or not, felt the obligation to have their boys circumcised. The prospect of deliberately exposing the newborn baby to a medically unnecessary genital operation is frightening on many levels. Although a non-complicated procedure, horror stories and castration fantasies abound. A set-back in the baby's postnatal adjustment is often reported. It may be particularly traumatic for less orthodox people who have heart-felt conflicts between tenets of their tradition (and parents) and tender humanistic feelings towards their newborn. Non-observant feminist mothers angrily challenge the archaic 'barbaric' practice inflicted on them by patriarchal or familial pressures. The procedure also invariably arouses unconscious ramifications and identificatory anxieties about paternal sadism in new fathers. In this era of greater choice, deliberating parents may need counselling to talk through their dilemmas during this difficult time of decision-making and if they do decide on circumcision, supportive follow-up may be necessary during the period of observation for post-procedural infection or complications.

22.7. FACILITATORS/REGULATORS:IDENTIFICATIONS

Close encounters with the new baby during these first days threaten to disarm the new mother of her usual adult protective 'veneer', stirring up and heightening primitive emotions. A Reciprocator who has been able to consolidate her own subjective identity before the birth of the baby, can realistically recognize the infant's subjectivity. Comfortable with her own ambivalence she is less threatened by responsibility for another sensitive human being, empathising with her baby, recognizing him/her as separate and different from herself yet sharing similar human states of mind. Fortified by inner confidence in her selfhood, a Reciprocator finds her resources suffice both to sustain her own individuality and to validate and foster the baby's individuality. In general, a woman who recognizes her own agency welcomes the infant's assertiveness, attuning her responses to the infant's communications and respecting his/her rhythms. However, she also feels entitled to initiate interaction, to express her own feelings and establish her stimulating presence. Thus, affirmation of the baby as a separate assertive person does not imply that the mother negates her own subjectivity. Indeed, self-effacement may be as damaging in an ongoing relationship as prolonged absence or withdrawal. Mutual delight requires both partners to be fully present, each contributing to and sharing an enjoyable experience. As we shall see, both the extreme Facilitator who dedicates herself selflessly to meeting her infant's perceived needs at the expense of her own adult being and the Regulator who regulates these needs out of fear of being taken over by the infant's 'insatiability' (which is a projection of her own unmet infantile demands), may vicariously use the baby to express their own repressed baby-selves rather than acknowledging both self and the baby as people each entitled to respective needs and personhood in their own right. However, given our cultural denial of female subjectivity and strong social pressures towards maternal devotion, sadly, many women forego reciprocity. Threatened by the emotional struggle of recognizing self and baby as equally present within the mothering context, many women avoid the issue either by escaping into self-denial and merger of facilitation or by reinforcing separateness in regulating a battle of control. Therefore, once again, the model of Facilitators and Regulators can serve to demonstrate two easily recognizable poles of the mothering spectrum, and provide guidelines for extremes. The majority of mothers oscillate along the continuum, according to their own moods, the baby's personality and responsiveness and the fluctuating supportiveness of their social milieu.

In the early days following the birth, the Facilitator is 'high': blind to imperfections in her state of post-birth exhilaration she tends to infuse her infant with a special idealizing aura by denying her own natural feelings of ambivalence. Encircling the newborn in her arms, the Facilitator mother tries to recreate the magic bubble of the containing womb, this time enclosing herself too within the enchanted circle, in a series of interchangeable identifications such as she experienced during pregnancy. She is both mother and infant; she identifies the baby with her own baby-self as in her fantasy she becomes a glorified version of her own mother mothering herself as baby. Voluptuously luxuriating, she operates on a primitive level of sensuality. Conscious of her baby's attraction to her bodily odours, she uses neither perfumes nor deodorants. Breathing in the baby's fragrance, which she imagines still smells of her own inner world, she emotionally invests the infant with her own ideal image, replicating idealized uniqueness. To her this is the best, the only baby in the world, and she feels she is the best mother for this baby, the only one who truly understands what the baby wants.

By contrast, having recuperated somewhat from the ordeal of birth and after-effects of anaesthesia, the Regulator (who may have had the baby transferred to the nursery for the first night), warily begins a tentative inspection of her unknown infant. She is helped if a sensitive nurse gradually introduces her to holding and establishing eye-contact with the little stranger, and gauging the woman's pace determines when and how long to leave the hesitant new mother alone with her unfamiliar baby. A competent nurse may not realize the enormity of impact such a tiny baby can have on his/her seemingly unruffled mother. Threatened by the upsurge of unruly emotions in the wake of the birth and contact with her fragile closest relative, a woman who is used to feeling in control needs time to compose herself for fear of being overwhelmed by conflicting experiences of her churned up dependency needs and her inner dictates to be efficient and strong. On an unconscious level, having invested the baby with weaknesses that she has repudiated in herself, she will now try to disassociate herself from these.

These different early postnatal experiences indicate the degree to which mothers' impressions of their babies are determined by specific internal ascription of characteristics to the baby rather than by an external reality alone. Studies have shown that although mothers agree with professionals when asked to categorize 'difficult' behaviour in babies (defined by persistent crying, poor soothability and poor organization of feeding/sleeping routines), their observations and category assignment of their own newborn's actual behaviour have been found to differ from that of the nurse [28]. This discrepancy confirms that even observant mothers' impressions of their own babies are determined by their own specific subjective orientation and attributions rather than objective measures.

22.8 INFLUENCE OF BABY'S SEX ON FACILITATOR AND REGULATOR MOTHERS

As has been shown, Facilitator and Regulator orientations towards mothering and bonding are usually set during pregnancy when knowledge of the fetus is minimal and the woman's unconscious fantasies are allowed free rein. However, in the same way that mothering is gradually modulated by the real baby's responses and personality traits, so each woman is also influenced by the sex of her infant.

Giving birth to a girl baby, the Facilitator is able to merge her own identity with that of the female newborn, identify with her helplessness and dependency and vicariously enjoy her own loving gratification of all her daughter's needs. A son, by contrast, forces his male difference upon her, and makes it more difficult for her to merge and identify fully with the baby as if it were herself.

Conversely, having a boy infant enables the Regulator to separate herself off clearly from her son. He is the weak and needy one, while she is the strong mother. By contrast, a girl baby poses the threat of being drawn willy-nilly into identification, a reminder of her own painful early experience of vulnerable infantile helplessness when she feels she was frustrated or neglected or engulfed by her own mother. Given her current desire to remain independent, it is more difficult for the Regulator to come close to her new daughter for fear of being sucked into the turmoil of loving, and turbulent re-arousal of tender, dependency needs and raw primitive feelings she has struggled to stave off in herself.

22.9 PHASES IN ASSUMPTION OF MATERNAL RESPONSIBILITY

An overview of the transition of puerperal change and restoration has been roughly divided into three, defined as the phases of taking-in, taking-hold and letting-go [29]. During the taking-in phase of the first 2–3 days, the average new mother is much preoccupied with her own needs, is rather passive and initiates little activity but is eager to talk about the birth. As she enters the taking-hold phase the woman tries to take control both of her body and her new situation yet feels intolerant of her own difficulties in acquiring the new mothering skills. Her essential needs at this point are seen as nourishment, elimination, comfort, rest and the presence of a supportive figure. In the hospital context, warmly reassuring non-patronizing help can encourage the mother's confidence and utilize her natural curiosity and desire to learn in this second phase which for many women coincides with experiencing the 'blues'. The third phase, dated in the original study from about ten days postpartum, involves some grieving work of accepting the baby as separate from herself and her previous life as changed. (In the present age, this phase is clearly accelerated with arrival home and women who partake of early discharge may have to condense the first phase as well).

22.10 BIRTH OF THE 'BLUES'

Between a half and two-thirds of newly delivered women suffer from the 'blues', a transitory syndrome of weepiness on the third or fourth day. The tears are usually accompanied by despondency, an anxious feeling of difficulty in coping and subjective impairment of concentration and memory [30]. With the incoming milk there are rapid physiological changes within her body, and corresponding alteration of body-image from 'pregnant' to 'matronly'. Unfamiliar bodily experiences fluctuate rapidly; lactating breasts leak, 'let down', become hard, swollen, painfully engorged, heavy, flabby, lopsided . . . While hormonal changes in parturition, the powerful experience of childbirth and onset of lactation all contribute to the disorder, it is likely that the 'blues' (which are also known to be experienced by adoptive mothers) hinge to a large degree on the emotional upheaval of becoming the mother of a tiny infant.

As we have noted, exposure to a fragile naked newborn and the intensely intimate contact with the baby sucking at her breast arouses buried feelings in the new mother that have been repressed or forgotten until now. Suddenly, she finds herself flooded with unfamiliar emotions, fantasies about her own infancy and birth, images of her own experience of being mothered as an infant. Feelings of confusion relate to a multitude of potent factors: dispossession of her previous self, disappointment with the birth or with her baby's gender or his/her persistent crying; dissatisfaction with early motherhood in hospital or with her own maternal inadequacies compared with the ideal she had visualized; jealousy of the baby showered with presents by excited visitors who appear to ignore her now that the baby is no longer in her. She may feel neglected and lonely, saddened by loss of the cosy feeling of having the baby inside, now replaced with emptiness and the sharp uterine after-pains triggered by feeding. Her inner depletion may be compensated for by the closeness to the baby sucking at her breast. However, for some mothers, in these early days, this suckling is the wrong baby: loss of pregnancy evokes poignant loss of her fantasy baby as well as dissolution of her glorified fruitful self, now no longer the focus of attention and promise. This anticlimax is for women unconsciously experienced as a sense of rejection, feeling deserted by the inner baby as they imagine themselves to have been by their mothers. Women who have recently lost their own mothers or those who, bereaved before puberty, felt abandoned before they were able to assume their adult sexuality in close proximity to a maternal female, are particularly prone to blues which might subsequently be intensified to full-blown postnatal depression.

Nurses on the postnatal ward will be aware of mothers who are inordinately depressed. These women need warm human comforting and possible referral for psychotherapeutic treatment rather than sleeping pills or 'bucking up'. Soon to be discharged to nuclear family isolation, many mothers feel that the supportive contact with the nurses and other mothers on the ward are the only rays of light in a dark tunnel. A weeping mother may need to be reminded that this seemingly unending over-whelming experience does eventually pass, but rather than jollying out of her tears she may want a motherly cuddle and a shoulder to cry on. Some women feel suicidal or murderously angry with the demanding baby. Others are apathetic and unable to function. Where feelings of hopelessness prevail coupled with severe depression, persistent anxiety and irrational fears about the baby or her own safety, specialized professional help is likely to be needed and the sooner it is offered, the shorter the duration and the less implacable the disturbance is likely to be. Postnatal emotional disturbance as it is triggered differentially in Facilitators and Regulators will be dealt with in Chapter 24. The general issues of postnatal depression and puerperal psychosis will be treated separately in Chapter 33.

KEY POINTS

*In order to assume her new emotional identity, a woman feels the need to establish a bridge between her pregnant self and the mother she is becoming by talking over the labour, working through traumatic aspects of the birth, imposing meaning on the confusion of her current maternal experiences and integrating these extraordinary happenings into her ongoing life.
*Early encounters with the newborn and bonding patterns are influenced by the parents' gender, the unconscious representation of the baby for the mother and father, as well as the specific characteristics of the baby, and these may be reflected in choice of name.
*In our model, the Facilitator emotionally imbues the infant with her own ideal image, whereas the Regulator invests her baby with repudiated weaknesses in herself, from which she now tries to dis-associate herself.
*Gender differences also influence maternal relationships, with the Facilitator finding it easier to fuse her own identity with that of a female infant while a boy baby enables the Regulator to separate herself off clearly from his maleness. Gender stereotyping begins at birth, its content being dependent on social influences and the parents' own personal gendered history.
*The three day 'blues' experienced by many women may be attributed to hormonal changes in parturition, the powerful experience of childbirth and onset of lactation and, above all, the emotional upheaval of new responsibility for a helpless infant.

Chapter 23

Postpartum professional care

For the woman giving birth in hospital, professionals with whom she comes into contact on the postnatal ward are invested with many of the qualities attributed to 'wise-women' in the traditional home birth situation. She expects advice on physical matters such as breast and episiotomy treatment, and reassurance about clots in the lochia or moulding of the baby's head, or postoperative nursing care if she has undergone a caesarean section. In addition, she also needs validation and guidance in assuming her new identity as mother and often expects magical formulae to produce the results. To provide such guidance, the nurse must be aware not only of the physical changes taking place but of psychological processes and transferential expectations of the woman herself as well as the complex alterations in family dynamics following the birth.

23.1 INTEGRATING LABOUR

During the first hours or days, most women need an opportunity to talk over the birth with someone who was there and can help fill in details. Quite apart from the desire for information is a need to relive this incredible experience and work through the frightening or particularly intense moments. When a labour ward midwife finds time in her busy schedule and makes an effort to visit a previous client now in the postnatal ward, she is often surprised at the warm welcome she receives as a very special visitor. The grateful mother may greet her as the staunch saviour to whom she clung at the height of the 'storm', the encouraging beacon at the end of the dark 'tunnel' of pain, the caring key-person in a room full of strangers or even the 'witch' or 'bitch' at whom she screamed then, and now needs to recognize afresh and be forgiven.

Not only does the midwife impose meaning on a confusing and possibly traumatic experience but she can, at a time of vulnerable uncertainty, provide continuity for the woman between her pregnant prebirthing self and the mother she has become. In addition, particularly when the parturient's own mother lives far away or is no longer alive, she can also offer maternal reassurance to a mother who feels she did not perform as well as expected during the labour and birth, approving her behaviour and function as admiring audience for the new baby so 'cleverly' produced. This is especially true for a woman who feels betrayed by the discrepancy between the actual experience of birth and the one she had led herself to believe she would have. Given that psychic reality dictates the meaning of the experience of birth rather than the external reality, she may regard as traumatic a delivery which professionals experienced as successful, and vice versa. The process of re-examining the birth, like a postpartum de-briefing, helps evaluate and integrate this extraordinary event into the parturient's everyday life experiences. The presence of a sympathetic co-traveller can enable her to work through this process which otherwise continues for weeks and possibly years as the woman recounts her narrative to friends and acquaintances, editing later 'transcripts' in her memory, subtly changing facets of it or in time revealing hidden, forgotten or repressed aspects, while inhibiting others.

23.2 FIRST FEEDS: BREAST AND BOTTLE

Whether a mother wants to breast- or bottle-feed her baby, depends not only on physiological and social factors but on a variety of conscious and unconscious psychological influences as well.

(a) Strangeness

In the West, many women have never watched a baby being breastfed. Although this is being remedied by a new generation of unselfconscious young women suckling their babies socially, and by the contemporary focus on breastfeeding and the heightened visibility of militant mothers demonstrating in 'feed ins' about lack of feeding facilities in public places. Nevertheless, many parturients have never had a close encounter with breastfeeding since their own infancy. Indeed, a whole generation of babies, now grown-up women, may not have encountered a lactating breast at all having been bottle fed in line with the baby care vogue at the time. One way to remedy the lack of exposure to breastfeeding is, in addition to videos in antenatal classes, to invite feeding mothers in parentcraft teaching classes, to demonstrate and answer questions.

(b) Sexuality

Current 'soft' media presentation of romantic visions of cherubs nestling at their Madonna-mothers' breasts conflict with the hard-core porn and media-generated male sexual-stereotype of high-breasted erotic women.

Many a parturient fears breast feeding may impair the attractive shape of her breasts. Underlying this conscious idea is the fantasy that body and love will be so monopolized by the baby that her sexual life will be depleted and her sex appeal reduced. This becomes a self-fulfilling prophecy in some cases where the breastfeeding woman views her full lactating breasts as off-putting or has the deep sense that her desexualized body no longer belongs to her or to her husband but is now the sole possession of her suckling. Indeed an ideational (and practical) conflict may exist. A recent study reveals that breastfeeders show greater impairment of sexuality at 4 months postpartum [1]. Frigidity has been found to result when the parturient has difficulty integrating her 'adult sexual pleasurable response with her maternal bodily response' [2]. This idea is found metaphorically represented in literature and myth in the symbolic split between mother and whore; between the nurturing devoted sexless woman and the other who dedicates her life to gratifying grown men. Case work reveals that some prostitutes feel compelled to live out this split, sacrificing their source of income while breastfeeding a baby [3]. Many traditional societies ban intercourse for the duration of suckling, which may last for 2–4 years. While this is clearly a means of contraception controlling nutritional intake and the interval between children, ideas that semen or menstruation poison the milk, or coitus weakens its composition suggest that the mother's lactating function and the child's nourishment and close emotional contact are seen during this period to conflict with the mother's sexuality. Recently, western women have been placed in a curious dilemma by being told that breastfeeding actually hastens their figure's return to pre-pregnant sexy slenderness.

(c) Breast eroticization

The image of the breast as an erotic object is so ingrained that many western subcultures retain a certain prudery considering public baring of the breast for feeding as a seductive or indecent act. To some, as reported in a classic study of patterns of infant care in urban Britain, offering the breast to a baby seems 'almost incestuous' [4]. Indeed, many women are disturbed by sensations akin to sexual excitation aroused by nipple stimulation during breastfeeding. Some husbands jealously fear erotic competition, particularly from suckling boy babies, especially if sexual relations between the couple have not been resumed. It has been observed that for women who have been sexually abused in a way that includes breast contact, breastfeeding may serve as a traumatic reminder of their secret shame, guilt and anger [5].

(d) Gender differences

Mothers experience different responses to breastfeeding their male or female infants, and find it difficult to consider or discuss these feelings. Variations in the perceived hunger of female babies are recognized with greater frequency by the mother than those of males [6]. Their partners, too, react in a variety of ways when watching a male or female baby fed at the breast, experiencing jealousy of the intimate relationship or a vicarious gratification in relation to a male baby. Others, re-experiencing early sibling rivalry and a sense of their own deprivation, envy the blissful gratification of male or female infant at the breast, resentful of all the tender maternal attention s/he receives seemingly at the father's expense. Yet others envy the woman her capacity to nurse wishing they too could lovingly produce a flow of liquid nourishment from their bodies to be taken in by the infant. Acutely aware of these gender differences and the complex historical factors underlying them, a woman may consciously decide during pregnancy to neutralize or equalize her share in childcare by introducing a supplementary bottle or unconsciously give up breastfeeding altogether with the birth of a boy.

(e) Commitment

Some women feel endangered by the emotional commitment and physical tie of breastfeeding. In our society, since shared breastfeeding is uncommon the mother has to be available at least intermittently for several hours a day and may be unprepared for and alarmed by the frequency of feeding in the early weeks (self-demand breastfed babies given free access to the breast have been observed to feed every two hours by the fifth day) [7]. For women intending to work outside the home, even scheduled feeding may appear impossible, although with good counselling and a flexible baby a mother may both breastfeed and hold a job. Even within the home, a mother who has other young children or demanding household obligations may find it easier to share the feeding responsibility by bottle feeding or bottle-supplementing.

(f) Intimacy

Letting another person suck out the juices of one's body arouses primitive feelings. Anxiety about the potential emotional intensity of the intimate feeding experience, may induce some women to forego breastfeeding altogether, while others dull the experience by detaching themselves, reading or watching TV while suckling, or finding themselves feeling bored, impatient and threatened, trapped or 'indifferent'.

(g) 'Wild' emotions

Some women fear the infant's 'cannibalistic' oral aggression or their own counterdestructive urges that may be released in this closed circle of primary exchange. A decision to bottlefeed the baby may reflect a mother's wish to protect the frail baby from the thrust of her own unleashed noxiousness. It may also represent an escape from the sinister projections or vampire-like leaching she imagines breastfeeding would entail. Her own unconscious aggression is projected in the fantasy of being devoured or attacked, while she also may fear poisoning/intoxicating/flooding/starving her suckling baby.

(h) Sustenance

Breastfeeding entails opening herself up and handing over her contents to somebody else. The mother is vulnerable to real or imagined criticism and rejection from her baby, who might not like her milk, might not thrive on what she has to offer, might demand more than she has to give. If she lacks confidence in her capacity to provide and replenish her stocks or doubts the quality of her inner resources, a woman might be reluctant to allow her baby to rely totally on her for nourishment. Ironically, due to the changing composition of milk during a feed (the fat content rises as the volume falls towards the end of a feed [8]), an anxious mother who terminates feeds early would significantly curtail her baby's calorie intake, thus creating a self-fulfilling prophecy about her capacity to nourish. Other mothers relish their bountifulness.

Clearly, complex issues underly the decision to breast- and/or bottle-feed. Not surprisingly, a large proportion of those who begin breastfeeding in hospital stop doing so once the ongoing neutralizing professional support ends.

23.3 'TEACHING' BREASTFEEDING

Breastfeeding is a highly emotive situation for an observer. Since the professional, too, was once herself a hungry infant bountifully given or frustratingly deprived of the breast, unless she is conscious of their implications, these unconscious influences will operate even in the professional situation. Likewise, she may or may not have had babies herself. Seeing a tiny tongue licking the nipple of a mother's rounded breast may naturally arouse envy in a childless nurse or one past her childbearing days. She may have to restrain herself from a contrary desire to sabotage the enchanted moment. From the very first feed on, analysis of feeding interaction reveals that even unexperienced mothers subtly adapt their tactile behaviour to the bout-pause pattern of their babies' sucking [9]. Any interference can disrupt the delicate timing of the exchange. Similarly, the mother's exclusive proprietorship of her newborn baby or the nursing-couple's mutual engrossment in eye- to-eye gazing, may leave a sensitive nurse feeling redundant, rejected or excluded. Although most postnatal-care professionals are understanding and generous with their time and efforts, if she feels offended by her expertise being slighted, a peeved professional may be tempted to leave the foolhardy woman to her own resources, to develop engorged breasts or cracked nipples.

The nurse or midwife who introduces the mother to the 'art' of breastfeeding brings her own feeding history into the situation. Consciously, she is the expert trying to teach a new mother to feed. Unconsciously, she may be enacting a recalcitrant baby determined to show the mother up. As everyone knows, a newborn who has been given some water between feeds or a feeding 'lesson' conducted with a sleepy or fractious baby or a mother made anxious can easily result in engorgement, selfconscious fumbling, poor timing between reflex rooting and nipple placement, and a sense of fundamental inadequacy, all of which subtly conspire to produce unrewarding feeding experiences and discourage an ambivalent mother from breastfeeding. Conversely, a nurse whose own experience of being fed enables her to be generous towards the mother can respect both the baby's and the woman's feelings and fine-tuned timing, offering them both the quiet space in which to savour the feeding interchange rather than turning it into a regimented means of getting milk into the baby. In effect, the facilitating nurse/midwife becomes a comforting mother substitute, 'feeding' the often deprived and needy mother and mothering her, which in turn enables her to feel replenished and full enough to feed and mother her own baby.

23.4 EARLY DIFFICULTIES WITH BREASTFEEDING

It takes maturity and compassion to sympathize with a new mother's self-inflicted problem, or to understand her confusion and tension around breastfeeding. Many mothers find the simple act of visually exposing their breasts to a series of strange nurses inhibiting and shameful. When she is also surrounded by other women, with larger or less droopy or seemingly fuller breasts her sense of embarrassment and feminine inadequacy is likely to increase. When, to top it all, the busy midwife casually touches her breast to illustrate milk-expression or gropes for the nipple to pop it in the baby's mouth, the mother may feel violated in herself and resentful at the interference between herself and her suckling infant. Thankfully, such insensitivity is rare. However, on the postnatal ward negative influences often take a much more subtle form. Artificial milk advertising is still rife (contravening the WHO code on infant feeding [10]). On many wards, mothers are offered inconsistent advice by different midwives and nurses who hold a variety of opinions on the best way to support the baby, the number of cushions needed, how to reduce the flow, and their own special expertise in 'latching', burping and breast care. Nurses, like Health Visitors, may also advocate a particular trend in feeding-lore which is at variance with the individual mother's or baby's own ideas. Facilitators who wish to feed on demand or Regulators who wish to establish scheduled feeding may find themselves at odds with hospital policy or the current vogue for feeding. Furthermore, terminology varies. Recent research conducted in Oxford on the policy and practice of midwifery found that while 97% of the 220 consultant units researched had a policy of 'demand feeding', interpretations ranged from free-feeding to restrictions over duration and frequency of feeds and necessity for night feeding [11].

Some new mothers demand to be told exactly what to do so as to have a scapegoat to blame if they fail. The mother may be embarrassed to confess her fear that she will smother the baby with her breast or starve or make her baby ill with milk that is bad or too 'watery'.She may be afraid to breastfeed, finding the uterine afterpains painfully distracting or her sore nipples too distressing. The midwife is thus in a most difficult situation, having to gauge each mother's needs, having to accept both idealization and anger from her clients and having to face her own inadequacies. In addition, she is often ill-equipped by training. Unfortunately, many of the interventionist practices taught in midwifery textbooks have been shown to be ineffective, untested or even harmful. For instance, the Oxford midwifery study found 32 treatments in current use for cracked nipples; among the six most common methods of these (resting nipple and expressing the milk; nipple shields; Rotersept spray, tincture of benzoin; creams; repositioning baby at the breast) only the first and last were found effective in trials. The same is true of the often conflicting 38 methods for treating engorgement [12]. The Royal Society of Medicine's forum for maternity and the newborn meeting at which these findings were reported urged members of the Royal College of Midwives to convene a working party with broad representation from other bodies (NCT, La Leche League, Health Visitors, etc.) to pool and update information [13].

When breastfeeding is regarded as synonymous with good mothering, a woman who has difficulties and eventually fails to feed her baby inevitably feels guilty, inadequate, depriving and egocentric. The modern-day assumption that 'breast is best' concentrates on the infant's needs, yet often neglects to take account of the mother whose breast it is, and who may be able to offer far more relaxed and contented mothering while bottlefeeding. As Winnicott said, many mother–infant struggles could be avoided if 'religion were taken out of this idea of breastfeeding' [14].

Professionals involved in counselling mothers about feeding must be aware not only of the many complex practical and physical pros and cons of breast- as opposed to bottlefeeding, but also of the psychological impact on the mother of the feeding situation as a releasing agent for powerful repressed emotions. Only the woman herself can be the judge of her ability to withstand the risk of emotional arousal and psychological disturbance during the period of intimate contact with a feeding baby. However, given her heightened sensitivity, her early incompetence coupled with her worried responsibility for the baby, and given her institutionalized dependence on hospital authority figures, it is often very difficult for a new mother to go against the expert's advice even when it conflicts with her own feelings. Only unhurried sessions and a reciprocal relationship of trust patiently built up by a tolerant encouraging midwife, can foster them other's uninhibited disclosures, allay her fears and enable her to try and overcome these. The very difficult task of the professional is to offer non-judgemental support, helpful encouragement and practical assistance and to create an atmosphere of acceptance which enables the new mother to make her own decisions without prematurely closing off the options.

In conclusion, as the chart in Appendix 1 shows, breastfeeding must be seen as a systemic product of many interacting factors rather than dependent on individual behaviour alone. Processes of 'positive feedback' encourage breastfeeding whereas negative feedback may dampen the process and lead to alternative methods of feeding.

23.5 HOSPITAL REGIMENS

As in most institutions, hospital regimens are often run more for the convenience of the staff than the clientele [15]. Unfortunately, in some units, many of the routines are at variance with the physical and emotional needs of the recuperating parturient during this vulnerable period of establishing her new identity as a mother and making the acquaintance of her infant:

1. **Sleep** is disrupted by ward-cleaning procedures, shift changes of staff, doctor's rounds, meal times, presence of other patients in addition to the mother's own disturbed physiological rhythms and new baby's needs.

2. **Food intake** is determined by the often unbalanced and unpalatable menu offered. Patients usually have no access to tea-making or snacking other than that supplied by visiting relatives. A breastfeeding woman is particularly prone to needing extra replenishment of her own resources; at home, many mothers will not begin a feed until they have made themselves a cup of hot chocolate or tea; others follow a feed with a

binge. Whether this reflects a physiological depletion or a psychologically experienced imbalance is an issue secondary to the unavailability of 'comfort-food' in most hospitals.

3. **Privacy is restricted**. The tentative and intimate nature of the budding interchange between the mother and her newborn is open to scrutiny of professional and maintenance staff as well as fellow parturients. Whereas some mothers welcome the dormitory-like atmosphere and bonhomie of some wards, to others, the priority is one of getting to know a unique baby rather than making friends with other women, and drawing comparisons with their experience. Ideally, facilities should be such as to enable each mother to partake of the supportive cameraderie when she wants it and be private when she wishes.

4. **Feeding practices** vary between hospitals where water, glucose, or dextrose is routinely administered to all babies and those in which the mother's discretion is respected. Some hospitals still advocate scheduled feeding of a fixed duration, encouraging a mother to wake her sleepy baby and break the 'suction seal' after 2–10 minutes; other places encourage the mother to feed at the baby's request. In most hospitals the double-blind of frank advertising of artificial baby-feeding products has now been prohibited but subtle commercial influences persist.

5. **Visiting policies** vary from an open-ended system to restricted times. In some hospitals, the number of visitors in a mother's room is restricted on the grounds of concern about infection, 'over-excitement' or noise. While the mother's fatigue is a consideration it must be balanced against her emotional need for access to familiar, loving representatives of her 'real' life outside the institution. Contact with her husband or partner may be a demanding drag on her meagre resources or else may offer a special source of comfort and emotional support for the inexperienced mother undergoing a new experience in a strange environment. He in turn may feel excluded, neglected and dumped or may desperately need her encouragement, having been left in a bewildering new role of total responsibility for the household and/or other children. He may be overflowing with unfocused fatherly emotions and loving feelings towards his child-bearing woman. The need to get close to this baby may be shared by the rest of the family. Hospitalization of the mother for childbirth curtails opportunities for satisfying her children's curiosity about their new sibling and desire to evolve a relationship with the newborn. The multiparous woman is often torn between her desire to have an uninterrupted period of close contact with her neonate and concern about her children left at home. Flexible visiting hours which enable young children to have easy access to their mother and new sibling can modify some of their sense of abandonment and reduce inevitable rivalry (Chapter 26). Grandparents and friends may not wish to wait until mother and baby's homecoming to greet the new arrival. Their

presence in the hospital may be a source of joy or a burden to the new mother. A sensitive midwife or nurse may, at a cue from the mother, use her authority to intervene and 'rescue' the woman from an emotionally overbearing situation, or adjust the visitor-flow; however, this presumes a close understanding between the mother and herself.

6. **Availability of baby**: some hospitals still operate central nurseries where babies are kept automatically or if the mother prefers not to have her baby with her. However, most places offer a rooming-in system which gives the mother continuous access to her infant yet the flexibility of knowing she may be relieved of her baby temporarily, which eases the transition between pregnancy and total responsibility for a newborn.

7. **Staff–patient ratio**: availability of professional help is curtailed in many hospitals where cuts have led to staff shortage. Overworked nurses are less able to attend to the psychological needs of new mothers, when they themselves feel like busy mothers at the beck-and-call of their own charges. Professionals too need support and care, from their peers and seniors as well as partners and friends outside the hospital. Respect for their professional knowledge and competent skills by both patients and medical colleagues enables postpartum midwives and nurses to make a significant positive contribution to the hospital experience of child-bearing. Conversely, nurse dissatisfacton can colour the crucial emotional experience of these early days, leaving the parturient feeling wretechedly inadequate as a mother, or aggrieved in her subjective sense of having been bossed about or disregarded. Flexibility is of the essence as the postnatal nursing needs of new mothers differ considerably, as shown by the Facilitator and Regulator model.

8. **Discharge policies**: many options are available to the parturient. She may choose to have a 'domino birth', leaving hospital shortly after the birth in the custody of her local midwife who brought her in, or else she may arrange to have a 48 hour discharge, or a six hour one, followed by the services of a community midwife for at least ten days following the delivery. Alternatively, she may stay in the hospital for the duration of her confinement as defined by the hospital or determined by her own needs. From a legal point of view, a woman can discharge herself and her baby from hospital at any time and does not need the consent of doctor or midwife. She is not obliged to return home in an ambulance. Equally, she is under no obligation to sign a form stating she has discharged herself against medical advice [16].

23.6 FACILITATORS AND REGULATORS IN HOSPITAL

Women differ in their needs, and this variety of options allows for individual choice. In the hospital situation, the Facilitator is usually disinterested in other women and their babies and longs for privacy and unintruded leisure in which to devote herself entirely to her special infant, without onlookers, well-wishers and 'busybodies'. Many Facilitators, finding these early days in a busy hospital unenduringly damaging, desperately wish they could be in the secluded comfort of their own homes and some discharge themselves early, at times against staff advice. Multiparous Facilitators often anticipate these feelings and plan a 24 hour or even 6 hour discharge. They are also concerned to resume unencumbered early contact with their partner and other children at home and try to keep visitors at bay.

By contrast, a Regulator often wishes to stay in hospital as long as possible. She may be terrified by the prospect of 'shapeless' unstructured days on her own with her baby and dreads being unable to cope at home alone. While adjusting to her new role and acquiring practical mothering skills in the security of the ward, she is also benefitting from the caring assistance of midwife/nurse and befriending room-mate(s). She needs to know that she is doing things in the 'right' way and values their acknowledgement of her growing competence. When pressurized to return home by her partner or other children, a Regulator might resolve her dilemma by employing a home help or nanny to help her through the first few weeks and looks to the health visitor or childcare manuals magically to provide the answers.

23.7 POSTNATAL PROFESSIONAL CARE AT HOME

The breastfeeding counsellor and community midwife have an important role to play for the mother at home. Following early discharge the community midwife takes responsibility for the physical welfare of both mother and baby for the first 10 days following a home birth or early discharge. The health visitor(s) will continue to visit for many months. How she is received will depend not only on the mother's emotional needs and the family set up, but very much on the manner of the professional involved. Sadly, all too often, the parturient is visited not by one regular person, but a succession of different professionals and students, all of whom enter her home when she is at her least presentable and feels most vulnerable, seeming to make demands on her time and to question her practices. Others want to see her stitches and each need to be informed afresh about her obstetric history and toilet habits. While some mothers tolerate this well-intentioned 'invasion' with good grace or gratitude, others may feel that home and privacy are violated by all these people intent on 'checking up' on her. Far from being grateful for their help, she may feel uncared for and taken for granted, patronized by 'do-gooders' and distracted from the very important intimate business of building up her relationship with her baby for which she discharged herself from hospital. However, many new mothers feel desperately in need of a knowledgeable woman to depend upon and turn to in times of confusion and stress. If the professional, whatever her position and title, can assume this role by earning the mother's confidence, she will be rewarded by seeing her care appreciatively received. Equally, given the unrealistic expections of some mothers, the health visitor will inevitably sometimes find herself blamed unjustly when her 'magic formula' for inducing sleep, or regulated feeds fail to work.

The professional's dilemma of protecting the rights of both her clients and attending to their seemingly divergent needs may be eased by regarding mother and baby as an intermeshing 'system'. If one is tense or unhappy, the other will inevitably be affected and react in some way that will in turn affect the first. Where there are several children and other family members involved, the whole family constellation may be seen as a system. Insight into why some clients seem to have difficulties in accepting changes while others seem to sail through these early weeks may only be gained from an overview of the family system, with its many complex and changing interrelationships. Various family members each have their different histories, needs, demands, responsibilities and relationships with the extended family and the community outside. The visiting professional usually offers advice in response to complaints or pleas only from the individual mother with whom she is in contact. However, awareness of potentially conflicting interests of other members of the family may allow the professional a wider perspective in her search for creative compromises in order to resolve conflicts and reconcile contradictions so as to benefit the family as a whole.

While early interventions can utilize the malleability of a system still in a state of flux following the birth, at times these same interventions may also hinder the family from finding their own equilibrium by using their internal resources. The professional needs to employ her skills to gauge each family's needs and capacities. If she can use her visits to activate the family into functioning healthily in her absence without her help, she will have achieved her goal.

23.8 CULTURAL VARIATIONS

In some ethnic groups, cultural traditions may be at variance with western hospital routines. Not only may custom deny the father access to the delivery room, he may also be forbidden to see his wife during the early postnatal period and be forbidden intimate contact with her for weeks or months. Where purdah is practised, the woman may need to protect herself from men visiting other women in the ward by drawing curtains round her bed [17]. Customs vary according to beliefs. Confinement may be regarded as purely a female domain from which all males are excluded or else the parturient herself may be considered a source of danger, unclean and defiling to men or virgins, and taboo to her husband. Vaginal discharge, like menstruation, may represent the source of contamination (a prolonged prohibition ensures the mother respite from sexual activity and the threat of a new pregnancy). If hospital confinement is lengthy, the family may wish to conduct postparum purification ceremonies on the ward. Clearly, however alien to the professional staff, these wishes must be respected and privacy provided. Similarly, celebration of the infant's arrival may constitute a joyful occasion for the whole extended family, involving singing and feasting which is not always compatible with hospital routines but hopefully can be accommodated in modified form, when confinement is prolonged for medical reasons. The home-visiting professional who is granted the honour of being invited to attend a domestic celebration will find herself in a privileged position to learn much from the experience. In some ethnic communities, such as Punjabi or Pathan Indians, a marked contrast is experienced by older women between such 'old-country' traditions as the practice of 40 day confinement with no work, bed-rest and a network of female relatives to cook special foods for the woman or care for the baby and the current experience of a dispersed social structure lacking practical close-family support [18,19].

Most cultures have protective rituals or superstitions and beliefs about a dangerous cannibalistic murderous woman, reflecting the mother's vulnerability to the envy of other less-fortunate women, and the neonate's defencelessness against the dangerous overpowering female. Jewish folklore calls her Lilith (Adam's first wife), who endangers newborn girls until the twentieth day and boys until circumcision on the eighth day, unless protected by amulet [20]. Browbeaten by a bossy healthcare worker or in-law, a new mother may begin to feel that she is being taken over by a figure such as this and that her primary right to the baby is being threatened.

A professional, too, may tend to be either a Facilitator or a Regulator where her client is concerned. Like the Facilitator with her baby, the professional may believe that her task is to adapt to the woman's needs, or else, Regulator-like, that her client must adapt to her own procedures and become 'socialized' in the English manner. However, in the case of home visits, between which the woman is left to her own resources to cope with a new and taxing situation, all the professional can do is to help each woman to draw out the best of her own abilities to mother her own baby in her own way. She might believe her task is to impose 'good' rules but if the woman is loathe to keep these, or obeys them against her better judgement, all that has been done is to alienate the mother from her own natural capacities.

23.9 TRADITIONAL CUSTOMS: BIRTH AND PLACENTAL CEREMONIES, FEEDING PRACTICES AND FOLK BELIEFS

Most communities have evolved their own traditional customs. If these conflict with the professional's own training, it does not automatically mean that they are wrong. Practices differ around the world, and even within the same Area Health Authority. A case in point is that of the afterbirth. The placenta may be incinerated unceremoniously in a hospital that regards it as waste matter, deep frozen and sent for withdrawal of some blood substances or dispatched lucratively to cosmetic manufacturers for face-packs and beauty creams. Alternatively, it may be lovingly preserved by people who regard it as a precious counterpart of their baby. Treatment of the placenta as sacred or belonging to its genetically related newborn from which it has been severed, bring in their wake various rituals. It is most important that birth attendants, in showing each mother the placenta, make it known that it is hers and available should she wish to have it, to enable these time-honoured customs to be respected should deference prevent her from asking for it. Increasingly, a new generation of young people 'going native' or seeking their 'psychological roots' in a return to 'natural' life wish to practise their own birth-ceremonies. Ritual has even more poignancy in the case of immigrants who feel themselves to be detached from their homeland and deprived of their own 'placental roots'. Being unable to cook the placenta and feed it to the mother to strengthen her, or to throw it into a river, bury it intact in the ground, plant it under a tree or preserve it whole for the baby's future success, may cause great distress to a family bereft of their ancestral home and own placentae.

Attitudes towards infant feeding also vary in different societies and people who were born elsewhere may wish to feed the baby as they themselves were fed. While professionals may have very strong views about the 'right way' to feed a baby, it is as well to remember that our own 'feeding fashions' have changed dramatically and styles have fluctuated quite frequently over the last few years, with each claiming to be the way. In non-industrialized countries the very survival of infants depends on breastfeeding. Even so a range of variations exist, in terms of position of holding, frequency and duration of feeding, initiation by mother or infant, each adapted to climate, shape of the breast, clothing, maternal nutrition and work habits. Although the climate may have changed with migration, the diet of many ethnic minorities in this country remains consistent with that 'back home'. In immigrants from hot climates or cultures where exposure of skin is considered immodest, vitamin D deficiency may result. Specific nutritional deficiencies may result from lack of unobtainable culinary ingredients; a recent study found that Asian toddlers are prone to iron deficiency [21]. Clearly intake must be monitored.

However, infant feeding follows maternal dietary considerations and caregiving practices. The way the infant is suckled and weaned rests on cultural beliefs defining manner of dress, daily activity and childcare practices woven together in an intricate pattern, so that no part of it may be changed without affecting the whole fabric of life. Thus considerations of feeding have to take into account whether the infant is exclusively looked after by the mother or relegated to another woman in the extended family; whether culture dictates that the mother dresses and carries her baby so he/she can suck at will or insists that like adults s/he has set 'meal times'; whether curry, coffee or garlic infused milk, via the mother's diet, is the required norm or is said to create 'wind' and colic; whether the baby sleeps with the mother or apart; whether the husband shares the same bed; whether the woman works in her home or outside it; whether 'dummies' and other forms of pacification are acceptable, including thumb sucking, and so on. The mother, equipped with 'new-fangled' expertise in hospital, may fall foul of her mother-in-law when she is discharged back into her family and be in conflict with members of her own community, thus inducing anxiety and divergence when none need exist. The highly impressionable balance of breastfeeding might be upset by 'foreign' intervention, with its failure attributed to medical disapproval of 'strength giving' ethnic foods or folk beliefs blamed for causing the milk to 'dry up'. Similarly, a home-visiting professional who does not respect the customs of the household is placing the new mother and baby in danger of being ostracized for collaborating with alien practices. Sensitivity is required, as well as humility which can question why things are done in a particular way by both the professional and the mother whom she is serving. In some cases of social isolation and inability to communicate, maternal self-image plummets resulting in inexperienced mothers feeling insecure and anxious which may in turn lead to difficulties and failure to thrive [22]. For many isolated women, the professional entering their home may be their most important social interaction with anyone or their main direct contact with the health services, as observation of purdah, language restrictions or shyness about excursions to the public sphere might restrict medical treatment to consultations by proxy [23].

23.10 INTERPRETATION FOR NON-ENGLISH-SPEAKING ETHNIC MINORITY CLIENTS

Where translation is required, the professional should carefully consider who to employ as interpreter. Many postnatal issues may be too delicate to relegate to husband or even bilingual female friend. In addition to content-unsuitability, it is unwise to use children as this role places on them a burden of responsibility that may skew family roles. Confidentiality may rule out various community officials and use of other bilingual case workers places an additional unpaid burden on already busy shoulders. In addition to the interpreter's interpersonal communication skills, their availability, confidentiality and knowledge of the area discussed, considerations of their dialect, religion, class (caste), age and gender must be tallied with the client's own needs. Short of multilingual health service provision a good solution might be found in 'link'-worker schemes such as that developed by the Asian Mother and Baby Campaign (and DHSS) which allocates one specific bilingual woman with nursing training to each mother throughout antenatal care, birth and postnatal follow-up. Another bicultural advocacy scheme is the Multi-Ethnic Women's Health Project (City and Hackney's Community Health Council, London). Where such schemes are unavailable, local community groups (e.g. The Pakistani Women's Welfare Association, The Turkish Cultural Association, The Chinese Community Centre) may be a source of suitable bilingual volunteers who could be trained specifically for this purpose [24].

KEY POINTS

*Healthcare personnel carry not only the responsibility for physical care but are subject to transferential projections from their clients, who treat them as 'wise-women' and mothers. Midwives have a focal role in 'debriefing' following the birth.

*On the postnatal ward, professionals play a crucial role in establishing healthy feeding patterns, which must involve not only teaching the techniques of breast- or bottlefeeding but an understanding of some of the intricate emotions underlying this delicate exchange.

*The early days in hospital form the foundation of the mother–baby interaction but hospital regimens may be disruptive to good early bonding. Sleeping arrangements, visiting hours, feeding practices, maternal cuisine, provision of privacy, policies about supplementary feeding all combine to determine the consumer's postnatal experience in hospital. Attention should focus on providing a variety of choices that can meet different women's needs.

*Once the woman returns home, the health visitor and GP fulfil the function of a traditional expert, however, at times, without knowledge of or contact with the rest of the family. Treating the mother and baby as two members of a larger 'system', in which actions of one create repercussions in the others, may enable the professional to consider the wider needs of the whole family.

*Professionals working with ethnic minorities (of whom they are not a member) need to concentrate their efforts on increasing their client's natural competence rather than implanting foreign practices, while ensuring the baby's healthy growth. Careful selection of interpreters and respect for time-honoured traditions can promote a two-way understanding of the needs of babies and mothers in the early weeks, leading to mutual enrichment of this period of postnatal care.

Chapter 24

First six weeks: differing patterns of maternal and paternal adjustment

'The mother [however] having been a child and having introjected the memory traces of being fed, nursed, cared for, in her own mothering experiences relives with her infant the pleasures and pains of infancy' . . . '. . . Parents meet in their children not only the projections of their own conflicts incorporated in the child, but also the promise of their hopes and ambitions'. (Therese Benedek, *Parenthood as a Developmental Phase*)

24.1 MATERNAL ADJUSTMENT

Each of us has been through an experience of babyhood and resolved the inevitable issues of dependency and separateness to a greater or lesser degree. Much of this early phase consists of preverbal states of mind which have no name and remain undefined in words. Inexplicable yearnings, bodily cravings, primitive furies and traumatic experiences of frustration, failure, humiliation, or emotional injury have been retained encapsulated in undigested form, never shared with anyone or transformed internally into part of life's experiences. These elusive unprocessed feelings continue to simmer below the surface of our civilized selves, erupting at times of greater permeability in dreams or fantasies or emerging when we encounter resonances in other people or art forms. Exposure to the raw emotions of an infant constitutes such a catalyst, and the new mother is particularly susceptible to revival of these wild residues, both because of her own post-birth vulnerability and her continuous unmitigated contact with the newborn.

24.1.1 Emotional permeability

During the early weeks of motherhood at home, the new mother is plunged into a state of inner disequilibrium and external upheaval quite unlike any other encountered in adult life. Still 'wide open' from her expansive physical and emotional experiences of pregnancy and giving birth, she also suffers from frequent rude awakenings, disturbed dreams and insufficient sleep. Tiredness, hormonal fluctuations, drastic bodily changes, painful stitches and lactation neither fully established nor suppressed, all add to the emotional turmoil evoked by contagious exposure to the primitive needs of the baby. As primary caretaker, the mother is dealing with bodily fundamentals – her own secretions and those oozing out of every orifice in the baby's body. Despite her own vulnerable and hypersensitive state, she is rarely designated space and time in which to recuperate her emotional balance, but is expected to be on call – to process reality for the baby, to be the recipient of her infant's unbearable feelings; to provide comfort, containment and care; to protect the baby from impingements and to dispose of the mess. In addition to emotional signalling, one way in which the preverbal baby com-municates with his/her mother is by making her feel what s/he is feeling. By activating maternal empathy, the baby can both evoke the hoped-for response in the mother and rid him/herself of intolerable feelings. If in her maternal 'reverie' she is receptive and responsive to these communications, she in turn can contain and process the baby's feelings, ameliorating emotions which are too intense or excessively frightening [1]. By sharing these with her infant, by linking experiences and structuring his confusion, the mother can create a shared body of knowledge between them. Her playful interactions of repetitive, imitative cooing, rocking, singing, calling, grimacing, jiggling and talking all create a sense of shar-ing – a social communality which the baby and parents (if there are two) elaborate and build upon minute by minute, day by day. However, all this must take place while the permeable mother herself vulnerable is being bombarded from without by worldly pressures in addition to those coming from the baby, and from within by a resurgence of wild inchoate preverbal emotions in herself, against which she has defended herself over many years [2a]. As each mother is plummeted into the powerful passions of infancy, her own repressed emotional reservoirs of frustra-tion, rage, anguish and desolation are tapped – a crying baby inside her echoing the emotions she attributes to the crying baby.

During the vulnerable first six weeks of motherhood, much of her energy is spent defending against these deeply disturbing early feelings, either Facilitator fashion by hiving off all the painful experiences in both herself and her baby through denial or erasure of their existence, or else, like the Regulator, by distancing herself from the baby, physically and psychically in the recesses of her conscious mind.

24.2 FACILITATORS AND REGULATORS: EARLY APPROACHES TO MOTHERING

The basic observable difference between Facilitator and Regulator mothers in their approach to the baby is that the Facilitator adapts to her baby: the Regulator expects the baby to adapt to her.

This model may be envisaged as circular – Facilitators and Regulators with Reciprocators as an intermediate group, and in the other direction of the circular continuum, the two extreme poles with a 'conflicted' group between them. Many mothers find themselves oscillating between two styles, struggling to maintain the orientation of their choice yet confronted by a reality that engenders compromise. The description of the Facilitator and Regulator orientations, therefore, applies not only to mothers who are strict adherents of these positions, but to various intermediary points where the orientations coexist with greater or lesser integration in mothers engaged at times in the unconscious fantasies underlying each of these stances. *The contrast between the two polar orientations may be accentuated by observing that on an unconscious level the Facilitator is afraid of hating, whereas the Regulator is afraid of falling in love with her baby.* In this chapter, the various permutations of mothers and their cohabiting partners are described. The model applies to single mothers too, although Facilitators, particularly those with other children, find it difficult to maintain their Facilitator orientation unless 'covered' by the support of a devoted partner or mother, while Regulators need a co-carer. A Facilitator may be determined to be the *sole* source of goodness for her baby for whom she wishes to provide the ideal infancy. In these early days, she jealously guards her exclusive contact with the baby, believing that only she possesses the intuitive understanding to interpret the baby's non-verbal messages, a capacity developed during pregnancy. She feels that she and the baby are in perfect rhythmic synchrony based on their intimate connection *in utero* and in breast-feeding and any external interference will distort their delicate harmony. Her partner may consequently feel excluded. A Facilitator maintains close proximity at all times, believing the baby 'knows best', communicates his/her needs in subtle ways which she, the mother must be on hand to decipher. To do this, she has to be constantly attentive to the infant whose every cry, coo, gurgle and grimace are received by as communications.

24.2.1 The Regulator's experience

Regulators distinguish 'real' cries expressing needs and 'niggling' or 'fussing', treated as 'noise'. Unlike the Facilitator, the mother believes that she 'knows best'. To her, the baby is a pre-social (or even asocial or anti-social) being whom she must socialize, a bundle of needs and drives which must be regulated to make them predictable.

(i)Routine

Returning from hospital with the new baby, she strives to establish a routine, by reinstating the regimen she learnt on the ward, or defining one of her own. This is designed to structure their existence together, to increase predictability in an indeterminate situation where breakfast seems to run into lunch and hours pass without any apparent achievement. The routine enables the mother to look after her baby and create time and space to meet her own adult needs, e.g. read a newspaper, talk on the phone, wash her hair, and recapture a sense of the person she was before the baby arrived. On a deeper level, the routine fulfils other functions as well. It can provide the containing structure for modifying and regulating the baby's seemingly insatiable urges. It provides continuity if the mother introduces other caretakers, and simplifies the changeover of carers.

(ii) Shared babycare

Regulators who can afford to do so employ a nanny or au pair to help with the baby. If married to a Participator, the father may take an equal share in caring for the neonate; in some families the Regulator's mother or a neighbour might also lend a hand on a regular basis. The Regulator believes that the neonate does not distinguish between caregivers, therefore, she tries to introduce her co-carers early on, once she has established a routine that ensures interchangeability of caretakers and provides the baby with the security of a predictable schedule. Sharing childcare is very important for the Regulator who fears that as sole provider she would become depleted by the baby's demands. She also fears being sucked into the whirlpool of infantile dependence, becoming so enmeshed that she would not be able to disentangle herself. The routine protects her from being ensnared while also clarifying the ambiguity of the baby's requirements since she cannot afford to succumb to empathic intuition. Sharing caregiving enables her to function part of the time as a competent individual in the non-domestic adult world, while also protecting her from the blame that is levelled against mothers for any wrong that befalls their babies. If she has a helper she is no longer solely responsible for the current and future physical and mental welfare of her offspring, nor can she be singled out by the baby as the cruel frustrator. ('I have this deep wish for set order. I want each day to be the same and to know just what the baby needs. When she won't have her nap I feel like such a failure. I should be able to control things. Other people's babies go to sleep on time. That's why having a nanny is great – she can really get things straight and I'm not the only one responsible'.)

(iii) Holding

Close contact with the tiny newborn might be frightening to the new mother. Not only does the infant seem fragile and breakable with its overlarge lolling head and little stick-like arms and legs but she is unsure of her own capacity to hold 'it' securely. The reflex gripping of the tiny hand tightly grasping her finger feels like an iron claim upon her heart. A mother who is trying to maintain herself as separate from the appealing infant may resist the temptation to cradle her nestling baby, fearful of being 'touched', of sucked into devotion, of 'spoiling' the infant or of being landed with having to hold a demanding child for hours on end. Every startle response and jerky over-reaction is experienced by the baby-carrying new mother as an accusation about her inability to reassure the infant that she will not drop him/her. The tense mother sets up a cyclical pattern: the sensitive baby stiffens in response to the mother's rigid contact as she fearfully tries to hold him/her while yet clearly relaxes contentedly and 'moulds' into a relaxed contentment in the nurse's or father's arms. Feeling rejected, the offended mother becomes hypersensitive to her baby's refusal to settle in her embrace which in turn increases her own tentativeness in holding the infant and reluctance to cuddle him/her, at times to the point of aversion and avoidance. There is now some research evidence that extreme cases of aversion to physical contact with an infant are related to the mother's own physical rejection in childhood by her own parents [2b]. For some mothers, one solution is reduced physical contact, swaddling the baby in a shawl, cradling the baby while sitting in a rocking-chair or getting someone else to do the holding. Mothers who are particularly awkward at holding the baby can be shown soothing supportive positions and secure means of carrying the infant which allows the baby freedom rather than restraint, and encourages friendlier non-threatening interaction between the two.

(iv) Feeding

Although these days many Regulators breastfeed as it is said to be beneficial for both mothers and babies, clearly, it is advantageous for the breastfeeding Regulator to introduce supplementary bottlefeeding so her fellow caregivers can share in nurturing the baby. In addition, many Regulators feel unnerved by the intimate sensuality of breastfeeding while others regard it as somewhat cannibalistic. Seemingly the insatiable baby is sucking the mother dry, draining her vitality with the milk, and potentially devouring. The mother might feel her own greedy feelings well up inside her during feeding. Irrationally, she may actually envy the baby at her breast, jealous of the special care this baby is getting which she herself feels she missed out.

As they make eye contact during the feed, the mother may experience her baby silently accusing her of withholding her breast, giving too little or producing bad milk that is not rich enough or brings on colic. She might feel that the insatiable baby selfishly takes no account of her own tiredness, demanding feeds in the middle of the night, raging and screaming when the breast is not available, or guzzling away with little regard for the woman on the other end of the nipple. The breastfeeding Regulator may feel herself held to ransom, always on demand for the hungry baby, her body restricted, as in pregnancy, prohibited excessive drinking, aspirins, curries, garlic or whatever is currently deemed bad for the suckling. Bottlefeeding seems to her so civilized by comparison, no restrictions, no horrid nursing bras and leakages, no lopsidedness, no expressing, no guessing if the composition is right or whether the baby's had enough. Making up the formula may give the mother a sense of purpose and precision, and washing out the lustily emptied bottle provides a sense of achievement. She knows just how much her baby has taken whereas with breastfeeding, except for timing each 'side' accurately or test weighing the baby before and after feeds she is not sure how much s/he has taken. Professionals working with a Regulator who is clearly finding breastfeeding distressing may advise her to supplement or bottlefeed entirely. As long as the baby is held while being fed rather than propped with a bottle, and close contact is maintained (skin-to-skin if the mother favours it), the infant can imbibe the mother's (or father's) smell and presence with the milk, engage in eye-contact and play games in between feeding. Whichever method she chooses, the Regulator will usually try and get her baby to adapt to a routine of 3 or 4 hourly feeds during the day, and eliminate night feeds as soon as possible.

(v) Burping
Bringing up the baby's wind may become an activity in its own right. It can range from simply allowing a pause between breasts to stroking or vigorous back-patting in several successive episodes during any one feed. The extensiveness and duration of the rhythmic pummelling and its occasional resemblance to hitting suggests unconscious determinants such as a displacement of the wish to beat or a need actively to overcome the passivity of the feeding situation or discharge emotional tension through busy contact with the baby's body [3], while also indicating something about a belief that unexpelled 'badness' from the milk will cause internal disturbance.

(vi) Sleep
Many Regulators report their babies sleeping through the night by 5 weeks, although it is possible that the mother has learned to do so irrespective of the wakefulness of the baby. However, there is evidence that suggests that babies can be conditioned to put themselves back to sleep upon wakening between different levels of sleep during the night if the parent does not intervene [4]. Likewise the routine, separate bed and/or bedroom and ritual of regular bedtime eliminate changes which may be disruptive to sleep patterns. A Regulator mother might also wish to introduce solids at an early stage, as a means of prolonging sleep, thereby reflecting her unconscious desire to have the baby grow and become independent of her.

24.2.2 The Facilitator's experience

In her empathic identification with the baby into whom she has projected her ideal self, the Facilitator vicariously enjoys infantile bliss, as she symbolically merges with her baby, intuitively deciphering and spontaneously meeting all the baby's needs as they arise. To do so she must be attentive at all times. ('I dreamed I was swimming underwater with the baby, completely sealed off from the world . . . Other people feel like intruders – directing me with their prattling conversations. I so enjoy this time of mooching around at home, just the baby and I, no pressures, no people, no outside world.')

(i) Proximity

Whereas the Regulator's baby spends time in 'containers' of various kinds, such as pram, carry cot, or bouncy chair, the Facilitator keeps her baby in a sling on her body, or in close physical contact. I have defined their proximity in terms of a fantasy 'umbilical radius', as if, still tied by an imaginary cord, they are psychologically tethered together for the duration of the period of 'fusion' until the mother gradually allows the cord to be cut. Some Facilitators gradually begin lengthening the umbilical radius after four months when the child begins to differentiate, while others prolong the early mirroring closeness, reluctant to give up her illusion of merger. Where the mother has not resolved her own childhood separation anxieties she may become oversolicitous and overprotective, gratifying the infant to compensate for her own sense of deprivation, clinging to the baby in a denial of separateness, unable to leave the baby at all, feeling empty, lost and 'hungry' when s/he is asleep. In pathological cases the mother cannot emerge from the illusion she is trying to maintain and her interaction with the older individuating infant becomes tinged with hidden anger about his/her growing 'rejection' equated with that of her own early mother.

(ii) Crying

Unlike the Regulator who distinguishes between 'real' crying that must be attended to and 'noise' which can be ignored, the Facilitator experiences every cry as a poignant appeal for help or urgent message. She is deeply upset by each wail that cuts right through her and continues to ring in her ears long after the crying has ceased. Research has shown that babies whose early crying is ignored tend to become increasingly more insistent and cry more frequently from the third month on [5]. A divergence is thus likely to develop in crying behaviours between Regulators' babies and those of Facilitators. To the Facilitator, crying spells failure – her failure to pre-empt need and her insufficiency in instantaneously providing a perfect environment for her tender babe. Whether the infant's cry signifies hunger, pain, cold, wet, colic, overstimulation or startled fear, the Facilitator guiltily feels she ought to have prevented it before it arose. Forever vigilant, she anxiously reads her baby's smallest expressions, paradoxically both following the baby's lead and trying desperately to anticipate needy expression. In extreme cases, one can observe Facilitators' babies compliantly converting the 'forbidden' cry into a whimper and quickly mitigating their mothers' heartfelt anxiety with a reassuring smile.

(iii) Feeding

The Facilitator feeds her baby on demand, whenever and for as long as the baby wishes to be fed. Whereas the Regulator times her feeds and breaks the 'seal' after 5, 7 or 10 minutes as advised, the Facilitator feeds on until the baby falls aleep at the breast or stops sucking of his/her own accord. As a result, Regulators' breasts become 'accustomed' to let down at set intervals, whereas the Facilitator mother may find herself leaking in public or spurting milk at any sound from her infant. She often continues frequent breastfeeds throughout the day and night for the first year whereas most Regulators wean by 6 months, when they go back to work or on the appearance of the first teeth. Facilitators who do not wean their babies before a year may find themselves unable to wean until around two years because of the baby's need to control the mother and avoid separation from the breast. However, despite their strong intention to adapt to the baby's needs, some Facilitators may be seen to misinterpret some of the baby's desires because of their own eagerness to feed and its symbolic significance to themselves as bountiful providers. In some cases, babies may be dissuaded from thumb sucking and offered the breast for comfort at any sign of distress, and some may become overweight or excessively dependent on feeding as a distraction or comfort.

(iv) Sleep

To a Facilitator, the night feeds, far from being a disturbance, may offer an opportunity for close quiet intimacy in an otherwise busy household. A multiparous mother may find this is the only time when she can dedicate herself completely to the baby, free from interruption or worry about other children. Alone in the dark with her sweet smelling, cuddlesome infant, she may actually prolong this feed, experiencing a profound sense of fusion and 'communion' between the baby and her own baby self. At times, in her intense symbiotic involvement with the baby, when he or she falls asleep during the day, she feels somewhat abandoned, left behind by the child who has drifted off elsewhere. One rather 'manic' means of denying the separation that has occurred since pregnancy, she may artificially prolong their physiological connectedness by taking her pace from the infant, synchronizing their breathing patterns, sleeping when s/he has a nap, living in a timeless infantile world of gratifying sensuality, cuddling each other, bathing together and feeding self and baby simultaneously. Such far-reaching identification usually wears off as the mother gradually responds to her baby's need to differentiate by regaining a sense of herself, although many Facilitators continue to have their infants sleep in their bedroom or bed throughout the early months (which invariably affects their sexual activity), and night waking may continue well into the second year. (Sleep difficulties have been found to punctuate developmental phases, relating not only to baby's anxieties but those of the mother and parents as a couple [6].)

(v) Excretion

The mother's attitude to her baby's defaecation is complex and determined by conscious and unconscious factors alike. A breastfed baby eliminating the waste products of her/his mother's milk may be seen to be 'rewarding' the mother for her goodness with this 'gift', like 'change' being given from inside the baby's body. To some mothers, the mustard-coloured stool may become concrete evidence of the unseen flow of maternal nutrients sucked in by the baby. A series of unsoiled nappies may cause the breastfeeding mother to feel cheated or rejected. Conversely, 'too much' or too frequent elimination may seem like a judgement on the poor quality of her milk. While a breastfeeding Facilitator may experience a fondness for her baby's excreta as a substance uniting them, to the Regulator, this process of intake, retention and elimination has negative connotations. A mother who is unconvinced of the 'goodness' of her milk may feel compelled to 'read' the stools for evidence of 'food poisoning' originating in herself, due to 'forbidden substances she has eaten or her milk being affected by her ambivalent thoughts. She may feel offended when what is excreted appears more substantial than what is retained by the infant. To her the baby's tangible excrement may assume the form of her fantasied internal badness or represent revolting messiness of the infantile in herself as well as the baby. The Regulator may be as repelled by the smell of her own baby's excrement as is the Facilitator by the smell of that of a strange baby. Conversely, she may find the similarity between her own stools and those of her bottlefed baby much easier to tolerate than the breastfed 'cottage cheese' variety. The similar solidity and relative infrequency of both may enable her to feel that the baby is a person like herself, and elimination merely the physiological function of disposing of waste products. Similarly, constipation or diarrhoea in a bottlefed baby can be blamed on the formula and remedied by adjusting the baby's intake. The mother herself is not implicated, other than as a preparing or sterilizing agent.

(vi) 'Diapering'

Nappy changing, too, may appeal to the Regulator as a clear-cut function which she can fulfil and 'tick off her list', and regularity of elimination confirms the baby has become regulated. Although disposable diapers are available, the Facilitator may actually love doing her baby's washing, preferring to use terry-towelling involving her in 'purification' activities. Accepting the baby's soiling, washing, sterilizing and softening the nappies, then drying, folding and finally fixing the sweet- smelling cloth against her baby's skin. Such seemingly 'selfless' acts of extra indulgent attention are lovingly offered as gestures of unconditional devotion to the infant, and by proxy to the idealized baby-self s/he represents while attempting to preserve the 'unsullied' purity of their connection

24.2.3.Lone -mothers:

Older single mothers-by-choice tend to be more mature and confident, falling into the flexible Reciprocator orientation. Their situation differs from newly divorced or widowed motherhood complicated by grief. Sole responsibility for childrearing without the backing of a co-parent may induce a facilitating single mother to regulate against her predilections, as material as well as emotional provider for her child. A single Facilitator is cheated of dedicating herself exclusively to 'on-tap' mothering. For some the enforced shift from antenatal expectations engenders postnatal depression as practicalities compel her to accept the help of another caretaker. However, a woman with supportive parents (or a non-cohabiting partner) or one lucky enough to have the professional and/or financial means to devote herself to her baby without having to leave home, can luxuriate in being a Facilitator. Indeed, if her maternity grant is sufficient, during the early postnatal weeks her very singleness allows uninterrupted adaptation to her baby, sleeping when s/he sleeps, bathing, feeding together, living in a timeless nursery space, spontaneously indulging herself and the baby through identification and intuitive gratification of their mutual needs, without consideration for worldly adult demands. For others, the complex reality of a lone parent's life favours regulation. An organised (and well-paid) Regulator can return to work in the knowledge her child is well-minded. An unemployed Regulator may become depressed as sole carer. A young lone mother may feel lonely, unsupported and crave teenage pursuits of peers. Outgrowing the early 'symbiotic' phase is complicated for a single mother by the absence of an intervening other parent to act as the third corner of the triangle. For a Facilitator, the intensely intimate relationship may be prolonged, producing inappropriately protracted regression in herself, enmeshment, infantilisation, and difficulties in the child's individuation/separation from her. Conversely, an unsupported Regulator mother is threatened by the exclusive closeness, fearing the temptation to relinquish responsibility for maintaining them both single-handedly. In addition, the child of a single parent may experience difficulty in expressing negative feelings for fear of alienating his/her sole source of comfort;   in addition, in the absence of a sharing spouse, the child can be burdened with inappropriate emotional demands. Lack of baby-sitting provision hinders socializing or forming new adult relationships. Many single mothers and babies have healthy relationships and well-organized lives. However, additional support from 'gingerbread' groups or professionals who can serve as allies and mainstays may be welcome in what is inevitably a difficult situation.

24.2.4 Postnatal disturbances: Facilitators and Regulators

Postnatal distress has been attributed to a variety of combined physical, hormonal, social, economic and cultural precipitants, such as lack of employment, poor marital harmony, instrumental births, poor housing conditions, maternal idealization [7–9]. I have suggested that universal or isolated causes of puerperal distress cannot be specified but they must be linked to each mother's own orientation towards motherhood and particular vulnerability factors. To my mind factors are distressing when they conspire to prevent the new mother from actualizing her own specific expectations about motherhood [10].

(a) Facilitator postnatal distress

To the Facilitator, inability to fulfil her ideal of exclusive continuous mothering is distressful. A Facilitator lacking the necessary backing to sustain full-time mothering is at risk for postnatal distress. Her specific vulnerability lies in her need to provide irreproachable care for her infant. To her, failure to sustain the perfect environment for her baby causes the mother anguish as she feels she has irredeemably let the baby down by allowing technological interventions at birth, by developing cracked nipples, by being unable to soothe the colicky baby, or inadvertently leaving the infant to cry, or having to place her child in someone else's temporary care. 'Spoilt' imperfect experiences remain with her, provoking deep-seated feelings of guilt and despair, arousing her depression, anxiety and a desire to make magic reparations. The Facilitator wants to be protected from unnecessary interruptions in her attentiveness to the baby as she in turn protects the baby from intrusions into their symbiotic 'bubble'. When Facilitators, for whom early separation is felt to have irreversible effects, are forced to separate from the young baby by economic pressures or for medical reasons (prematurity, special care, hospitalizaton of the mother or urgent needs of other children), postnatal distress may be acute and prolonged. In order to mother she needs to be mothered, but all too frequently her own mother is absent or unwilling to fulfil this role, her partner is unsupportive and other children, social or professional demands create distractions leaving her torn and unable to dedicate herself to facilitating her new baby's well-being.

(b) Regulator postnatal distress

Whereas the Facilitator welcomes her baby's intense dependence and the intimate exclusivity of their contact, the Regulator feels threatened by the baby's fragility, helplessness, messiness and greed. She fears that her own hard-won independence will be jeopardized and the baby's defencelessness will endanger her by reawakening her own unresolved dependency conflicts. Feeling consternation at the infant's incessant demands upon her as sole provider she wishes to enlist her partner's help in providing childcare or to employ some help. In one study I conducted where women had no financial restrictions, 75% of the middle-class Regulators interviewed employed a full-time nanny or au pair whereas no Facilitator did so [11]. However, partners may not wish to participate in childrearing and only a few Regulators can afford paid help. Thus many Regulators find themselves 'trapped'; not living their 'real' adult lives in the world but confined to domesticity and full-time mothering of a baby who severely restricts freedom of action and movement. For such a woman, self-esteem is undermined by her lack of personal productivity and inability to maintain her previous self-identity. Given current career structures, 6-weeks maternity leave at 90% pay, and a social climate advocating maternal primary-care, it is the unemployed, unsupported Regulator who is most at risk for depression during the first six weeks. Faced with total responsibility for crucial maintenance of an unpredictable baby with whom she experiences little rapport, she finds few rewards. During the same period, it is the Facilitator who has raised her idealized expectations to heights which cannot be maintained, and those who face enforced separation, who are most liable to suffer postnatal distress.

(c) Precipitating factors

What we find then, is that the self-same factor, such as a employment or separation, has very different meanings for the two types of mothers. Employment spells freedom for the Regulator and lack of it means financial dependency, lowered self-esteem, entrapment with her baby and inability to exert her adult competence. To the Facilitator employment means interruption in the continuity of contact with her infant, possible separation and inability to fulfil her role as devoted mother. Similarly, enforced separation and obstacles to realizing her full potential as mother are precipitating factors to the Facilitator whereas enforced togetherness and obstacles to maintaining her previous identity and skills expose the Regulator to depression and lowered self-esteem. An instrumental birth is distressing to a Facilitator who had planned a perfect natural birth, but is likely to be acceptable or even procured by a Regulator. To both,

Table 24.1 Early maternal orientations

	Facilitator	Regulator
Daily babycare experience		
	Adapts to baby	Baby adapts to mother
Feeding	Permissive, frequent	Schedule, limited duration
Crying	Communication/appeal	'Real' vs. 'fussing'
Sleep	Parental bed/room; night feeds	Own room; sleeps through night
Proximity	Close physical/spatial contact	Baby in own 'container'
Excretion	'Gift'	'Mess'
Maternal beliefs		
re Newborn	'Baby knows best'	'Mother knows best'
	Newborn is alert and knowing	Newborn is undiscriminating
	Newborn is sociable	Newborn is asocial
re Mothering	Mothering = intuitive 'instinct'	Mothering = acquired skill
	Mothercare exclusive and monotrophic	Babycare shared and interchangeable
	Security = mother's continued presence	Security = continuous routine
	Babycare should be spontaneous	Babycare should be predictable
	Mother must gratify baby	Mother must socialize baby
Underlying unconscious fantasies		
	Baby = mother's ideal self	Baby = split off weakness own mother denigrated/ dismissed
	Wish to recapture idealized state of 'Fusion'	Mother threatened by lack of separateness
	Fear of hating	Fear of loving
Maternal defences		
	Idealization/vicarious compensation	Dissociation/detachment
	Altruistic surrender	Excess control/rigidity
	Manic reparation (guilt denied)	Defence against fantasy
Precipitants of postnatal distress		
	Enforced separation from baby	Enforced 'togetherness'
	Obstacles to being 'mother'	Obstacles to being 'person'
	Non-supportive partner	Non-egalitarian partner
	Deep disappointment re-birth	Reduced adult competancy

a partner who is mis-matched in the sense of being unprotective towards the Facilitator or non-egalitarian towards the Regulator increases the likelihood of depression. Of prime importance is each woman's subjective representation of having been mothered herself, and her current sense of internal resources, as replenished or in danger of being depleted through the experience of mothering her baby. A detailed account of severe postnatal disturbance, is given in Chapter 33.

KEY POINTS

* Exposure to primal substances (amnion, milk, blood, urine, feces), to primitive emotions of the newborn and the unrelenting intensity of demands threaten reactivation of suppressed infantile experiences in the mother
* A Facilitator copes with this experience by identifying with the infant and vicariously gratifying her own revived needs. The Regulator dissociates from archaic stirrings by distancing herself emotionally through shared babycare and a fixed routine. Reciprocators empathize with the infantile feelings while maintaining adult separateness. In behavioural terms, Facilitators adapt to the baby while Regulators expect the baby to adapt. Rather than a set pattern of adaptation Reciprocators negotiate each incident in its own right. Feeding, sleeping and holding patterns differ accordingly.
* Postnatal distress occurs when women cannot fulfil their own specific expectations of motherhood. The Facilitator is vulnerable when she cannot be the perfect mother or maintain her ideal of babyhood because of personal failure or enforced separation. The Regulator suffers disruptions in her sense of personal identity and lowered self-esteem due to enforced togetherness, no employment and few opportunities for self-replenishment.

24.3 PATERNAL ADJUSTMENT

24.3.1 Social role of the father 'Is you is or is you aint my baby?'

Because paternal status is not defined by biological changes, it depends on declaration of a social relationship with the baby and his/her mother. The father's position arises out of the 'knight's move' interplay of two biological relations – that of intercourse between man-and-woman and that of gestation between woman-and-infant. It has been suggested that, precisely because of the abstract nature of paternity, being based on a premise rather than a biological immediacy [12a] and being defined culturally rather than a direct blood connection, fatherhood may be regarded as the paradigm for our capacity to regard any relationship from a psychological point of view [12b]. Indeed, social definitions of the paternal role have tended to focus on external 'instrumental' activities, the basic function of which has been assumed to be introducing the child to the World, with the father forming a bridge between mother and domesticity on the one hand, and the public arena on the other [13]. In psychological terms, the father, as earliest representative of the 'non-mother' realm presents an exciting fascination [14], serving to draw the child out into the world towards discovery of new knowledge and new people. Thus, symbolically, the father is seen to introduce the child to the Word, language signifying abstraction and patriarchal culture, with the metaphorical 'name' of the Father called upon to represent paternal

Law [15]. ('Just wait 'til your father gets home' is a common threat of disempowered mothers.)

In western countries, following the powerful impact of the Women's Movement and ideologies advocating personal choice for all, mothers and fathers alike have begun questioning traditional expectations and the fixed gender roles attributed to them by childcare experts and governmental policies, with broadening public opportunities for women reciprocally mirrored by increased male domestic involvement. Nevertheless, a contradiction is often found between expressed egalitarian accounts of childcare and shared domestic workload and the real practice of differentiated roles which still define childcare as essentially the prerogative of mothers. Thus, a recent English study across classes found that by the child's first birthday, 40% of the fathers interviewed had not changed a nappy and even fewer had bathed their babies [16]. An American study of middle-class couples interviewed in their homes with their year-old first-born child, found that when the wife is employed outside the home, fathers reported more participation in childcare and household tasks. However, on observation there was little difference in caregiving interaction from their male counterparts with 'home-maker wives [17].

The quality of early fatherhood across countries is clearly influenced by availability of paternity leave. In Sweden, for instance, fathers, like mothers, can take parental leave for the first 18 months of the child's life, of which the first 9 months are almost fully remunerated [18]. In other countries, the minimal acknowledgement of a father's emotional need to be with his family around the time of birth reflects not only political trends but societal ideologies about maternal primacy during this early phase and devaluation of the father's nurturing contribution. Financial considerations at this very time of increased expenses and reduced income (if the wife has stopped earning) induce some fathers to take the bare minimum by way of unpaid leave after the birth and some may even step-up their work activities to cope with the extra burden.

Interaction of father and infant in the early weeks is determined not only by his own emotional capacities and social expectations but also by the degree and quality of access to the child that the mother grants her partner. Fatherhood can only thrive with the mother's permission and support [19]. Her evaluation of the father, absent or present, is crucial [20] and she mediates his image for the baby, establishing positive or negative attitudes to the father through her own subtle body language and relationship to him [21]. Whatever the degree of their daily contact with the newborn, like mothers, fathers too have an adjustment to make. Survey studies have found that about a third of fathers experience mood disturbance in the early months postpartum and paternal strain appears related to the father's own general stress levels and negative attitude towards the pregnancy rather than marital disharmony [22]. Similarly, men's general health 'status' has been found to decline over the first eight months of fatherhood, linked to subjectively perceived negative life events, lowered self-esteem and mastery, depression and anxiety [23].

24.3.2 Psychological role of the father

From Freud's day until recently, psychoanalytical theories focused on the oedipal role of the father, and overlooked his importance in early infancy and childhood. Recent research with neonates has revealed that not only do babies recognize their fathers as well as their mothers, but they relate differently to each. It is difficult to identify the various interactive strands, but it appears that fathers are more playful, exciting and physical in their handling of babies than mothers (who are seen as more modulated, enveloping, secure and controlled) [24,25], although fathers and mothers have been found to be equally responsive to cues from the newborn [26]. In addition to being more arousing and stimulating in their spontaneous handling of all babies, fathers have been found to relate in a more 'sex-typed' way to newborns [27], have been found to show a stronger interest in boys [28] and concerned with fostering assertive behaviour in them [29]. Babies, in turn, have been found to show more positive responses to fathers' rather than mothers' play, and toddlers prefer the exciting stimulation of male adults, although girls, who have been found to show specific attachment to their fathers earlier than boys, are also more wary of strange men [30].

Thus it seems that far from being only the inhibiting father of Freudian theory, the father is also a stimulating and exciting figure, inviting 'self-articulation', independent expression and, a way out of the emotional entanglement with the mother [31] for both sexes [32]. Put differently, we may envisage four interlacing relationships in early childhood – the positive one with the nurturing mother and the dread of sinking back into womb-like dependence, a positive one with the stimulating father and a dread of his authority. A man who fulfils his unique position as father can serve both as a support for the mother and as a shield for the child against prolonged symbiosis [33] while also stimulating independence and creative endeavour in children of both sexes. Emotional or physical absence of a father during the critical period of the early months of a child's development has been found to be associated with difficulties in forming affectionate ties [34], increased incidence of juvenile delinquency [35] and disturbances in separating and in establishing sexual identity [36].

24.3.3 Paternal subjective experiences

Fathers are not merely experiencing parenthood, but have also made that transition via the birth. I have found that some men find labour disturbing and their personal experience, whether of being absent or present at the delivery, might prove quite traumatic. Labour heightens awareness of the female–male differences, and the man may emerge from the experience feeling inadequate or threatened in his masculinity, astounded at his wife's awesome capacity to produce a live human being or enviously belittling of it. He may be critically dissatisfied with her 'performance', or scandalized by her uninhibited behaviour in labour or physical abandoment during birth. The main problem he faces in the delivery room is how to establish his place and connection to the baby who is so obviously physically connected to the mother. On an unconscious level he may be deeply shocked by the sight of all that 'inner stuff' pouring out and her expanding genitalia. A man may experience disturbing fantasies stirred up in him by unconsciously equating the arousing birth scene with a 'primal scene' of intercourse between his parents, imagined or actually witnessed in his childhood.

Like the mother, the father too has to reconcile his fantasy image and preferred gender of the imaginary baby with the real one they have been 'given'; he too, may feel disappointed, or neglected and overlooked in favour of the new arrival. Unable to comprehend his wife's exhaustion or maternal preoccupation curtailing their social life, her lack of erotic interest may make him feel sexually redundant and 'spare'. Extra demands on him to help with housekeeping or the lowered 'standards' of tidiness in the home may irritate him beyond comprehension. Now that they are all home together, the father too may be catapulted back to his own childhood days when his mother brought home a new baby rival or when he became disillusioned of being cared for without concern about the source of care. On a babycare level, he wishes to become the father he would have loved to have had and yet is also poignantly aware that his son or daughter might prefer the mother to himself – painfully reactivating the old 'who do you love best, Mummy or Daddy?' question. In order to be a 'loving father', the man must be 'able to accept that it is the baby's right to bring him all his/her needs, fantasies and feelings' without expecting the baby 'to deal with his own mainly unconscious needs, wishes, fantasies or feelings that are inappropriate to that relationship' [37].

Fathers, too, have a need to talk through their excitement, elation, fears, guilts or horrors associated with the birth, as well as airing their anxieties, sense of emotional upheaval, disappointments and possible revulsion. The male partner, who often feels he cannot inflict his emotions on the vulnerable or preoccupied parturient but lacks a confidante, may seek other outlets for tension release. A professional visiting the home or the GP may find themselves presented with such material overtly or in behavioural, symptomatic or psychosomatic disguise. Most fathers need reassurance that their feelings are normal and common; those in need of further assistance may be referred for counselling or psychotherapy.

24.3.4 Renouncers and Participators: a model of paternal approaches to early fatherhood

This model is merely a vehicle to illustrate two easily recognizable extreme points on a continuum, rather than 'types'. Here too, as in the Facilitator/Regulator model, no value judgement is being made.

(a) Renouncer

The Renouncer is not unduly put out by limited paternity leave. Indeed, given his freedom of choice, he might vanish for the duration of the early weeks on a business trip or walking expedition. Many Renouncers find exposure to the newborn deeply disturbing. The fragile baby reactivates his own early experiences of helplessness, and re-arouses repressed rage about frustrated dependency. Birth of an infant may revive old sibling rivalries in men who unconsciously equate the new baby with younger siblings born during his own childhood. A male baby is jealously regarded as heir to the intimate contact he himself enjoyed with his own mother, and with his wife, mother of this baby. A girl baby too may be seen as a rival for his partner's attentions, particularly with a Facilitator spouse who becomes so absorbed in identification with her little daughter that he feels superfluous. In addition, he is worried by increasing domestic demands upon him which combined with babycare requests, seem to threaten his sense of masculinity. To protect his familiar identity, the beleaguered Renouncer may be tempted to flee his home which has turned into a nursery, full of baby equipment, nappy-sterilizing buckets and advice-giving crones. When flight is not feasible, he may compromise by confining himself to his newspaper or the front room where he can engage in masculine activities, or else may agree to participate in a minimal way by cooking or running baths. If his partner is a Regulator who asks him to engage in primary childcare, he may find himself loathe to change the baby or even hold 'it' for very long, afraid of his own roughness and incompetence as well as the enticing proximity of the snuggling little creature. However, he may be able to provide a protective barrier around his Facilitator partner, grateful for her mothering presence although missing her wifely attentions. Studies have found that new mothers may expect their partners to fulfil a 'fatherly' role towards them, by approving and encouraging their new skills and through an emotional alliance, helping them differentiate from their own mothers. Some Renouncers, although unable to 'mother' their wives, are particularly capable in this supportive paternal role, admiring their woman's 'feminine' capacities and motherly skills. With time, many Regulators become more involved in their babies, especially with a first-born male, offering themselves as a 'solid rock' upon which the child can rely. Others, beset by multiple unconscious conflicts and threatened by all the new demands, experience a 'dread of paternity' and opt out of the family circle, seeking male comradeship in the pub or club, or female succour in an extramarital affair.

(b) Participator

With a hospital birth, the Participator cannot wait for mother and infant to return home. He may feel somewhat jealous of the 'instant' relationship the mother has established with the baby who was inside her, and now suckles at her breast. Determined to catch up, he hopes to build his own relationship with the newborn through holding and feeding, bathing and caressing, doing for the baby what his own responsive body 'remembers' his mother doing for him. He feels a desire to be a 'receptacle' for all the baby's feelings and wishes, hoping to envelop his baby in warmth and soothe away unpleasure. If his partner is a Regulator, she will be pleased to hand over the baby to his ministrations while she sees to her own adult needs. Much of the research on fathers as primary care-takers has been biased by being conducted on one-parent families, hence reflecting the absence or loss of the mother, or her incapacitation [38]. However, recently, a psychoanalytically orientated clinical study was conducted of intact families in which the father had the primary nurturing role. The children thus raised were found to be 'vigorous, competent and thriving infants' . . . with a 'heightened appetite for novel experience and stimuli'[39]. These advantages may possibly be explained by the father's primary caregiven greater involvement in a role of his choosing as opposed to many mothers' sense of little choice in fulfilling a lifelong role-expectation. Interestingly, some of the differences between maternal soothing and paternal rousing of infants [40] are found to vanish when the frather is the primary rather than secondary caretaker [41].

Espoused to a Facilitator, the Participator may be agreeable to nurturing her instead of the baby, thus establishing what I've called a 'hierarchy of mothering' [42]. Alternatively, he may try to set himself up as primary caregiver in competition with her own desires. Such rivalry can cause the Facilitator great distress as she finds herself caught between her wish to gratify her husband's need to 'mother' the baby and her belief in the necessity for her own exclusive nurturing. A Participator may be resentful of having to leave the baby at home with his wife and go out to work each morning. While still a relatively new phenomenon, it is increasingly acceptable in western societies for the couple to share both childcare, domestic jobs and work outside the home, an arrangement that also may suit less extreme Facilitators and Regulators and 'intermediary parents'.

24.3.5 Interactions and balance of power: Facilitator/Regulator and Participator/Renouncer permutations

With the birth of a baby new issues of responsibility and care emerge, which necessitate the reconceptualization of family roles and renegotiation of the couple's previous mode of coping.

(a) 'Conventional' family

In this set-up (Facilitator mother–Renouncer father), the mother becomes increasingly housebound and economically dependent while the father takes on greater expenditure and administrative responsibility. The woman may need her husband to become more 'dominant' at this juncture, and free her from worldly decision-making and enable her to 'regress' in her empathic identification with the baby. Fulfilment of this expectation depends on the degree to which he has established an internalized model of a protective, effective father, without which he may go through the rule-bound motions but feel inadequate and resentfully competitive with the baby or become aggressively dominant, devaluing her maternal role and confining the mother to a helplessly dependent, denigrated position of social invisibility.

(b) Adult self-realization

In happy 'dual-career' type marriages (Regulator mother–Renouncer father), both members of the couple are in agreement that the baby be 'mothered' by someone else part of the time while they both continue to pursue their own activities. Often these arrangements are motivated by healthy development. However, in some cases where their own involvement with the baby is intended to be minimal, the decision, however intellectually phrased, is a product of their early backgrounds – either one or both have been brought up by nannies, or other caretakers or in families where the parental couple took precedence over children. In other cases, their own early maternal deprivation makes it difficult to tolerate a symbiotic union between mother and baby.

In some malfunctioning families, an infant may be scapegoated as the representation of the parents' split-off weakness and neediness of which they each feel ashamed and helpless to confront or change. Conversely, the treatment of children in one or both of their respective families of origin may have been one of overindulgence which has left the new parent narcissistically unable to be subservient to the needs of another. Where only one member of the couple has had this upbringing, he or she may insist that the other play the role of doting mother or that of an incestuously involved father within the couple's relationship, keeping the baby as an excluded envious spectator, representing a rival sibling or same-sexed parent in childhood.

(c) Role reversal

In this type of relationship (Regulator mother–Participator father) where the man 'mothers' the baby in identification with his own mother while the woman behaves like her internalized non-domestic 'father', each feels enriched by their preferred role, and utilizes emotional strengths. However, in couples where the original models do not dovetail, each may try to induce their partner to behave as the parent of that sex did in their own family of origin, causing bitter arguments or critical discontent.

(d) 'Dual nurturer' family

Finally, where both parents are primarily caregivers (Facilitator mother and Participator father), if each is identified with a loving, generous parent, what previously was played out between them can now be focused in nurturing the real baby. However, if the issue becomes a competition to lay claims to being 'the best', 'most loved' 'really devoted' 'true' mother, not only will the baby be overindulged at times by two self-idealizing parents outdoing each other but the couple's adult relationship will become non-existent in the bid for exclusivity.

Needless to say, these permutations represent four static positions whereas, in reality, most couples oscillate between these different modes. The next chapter focuses on the dynamics underlying some of the complex changes in the family constellation and marital interaction.

KEY POINTS

*Fathers, too, are affected by exposure to a newborn and have to adjust to the changes in their relationship to their partner.
*While Participators actively engage in childcare, at times in competition with the mother, Renouncers may feel their masculinity threatened by the intensity of feelings, trying to continue life as usual yet stirred up by the inevitable changes.
*Four possible combinations of Facilitator/Regulator mothers and Participator/Renouncer fathers provide a framework for broadly defining parental interaction.

Chapter 25

First six weeks: dynamics between the parents

'The balance between individual autonomy and couple mutuality that develops . . . may be important in establishing a pattern that will later affect the quality of the parent–child relationship and the extent of the sex-role segregation of duties between the parents. It is only in the context of a growing egalitarian base to the marital relationship that one could find . . . a tendency for parents to establish some barriers between themselves and their children, a marital defense against the institution of parenthood . . . (which may) eventually replace the typical coalition in more traditional families of mother and children against husband-father'. Alice Rossi, 1968. (Transition to parenthood).

25.1 RESEARCH INTO EFFECTS ON THE COUPLE OF THE TRANSITION TO PARENTHOOD

Once the first child is born, the parental couple's relationship inevitably undergoes a change. Once defined as a 'normal crisis', the phrase 'transition to parenthood' was coined to describe the postnatal reintegration of personality and social roles. The impact of a first birth is determined by its timing in the life-cycle of the couple's relationship, and is affected by irrevocability of the birth, paucity of preparation and abruptness in taking on full responsibility in an isolated family with little access to guidance [1]. Research on the couple's transition to parenthood has focused on psychological processes, socioeconomic patterns, reconceptualization of sex-roles and changing marital power-structure [2]. Often described as a postnatal 'deterioration' in first-time parents' relationships [3], it may be more accurate to say that studies have demonstrated changes in the quality of affection and decline in satisfaction between partners with the arrival of their first baby. This qualitative change includes mutual dependence, decreased sexual contact, reduced shared leisure time and social activities, and both men and women receiving less nurturance than they needed from each other. However, the finding that 'affection levels' remain constant between partners who already had a child, suggests that once the transition to parenthood has been made further pregnancies and additional children do not repeat or exacerbate the process [4]. It is difficult to reconcile the many conflicting findings. A 1966 study distinguishing between couples who reported improved as opposed to declining postnatal marital satisfaction found that a more 'differentiated' rather than companionate marriage increased the likelihood of satisfaction [5]. Others have found that many couples gravitate postnatally towards a 'segregated' traditional role structure [6] in spite of egalitarian attitudes [7,8]. In our model, 'segregated' couples belong to the Facilitator/Renouncer type solution common in the 1960s and still prevalent in the late 1980s despite egalitarian changes. I would stipulate that a good marriage is one in which each member feels comfortable with and supported by the partner in the parental role of their choice, and yet retains a sense of connectedness to the intimate relationship with the other. Many studies attribute marital satisfaction to agreement between the couple. All but 7.5% of female and 5.5% of male respondents in a study of 511 couples reported improvement in their marital relationship since the baby's birth, with the couple's adjustment attributed to their communication pattern, high commitment to the parenthood role and a lengthier pre-pregnancy relationship [9]. Other research attempts to tease out the positive effects of childbearing (emotional benefits, self-enrichment, family cohesiveness, identification with the child) from negative factors (physical demands, strain on the relationship, emotional costs and restrictions) [10]. Clearly, it is difficult to generalize since each individual couple will experience the impact of parenthood in their own way, determined not by external criteria of 'normal' adjustment and 'role satisfaction' but involving daily fluctuations as the 'marital pendulum' stabilizes between the conscious and unconscious vectors of the expectations of each member of the couple, both in relationship to each other as partners and as parents to their child(ren). These subtle dynamics, difficult to tap with questionnaires, are revealed on the analytic couch, during marital therapy and in parental discussion groups.

25.2 DYNAMICS IN THE COUPLE'S RELATIONSHIPS AS PARENTS

Parenting is a process which is internalized in infancy and early childhood. Each member of the couple has had a mother and a father in his or her family of origin, even if they did not consistently live together or know each other. Each partner brings to their parenting relationship an internalized model of parenting [11] as he/she experienced and fantasized it – an internal reality rather than an external one. Parts of this model may have been consciously rejected in adulthood by the man or woman determined to act differently from their own mother or father, yet the rejected parts live on in the unconscious to emerge at times of stress or pressure ('I sound just like my mother when I lose my temper'). Part of the original model may have been denied or repressed because it was too painful, violent or sexually disturbing to hold in mind. As we have seen, unconscious aspects of the internalized model exert a powerful influence on choice of marital partner and on the daily interaction between them and with the child of this union.

In a first birth, the adult twosome now incorporates a third who may be the product of them both. The mother and the infant who has emerged from inside her now form a potential primary dyadic unit. Whether or not the partner is the baby's father, he will feel excluded from the physical primacy of the mother–baby pair. In a couple where the wife has been cast in the role of mother to her husband, enacting his internalized parental model of his own mother who indulged him at his father's expense, she may be so conscious of how painful it is for her partner to be displaced that she decides to forego breastfeeding and other intimacies with the baby so as to maintain the couple's special relationship. Threatened now by a direct repetition of this original scenario with the birth of his own son, the irate husband may induce his wife to maintain her primary loyalty to himself as 'child' rather than to the actual baby. She may collude with this because it dovetails with her own early experience in her family of origin, where children were neglected and father overidealized and indulged. Conversely, where the wife had in the past cossetted her husband to fulfil her own frustrated mothering needs, the birth of a real baby induces her to focus her motherly feelings on the infant and to expect her husband to 'grow up', thereby creating a shift in their 'unconscious contract'. He may in turn respond not only by becoming even more demanding, but possibly with the violence his own father displayed at his wife's overpossessive relationship with her son. . . Clearly, parenting is a three-generational process, with the new family being influenced by the individual past parental model of each member of the couple, as well as their shared or complementary transactions.

25.3 PARENTHOOD AS A DEVELOPMENTAL PHASE?

Parenthood not only makes demands for new role adjustments and formation of bonds with a new baby, it also stirs up old feelings. Seen from a psychoanalytic perspective, parenthood has been described as a 'developmental phase' [12], like those of childhood and adolescence. During parenthood the mother and father relive their own early experiences in conjunction with their baby, this time finding themselves in the active position of parents rather than infant-recipients. ('Developmental phase' may be an unfortunate formulation, since it hints unrealistically at universal phase-specific behaviours essential to parenthood [13].) It is suggested that parents who have themselves failed to master particular developmental tasks during the developmental phases of infancy and childhood are unable to guide their offspring skilfully through these. Thus, for instance, a parent may not have resolved his or her own conflicts regarding very early splitting of the world into good and bad, or treating people as untrustworthy objects to be exploited. Unresolved developmental issues from the oral phase may focus on issues of greed, envy, dependency and insatiability. Anal phase preoccupations of power-submission, acquisition and mastery, or 'phallic' competitiveness, erotization, voyeurism or exhibitionism may not have been surmounted [14]. Transactions between parent and child evolve relatively smoothly until the child reaches the developmental level at which the parent, because of his own early deficits, is unable to respond to the child, who senses his insecurity or inappropriate response, interprets it as a weakness which diminishes the child's sense of being protected which in turn increases his anxiety. The child's ego will therefore be weakest in areas which correspond to the unresolved conflicts of the parent or his/her surrogate [15]. Thus, the original fixation or omission is shown up in parenting the next generation, and perpetuates an area of difficulty in the new generation. Nevertheless, I have found that in some marital (or cohabitee) relationships, the new partner-combination and actual experience of mutual parenting of a child also provides fresh opportunities for healing and growth as each member of this couple offers the other solace and support, using his/her mothering and fathering strengths to mitigate the other's weak spots and meet the partner's infantile needs as well as adult ones. In less healthy relationships, destructive envy or competitiveness with the child or rivalry with the other partner over the child's love can create a pathological stronghold which affects all other interactions and may require marital or family therapy to disentangle the participants.

25.4 MID-LIFE PARENTS

The experience of having a baby, particularly a first baby, later in life, has been found to have a greater impact on the lives of women than on men. A detailed study of timing of parenthood among 86 (American) couples in 1980 found that whereas the reaction of older men was fairly uniform, women's adaptation to mid-life motherhood was varied, taking the form of three distinct versions which the researchers called: the 'supplement' experience, the 'new chapter' and the 'crunch'. Most of the men interviewed regarded fatherhood as a supplement, an 'extra' to their lives, with career decisions and priorities largely insulated from 'the daily press of family life'. Their comparative financial stability and job security mean that, unlike younger fathers, they did not feel the need to intensify their involvement in provision for the family. Whereas young fathers found themselves 'jolted' out of 'the egocentric self-absorption and identity confusion of late-adolescence' into the activity of supporting a family, older fathers (late 30s to 40) felt 'recharged' by fatherhood and propelled with new energy to live up to commitments at work and at home. Finally, in men becoming fathers for the first time in mid-life (40+) 'parenthood seems to bring a glow', as if 'their generative circuitry, fashioned and in place, could now light up and be displayed for anyone to see'. About half the mid-life mothers in this study reacted as did the fathers. They did not undergo a radical shift but 'incorporated motherhood and the baby into the structure of their ongoing lives'. Some women becoming mothers at 40 had a sense of a 'new chapter', in that their identities and priorities became reorientated around the child and child-rearing activities, involving a shift of acquaintances and interests as their current lives were out of phase with their peers. A final group of mid-life mothers experienced 'the crunch' – a critical situation, resembling 'overload' phenomenon, in which reality differed from their fantasies and expectations, and they felt that both inner and outer demands exceeded their capacity to respond competently by their own standards [16]. In these reactions there are some similarities to our own Facilitator/Regulator–Renouncer model, and although Participators seem absent among the mid-life fathers, this may be a function of the upbringing of older men, as nearly two-thirds of fathers of children born in the 1970s had some parental 'hands on' daily care as opposed to offspring born in the 1950s and 1960s. So rapid have changes been over the last decade that it is likely a similar study conducted today would find a greater shift towards paternal nurturing. In sum, becoming a parent in later life involves adjustment to a whole new range of emotions and activities, which in many ways older parents are better equipped to tolerate. Having postponed parenthood voluntarily or because of prolonged infertility, they have a sense of having made the most of adult freedom, and now feel their 'ripeness', accumulated life-experience and inner resources stand them in good stead. The same applies to what the aforementioned study called the 'caboose' sequence of having another child very much later than his/her sibling(s). Parenthood then straddles two family stages, each with its own dynamics and momentum, necessitating revision of priorities and accommodation, with the baby welcomed as a 'treat' or initially experienced as a disruption of plans, yet brought up by two sets of older people, parents and siblings, who can serve as models and intermediaries between the generations. Birth of a baby in later life can restore vitality and help the parents overcome some of the losses ageing involves. Among older parents concerns for the future focus on how their children will deal with the 40-year gap between them, how they, the parents, will cope with adolescents, and the age-related drawback of a lower energy level [17].

25.5 SEXUALITY, BREASTFEEDING AND EPISIOTOMY

Through their sexual contact, partners confirm their special intimacy with each other, one entering the other's body, the other allowing herself to be entered, both coming together in momentary mutual loss of separateness before reaffirming their respective autonomies. Following the birth, sexual intercourse is often delayed although close physical contact may be maintained. The point at which the mother resumes her sexual relationship with her partner will depend not only on her physical recuperation from the exertion of pregnancy and birth but psychologically on many factors in her new state of motherhood. Regulators, affirming the partner relationship, resume their interest in sex earlier than Facilitators, for whom the mother–baby dyad continues to be the prime unit of intimacy for some months. Breastfeeding, which has been associated with 'impairment' of sexuality in the early months postpartum [18], may inhibit the mother's sense of her erotic self if she experiences a conflict between her maternal role and that of a sexual being. She may feel her lactating body is at the beck and call of her infant and she can tolerate no more demands upon her. If she is scared of leaking milk during intercourse, or believes her breasts belong to the baby, oral stimulation or caressing of her enlarged breasts by her partner may feel particularly 'wrong'. To either member of the couple, genital contact with the place from which the baby emerged may now seem forbidden and 'perverse'. Her episiotomy usually remains tender for many weeks and a woman might continue to feel so mutilated or humiliated by this procedure that she cannot bear to be touched there. Her mate, too, may be afraid to penetrate for fear of hurting her or displacing stitches.

Although stitches do heal, the cat-gut dissolves or the 'green string' is eventually removed, there is a sad irony when during the first precious early days of a baby's life his mother is in agony every time she sits on anything other than an air-ring or in a tub of warm salt-water, due to an unnecessary artificial infliction of suffering from the very people who seemed so concerned to promote pain relief for the natural process of birth. Equally ironic is that common excuse of episiotomies done 'for the sake of the husband' to tighten a vagina stretched shapeless during birth. Far more sexual difficulties are reported due to the mutilation of episiotomies and their long-lasting unconscious psychological effects than due to slack saggy vaginae. Many women continue to suffer from a tender scar and pain on intercourse for years after the birth, which may in extreme cases necessitate stretching or a secondary operation to relieve the tightness. However, women complaining about pain or expressing anxiety about scars from perineal trauma are often obliquely referring to psychosexual implications of this operation, a delicate topic which GPs, midwives and health visitors may be nervous to discuss. Her throbbing clitoris, aching pelvic floor, urinary incontinence and other symptoms which persist for weeks after the birth, all combine to make her doubt that she will ever regain her exuberant sexuality. Failure to respond to her plea for help may result in a collapse of the sexual relationship, already so eroded by fatigue and the overwhelming demands of early parenthood.

Research comparing parturients who have or have not had episiotomies indicate resumption of sexual intercourse is often postponed far beyond the 6-week postpartum examination in the episiotomy group [19]. Clinical evidence suggests that in addition to her having become in unconscious fantasy a 'Madonna-Mother' with all the sexual taboos implied, both partners may have the unconscious idea that her episiotomy 'scarification', like loss of virginity, is an assertion of ownership over the body, both by the emergent baby or the knife wielding father/obstetrician. The woman's sexual pleasure is often curtailed for similar reasons of feeling that her body is not her own to enjoy sexually but belongs to the baby she gave birth to whose home it was. With every visit to the toilet, the episiotomy scar serves as a constant reminder that she is no longer the sexual-being she once was. Encouraging the woman to massage the area and touch her scar helps her reclaim it as her own as well as helping the healing process through increased circulation [20].

Her partner's sexual responsiveness may have been adversely affected by watching her give birth and she too, may feel sexually unattractive, embarrassed by her scar, stretch marks and post-pregnant flabbiness. Psyche and soma combine intricately in sexuality and minute variations in each partner may affect the delicately balanced process between them. Genital tissue takes time to regain prenatal sensitivity and hormonal fluctuations, too, affect sexual desire. Supersensitivity of the perineum following birth (and nerve endings affected by the episiotomy) as well as lochia and, later, fear of pregnancy add to the confusion. Fairly common post-episiotomy physical complications may include a discharging infection, a too tight vagina (either due to reflex muscular contraction on painful penetration or overenthusiastic stitching or tightness in healing) or else, a slackened too lax vagina (from excessive stretching during delivery or incompetent stitching). Vaginal secretions are affected by the hormonal changes and episiotomy; lack of lubrication causes chaffing. The male partner may interpret her dryness even after considerable foreplay as lack of erotic interest. He may wryly assume that now she is fulfilled by the baby, he is redundant. She may stiffen at his touch, rejecting affectionate caresses in the fear that intercourse will follow. All these intricate feelings, occurring at a time of tiredness, broken sleep and infantile demands and physical changes, may result in an indefinite postponement of love-making after a few painful attempts, or a reluctance to begin at all.

25.6 PARENTS CAN BE LOVERS

While sexuality is but one aspect of an intimate relationship, it serves to affirm and renew the couple's mutual closeness and can act as a barometer of emotional difficulties. A sympathetic visiting professional, alerted to hidden anxieties, can broach the sensitive topic, possibly through questions about contraception. When neither member of the couple has any other confidante, one or other may turn to her in despair. If the couple have been unable to discuss their problem with each other, the Health Visitor or GP may be used as 'umpire' to open-up and guide them through the taboo subject. Sometimes, the visiting professional may be able to offer practical tips to alleviate some distress, always emphasizing the importance for both members of the couple to talk together about their feelings and try and share them by expressing their conflicts openly. There are many ways of showing affection and laughing together, cuddling and kissing can refresh the couple's closeness even if sexual intercourse is postponed for a while. They may need advice on artificial lubrication or some medical intervention. They may just need permission' to revert to being the sexual-pair they once were despite being parents. Sleep deprivation and apprehension about being inter-rupted by the baby's crying are common dampeners of ardour. A rearrangement of timetable may be suggested, with parents getting together as soon as the baby has a nap rather than late at night. The baby's noctural presence in the parental bed or bedroom may inhibit love-making or conversely, lend voyeuristic fantasies to coitus, now playing out an archaic 'primal-scene' of their own parents copulating during their childhood.

Where the couple is unable to talk about their inhibitions and resort to seeking professional advice, brief marital therapy or pair-counselling may be necessary. Sexual dysfunctions can be helped by sex-therapy. However, in some cases individual psychotherapy may be required to alleviate unconscious fantasies which have become activated postnatally. In some ways, a member of the couple may be attracted to the other, no longer only a lover and partner but now a mother or father, like their own other-sexed parent in childhood. Sex may be unconsciously 'prohibited' for the couple now become mother and father. Their abstinence might be dictated either by identification with their own 'asexual' parents ('my mother never did that! well, perhaps just once') or by unconscious fears of 'incest' as the partner concretely becomes a mother or father. The arrival of the new baby also arouses old fantasies of merging with mother. In some people this may exacerbate early anxieties about loss of identity and fusion which inhibit full surrender to intercourse resulting in semi-abstinence, or symptoms of impotence or frigidity. In couples where one partner has suffered actual incestuous abuse in childhood, sexual problems may develop now, not only in relation to the other partner become parent, but in relation to their own baby (see Chapter 33). Postnatal sexual difficulties within the marriage cannot but have their effect on the baby and older children who unconsciously sense the tensions between the couple, or are put in a false position in the family circuit, having an emotional current directed at the child which is intended for an adult partner.

25.7 EXTRAMARITAL AFFAIRS

During his partner's pregnancy and early parenthood, it is not uncommon for a man to resort to an affair, justifying this to himself on the grounds of his reluctance to 'bother' her sexually or because of her withholding sex from him.

On an unconscious level, his affair may signify various motives:

– a simultaneous attempt to deny yet express the loss of exclusivity that parenthood inevitably entails. ('We were two peas in a pod, now she's the pod')
– an effort to split the good and bad aspects of his archaic mother, preserving the ideal in his partner and projecting badness on to his mistress, or vice versa.
– a means of avoiding the transition to parenthood by prolonging an adolescent type sexuality. ('The wife's no fun anymore, but I still lark about')
– If he experiences his own sexuality as aggressive or destructive, avoidance of his wife and his endeavour to divert these forces elsewhere may be protective towards his partner or their baby.
– The man may be loath to have intercourse with a womanly body that is so clearly maternal, recoiling from the incestuous aspects of his sexual relationship with his wife, now become or about to become a mother.
– A further fantasy may revolve around the element of secrecy – clutching his precious secret to himself as she holds her pregnancy or newborn, unshared with her, his very own thing. (She's besotted with that baby. I've got mine!)
– If his affair is a homosexual one, the heterosexual oedipal triumph may be displaced into another kind of victory – gaining forbidden access to the same sexed parent to spite the other 'parent', his wife.

Clearly, 'playing the field' involves playing many different games in which the female partner may be collusively participating or an unknowing victim. Discovery of an affair may cause untold damage to a woman already feeling vulnerable in her altered body and sexual image. Marital therapy is indicated where the husband has 'confessed' during the crucial early weeks of parenthood. Already having to cope with the major reorientation entailed in having a first baby, the marriage may not survive the impact of disloyalty, however 'considerate' his motives appear to have been. She may feel not only betrayed and devastated by his sexual faithlessness at this particularly intimate stage of their relationship, but also dismayed at his capacity for double-dealing and duplicity. Suspicion inevitably infiltrates all activities, as she deems him to be untrustworthy until proved otherwise.

While much of this applies to any marital infidelity, the woman's greater emotional sensitivity during pregnancy and early motherhood and her increased emotional, economic and practical dependence on the father of her child, render her vulnerable at a time when her own inner resources are taxed to the full by her new condition. The relationship, too, is often taxed, when emotional resources are scattered outside the home, and when positive internal figures are displaced onto 'outsiders' rather than reinforcing and revitalizing the relationship in its new phase of parenthood. Revived 'sibling' rivalry with the new baby may underlie infidelity. If a parental partnership is to be established, one or both members of the couple may require ongoing therapeutic help aimed at stabilizing and reintegrating the sexual and emotional forces of the relationship.

25.8 THE SIX-WEEK CHECKUP

Many couples postpone intercourse until they have the 'go ahead' of the doctor following the six-week postnatal checkup. This can result in the pair's discovery of sexual problems only after the appointment, so that few of these get reported to professionals. If, in trying to discuss her sexual inhibitions, the puerperal woman meets a 'what about your husband, poor chap'-type of response from her doctor, she may clam up and battle on unrelieved, or foster a grudge against men, including the male doctor and her husband, who cannot see it from a woman's point of view. Women doctors can be equally insensitive to the momentousness of the postnatal checkup. Unconsciously, it takes on the significance of a rite of passage – the point of return from which the woman begins to re-enter 'ordinary' life. The doctor may unconsciously be allocated the role of 'high priest'(ess), or 'shaman' who can proclaim her internally 'back to normal' after her strange corporeal ordeal. In some ways, the first six weeks are an extension of pregnancy, with the checkup signifying another form of birth for the mother and official recognition of her established new status. Casual or unnecessary postponement of this date by the professionals involved may make her feel she is being put on 'probation'. Delay may prolong the period beyond the point the woman has been geared to sustain herself. Conversely, delaying tactics and excuses from the woman may indicate her own wish to postpone 'waking up' from the 'honeymoon dream' or fear of 'flunking' the test of official recognition as a fully fledged mother. By contrast, attempts to be seen earlier than six weeks not only reflect the anxieties she brings to the appointment but may illustrate her desperate need for emotional acknowledgement, practical help and/or rescue from her isolation with the baby.

Time should be set aside for this checkup to be more than a cursory examination of blood pressure, weight, breasts, stitches, abdomen and cervix. Contraceptive advice has little meaning where no clear picture of the woman's sex-life exists and, like feeding advice, can only be heeded if related to her own particular lifestyle. The woman is a whole person, often being torn apart in different directions by the conflicting demands of her various dependants. She looks to the doctor as the highest authority who can give her permission to find time for herself, relax her high standards and regain her sense of feminine sexuality. Often, the doctor may be the first male she has encountered since the birth, other than the postman and milkman. In their intimate physical contact, he is inevitably a sexual presence. If he is also the doctor who saw her through the pregnancy and birth, he forms a crucial link between her pre-conceptual body, her pregnant body and this postnatal changed one.

Although verbally asking for a prescription, what she wants is recognition – acknowledgement from this fatherly or motherly figure that she has become a full-blown adult woman in her motherhood and is being granted serious consideration as a person rather than dismissed as her baby's tired mother or her husband's plump wife. She may also be wishing to convey the disappointing and distressing aspects of her experience, and to be reassured of the normality of her depressed mood, that her tension, frustration and anxieties about mothering are a natural part of the adjustment to her new situation and above all, that her ambivalence towards her beautiful healthy baby is commonplace. She might benefit from establishing contact with other mothers through the well-baby clinic, a mother and baby group or local National Childbirth Trust postnatal group. Professional help is required for women who express intense feelings of helplessness, inadequacy and inability to cope or those who remain in bed and do not get dressed most days. Those who cry a great deal and experience insomnia unrelated to the infant's sleep patterns, lack of appetite or compulsive overeating, withdrawal or derealization and suicidal thoughts are suffering from depression which needs to be treated (Chapter 33).

KEY POINTS

*In the transition to parenthood, the marital relationship undergoes new stresses postnatally, due to assumption of new roles, bonding with the newborn and newly reactivated unconscious identifications.

*Parenthood may be described as a 'developmental phase' during which the participants encounter their own early experience again, yet this time in the capacity of active parents rather than passive recipients.

*Developmental deficits and unresolved conflicts are revealed in the parents and passed on to the child, unless rectified through understanding, current supportive relationships and/or therapeutic healing.

*Sexuality, often affected postnatally, may serve as a barometer for disturbance in the relationship and extramarital affairs at this time are indicative of failure to integate emotional, sexual and parenting resources with the family.

*The unconscious significance of the six-week checkup is one of a rite of passage, incorporating the parturient back into ordinary life, acknowledging the importance of the change that has occurred in her and granting her 'official' recognition as mother and mature woman.

Chapter 26

Siblings

' . . . In cases in which the two children are so close in age that lactation is prejudiced by the second pregnancy, this reproach acquires a real basis, and it is a remarkable fact that a child, even with an age difference of only 11 months, is not too young to take notice of what is happening. But what the child grudges the unwanted intruder and rival is not only the suckling but all the other signs of maternal care. It feels that it has been dethroned, despoiled, prejudiced in its rights; it casts a jealous hatred upon the new baby and develops a grievance against the faithless mother . . . *Nor does it make much difference if the child happens to remain the mother's preferred favourite. A child's demands for love are immoderate, they make exclusive claims and tolerate no sharing.'*
Sigmund Freud, (Feminity 1933, italics added)
'When other children appear on the scene *the Oedipus complex is enlarged into a family complex*. This, with fresh support from the egoistic sense of injury, gives grounds for receiving the new brothers or sisters with repugnance and for unhesitatingly getting rid of them by a wish . . . '
Sigmund Freud (Introductory Lectures 1916–17, italics added)
'The nature and quality of the human child's relations to people of his own and the opposite sex have already been laid down in the first six years of his life. He may afterwards develop and transform them in certain directions, but he can no longer get rid of them. The people to whom he is in this way fixed are his parents and his brothers and sisters. All those whom he gets to know later become substitute figures for these first objects of his feelings . . . ' Sigmund Freud (On Schoolboy Psychology 1914)

26.1 FAMILY REPERCUSSIONS

Birth of a new baby constitutes a family upheaval and need for realignment of relationships and positions within the family constellation. A couple becomes a family. Each new family member increases the number of inter-relationships considerably by a formula of $n(n-1)$. This means, for instance, that whereas three people have six relationships between them, with the arrival of a fourth this number increases to 12! Gender combinations abound: female mother, male father and either male or female first child; second male or female child means four possible sibling-combinations: male:female; male:male; female:female; female:male. Subsequent births and multiple births add to the complexity of permutations. An only child becomes one of a pair; the doted male singleton may become 'one of the boys' – either coupled with his Dad or with the new male baby. An 'abandoned' child by a first marriage will be threatened by the newborn's founding of a new family-branch which indicates consolidation of his/her mother or father's relationship with the new partner. However, such a threesome living under the same roof might feel 'blood-united' by the baby that carries all their genes, as may the assorted siblings of two step-families by their new common sibling. Arrival of a baby also unsettles ordinal positions: The second child becomes a 'middle' one, the little one 'big'. The newborn displaces the previous baby of the family who now becomes elder brother or sister, suddenly expected to help out, watching with fascinated amazement and envy as the infant is allowed bodily indulgences no longer permitted the older child. Parents having to rotate these relationships in their own minds find that adding another chld is more than a simple multiplication of 2×1 child, and much more than double the work.

It can be seen therefore that reactions to the new arrival must vary according to the family constellation, emotional development of the older siblings, the age-gap between them and the sex of each. Not only do each of the parents have to bond with their recent addition, but each other family member independently must forge their own emotional links to the new baby, for better or for worse. In principle, two interacting profound 'dynamic forces' have been identified as significantly shaping the sibling experience: the nature of parent–child mutual relationships and each child's developmental capacities [1]. A contributory factor to the complexity of describing sibling experience is that the developing interaction is not static but fluctuates with the daily experience of ongoing close shared contact with now 'un'-pregnant mother, father (other siblings) and the rapidly changing newcomer.

26.2 BECOMING A SIBLING: FIRSTBORN'S INITIAL RESPONSES TO THE SECOND BABY

Like new parents, most first children have only a vague idea about what getting a 'new baby' means. Little firstborns anticipating a playmate are disappointed with the unresponsive needy intruder-baby who arrives. They naturally feel displaced and jealous of the attention the infant receives. By comparison, the younger of two children, who has always lived in a family with a sibling, will be less conflicted about the birth of a new baby, gaining status in being an older brother or sister in proud alliance with his own older sibling. On a practical level, routines, rearrangements in the home such as rotation of bedrooms, new 'big' bed for the older sibling to release the needed cot, prominent new baby equipment, ecstatic grandparents and exhausted preoccupied parents all contribute to the confusing momentousness of the situation.

Studies of preschool first siblings report that the most common initial reactions to the birth of a new baby are hostility and rivalry with the infant, rage and possessiveness towards the mother, increased attention-seeking behaviours and, often, regression back to bed-wetting, thumb sucking, baby talk and use of dummies and nappies in the younger ones. In one study, distinctly negative reactions were found in 89% of 66 children under 3, but only 11% of those over 6 years. The sex of the newborn was found to affect sibling reactions, with the birth of a boy causing more difficult behaviour, whereas brothers of a female baby showed increased attention-seeking behaviour [2]. In another study of first-born siblings aged 1–3½, sleep disturbances were reported in 73% of cases, and an increase of temper tantrums and excessive activity, particularly in girls [3]. At the same time, developmental advances may be noted (my own daughter's first steps coincided with the birth of her next brother) and the initial desire to get rid of the baby changes with gradual acceptance of the fact that the newcomer is a permanent member of the family.

First-born school attenders are, as a group, less distressed by sibling birth, partly because of the greater internal resources of older children, and equally because of their own activities outside the home which provides them with an alternative personal domain and access to other adult sources of emotional comfort. However, in some seemingly accepting children, sibling rivalry may be concealed by its displacement onto peers at school. Information from infant observation studies and direct maternal reports indicates that the older child's partial absence from the home paradoxically 'refreshes' the mother to focus her attention on the child upon his/her return home from school. Nevertheless, the older child is inevitably envious of the new baby's close contact with the mother during his/her absence from the home and school phobia is not an uncommon initial reaction of children who are insecure about retaining their favoured place in the mother's affections.

26.3 MATERNAL SEPARATION

During these early weeks, disturbances, particularly among younger children, are more common when the mother has been hospitalized for the birth. The emotional effects of a prolonged separation of a child from his or her mother, particularly if she is the primary caregiver, are well documented. Although reversible, reactions of distress, detachment, rejection and angry responses may be noted after even a short separation for which the child is unprepared. In the case of a planned temporary hospitalization, such as the mother's for the birth, an older child should be forewarned and emotionally prepared for the separation. Ideally, a close caring relative should come to stay with the child in the home. In the event of a premature birth or unexpected complications which necessitate both parents being away for a prolonged period, the child requires the security of home and familiar routines even more. Far from avoiding distress, the well-known practice of sending a child away during a time of stress compounds it with separation anxiety.

During pregnancy, a mother can begin preparing her child for her hospitalization some time in advance of her delivery date, preparing meals together to be frozen and eaten in her absence, visiting the hospital in advance (or looking at books and brochures). While she is away, the caregiving adult who has become familiarized with home routines in the mother's presence forms a bridge to her in her absence. Talking about mother rather than avoidance of the subject, having her photograph available, speaking to her on the phone if possible, and activities which make something to be shared with her later can help alleviate some of the sadness. The mother, too, can be encouraged to leave something of her own with the child (a bed-jacket with her 'smell' on it or a coveted possession to be shared in her absence) and a stock of little drawings, mementoes or small gifts to be 'found' when the child seeks her. Fathers who attend the birth can report back to the child, demystifying mother's 'hospital activity' and modifying inevitable fantasies without burdening him or her with unnecessary details and additional strain[5]. Needless to say, effects of maternal separation are best modified by early discharge from hospital or frequent visits which centre on restoring the older child's relationship with mother rather than introducing the sibling to the new baby.

26.4 HOME BIRTHS

While home birth eliminates the problem of separation, the effects of actually being present at the birth have not yet been sufficiently researched. Granting the child freedom to wander in or out of the birth-chamber will allow him/her some measure of control in an inevitably frightening, as well as exciting situation. A few studies have focused on the sibling's behaviour during labour and birth. These observations were made in American 'alternative birth centres' (53% of which in a 1979 nationwide survey allowed children into labour facilities and 44% permitted children to be present at the birth [6]). Reactions noted were a heightening of the child's normal coping style – quiet ones becoming quieter and active ones more restless. After the birth, their excitement subsided as they 'resumed normal activities' or interacted with the newborn. Most reports stress the younger child's emotional need for his/her mother possibly distracting her during labour and delivery, and hence advocate provision for a specific birth attendant to care for the young child. Conversely the distressing experiences seeing maternal blood and watching her suffering have an acute effect on older children, who cannot help but associate this with morbidity [7]. While live births are featured on television and parental nakedness is a common sight to many young children, nevertheless, I feel we must not underestimate the momentousness of actually participating in the birth of a sibling and the disturbing nature for the child of the sight of mother in pain or observing the distorted, normally hidden maternal genitals.

In families where it is planned that a child is to attend a home birth she or he should be included by the midwife or childbirth educator in appropriate preparatory sessions. Parents should discuss the birth in advance with the child, using books with colour photographs and possibly videos, focusing on some of the sights and sounds of labour, the appearance of the newborn, and emphasizing that the cutting of the cord will not be painful to mother or baby [8]. According to his/her age, the child may benefit from being offered some preplanned necessary, varied yet relinquishable tasks to perform during labour, such as timing contractions or monitoring telephone calls. A carefully selected stock of self-engrossing activities, 'nibbles' and playthings should be on hand to enable the child to retreat and replenish him/herself at will. It is my strong belief that children must feel free to leave the birth chamber of their own accord during labour or birth and should be excluded from watching complicated births, episiotomies and perineal repairs. A special person, capable of being emotionally available, should be appointed as 'doula' to the child, prepared to anticipate needs and respond to questions both silent and asked, in a responsible, supportive manner that is sensitive to potential distress. Whether or not the birth is actually observed, the child should be included in a post-birth 'debriefing' and parents should encourage and expect questions and comments to continue for many weeks, months and years to come, as their cognitive capacities increase in complexity and the birth-experience is re-evaluated and reintegrated.

26.5 MANAGEMENT OF SIBLING RIVALRY AND AFFIRMATION OF BONDING

One advantage of homebirths or early hospital discharge is their provision of sibling's access to the newborn soon after the birth, while the neonate is still alert and interaction is as yet undefined by parental attributions. Once a relationship is established, although naturally ambivalent, inclusion in babycare activities may help the older sibling feel responsible and loving towards the baby, emulating parental nurturing. A firstborn will feel gratified as well as tetchy about 'parental lore' having been learnt from experience of his/her own 'guinea-pig' babyhood, and will wish to hear again and again what she or he was like as a baby, while observing the new baby, vicariously re-experiencing and enacting the babycare of those forgotten early months.

(a) Jealousy and rivalry

Parents who are excessively afraid of jealousy and focus exclusively on the older child to the detriment of attentive care of the new baby actually end up exposing their firstborn to a false impression of security, as s/he guiltily becomes aware of the baby's neglect. Parents are much helped by professional reassurance that siblings cannot but feel angry and displaced by the baby. Rivalry, the competition between siblings for exclusive possession of the parent, involves increased yearning for and fear of losing the carer's love while wishing to eliminate the rival [9]. The parents' capacity to accept these competitive feelings and yet continue to love the older child despite her/his hatred, helps the child to accept and integrate contradictory emotions within him/herself. This is particularly true when both parents are there and can remain emotionally available and responsive to the needs of both children, proving that they can survive the angry firstborn's aggressive attacks, withstand emotional 'blackmail' and yet continue to cherish him/her. Reassurance that despite mother having a 'new' baby, this infant is not a 'replacement' because the firstborn has been naughty or has been outgrown by the parents, also increases the older child's capacity to express feelings openly, reduces jealousy and proves that there is enough love to go around. Verbal appreciation of the older child's loving capacities, special 'private' time with the parents (treats, carefully chosen activities, or just wholehearted outings and undivided attention) reinforce the older child's undiminished ongoing relationship and confirm his/her unique place in their affections.

(b) Aggression

Parents who are inordinately afraid that the older sibling might hurt the baby may actually provoke such an attack by constant warnings, threats, watchfulness or overprotectiveness of the infant, leading to 'sneaky' assaults. Nevertheless, parental recognition of the child's entitlement to express angry feelings does not mean acceptance of angry actions as the baby must be shielded. For a while, this idea of the 'right to sibling rivalry' became so hallowed and entrenched in the modern family that some parents were found to 'show a tendency in their own behaviour to protect those rights', taking hostility for granted rather than helping the child find 'civilized solutions' [10]. Likewise,the older child needs protection from the younger's intrusions and destructive impulses. Enabling the angry 'displaced' child to vent his/her rage in words and time allocated for both serious and playful interaction with each older one on his/her own help alleviate murderous resentment.

(c) Interaction

For a child, encouragement to teach the infant from his/her own repertoire of know-how is a source of great pleasure and babies often seem to respond differentially to the games and activities generated by a child rather than an adult. Indeed, when the age difference is slight, the older child, attuned to similar feelings and closer in experience, often seems to fathom the baby's needs and can 'interpret' non-verbal communications for the parents. The sibling can also benefit from being alerted by the parents (or visiting professional) to the baby's considerable cognitive capabilities, taking pleasure in the little one's ability to imitate his expressions and respond with interest and a smile to his/her advances. Parental acknowledgement of both the older child's generosity and the younger's admiration, affirms the special interaction between the children, creating respect for the sibling-relationship as a bond in its own right rather than something fostered by themselves or subject to their own constant intervention.

(d) Sibling experience

Although often seen by experts as a relationship coloured by parental unconscious expectations, or even 'subordinated' to the parental relationship and a function of it [11], the sibling relationships can be rich, intense and is uniquely endowed by the young participants themselves. Their common background and closely shared experience provide opportunities for companionship, mutual support, experimentation, community of interests and imaginary play in a home-based 'playground' sheltered from the outside world. The sibling-bond can offer a stage on which to 'rehearse and act out scenes of their inner lives', and the rivalry between them over parental resources has been defined as the catalyst to a sense of justice, group spirit and social sharing [12]. A spin-off of overlapping babyhoods may be the prolongation for the older one of the pleasures of infancy while the younger is spurred into precocious development. However, siblings might also stimulate each other psycho-sexually out of synchrony with their own developmental phases and beyond their ego-capacities [13].

In larger families, subsequent babies may be regarded as 'belonging' from the start to the other children rather than the possession of the mother. Siblings may be eager to be consulted and participate in every minor decision concerning the new baby, even getting up for nightfeeds or taking over aspects of the physical care. Professionals may feel the need to intervene if reliance on older siblings appears to be becoming exploitative.

26.6 REVIVED PARENTAL-SIBLING EXPERIENCES

During the course of pregnancy and early parenthood emotional residues of early significant relationships are reactivated and unresolved conflicts resurface. The mother or father usually identifies with the baby in the same birth order as him/herself [14], however the sex of the baby may change the attributed identity of the new infant. When their own sibling rivalry has been intense and unresolved, these feelings may prevent the parent from adequately preparing the child for the arrival of a new baby; conversely, a positive sibling experience can enhance the mother's anticipation of the birth [15]. As noted in the section on early reactions to the newborn, parental unconscious fantasies about the identity of each of their children affect their interaction with them. These subtle differences are unconsciously conveyed in tone of voice, gestures, facial expressions and attitudes, and are incorporated by the children who unconsciously read and respond to such communications in relation to their siblings and to themselves. Parents often idealize a firstborn and later, when expecting a second child, idealize not the baby but the relationship between the siblings [16]. Such idealization vies with their fears of the impending competitive demands of the children on them and may also reflect a denial of their own early rivalry. Equally, a second or subsequent child might be awaited with less trepidation and more confidence by the now experienced parents. Where the relationship to the first child has been fraught, birth of a second offers a 'second chance' to do things differently.

Undoubtedly, very real changes occur in the parents' relationship to the older child once the baby is born, and even before, as the mother, engrossed in her pregnancy and relationship to the fetus, inevitably removes some of her maternal preoccupation from the child. She is also concerned with her dilemma of how to love two babies, and how to love them differently. These preoccupations inhibit her availability to her firstborn if she is identified with the second, or poignantly enhances her sense of lost exclusivity if she herself is identified with the older sibling about to be usurped by the new baby. During the early weeks before the baby's responsiveness and unique identity assert themselves undeniably, parents may often be observed to be unconsciously recreating their own families of origin, enacting their parents or selves as children, casting their children in the role of their own siblings and silently dictating the 'script' to be followed.

In some cases the older sibling may be used unconsciously by the parent to express his/her own feelings of resentment about the arrival of the new baby (this one or a remembered rival in childhood). Where a professional observes parents tolerating excessive aggression or turning a blind eye to vicious attacks on the baby, crisis intervention or family therapy should be considered, possibly conducted by a team of professionals in the home.

26.7 PREMATURITY OR NEONATAL ILLNESS

When the birth of a sibling is further complicated by the baby being ill or at risk, the older sibling has to contend with added burdens, and, in the context of her/his worried parents' preoccupation with the newborn baby, is in danger of becoming the 'forgotten family member' at the very time of needing support [17]. Professionals caring for the baby are in a position to encourage parents to be aware of this danger, and avert it by sharing with the child, however young, some of their concerns. The puzzled child needs to understand why their happy pregnant anticipation has been soured by the birth, and what is wrong with the baby. Because most children have ambivalent feelings about the birth of a sibling, when things go wrong, they need to be reassured that it is not their fault, and that the same thing will not happen to them. Explanations about prematurity or congenital abnormality must exonerate the child from these fears, however, to do so, parents too, may in turn need to be reassured by professionals that preterm labour was not instigated by running after or lifting the toddler. Otherwise, their erroneous beliefs will filter through as silent blame that the abnormality was caused by activities of the sibling, whether a twin in utero or the older child's romping or rage. The sibling of a congenitally handicapped baby will inevitably require ongoing discussions with the parents (now and during each new phase of development) as guilt over her/his own normality may inhibit healthy developmental skills. It is important for the older sibling to visit the baby if possible as the imagination can conjure up monstrous features which sight of the baby immediately dispels. However, complex feelings do take time to be sorted out and working through them can be helped by drawing pictures and talking about the new baby to parents, friends and nurses. Special attention from the staff can help the healthy sibling(s) to feel recognized, supported and appreciated during this time of stress, and this may include being allowed to make a contribution to the baby's welfare, however modest, in the form of a gentle caress or the gift of a toy, a drawing or snapshot of themselves to be kept with the baby. Once home, fears of injuring the fragile afflicted baby may prompt self-condemnation and suppression of normal aggression, which, unmodified by parental reassurance or therapeutic help, can result in an overly harsh conscience and passivity. Parents, too, may collude by encouraging the healthy sibling to be exceedingly protective of the handicapped baby thereby stultifying a robust sibling experience. Envy of each other's special treatment received from the parents may exacerbate the already complex interaction between the growing siblings. Parents may also expect the undamaged child to compensate them for their 'failure' or disappointment by being especially successful. A younger child too, born into a family with a mentally or physically handicapped older sibling, will encounter residues in the form of idealizing pressures or emotional withdrawal from the already burdened parents. It has been noted that the difficulties of growing up with a chronically ill or handicapped sibling can involve the healthy child in bitterness over extra favours and attention lavished on the disabled child and social discomfort including stares from strangers or teasing and taunting from friends [18]. Parents and/or the child may need counselling or therapy.

26.8 TWINS AND MULTIPLE BIRTHS

The leap from being childless to parents of two or more babies is an extraordinary one, particularly for a couple following prolonged childlessness. Since multiple gestations are often associated with clomid treatment for infertility and implantation of several fertilized ovum in IVF treatment, the incidence following infertility is higher than expected for the general population. While some relish the idea of having a family in 'one go', others find the idea of relating to so many new people all at once quite daunting. In other families, twins follow on older siblings or even other sets of twins.

If bonding is centred around forming an intense relationship with another individual, having two or more babies at the end of a pregnancy creates difficulties in attachment. Even with babies a pregnancy apart, parents find it difficult to meet the needs of two infants at the same time. When they are the same age, finding the emotional space and 'reverie' for two neonates and enough loving resources to discover personal differences and respond appropriately to each is a feat many parents are unable to achieve. When babies are identical in looks it is tempting for parents to assume that they have identical personalities and needs and can be treated as 'two-times-one'. Monozygotic twins pose particular bonding problems in physically distinguishing between the babies. Treating them both (or all in the case of triplets) as 'one' and dressing them alike may resolve some of the immediate parental conflicts but such blanket relating must complicate development of the babies' individual identities. Advising parents to keep wrist name-tags on their babies for some time after the birth may aid a gradual process of differentiation, and professionals can help parents to observe minute physical differences or perceived behavioural trends.

In such closely interconnected feeding and play situations, parents may induce unfair competitiveness between the babies or exacerbate existing differences. When one twin is more robust at birth, s/he may be invested with lively qualities that the other, needier baby seems not to possess. The latter may be cossetted and receive more handling and care from the worried parents, or be neglected in favour of the more appealing, less anxiety provoking twin. Using detailed baby-observation methods, subtle differences in parental handling and interaction with twin babies may be traced [19]. As with singletons, differentiation between twins may be achieved through unconscious identification of each baby with characteristics borrowed from elsewhere, parents and other siblings 'transferring' vestiges of previous relationships into the new ones. An interesting example of differential treatment of twins reported in the literature employed through micro-analysis of video taped interaction with fraternal twins. The observing neonatologist Stern located the mother's ambivalence about her husband and her twins in a split emotional reaction – one twin receiving her positive feelings and identified with herself, and the other, towards whom she was found to behave quite differently on an unconsciously motivated level, targeted with negative feelings and identified with his father. These almost imperceptible differences in her interactive behaviour, highlighted by video analysis, nevertheless were found to induce a mutually unsatisfying repetitive cycle of reciprocal activity with one twin, while the other remained free to terminate contact with his mother at will, was less controlled by her at 3½ months and on observation after a year was found to be more independent and secure [20].

Twins offer a unique opportunity to explore the interaction of nature–nuture in the development of individual characteristics. Observations conducted on twins prenatally with the use of ultrasound and after birth, have revealed clear individual temperamental differences between members of a pair of twins in utero, early markers of distinct endowments which persist after birth. Thus, unless we postulate maternal attitudes operating selectively on each twin, these observations of prenatal differences in twins sharing the same mother and womb suggest that a cautious approach to the degree of influence attributed to the mother's fantasies and emotions on fetal personality. In addition, these prenatal observations reveal differences in the interuterine environment for each twin determined by their respective position, and in some cases individual placenta, cord and amniotic sac. Relationship of the twins to each other also varies from an active withdrawal to an apparent search for contact [21]. The mother may feel excluded from her twins inter-relationship.

If twins are complex, triplets pose many more problems. After the birth, not merely is the mother faced with the sheer practical difficulties of feeding and holding more babies than she has arms or breasts but on a very primitive level she may feel that her own primary relationships with her parents geered her to loving no more than two people. Klaus and Kennell have taken up Bowlby's idea of 'monotrophy' (a baby forming an attachment with one figure, the mother) suggesting that maternal bonding too may be governed by monotropic attraction to one person. They bring evidence of nurses in premature units becoming attached to only one 'favourite' infant at a time. Likewise, observations of battering occurring selectively in cases where one of a pair of twins had been discharged from hospital later than the other and became the target of maternal abuse. To combat such discrimination, these two professionals suggest keeping twins together and discharging them at the same time to enable simultaneous attachments to occur [22]. Nevertheless, reviews of research studies indicate that most babies do form intense relationships to more than one person if they are exposed to various loving caregivers during infancy [23] and often siblings increase our primary love relationships to more than two. In the case of twins, the intriguing question of their interaction in the womb raises the issue of whether the nucleus of a relationship already exists at birth, and what the implications of this are for separation of incubated premature twins?

Finally, as we have seen, differential bonding is often the result of parental attributions rather than reality considerations. In the case of twins and multiple births, parents may be assisted in their prenatal bonding by detailed ultrasound commentary, prenatal naming and counselling. The latter may help with feelings of bewilderment and rejection experienced by the mother in being excluded from the relationship between her fetuses, and concern about their interaction which she may regard as too close or too competitive. After the birth, both parents and other siblings may continue to experience themselves as secondary to the primary strong bonds between the babies, sometimes feeling jealously excluded or superfluous. New evidence of prenatal interaction may lead us to pose the question whether it is possible that with twins there is a precocious activation of 'triangulation' – the realization that the dyadic-'other' has an intimate relationship with a third. And in this case, is it the mother/primary caregiver who is located in the third corner, usually occupied by father or siblings?

26.9 PERINATAL SIBLING LOSS

When an ill baby dies or a still-birth occurs, a common parental reaction to the perinatal death is to try and protect the dead baby's siblings from their own feelings, by hiding their grief or attempting to be cheerful in their presence. The young children may be still undergoing reactions to the separation from their mother hospitalized for the birth, and find parental tears or lack of them quite bewildering. In addition, they too are going through a mourning process of their own for the baby who never came home, or the one they knew so briefly, a process which may be exacerbated by feelings of real guilt. Young children often have murderous and hostile feelings about new siblings, and with the magical belief that thoughts can harm, may be suffering under the impression that they have caused the death. In addition, the intrusion of death, something which only happens to others out there, into the little circle of their own immediate family, raises doubts about their parents' capacity to keep death at bay, increases their own fears about personal safety and survival of retaliation. In some families children may have been sent away to protect them or the parents during this difficult time, particularly if the mother and father have wanted to spend as much time as possible in intensive care of the very ill baby. Under these circumstances, in addition to the pain of separation from home and the baby's unreality, lack of opportunity to share in the process of mourning forecloses an experience before it has run its course. Children's unexpressed fantasies about the baby's birth and death may become floridly unrealistic when uncorrected by parental explanations and reassurance. In families where mourning is hidden from the child, his/her own grief may be repressed along with secret unresolved guilt. A 'pocket' of unverbalized emotion remains, to erupt in action, symptoms and enactment over the years, a phenomenon which can be traced in Freud himself following the death of his infant brother while he himself was only 23 months old [24]. Fear of dying, blaming the parents for the death or losing faith in their capacity to prevent tragedy, dread of separation and abandonment and nocturnal anxieties are all common reactions to the 'invisible loss' of an unknown baby. Surviving siblings, however young, need some evidence that there has been a baby: a visit to see the ill newborn in the incubator, or a photograph of the still-born, or a chance to participate in the funeral or to mark the death of the baby in some way. Therapy, either during the stressful period of intensive care and death or years later, can help the surviving child to come to terms with the loss [25]. It has been noted that in many cases children will reserve their reactions until their parents regain their emotional strength. Others become anxious during the following pregnancy although presumed to have been too young to know what had happened previously [26]. After a neonatal death, other children in the family may become emotionally neglected or inappropriately overprotected, or one particular child who unconsciously reminds the parent of the dead baby may be avoided or be singled out to comfort the parents and replace the idealized baby.

The childhood mourning process itself varies from that of adults and is also determined by the developmental level of the surviving sibling. Both immediate and long-term reactions will be affected by the quality of their previous and ongoing relationship to the parents and other siblings. While it was previously held that little children were unable to mourn, recent psychoanalytical investigations have shown that given accurate information and clarifications, and being granted family permission to grieve within a secure pre- and post-loss environment, mourning is evident as early as the age of three [27]. In addition to the immediate loss, the bereaved child, unlike the adult, must also deal with the impact of this loss at subsequent stages of development. However, denial and inability to tolerate painful effects may interfere with resolution of childhood mourning [28]. Secretly held fantasies about the continued existence of the dead sibling are not uncommon, particularly when the death occurred at an age when the surviving sibling was unable to comprehend the meaning of death. The child's distorted interpretation of perinatal death and their maladaptive consequences may be understood as the product of:

a. Infantile intrapsychic limitations due to magical thinking and blurring of fantasy and reality;
b. Family influences of inaccurate information, reinforcement of the child's fantasy and heightened parental emotions of rage, guilt and anxiety [29].

Thus the parent's inability to cope with the child's sense of loss, their own self-blame or scapegoating of a child and inability to deal with their own grief, all prevent them from helping the child deal with his/her own feelings about the death. Depending on his/her age at the time of the loss, each child will muster the capacities they have to respond to the bereavement. However, unlike an adult who may accomplish mourning within him/herself, the child will need an adult to serve as focus and facilitator for his/her emotional reactions [30]. When parents or their substitutes cannot provide this outlet because of their own mourning reactions, professional help may be required for the child, parents or family.

KEY POINTS

*The birth of a baby necessitates realignment of family relationships. Reactions to the new arrival vary according to the family constellation, emotional development of the older siblings, the age-gap between them and the sex of each.
*Rivalry between siblings over exclusive possession of the parent involves increased yearning for and fear of losing the carer's love while wishing to eliminate the rival.

*Parents are helped by professional reassurance that siblings cannot but feel angry and displaced by the baby. Their capacity to accept competitive feelings and yet continue to love the older child despite her/his hatred helps the child to integrate ambivalence, and trust in love.

*Nevertheless, parental recognition of the child's entitlement to express angry feelings does not mean acceptance of angry actions as the baby must be protected, the parents trusted to provide boundaries and the older child needs to learn to channel aggression while having his/her rights safeguarded too.

*Positive aspects of sibling experience include companionship, emotional and intellectual stimulation; interchange of experience, mutual interests and imaginative experimentation; development of empathy, justice, confidence, caring, generosity and sharing.

*Twins pose complex bonding problems pre- and post-natally. Living with a chronically handicapped child takes its toll on both parents and siblings. Other complications are caused when parental sibling rivalry is intense and unresolved, and the ensuing identificatory spill-over into current relationships with the children necessitates therapeutic intervention.

*Following a still-birth or neonatal death, surviving siblings need help in adjusting to the loss, a process that will involve further articulation and enlightenment at different stages of intellectual and emotional development. In the process of parental mourning, children in the family may become emotionally neglected or inappropriately overprotected, or one particular child may be scapegoated or singled out to comfort the parents and replace the idealized baby.

Chapter 27

Adolescent parents

'The relation to one's own parents is repeatedly re-enacted by repetition or by avoidance. In parenthood the psychological life cycles of two generations overlap and a third one is regularly involved' (Rose Coleman, Ernst Kris and Sally Provence, The study of variations of early parental attitudes. *Psychoanalytic Study of the Child*, 1953).

Adolescence is a time of maturational turmoil when the young person is physiologically mature but as yet psychologically poised between childhood and adulthood. In the usual course of events, a to-and-fro intrapsychic process of regression and progression enables the teenager to rework earlier conflicts and gradually relinquish childish sources of emotional security by replacing these with age-appropriate goals, realistically tested self-esteem and new intimate relationships outside the family.

Although the adolescent has attained adultlike physical stature, sexual powers and a capacity for truly abstract logical thought, there is a healthy requirement for delay before reaching full adulthood, a need for a phase of partial denial of both his/her strength and weakness, so as not to have to face prematurely the full consequences of physical maturity and emotional lag.[1] Becoming a parent during this phase superimposes all the problems experienced by most first-time parents establishing their identities as mother or father onto the adolescent's already existing struggle to establish his or her individual identity as an autonomous person.

27.1 TEENAGE MOTHERS

While some female adolescents are sufficiently mature to cope with the responsibility and emotional demands of rearing a child, others will have precociously become pregnant in an attempt to try and resolve problems of feminine identity and ambivalent feelings towards their mothers. In some cases, a girl may have used her pregnant body to establish a differentiated sexual identity separate from her mother's while also thus expressing infantile longings to be a baby once more and the wish to be mothered herself [2]. Others may wish to punish the mother, escape from an unhappy family life, repeat the mother's own teenage pregnancy or give her mother a baby. Thus, becoming pregnant need not imply wanting to have a baby. In fact, for every two teenage mothers who have their baby, one has an abortion and an investigation of adolescent mothers of 4-month-old babies found that 13% of these had considered abortion of their unintended pregnancies, some had discussed this with their doctors while others had not pursued it out of inertia, fear, ambivalence or embarrassment [3a]. Over the years, studies have attributed teenage pregnancy to rebelliousness, loneliness and poor self-image. Significant preconceptual experiences of loss have been cited, along with a high incidence of separation from primary caregivers, parental divorce and death in the girl's early family life. Many researchers have focused on the pregnant girl's intensely complex relationship to her own mother, isolating hostile or rivalrous feelings, and overdependence. However, sexual mores and contraceptive patterns have changed so rapidly over the last decade that findings from earlier studies may no longer apply across the board. Indeed, a recent study comparing three groups of 'unwed' adolescent girls found no differences in the ways pregnant and non-pregnant teenagers perceived their mother's nurturance. Nevertheless, sexually active non-pregnant girls expressed more security in their relationship to their mothers than either the abortion group or those intending to keep the baby. A higher percentage of the latter third group was found to come from divorced homes [3b]. Findings such as these do seem to suggest that a secure mother-daughter relationship may offer better contraceptive understanding as well as protecting the girl from an unconscious need to conceive. Also, that girls in whose lives early parental separation and possible single parenthood occurred, are more liable to risk single motherhood and have the emotional motivation to do so. (Also see section 29.3.)

When a young girl has a baby, she requires support. Ninety per cent of a national sample of 533 teenage mothers interviewed in England and Wales reported finding their health visitors helpful, although a small proportion found problems of communication and a need for more reassurance and advice [4]. However more than health care support is required. If the girl's mother is able and willing to look after her, or if she has a loving partner who will provide nurturance and mother her so she can mother her child, she may be able to utilize the experience of parenting a baby to grow up herself, vicariously enjoying the love she lavishes on her baby. In the absence of these an immature girl may experience 'sibling' rivalry and competitiveness towards her own baby, feeling that resources are scarce and that there is not enough for both of them. Her own dependence and unresolved hungry need for mothering will prevent her generosity towards the infant.

Other adolescents may use pregnancy as a means of filling an old dissatisfied emptiness inside themselves, carrying the hope of self-renewal and a chance to change everything. On giving birth the girl may feel resentfully disillusioned as life becomes more difficult rather than easier. Her life is restricted – many schools refuse to keep a pregnant pupil on their registers and few educational institutions have creche facilities available for mothers of young infants. Simple outings and shopping expeditions involve planning and transporting baby and paraphenalia. She is unable to take the baby to teenage haunts and baby-sitters are expensive. Social Security and supplementary benefits are insufficient, and even if married, very young couples are likely to have low income. Travelling by public transport is complicated with a pram or pushchair. Her old friends pursue their own interests which are no longer identical to her own; she may feel socially ostracized or abandoned by her friends, virtually isolated, cooped up with a baby and a pile of dirty nappies. How she spends her time is dictated by the baby, any available attention is focused on the infant and she feels further left-out if her baby becomes the centre of attraction. If breastfeeding, her body is no longer her own to do with as she pleases, and sexuality may be curtailed if she lacks a partner and the freedom to meet her peers. Sorely disappointed with the reality of a baby who changes things for the worse, who is a real person making real demands and needing full-time attention, the irritable hurt mother may resort to teasing the baby, rebelliously neglecting him/her or actively becoming the sadistic uncaring mother she has internalized, in impulsive acts of punitive emotional or physical cruelty. (Chapter 33)

27.2 PROFESSIONAL ASSISTANCE

The difficulties in coping with mothering a baby while still in need of mothering herself necessitate extra professional attention for the adolescent mother. Special supportive programmes have been developed in the United States in response to the growing social problem of teenage pregnancies. During pregnancy, these emphasize parenting skills and health care practices to counteract the higher incidence of low-birth weight and premature babies among adolescent parents, and the greater risk for child abuse [5]. Much research has been focused on improving professional support for adolescent mothers in the form of parenting advice and classes [6] and investigations have attempted to determine the quality of support systems that would decrease stress and foster positive functioning during pregnancy and postpartum [7]. As indicated, the health visitor and often, the social worker, play a crucial role following the birth.

However, there are teenage mothers whose deep-seated problems require personal therapy to enable them to relate as 'good enough mothers' to their infants. In cases where the adolescent mother's own family have been unable to help by providing ways of resolving the normal teenage conflicts of attachment/independence, these conflicts may be mirrored in her relationship with the baby, with exaggerated and prolonged dependency or inconsistent reliability. Likewise, when universal struggles of adolescence become distorted by personality disorders and familial conflicts, the interlocking crises of puberty and motherhood affect the mother–baby interaction. Babies in these disturbed relationships are inevitably neglected, impoverished in human attachment and subject to distorted interaction with their mothers. For example, where the normal adolescent process of detachment from her oedipal love has not yet been completed, the pregnancy may unconsciously be imbibed with a forbidden and dangerous fantasy of being the love-child of her own father, leaving little emotional availability for a relationship with her sexual partner if she has one. Once born, the baby becomes in fantasy the embodiment of this 'shameful' secret and a make-believe baby rather than flesh and blood.

Inappropriate affective exchanges serve as indicators of emerging problems in the relationship. Whereas a normal positive interaction would be reciprocal, animated and affectionate, reflecting emotional availability and attunement of the mother, these negative exchanges may fall into three patterns:

1. Bland interaction – mother and baby each in their own world and unable to reach out to the other.
2. Angry exchanges – the mother's frustration mirrored by aggressive relating in the child.
3. Mixed negative affects, where the mother and baby are out of synchrony with each other or the mother uses 'double-blind' type discrepancies between contents and tone of voice [8].

27.3 PSYCHOTHERAPEUTIC TREATMENT

Psychotherapy can provide the adolescent mother with psychological nurturance to sustain her in her difficult task and to heal some injuries from the past. It can provide her with a sense of worth as a mother, and by cherishing the baby, undo some of the shameful social stigma or the forbidden aura lent to it by fantasies of oedipal romance. A successful model of intervention in cross-generational maladaptive parenting was pioneered by Fraiberg who developed a therapeutic programme to tackle disorders of attachment and failure to thrive in babies of adolescent mothers [9]. This type of therapy in the home attempts to solve the developmental disorders of two clients, by providing support and emotional guidance while working with the mothers on their own developmental conflicts thereby releasing them emotionally to mother their babies. Mother–baby pairs may also be admitted to special units such as the Cassel Hospital in London which focus on the essential experiences of mothering.

In addition, psychotherapy can provide the adolescent mother, as other teenagers in need of treatment, with an opportunity to work through this second individuation process (as opposed to the first one of relinquishing dependence in early childhood) by achieving independence from their internalized parents. Many adolescent disturbances, both emotional and behavioural, may be seen to be related to this psychic 'restructuring': such as swings from avid hunger for company to emotional withdrawal; from motoric impulsivity and 'action craving' to indifference and passivity; from self-sufficiency and arrogance to dejected states of shame and guilt [10]. Psychotherapy can ameliorate these disturbances by providing what has been termed a forum for 'regression in the service of development' [11], which when provided for the adolescent mother enables her to work through her own revived conflicts about individuation and independence so that she can foster development of healthy individuation and separation in her infant.

27.4 YOUNG FATHERS

Although most research has focused on the easily detectable and readily interviewable housebound teenage mothers, many girls have male partners who have also become parents while very young. Like their female counterparts, they have also had rapidly to achieve the leap from being a kid to seeing oneself as a caregiver and protector of a baby. This change in self-image necessitates an internal reworking of his own relationships with paternal figures. It is here that male professionals such as GPs can have a great positive influence, by serving as a caring model and encouraging nurturing qualities in a young man who has not had a loving father. We tend to have a stereotyped idea that teenage fathers are irresponsible, partly because they impregnated the girl when effective contraception is available. Indeed, in one national survey which located 59% of the partners of 623 mothers aged under 20 years in England and Wales, only 20% were found to have used birth control. A fifth of these men were teenagers and a further two-thirds aged between 20 and 25. Of the sample, 87% were classified as working class, 56% had no further training after leaving school and 12% were unemployed. Four-fifths of those interviewed were married, but comparison with the Office of Population Censuses and Surveys data about births to women under 20 years suggested the researchers had failed to reach less-stable relationships and less positive fathers. Surprisingly, those fathers interviewed expressed a high degree of satisfaction with marriage and fatherhood despite economic adversity, curtailment of social activities and greater responsibilities. Although three-fifths of the marriages took place because of the pregnancy, 40% of the men said they wanted a baby, 75% were pleased when they realized their partner was pregnant and four out of the five had stayed for at least part of the labour. For the majority of the men interviewed, marriage had offered a means of getting away from overcrowded home conditions as most had come from very large families, and nearly one-third of their own mothers had been teenage mothers themselves. Changes in their own life styles following the birth included a sense of responsibility towards the baby (although a small proportion of the men expressed indifference and did not see their offspring). Fathers living in the same household with the baby reported enjoying watching the baby develop, fed the baby at least occasionally, and liked having 'something that belongs to you'. Bathing the infant was the least frequent paternal activity, and noise and nappy-changing were mentioned as the most disliked features of fatherhood. While three-fifths agreed they had matured since having the baby, not all approved of the changes in their partner, and cited tiredness, moodiness, preoccupation, bad temper and possessiveness in the new mother. Nevertheless, achieving rapid maturity was highly regarded in this largely working-class sample as it might not have been among middle-class youths eager to preserve prolonged adolescent freedom [12]. While this survey admirably attempted to focus on both activities and feelings, it reflects the conscious attitudes and experience of the largely working-class sample of fathers interviewed. The procedure of contacting fathers via their female partners means that those fathers who had ambivalent or largely negative feelings towards the baby, the mother and/or fatherhood were unlikely to be reached and deeper unconscious feelings are difficult to determine in a one-off interview. In addition to socioeconomic factors, the nature of a young father's deeper feelings about paternity are determined (as are any father's) by the degree of his own emotional maturity, self-esteem and independence; the quality of his own experience during adolescence and earlier with his father and/or parental figures; and his relationship with the mother of the baby. An overload of responsibility may trigger an emotional crisis.

KEY POINTS

*The juxtaposition of adolescent turmoil, pregnant vulnerability and now, new parenthood, may constitute a great load for a young, unsupported person, particularly when the baby is unplanned.
*Special professional support is needed to help the mother cope with

mothering the baby and fostering his/her growth while herself continuing to develop her potentialities and capacity for self definition.

*Pregnancy imposes additional strains on a teenage couple who are confronted simultaneously with adjusting to the new experience of living together and achieving emotional detachment from their families of origin, while sometimes still sharing the same household. Not only are their individual boundaries threatened by the intimacy and interdependence of close relating to each other, but birth of the baby may further undermine a fragile sense of identity and maturity.

*When family relationships are fraught or distorted, mother and baby, (and possibly the young father too, if he is in contact with them) may need therapeutic intervention, to undo current difficulties between them, and by work on their own underlying developmental conflicts enable the young people to release their emotions from their families of origin for use in the new family they have created.

Chapter 28

Adoption

There are three parties involved in adoption – the birth-mother (parents), the adoptive family, and the adopted child. For each, this contractual solution inevitably brings a lifelong process of adaptation to loss. For the biological mother separation from her child, for adopters, loss of a fantasy child and ideal self, and for the adoptee, the painful fact of having been given away. Professionals can play an important part in facilitating this adjustment.

28.1 THE BIRTH-MOTHER: PRE-ADOPTION COUNSELLING

When abortion has been ethically unacceptable, unavailable or delayed beyond the point of safety, or when emotional, physical or practical factors prohibit mothering, the baby may be offered for adoption. If the decision is made during pregnancy, it is beneficial for a contemplative woman to have counselling or therapy to enable her to work through her feelings about relinquishing her baby, and examine various options while these still operate. However, a woman who feels she has no choice but to give up the baby may not wish to dwell on her loss, fearing that 'opening the floodgates' will complicate her decision. Paradoxically, with availability of contraception and abortion, the stigma of illegitimacy and unmarried motherhood has lessened and increasingly pregnant women decide to become single mothers rather than give up the baby. As a result, the demand for babies far exceeds their availability for adoption, and the double standard of encouraging adopters while ignoring or denigrating the biological mother can no longer operate, as pregnant young girls are wooed to consider relinquishing their babies for adoption [1]. In the United States for some time, and recently in the United Kingdom, adoption agencies and centres are exploring new possibilities in considering the needs of birth-mothers and offering counselling (at her discretion) to herself, her partner and/or parents during the pregnancy to consider the variety of options available. If a decision to relinquish the baby for adoption is reached, the expectant mother is encouraged to think of the process as a preliminary one, to be reviewed after the baby is a reality. Further recognition of her predicament, the solution of which may entail painful self-sacrifice, can be furthered by exploring her feelings and needs in therapy, as well as the practicalities of implementing her decision in the way which best reflects these.

'Open adoption' is a consideration, empowering the mother to have some say in choosing the adoptive couple and possibly meeting them; preparing an information profile on herself for the baby, knowing her child's general whereabouts, receiving non-identifying reports and possibly maintaining some form of future contact through updated photographs, letters and even visits. It has been suggested that the process of pre-placement information collation should involve the active participation of the birth-family, in both contested and uncontested adoptions. The format could include basic factual and chronological information about the child and extended family; full photographic documentation of the wider family and places of significance; medical documents; self-descriptions by family members with particular attention to their positive qualities, attributes and aspirations. Tape recordings and video material may be an adjunct [2]. In addition a birth record of maternal or staff impressions of the labour and delivery might be of interest.

During childbirth and the postnatal period, nursing staff at the hospital play a critical role in creating an emotional environment that may be either tolerant and supportive or moralistic and destructive for the mother surrendering her baby for adoption. Some places recognize the similarity to other painful processes and encourage the mother to spend time saying goodbye to her baby [3]. A facilitating professional can help negotiate this phase, by reassuring the parturient and her family their grief is normal and that the final decision should be postponed until after the period of intense mourning. Some adoptive agencies enable the birth-parent(s) and adoptive parents to meet before placement to help them form a positive realistic image of each other, thereby reducing the potential for fantasy and/or denial [4]. Such a meeting constitutes recognition of the handing over of a baby to be treasured, rather than the baby 'vanishing into thin air' from the birth-mother's point of view, or 'materializing out of the blue' for the adoptive parents. Individual counselling by someone totally unlinked to the adoptive family during the interim stage between placement and finalization of the adoption, could help the mother review her decision and move on in her life.

In some cases, the pregnant woman might be reluctant to engage in exploring her feelings at all, resisting any form of introspection which might weaken her resolve to surrender the baby for adoption. She may defensively prefer to continue her life as if pregnancy were but a temporary medical condition, blotting out awareness of movements and symptoms and even expressing a wish to have a general anaesthetic during labour and birth. After the birth, she may persist in her desire to know as little as possible about this 'unfortunate episode' before resuming her 'real' life. However, even in the most clear-cut cases, for instance, of an unwanted baby following rape, the memory of this life event cannot, in the long run, be wiped out and in years to come the knowledge that someone who was part of her is breathing and growing somewhere in the world, unknown to her yet possibly seeking her, remains a potential torment, revived during subsequent pregnancies and motherhood.

28.2 BIRTH-MOTHER: POST-ADOPTION COUNSELLING

Psychotherapy or counselling may be promoted at a later date to work through these unresolved feelings about the adoption. Indeed, the Post Adoption Centre in London have found their workshops and groups for birth-mothers attended by several hundred women, some of whom had given up a child for adoption as long as 40 years previously, and many of whom had never disclosed or discussed their loss before. All the women seen had suffered varying degrees of mental stress following their relinquishment. These were experienced as 'physical ailments, relationship difficulties, mental breakdown, infertility, reactive depression and sexual problems' [5]. In addition to the therapeutic benefits to themselves in 'de-compartmentalizing' their secret, relinquishing defences and expressing pent-up grief, anger and loss, and retrieving self-respect, these groups contributed further to understanding about counselling needs of such women. Three themes are found to be of central importance in helping women face and integrate their past:

(a) The traumatic effect of the pregnancy and relinquishment of the child

These include failure to grieve; total amnesia or selective recall; repression of the pain of loss, resulting in psychosomatic conversion; low self-image, guilt and inability to engage fully in adult relationships; unresolved feelings of resentment, anger and blame towards the baby's father and her own parents or persecution where her rights were terminated involuntarily; morbid fear of sex and pregnancy, resulting in possible psychogenic infertility; overprotectiveness or unrealistic expectations of subsequent children.

(b) 'Universal need to know' if child is alive and well

Absence of knowledge results in a 'reality' based on fantasy. The desire to know and to reclaim may become an obsession overshadowing the realities of life. Transracial adoptions may be accompanied by persistent fears of prejudice. There is a need to know whether their expectations for a 'better deal' for the child have been met; whether the child is physically and mentally well and knows s/he is adopted; what s/he looks like, whether s/he has children, and what would happen if s/he was orphaned. There is a desire to know whether the placing agency would be willing to facilitate contact, to update records, and allow non-identifying information, and to inform parties involved of the respective deaths of birth-mother, adoptive parents or adoptee.

(c) Preparation for being traced

Once work has been done on separation and loss, exploration can centre on conflicting concerns about being sought by and/or rejected by the adoptee, being wrongly perceived in the past and after a possible reunion; concerns about an unexpected reunion and consequences of sharing their secret with partners, subsequent children, parents and significant relatives [6].

When the decision to have the baby adopted is taken after the birth due to the mother's mental or physical incapacity or when separation has been delayed and caregiving of the baby prolonged despite intended relinquishment, the mother will require special therapeutic help.

28.3 ADOPTIVE PARENTS: PRE-ADOPTIVE PROCEDURES

The decline in the number of babies for adoption after the peaks in the 1960s and 70s resulted in close scrutiny of would-be adopters, prolonged assessment procedures and fluctuating policies of 'matching' baby and parents for race, appearance, class and religious background. This policy was later reversed by the British Adoption Project (BAP) who placed black babies with white families, followed by the Adoption Resource Exchange (ARE) founded to coordinate homefinding efforts for black children and those with special needs. The Post Adoption Centre in London has utilized feedback from over 1600 adoptees and some 450 adoptive parents to conclude that matching fulfils a function both for the child who wishes to identify with the adoptive parents and the latters' need for some congruence between the child placed and the fantasy one hoped for. A cultural, social or racial gulf may result in unrealistic expectations and cause children to feel out of tune and cut off from their heritage [7]. Recently, the policy of racial matching of adoptive parents and baby has been reinstated.

The process of assessment can be a difficult one for would-be parents, particularly following prolonged unsuccessful treatment for infertility. Adoption is a compromise to which they feel driven by circumstance rather than choice. At the very time of needing a receptive ear for their ambivalence and sorrow, the assessment worker appears to be wanting whole-hearted commitment and joyful anticipation. Feeling scrutinized and in danger of being considered ungrateful for this rare chance to adopt, would-be-parents may present the false image they assume is required. Others truly work themselves up into unrealistic expectations that the adoption will erase their sadness at not having a baby of their own. Such unresolved idealization leads to inevitable disillusionment, since the replacement child cannot live up to the ideal and the narcissistic wound of being unable to have a baby cannot be healed by getting a baby, which does not replace carrying one. Once again, the unfulfilled yearning to be pregnant must be distinguished from the desire for a child which adoption meets. Paradoxically, the taboo on explicit preconceptions of an ideal child is conveyed by the agency's covert message that the parents should love whomever they get. It is recommended that adoption agencies may help prospective adopters to express and understand their mixed feelings by acknowledging their need to grieve their lost hopes, encouraging them to perform tangible tasks such as preparing a life-story including their infertility (to mirror the life-story work done with older adopted children), preparing them for the placement reopening old wounds (even with a second child), and by keeping in touch while awaiting placement, thus promoting realistic expectations rather than fantasy [8]. Support groups help negotiate the transition to parenthood. ['At the adoption support group, it was just wonderful. I felt uplifted being in a room full of people sharing my experience of pain and frustration and differentness, anger and now, hope – like a hungry person, I've been longing, yearning to voice these feelings that my husband doesn't seem to understand at all. But I find I have a right to my feelings. . . . I don't have a pregnancy. I don't have any of the visible signs but I'm going through something similar while waiting and have a lot of things going on inside preparing, dreaming, planning for my baby. My sadness is that I'm doing it alone but I suppose if I was pregnant, he couldn't really share that experience either. But I'm not alone or crazy – there are other people who understand and feel like me so I'm entitled to feel sad without feeling bad or mad'.] The adoption procedures themselves may magnify the risks inherent in any adoption by serving as a receptacle for persecutory feelings and encouraging the couple to believe that obstacles (in the form of bureaucratic difficulties) lie outside themselves rather than enabling them to explore their own difficulties with each other and their internal parents [9].

28.4 ADOPTIVE PARENTS AND GRANDPARENTS: BONDING

The bonding process in adoptive families is hampered by lack of a defined period of waiting, analogous to pregnancy. Parents may be on 'red alert' for prolonged periods of time, or have a baby sprung on them without much warning. Time is not punctuated by preparatory physiological changes and gradual build-up of rhythmical interactions with the baby, and acquaintance with the infant must be made from 'scratch'. However, unlike the adopting mother, the baby has experienced pregnancy. The child-in-the-womb has built up a rhythmic biological bond with a woman who will not be his/her mother. Prenatal psychologists believe the adopted baby has to learn to separate from the mother s/he has known *in utero* and form an attachment to a new set of parents [10]. Some parents believe this too. They feel that their newborn baby has already had intimate prenatal and birth experiences and possible memories from which they are excluded. These parents interpret the baby's cries or discomfort as pining for the birth-mother's smell, her touch, the sound of her voice or her naturally synchronized rhythmicity. Such hypersensitivity and fear of rejection by the baby may reflect the adopting parents' own unconfessed preferences for a 'natural' child of their own.

Infertile couples who have not yet worked through their sense of inadequacy and injury to self-esteem in being unable to produce a child of their own may inflict their disappointment onto the adopted child who cannot compensate them for their loss. Both blame and 'defect' may be shifted to the child, thereby exonerating the infertile couple, and homing in on the baby's inadequate genetic endowment [11]. Following a prolonged experience of unsuccessful treatment for infertility, couples often have a double sense of failure, feeling they failed to conceive both naturally and with sophisticated medical help. Despite their efforts to adopt, they may unconsciously continue to feel that they are 'forbidden' to have a child as their parents did or feel that their own parenthood is 'not meant to be'. These unconscious beliefs are probably related to unresolved oedipal or incestuous conflicts with figures in their internal worlds. Arrival of an adopted baby revives the sense of having 'stolen' a child they are not entitled to have. In addition, fantasies about the baby's unknown conceptual and genetic history contribute to difficulties in falling in love with the little stranger who is to be part of their lives. Similarly, the danger that the biological mother may change her mind and repossess her baby may engender further reluctance to become irrevocably attached until the six months 'probation' period are over. Parents may indeed feel 'on trial' and open to 'inspection' during this initial period, which, as we have seen, is a difficult and demanding time for all new parents. However, the adoptive mother may find it particularly difficult to establish a meshing of reciprocal interchange with the adopted infant because of her belief that the biological mother, whom the baby was once part of, could have done it spontaneously and better. Emotional signalling between the infant and caregiver may become distorted if adoptive parents attribute meanings beyond those implied in the communication.

If the adopted child is felt to emphasize the mother's infertility (i.e. her instinctual incapacity) she may find it difficult to accept the infant's instinctuality (such as soiling, sexual curiosity, aggression), seeing this behaviour as a reflection of the baby's 'bad blood', and a throwback to the birth-mother's imagined heightened sexuality and promiscuity. In cases such as these, the mother's internal representation of the child may consist of two disconnected parts, one acceptable and the other unacceptable, a division which must influence her child's developing sense of identity [12].

As we have seen in previous chapters, becoming a parent reactivates old parent-child intergenerational conflicts, yet also offers an opportunity to repay an old debt and make reparations through the grandchild by symbolically renewing procreation and perpetuating the family line. However, adoptive parents may sadly feel they have not fulfilled their parents' expectations and are unable to identify with their fertile pro-creating parents. Guilt may be exacerbated and the bonding process hampered in adoption if the grandparents' quest for immortality and concern about the bloodline overrides their joy at greeting their own children's adopted baby. Disappointment about lack of genetic continuity may be subtly expressed by the grandparents treating the adopted child differently from other grandchildren or regarding him/her as an 'out-sider', unconsciously condemning him/her as a 'bad seed' and product of 'sin'. These grandparental fantasies may be transmitted to the parents, mediated by unconscious communications and later shared by the child whose own initial experience of abandonment by the natural mother confirms his/her imputed 'badness'. Thus the conflicts of generations will have a positive or negative effect on the parents' attainment of parental identity, attachment and confidence while their reciprocal reactions will influence the child's concept of him/herself [13].

28.5 THE ADOPTED CHILD

That adoption poses special hazards for the child's development is borne out by a review of the literature which finds that adopted children are referred for psychological treatment two to five times more frequently than their non-adopted peers in countries as widely dispersed as Great Britain, Israel, Poland, Sweden and the United States [14]. Symptoms appear to follow a consistent trend, with behaviour characterized in the majority of studies reviewed, as: impulsive, provocative, aggressive and antisocial.

Three sets of deprivations and losses have been specified for the adoptee, each of which has to be mourned:

1. Overt loss of previous attachments (for children placed after 6 months or even earlier).
2. Status loss of being different from other children, and in appearance, from the rest of the family.
3. Covert losses – such as the fact of having been relinquished; lack of knowledge about the original parents; stigmatizing experiences [15].

Recent cognitive research has shown that, contrary to previous ideas, the child's understanding of being adopted does not grow by gradual accretion beginning in the earliest years but rather the early acceptance and understanding shifts between the ages of 6 and 8 years to a more complex attitude characterized by worry, questioning, withdrawal and acting out (such as stealing or seemingly gratuitous aggression). The child is seen to be going through a period of 'adaptive grieving' as she/he acknowledges the loss and pain involved in adoption and explores the two sets of parents' respective motives for relinquishment and for adoption [16]. At each developmental stage, therefore, children need clarifications and new explanations which are synchronized with their current emotional preoccupations and intellectual development to enable reworking and further working through.

In addition to a split representation of being unconsciously regarded as both the adopting parents 'chosen'/'good' child and the biological parents' 'thrown away'/'bad' one, the adopted child also faces an internal split in his/her parental images between the adopting parents who took him/her in and those who let him/her go. The latter may be seen as harsh and rejecting or mythologized as ideal. All children build fantasies at times about their preferred imaginary parents, which Freud termed 'family romances'. However, adopted children have experienced a reality which interferes with playful fantasy: their 'other' parents are not imaginary but real, although little or nothing may be known about them. Elaborate fantasies may be constructed to justify their abandonment, and casual contacts may be invested with a sense of mystery in the ensuing search for 'real' parents. Creative imagination may be impeded by painful associations, untested in reality because of the dangers inherent in investigating origins and a fear of disloyalty to the adoptive parents [17]. The factual basis of rejection by the biological parents is so painful that it is not uncommon for an adoptive child to set in motion a self-destructive cycle by repeatedly testing the commitment of her/his adoptive parents, demanding ongoing proof of acceptance while engaging in increasingly more unacceptable behaviour which eventually may provoke the very outcome of abandonment and rejection feared [18]. Adolescence, when young people begin to prepare themselves through sexuality for future parenthood, evokes many further conflicts about identity as the adoptee is torn between identification with the fertile biological parents and the infertile adoptive ones. In transracial adoptions the child will have to contend with additional complexities of physical and cultural differences. If the adoptive parents are insecure in their own sexual identities, their anxieties about the adolescent's budding sexuality compound anxieties about heredity and danger. Such 'mutually reinforcing anxiety' may lead to acting out and an extreme form of protest by the adolescent and rigidity and rejection by the parent, which results in adopted children 'exploding out of their families dramatically and prematurely', or refusing to take responsibility for themselves, with such conflicting behaviours as violent rebellion and demanding dependence co-existing simultaneously [19]. Sexual acting out may lead to another precipitous pregnancy and repetition of the adoption situation, with the child now as birth-parent.

28.6 HELPING ADOPTIVE FAMILIES

Adoptive parents are dealing with powerful conflicts and ambivalence in themselves and their child(ren), which, unresolved, may escalate and become embedded in their ongoing relationship. Individual, group or family therapy can help integrate the 'good' with the 'bad' aspects of both child and parents, and create a sense of 'wantedness' in a child who has to come to terms with having been rejected in reality. Furthermore, the burden of having been 'chosen' rather than just 'had' pressurizes the adoptee to do well. The parents themselves often continue to feel scrutinized by society and the child. Feeling on trial as parents, they have to live up to the adoption agency's assessment, to prove themselves worthy of the birth-mother's trust and of the child's internal comparisons. In addition they also have to gain awareness of their own causal relationship to their child without splitting off negative responsibility onto the 'bad mother' out there. The corollary is that the adopted child needs help in mourning the losses in her/his life, and must learn to forgive the abandoning mother. Help may be needed to keep a family dialogue going and for the parents to be alerted to their child's ongoing need for further age-appropriate clarification and support [20]. Although in many cases parents are able to provide for the child, at times, child-therapy might be indicated to help the adoptee work through personal dilemmas or conflicts which they wish to keep private or fear would hurt the parents. Such intervention can release the adopted child or adolescent from a sense of frustrated isolation or break a maladaptive pattern before it escalates. Adoptees wishing to obtain their original birth certificates and/or trace their birth-parents or other blood relatives may need counselling to tide them over this difficult period of deliberations, action, discovery, reappraisal of identity and possible reunion. Often, the urge to search for the birth-parents is renewed as a direct consequence of transitional events in their own life such as marriage or pregnancy.

Adoptive parents live with the burden of having to anticipate the child's needs at each stage of development and meet his/her right to know about their identity, to live with few secrets, to make sense of their experience, to develop a positive integrated self-image, to mourn their losses and to deal with curiosity and derision in the outside world [21]. The Post-Adoption Centre's experience with almost 2000 people has led them to stress the importance of post-adoption support, advice, counselling and workshops, in meeting adoptive families' need for both positive guidance and alleviation of the anxiety inherent in the ongoing process of 'explaining adoption'. They feel that families may be helped by professionals who can go beyond the focus on fact (such as the 'life-story book' compiled by workers for adoptees), to explore the many facets of fantasy through counselling, parents groups and workshops, with professionals giving 'permission' for 'the often sacred subject matter of adoption to become something that can be played with, handled, painted, embellished, dramatized, turned inside-out and transformed via puppets, poetry and pantomimes'. It is their belief that 'this sharing between professionals and parents, parents and children, of the sacred and profane, fantasy and feelings, provides the balance and symmetry that is required in explaining adoption' [22].

Lesbian adoptees [23], adoptive parents who subsequently fall pregnant, adoptees in a 'mixed' family with biological offspring, interfamily adoption, relinquishment of a child for adoption by a birth-mother who has other children aware of the birth, may require special consideration and longer-term individual treatment or family therapy. Since January 1988, Social Service Departments and Adoption Agencies have a statutory obligation to provide a counselling service to all parties involved in adoption. Adoptees, birth-parents and adopters may also benefit from joining a self-help organization such as NORCAP (a self-help group in Oxford), that not only provides counselling and group support but holds a register of adopted people and birth-parents seeking each other.

KEY POINTS

*To consider best the differing needs of all three parties involved in adoption – the birth-mother (and possibly foster parents), the adoptive family and the adopted child – separate specialized professional support should be made available to each.

*The birth-mother may need counselling during pregnancy with the process of deciding whether to relinquish her child. Unresolved mourning following adoption may have long-lasting effects, including psychogenic infertility or overprotection of subsequent children. As in all cases of loss, grief may be eased by forming memories and reducing opportunities for fantasy and denial, by working through separation from the baby, having some say in determining who the adoptive parents might be, providing some record of herself and maintaining some degree of feedback. Foster parents, too, may experience a wrench at the loss of the child they have cared for, particularly in an enforced transracial resettlement.

*The adoptive parents may need help in coming to terms with their reasons for adopting (infertility or perinatal loss), and preparation for the difficult task of bringing up someone else's child. Lacking the anticipatory period of pregnancy, engagement with an empathic professional can initiate a process of self-examination, including enquiry into aspects of their own experiences of being parented by people who bore them and how getting a baby rather than having one, differs. Assessment can be experienced as intrusive and persecutory rather than helpful, and a therapeutic opportunity will be lost if couples try to live up to expectations rather than explore their true feelings and work through their natural ambivalence. Difficulties in bonding may be exacerbated by disappointed grandparents, not included in the preparatory process.

*The adopted child has to come to terms with the loss of previous attachments, being different from others and the fact of having been relinquished. Identity problems may revolve around difficulty in integrating splits between aspects of the self which are identified with each of the two sets of parents, in addition to parental fantasies projected onto the child. Creativity may be stultified by painful associations and fear of investigating his/her origins.

*By virtue of the reality of their non-biological conjunction, adoptive families deal with powerful conflicts and emotions which flare up at nodal points of the adoptee's development, as issues are revitalized and need fresh explanations, reformulation and revised integration.

Part Seven

COMPLICATIONS

Chapter 29

Interrupted pregnancies: abortions

'It was painful and shocking. Not as painful as birth, but sharper, and where I couldn't get at it. I just kept saying, 'Bye bye baby, bye bye baby,' letting the pain out in soft moans as the instruments went in and, after an age, came out again. Afterwards I lay curled in the recovery room like a foetus myself, full of hurt.' (Lesley Saunders, *Hidden Loss*, 1989)

When the act of creating life is rudely interrupted by death or destruction, the depth and range of emotions is inevitably complex.

29.1 INDUCED ABORTIONS: MOTIVATIONS FOR CONCEPTION AND DECISON TO TERMINATE

An abortion not only interrupts the pregnancy by getting rid of a fetus, it interrupts a psychological process, and in so doing constitutes a trauma, whatever the reality of the social situation. What is interrupted by choosing abortion is fulfilment of an old wish to have a child. What is destroyed is not only that child, but something of the woman, who cannot emerge unchanged despite her counterwish to do so [1]. Even an unwanted pregnancy reactivates these feelings: her unconscious wishes, conflicts and anxieties bubble up uninvited in dreams and fantasies during the period of decision-making and may persist for a long time after the abortion. The reasons for conceiving in the first place are invariably complex and often overdetermined by ambivalent unconscious motivation in which the wish to conceive or be pregnant might not reflect the wish to have a child. These unconscious motives for conception and initial reactions to the discovery of pregnancy are underlying forces which affect the rational decision-making process. Abortion may be sought on any number of grounds which are consciously felt by the woman and/or her mate to outweigh desire to keep the pregnancy. Thus circumstances of each pregnancy differ according to the woman's life-experience, emotional support, age, parity, physical and mental health, conscious and unconscious motivation for conception and termination.

29.2 SINGLE WOMEN

The stigma of unmarried motherhood has lessened considerably over the past 20 years. In the 1980s an 'illegitimate' baby was born in Britain every five minutes throughout every day and night representing 14% of live births [2] and conditions for single parents have improved with socioeconomic tax benefits and recognition. Nevertheless, the emotional burden of being an unsupported single mother is more than some women can contemplate. With abortion still freely available to all, anxiety about illegally terminating a pregnancy has been removed, thus theoretically allowing women to make the choices that suit their lives rather than those that reflect their medical connections, ability to manipulate the system or to pay for an abortion. The number of abortions in the UK peaked in 1980 with an average of one baby being aborted every four minutes; 66% of operations being performed on non-married women [3]. American studies have found ethnic and socioeconomic divergences among women seeking terminations. Middle-class white women tend to abort their first pregnancies and to deliver later ones, while women of lesser financial and educational means, and those in some black ethnic minorities deliver their first but abort subsequent pregnancies [4]. Legalized abortion has revealed many emotional sequelae to the whole process of decision-making in addition to the psychological trauma of abortion, which were previously masked by the panic-stricken search and fears involved in securing an illegal abortion and relief on obtaining it.

Decision-making hinges on personal psychological, ethical, religious and socioeconomic issues. It is often further complicated by the attitude of the woman's parents and the man involved. Clearly, conception following a 'one night stand' differs from that in a long-standing or complicated loving relationship. 'Unwanted' conception may have been motivated by any number of factors such as reaction to loss, mistimed expression of joint creativity, hope of restoring a faltering love-relationship, proof-seeking of fertility or 'femininity', premenopausal panic at never becoming pregnant or an incipient fear of loneliness.

Going through with the mutual decision and painful experience of abortion may draw a couple together. However, on some level, unwanted pregnancy invariably causes an emotional rift between the female partner experiencing the abortion and the physically unscathed male who has impregnated her, an unseen 'fault' in the relationship which is not excised with the abortion. Her lover may impose abortion or oppose her decision to abort by upholding his genetic right to her child. She may withhold information from him, about both pregnancy and termination. Her parents may put pressure on her to marry, to keep the child, or to abort against her will, to have the baby adopted or hand it over to them. Finally, her decision may hinge on the lesser of two evils rather than being a true solution ('single motherhood makes me feel desperate – a life of hardships, the stigma and rough life, pinned down – but I'm going through with having this baby, I feel I must – I wish I'd had an abortion at 6 weeks – now its become part of me').

29.3 TEENAGE PREGNANCY

The pregnant teenager is often also single, although conception may also occur within an adolescent marriage or a stable young relationship. Nevertheless, the age of the girl is crucial – a child cannot easily mother a child, and having one would automatically interrupt the trajectory of her life. Although some girls do go ahead and have the baby as a source of love and a solace for loneliness, or as compensation for a deprived childhood, or need to emulate their mothers or other healthier reasons, some adolescents continue the pregnancy out of fear of the abortion, or ignorance of the symptoms, omnipotent denial of consequences or the hope of miscarriage. Yet others, ideologically against abortion, or neurotically engaged in acting out, will give birth then have the baby adopted or hand him/her to her own mother by way of unconscious reparation for an old wound. (Also see Chapter 27 on adolescent parents.)

Conception

In this age of contraceptive availability, media coverage and sex education in schools, few western teenagers can truly claim pregnancy to be the result of total ignorance about birth control. However, obtaining contraception requires some maturity and foresight and conception is often the outcome of contraceptive ambivalence or failure. Sexuality may be used to express rebellious acts of body ownership, bravado or tempting Fate by promiscuous teenagers 'living dangerously'. Some may rationalize that they cannot afford to buy condoms. Inadvertent pregnancy may also follow faulty precautions, mal-use of contraceptives or drunken carelessness. Since fertility usually ensues about 2½ years after menstruation begins, girls who have precociously commenced unprotected sexual activity during the infertile years are overtaken by fecundity, erroneously believing that pregnancy could never happen. Quite commonly, pregnancy is the result of a romantic 'fairy tale' attitude towards reality, in which 'adult' conception is irrationally separated from pubertal 'recreational' sex. On an unconscious level, impregnation may stem from a need to prove virility even as conception may reflect a desire to confirm feminine fecundity or desirability. It may constitute a means of acting out conflictual primary identification with her own mother as a sexually active maternal woman, or enactment of her own infantile relationship to her mother. It has been noted that some adolescents use their bodies to split off and deny painful emotional states by substituting bodily sensations. Although physiologically sexually mature, the body may be used to satisfy yearnings for an early experience of mother/baby closeness, substituting a boyfriend for the mother [5].

Abortion

Approximately one-third of abortions performed annually in the United States are obtained by teenagers. A study of non-pregnant adolescents' attitudes towards abortions and intentions to resolve a pregnancy should it occur finds, not unpredictably, that young women who hold a more positive attitude towards abortion show stronger intentions towards terminating an unwanted pregnancy; that perception of best friend's and mother's attitudes also influence behavioural intentions and that career-orientated teenage girls exhibit more positive attitudes towards abortion and those who feel closer to their boyfriends appear less disposed towards terminating a pregnancy [6]. A study in England and Wales found that a proportion of the national sample of teenage mothers given the choice may not have had their babies as 13% had considered having an abortion and did not seek it out of inertia, embarrassment or fear, whereas those who sought it had been turned down by their doctors on nebulous grounds. The study was conducted in 1979 when 60 000 adolescent women had their babies (a rate of 31 per 1000 women) and 30 000 had abortions (a rate of 17 per 1000) [7]. Many girls deny the pregnancy or are fearful of their parents' reactions and delay or avoid telling them. An early study of abortion gave a breakdown of teenage experience of pregnancy and abortion according to the stage of adolescence – early, middle and late. Very young girls lacking birth-control knowledge or even correlation between intercourse and conception (this was in 1973) may deny the pregnancy and disclaim responsibility for it. An older girl may still blame others for the pregnancy (non-birth control dispensing parents, doctors, etc.), externalizing the guilt and ridding herself of it by seeing pregnancy and abortion as forced upon her. The late adolescent takes the blame upon herself and might have conceived deliberately [8].

As in older couples, pregnancy among teenagers may also reflect the irrational hope of reinforcing a faltering relationship or an unconscious playing out of oedipal fantasies. In some particularly sad cases, abortion may be obtained to get rid of an actually incestuous conception by father, brother or cousin or an unwanted pregnancy following rape or gang-bang. In most cases abortion constitutes a complex decision reflecting the simple realization that she is not ready to mother a child yet although the decision may be rationalized in lofty ideals such as not contributing to overpopulation or physiological ones such as hating the experience of nausea. Pregnancy and abortion, like anorexia, might be used by the teenager to enact a desperate competition with her mother over ownership of her own body and its contents. It may also reflect her need to prove that her body is feminine and in procreative working order, a wish that is fulfilled by conception rather than a desire to have a baby. Whatever the reasons for choosing a termination, there is a poignancy about youth having to make irreversible life-decisions at a time when they are idealistic and supersensitive, and when the normal emotional storm and stress of adolescence is compounded by the turmoil of pregnancy. As in all operations conducted on children and teenagers, special attention to emotional preparation, ongoing support and aftercare are necessary, and counselling may be required to alleviate the long-term guilt. ('No success can wipe out what I did to my baby and home.')

29.4 PARTNERED ABORTION

As above, a pregnancy might be unwanted because the father of the baby is not the preferred partner. Infidelity, extra-marital conception and promiscuity pose the moral dilemma of whether to tell the partner that the baby may not be his, and whether to consult him about the abortion. Furthermore, abortion offers both punishment and moral solution unconsciously required in most such 'forbidden' sexual encounters.

In a partnership, abortion may be sought on economic grounds, either because of lack of resources, poverty and inability to give the baby the care parents would wish, or out of career considerations, long-term economic plans and other reasons of unsuitable timing or imperfect conditions. There may already be other children and insufficient devotion and emotional resources to extend to another baby. The decision to abort a fetus after having children makes it difficult for the couple to dismiss the aborted matter as a 'bunch of cells'. To parents, the embryo is a potential child, like their others, and their decision to destroy it takes on painful emotional and moral significance of a different order to ethical dilemmas of some childless women.

Conception may have been motivated by a desire to be pregnant rather than have a baby. An untenable pregnancy often occurs following a bereavement or notice of terminal illness in a grandparent, reflecting a sentimental desire to reinstate the loved one or to provide genetic continuity but not necessarily the wish to have a baby. Unwanted pregnancy following contraceptive failure will inevitably arouse anger and loss of faith in birth control. The woman may feel trapped in an unsatisfying relationship and dread the long-term commitment a baby would entail. Paradoxically, unplanned, unwanted pregnancy nevertheless may arouse mixed feelings of anger yet also relief and pride about her fecundity and functioning female body in an older woman and she may pathetically relish her brief pregnancy despite the necessity to terminate it.

Making the decision to abort reveals hidden chasms within the couple's relationship, with disagreements about whether to have children at all or at this time. A woman may rationally recognize her husband's incapacity to father any or more children, agreeing to the abortion out of consideration for him, despite her own deep desires to have the child. As well as unconsciously motivated contraceptive risk-taking, conception may be the result of one partner's decision to conceive, or thoughtless or drunken imposition; a broody man may withhold contraception to impregnate his unwilling partner or a woman may have removed her coil or come off the pill unbeknown to her husband in the hope that he would 'come round' to keeping the child once she conceived. In these unilateral cases, what is destroyed with the abortion in addition to the marital trust is her sense of inner value. She may feel raped, cheated or deeply humiliated: deceived by him or self-betrayed by her own attempt to seduce him – not only was he unmoved by her act of creativity, she has colluded with him in its destruction and in the attack on her body. Such diversive chasms may reappear years after a seemingly matter-of-fact abortion to which one partner agreed against his/her heartfelt desires out of love for the other. The reawakening of guilt and regrets about the vital sacrifice may be accompanied by silent or verbalized accusations of child-murder and blaming the spouse for aborting their mutuality. Termination resulting from a conjoint decision to remain 'childfree' may be followed by sterilization, or by a pregnancy at some later date during which many unconscious abortion-related hidden persecutory feelings may resurface.

29.5 FETAL ABNORMALITIES

These abortions are often particularly poignant, as they come late in a wanted pregnancy after the experience of motility and attachment. Some information, such as AFP (alpha fetoprotein screening for spina bifida and ancephaly) and amniocentesis results only become available at 17–20 weeks. Even if a woman has consciously withheld her affections from the fetus until receiving the test results, abortion still entails loss of the baby, loss of hopes, disillusioned trust in 'wholesome' conception, loss of her pregnant state and severing of an emotional process which has already artificially been held in abeyance. Irrespective of whether the reason for aborting is a developmental disturbance or a hereditary disorder, some of the pain at their helpless decision is deflected by the couple into irrational guilt at being the cause of abnormality, through their actions or inactions. Culpability may focus on parental infections during or before the pregnancy, falls, food, alcohol, tobacco or medication, dental

X-ray and other radiation, or simply timing – having brought about unification of that particular combination of sperm and ovum. They may deflect their guilt, projecting blame onto the hospital staff, erroneously assuming the tragedy could have been averted or feeling anger at having the dilemma at all or raging about the tardiness of medical test results. In addition to the normal reactions of shock, disbelief, blame, anger, guilt and sorrow, parents may worry as to whether their baby felt pain during the abortion and whether they may have made the wrong decision. Years later anniversaries of the due date may be marked as an uncelebrated birthday and self-recriminating doubts about having unquestioningly believed in the veracity of the diagnostic verdict or their own incapacity to cope, may suddenly flood the couple. In addition, a sense of unworthiness and feelings of inadequacy and inability to produce a healthy child pervade grief about the loss, and may also accompany the following pregnancies until reassured by the birth of a live normal baby. In some tragic cases, unresolved guilt over the termination overshadows the subsequent birth of a healthy child who can never replace the wanted aborted first. Not surprisingly, studies have shown a high incidence of depression following termination of a malformed fetus [9].

29.6 ABORTION AND SEX PREFERENCES

Prenatal screening enables selective termination in hereditary conditions which are gender-specific. However, one of the spin-offs of prenatal testing is sexing of the normal fetus. This knowledge is used by some parents as a reason for aborting the child of the 'wrong' sex. Some cultures have a strong bias in favour of male firstborns. In others, additional females may constitute an economic drain (in terms of work-restrictions and dowry requirements) in a family already stretched to its limits. Council housing laws which provide separate bedrooms for different-sex siblings may heighten the disappointment of discovering that the fetus is the same gender as other children in an overcrowded household. In many cases, be they patriarchs wishing a male heir, carriers of sex-linked conditions or lesbians who cannot tolerate a male fetus, the decision to abort may be the result of prolonged and heartfelt deliberations. In others, the decision may be rationalized by turning the fetus into a dispensable 'non-human thing' a 'mass of cells' or 'matter' and the operation into a casual semimedical procedure, like having a tooth out. Indeed, in their advertising, some private clinics collude with this idea, promising a brief in-and-out procedure in which the woman never even removes her street clothing.

29.7 ABORTION DUE TO MATERNAL ANXIETY AND ILL-HEALTH

While seemingly more justified than some so-called 'social' terminations done on flimsy grounds, aborting for the sake of the mother's health or peace of mind may leave the couple feeling guilty about 'selfishness' of their decision, particularly if pregnancy is not life-threatening. Abortion may be sought because of excessive anxiety, unpleasant physical side-effects of pregnancy, panic at parenthood, exacerbation of a pre-existing medical condition or the realization that chronic ill-health will affect the woman's ability to mother. For a long time after the abortion, despite her involvement in the decision to terminate, a woman may continue to feel deprived of her baby or incomplete in her femininity and reverberations of their action may destabilize the marriage. Abortion of a pregnancy that has caused concern, such as one occurring with an unremoved IUCD coil inside the womb or following exposure to X-rays, toxic chemicals or infections, often continues to haunt the mother with doubts about the necessity for her decision while blaming herself for her 'negligence'.

29.8 REPEATERS

With increasing social acceptance and legalization of abortion on the one hand, and disillusionment with many female-based birth-control methods on the other, many women have more than one abortion. Although prejudiciously held to be amoral or irresponsible, Scandinavian studies have found that these women were not psychologically 'deviant' compared with first timers or non-aborting pregnant women but in fact tended to be of higher professional status, had more children, more sexual partners, greater experiences with different types of contraceptives and more trouble with their previous pregnancies, e.g. they were at higher risk for pregnancy and more incapacitated by it [10]. However, the necessity for repeated abortions could be eliminated for many women with effective, better researched non-harmful contraception, post-abortion counselling, realistic support systems and better childcare, financial help and social service facilities to prevent socioeconomically induced abortions. For other women driven to conceive against their rational impulses, timely psycho-therapeutic investigation following the first abortion, of their complex unconscious reasons to be pregnant and abort, may prevent them becoming repeaters.

The emotional process of abortion may be subdivided into three stages – preabortion, abortion experience and psychological sequelae.

29.9 PREABORTION DECISION-MAKING

Coming to terms with the reality of an unplanned pregnancy and its consequences is the first step in deciding whether or not to abort. Some couples may spend long hours debating the painful issue. In others, the decision will be a foregone conclusion or, more rarely, an impulsive act. Some women may block out both emotions and awareness of options in an urgent need for resolution. Even when the abortion provides a woman with the symbolic means of evacuating unpleasant feelings along with the embryo, natural ambivalence may break through her matter-of-fact plan as she is caught unawares by twinges of loss. Knowledge of alternatives, understanding the consequences and availability of choice must underlie the notion of informed consent. The process of deciding to terminate and get rid of something from inside oneself is a complex one. The fetus may not merely be seen as the child of its mother and father, but also represent some aspect of the woman herself. Confusion can be eased by professional counselling in which the woman is given a breathing space to discover the meaning in her own mind of what is being terminated. On a rational level opportunity is provided to explore other avenues and weigh up the pros and cons and effects of each. Some time into the consultation(s), a client should be asked whether or not she would like to include her partner or parents in the conselling session, as their own views might need to be sounded out in the safety of a neutral space, particularly when discussions have been heatedly emotional or non-existent.

Where time allows, a delay between pregnancy confirmation and the abortion itself, even if it is only a few days, enables the woman to consider this vital decision in a less hurried way, on her home ground. Women who are unresolved should be encouraged to attend for further counselling or psychotherapy sessions. Where this service is not readily available, it has been suggested that the interviewing nurses may be trained to facilitate expression of the clients' feelings during the course of history-taking and imparting information about the method and experience of abortion, and by providing a caring, non-judgemental atmosphere, help her arrive at the best decision for herself by working through her alternatives [11].

29.10 ABORTION PROCEDURE

Depending on the woman's condition, current local trends and whether the abortion takes place in early or late pregnancy, methods will vary from menstrual extraction, vacuum aspiration, D&C, D&E, saline or prostaglandin induction, hysterotomy or hysterectomy. In each situation the client will need to be told in detail what to expect during and after the procedure, in the clinic and later at home. While waiting for the operation she will probably be scared and need reassurance and encouragement from her companion and/or staff. Once the operation has started the patient may have a pang of remorse and try and stop the proceedings. One means employed by some clinics to prevent this last minute panic when it is too late, is to give some women responsibility for actively conducting some aspect of the procedure for herself, such as a pill (placebo or tranquillizer) to take the night before it all begins. Thus she herself has to make the decision to initiate the process leading to the abortion, in her own space and time without experiencing the pressure of authority figures or relegating responsibility to them [12].

Some regret is inevitable even in the most clear-cut case and any slight atmosphere of moral disapproval in the clinic will exacerbate her guilt and belatedly retrigger ambivalent doubts. Painful procedures may be experienced as rightful punishment for her deed. They might arouse her anger at the man who 'got away with murder' and hurtful recriminations against him if he is present. Whether a partner or parent of a younger girl remains with her must depend not only on hospital policy but each individual's needs. In some American abortion clinics, the aborting woman is accompanied by a feminist patient-advocate who 'watchdogs' the procedure for dehumanizing aspects such as casual disrespect (staff chit-chat during the operation) or instruments (such as metal vs. plastic speculum and unnecessary large tubes) which serve doctor rather than patient [13].

Late abortions are both physically and emotionally more taxing. The prolonged procedure and its similarity to labour exacerbate guilt in a woman who has already had prolonged conflicts about the abortion as the postponement suggests, and possibly has felt the fetus moving. Hospitals vary in the care they offer and some still insensitively place abortion patients in with women having babies. In others, patients are left alone for long periods of time with insufficient information or pain relief [14] where pairing aborting women or providing each with a 'doula' might provide support. Some women may need a midwife present through labour and birth. Women having a late abortion have a particularly difficult time, in effect experiencing very painful labour with no prize at its end. Those who wish to see their fetus or ask to know what sex the 'baby' was, are indicating the poignant ambivalence of their decision, made with full awareness of a person being 'killed' rather than an 'it' or 'clump of cells'. Although some nurses prefer to keep the knowledge of gender from the mother, the question to be asked is whether, since the fetus is hers, she does not have a right to this information, and whether seeing the fetus will help her grieve its destruction or merely exacerbate her guilt. As we have noted, women or couples experiencing termination for abnormality are particularly vulnerable, having made the decision to abort a wanted pregnancy. Some parents may wish to have the fetus photographed or to hold their dead baby, however macerated. Some professionals regard this as a morbid interest, but to the parents it may be a necessary step in their mourning process, which may also include naming, baptizing or having a funeral for the aborted baby.

29.11 PSYCHOLOGICAL SEQUELAE

The initial feeling of relief of an elected abortion is often followed by a syndrome of grieving, regrets and tearfulness termed the 'post-abortion blues'. Where milk production has not been suppressed, women may suffer acute distress. Even in cases where no conscious sadness is experienced, feelings of feminine inadequacy may surface now or many months or years later, alongside unmourned loss and guilt conveyed in recurrent dreams of lost babies, operations or deaths. In some cases, when these conflicts have been sufficiently worked through in preabortion counselling, relief predominates over sadness, with a sense of having made the right choice. Long-term morbidity is rare following termination, but in a prospective study of 216 women, 7% still felt considerable guilt 18 months later [15]. The anniversary of the expected birth or the abortion date, a major marital disillusionment or the subsequent birth of a baby, can trigger earlier unresolved feelings and previously unknown emotional reactions, including anger at the parents, boyfriend or husband who did not intervene forcefully to stop the abortion, which with hindsight, she regrets.

Follow-up care allows the woman a further opportunity to express her feelings, for which, in cases of secrecy or reticence, she may not have another listener. Women who have had to overcome religious qualms may fear retribution and interpret any negative life event as a punishment. Others fear paying for the abortion with future infertility. Sexual inhibitions may arise as the woman fears a repeat impregnation or finds sex repulsive now it is associated with ending life rather than creating it. Women who have lost faith in birth control and appear currently disillusioned with sex need attentive contraceptive advice to prevent future repeat abortions. Severe depression, persistent guilt reactions, sexual problems or marital discord specifically related to the abortion may indicate a need for specialized help. It is at this point of follow-up that women who request or appear to require psychotherapeutic intervention should be offered an opportunity for referral. Parents who have aborted following diagnosis of fetal abnormality always need genetic counselling and post-mortem information. Prolonged sexual difficulties following such a termination are not uncommon, reflecting the painful contamination of procreativity and mortality [16]. They may benefit from being put in touch with other parents suffering similar losses.

29.12 PSYCHOLOGICAL IMPLICATIONS FOR
ABORTION CLINIC PERSONNEL

Working in an abortion clinic can pose difficult problems for people who have chosen a caring profession to help create rather than destroy life. Faced with the juxtaposition of a seemingly casual abortion and an infertile client or one battling to overcome habitual miscarriages, some professionals find themselves unable to maintain neutrality. While condoning abortions following rape, incest, fetal abnormality or due to maternal impairment, some nurses, midwives and doctors may feel that other abortions are immoral. Late abortions inevitably raise many ethical dilemmas, particularly with the decreasing age of viability for preterm births. Faced with a live, squirming and possibly viable aborted fetus should the caring nurse or doctor dispose of it or put it into an incubator? When professionals find they are identifying more with the fetus than with the woman aborting it, their bias will surface and the woman will experience it as disapproval. Members of some ethnic minorities or religious groups, among both staff and clients, may experience particularly difficult conflicts, as they grapple with religious taboos, racial prejudice and subcultural social mores regarding abortion. As in all stressful jobs affecting morale, professionals may benefit from a regular staff group-meeting as an outlet to vent their frustrations, to release emotions which have been stirred up by contact with people experiencing physical and emotional loss and to regain a sympathetic perspective towards women who have no choice but to make the sad choice, of aborting their babies. Staff may benefit from workshops run by counsellors focusing on the skills of listening to distressed people without hearty jollying or sedation, the art of conveying painful information to disbelieving clients and absolving parents from guilt and self-blame while strengthening the inner resources professionals require to cope with acute grief reactions and absorb the flack of irrational accusations and anger without personal affront.

KEY POINTS

*The decision to have an abortion is a complicated one, influenced by each woman's psychosexual history, conscious and unconscious motivation for conception, timing of the pregnancy, emotional and social support, age, parity and current circumstances.

*Pregnancies terminated because of fetal abnormality, maternal ill-health or partner pressure leave a residue of guilt and sorrow that, untreated, may affect future pregnancies.

*Women finding the idea of an abortion scary, need support, particularly during late abortions when labour and birth are simulated but produce no 'prize'.

*Follow-up care is an essential part of treatment as it allows the woman a further opportunity to express and abreact her feelings, for which, in cases of secrecy or reticence, she may not have another listener.

*Due to the pressures of working in an abortion clinic, professionals may benefit from a staff group in which they can offload their own feelings and workshops run by counsellors to foster listening and coping skills for dealing with distressed people.

Chapter 30

Prebirth loss and pregnancy complications

30.1 MISCARRIAGE

'Three times then/ Seeping loss/ And with each seeping/ A child becoming nothing/ An empty hollow pain/ A flushing away – / Then grief.' . . . (Miscarriage, Penny's Poem, in *Hidden loss – miscarriage and ectopic pregnancy*)

30.1.1 Spontaneous abortion

About one in six confirmed pregnancies end in miscarriage, 75% of these occurring during the first trimester and some 60% of these showing evidence of chromosomal disorders. Thus, the crisis of miscarriage often begins at home. During early pregnancy, spotting, cramps or pain may be disregarded until considerable bleeding or expulsion raise the alarm. This denial could be due to emotional ambivalence about the pregnancy, ignorance or a hope that if she ignores it 'it will go away'. With threatened abortion or gradual and prolonged miscarriage, the hopeful woman reaches an emotional watershed, after which she hopes the fetus will be miscarried as she cannot believe it would be born healthy after all the pain and profuse loss of blood.

These days of anxious uncertainty are particularly difficult for busy women and mothers who try to take bedrest in the hope of preventing the miscarriage, monitor the colour and clots in their bleeding, and blame themselves and silently question what they might have done to bring on the miscarriage, while being emotionally available to answer and appease mystified children. Nevertheless, the longer period of adjustment gives them time to 'deflate' the hopes and aspirations of pregnancy in a way that abrupt spontaneous abortion does not. After the latter, women often feel dazed and bewildered by the sudden unexplained change in their fertile status, and may be as disbelieving of the miscarriage as they were of the unseen conception.

A late miscarriage, heralded by bleeding or leakage, catches by surprise the woman who has begun to take her pregnancy for granted. The wide circle of concerned relatives and acquaintances who know of the pregnancy will enhance her precarious sense of being at the mercy of erratic fate, and although their support can be a comfort during the long helpless days of waiting for a threatened miscarriage to settle, if she does abort, she may feel she has let them all down. If miscarriage occurs in hospital, the aborted fetus may be unceremoniously removed, usually in a bedpan, and women are not generally asked whether they would like to see the baby. Bodies may be disposed of in the hospital incinerator or macerated and, according to some reports, flushed down the 'foul drain'. Staff may feel they are protecting the mother from the sight of a monstrosity. However, their attitude of dismissal and disposal is hurtful to the shamed mother, and implies that her baby is 'an object unfit to be seen, unfit to be loved, unfit to live and not worthy of mourning' [1]. The woman too may be unceremoniously 'removed', discharged from the ward, having become an embarrassment in a place that is dedicated to producing life not death. Questions about what happened to her aborted baby may continue to persecute her in waking thoughts and dreams.

Most women feel they would like information about the cause of the miscarriage, both to reduce the sense of guilt, mystery, confusion and unfinished business about this pregnancy and to ensure that this miscarriage does not preclude another full-term pregnancy. If it occurred at home, they arrive at the clinic clutching what remains of the 'products of conception', the expelled contents of their body which they have painstakingly collected, often having had to overcome squeamishness and trepidation to do so. In most cases a woman who has miscarried is simply given a check-up or D & C but no tests are conducted on the expelled fetus (which might not even be accepted from her) and she is blandly told that 'each pregnancy is unconnected to the one before' or to 'go home, wait three months and try again'. Justification for lack of routine examinations is expense and since over 50% of spontaneously aborted fetuses are abnormal, prevention of miscarriage without commensurate prenatal screening would lead to an enormous increase in the numbers of handicapped babies born. To the woman seeking information why her baby died and whether it will happen again, it matters greatly whether this was a 'blighted' pregnancy, a hormonal insufficiency or genetic abnormality. Above all she needs to differentiate a random event from one with a cause that can be cured; she wants to know how future pregnancies may fare and whether she herself is to blame in any way. A miscarriage, like a still-birth, is a non-event. However, unlike the latter, she may be granted little recognition of her emotional condition or entitlement to any legitimate grief by relatives or professional staff. Indeed, if she has not begun disclosing it, many people may not even realize she has been pregnant. She tries desperately to make sense of her tragedy.

('I feel like a cork bobbing at the mercy of dark forces of inevitability. There is no arbitrariness to Fate. When I lost the baby, in my mind it was clearly a punishment for the abortion I'd had when I was 19. You can't get away from what you've done. It catches you up in the end.') In reality, less than 4% of miscarriages are due to previous abortions.

('With the miscarriage it was as if my parents whisked me back to the past, breaking the illusion of freedom I'd had all these past years since leaving home. I'd been so lively and happy in my pregnancy but when I came to visit them, they felt I was flaunting it defiantly and the next thing I knew I was bleeding. They killed the life in me. This miscarriage was murder, a vindictive act, their revenge on me for wanting my own independent life.') Miscarriage can follow emotional stress.

Even early miscarriage means that on some level, a bereaved woman is burying her hopes for a baby, losing trust in her body's reliability and her special connection to her partner's genetic being. In a society in which 'people tend to stigmatize the bereaved as if their loss and suffering is catching', the depth of feeling and duration of grief are often denied yet the woman who has experienced a prebirth loss needs to be granted the right to mourn, not as a 'self-indulgence or weakness', but as a 'psychological necessity' [2]. The ensuing process of grieving follows the stages of all mourning – shock, pangs of grief and search for the baby, painful acceptance of the loss and gradual recuperation. Nevertheless, miscarriage is not regarded as a 'proper' bereavement ('not like losing a real baby is it?'), although as one woman who has had seven miscarriages writes years later: 'the lost babies never let go, I can remember exactly when each one was due' [3].

30.1.2 Missed 'abortion'

The bizarre situation when pregnancy technically ends and the fetus dies *in utero* but is not expelled for some weeks, is emotionally harrowing for the mother. She may disbelieve the diagnosis, experiencing hope with every movement of her guts. Denial may alternate with grief-stricken terror at carrying a corpse inside her. She may oscillate between acceptance that she no longer feels pregnant, impatience to abort yet a morbid desire to hold onto her baby a little longer. Gradually, she begins to feel her body has become her baby's grave. Nightmarishly, unbeknown to others, she walks around with a dead 'thing' inside her, awaiting a birth that is not life-giving. She herself has not been able to sustain life. Unlike a spontaneous miscarriage, it does not seem that the baby has chosen' to reject or leave her, but that she has failed her dead child and her mate who entrusted the baby to her. Stimulation of labour may not immediately succeed, and an exceedingly painful birth results in a macerated 'non-baby' after which she is shunted off to a side ward or 'dismissed' from hospital. She has become a 'non-mother', returning with empty arms to her home with its painful reminders of joyful anticipation.

30.1.3 Resorption

This experience raises strange fantasies in the mother: she may feel she has selfishly 'digested' her baby for her own growth, or that the loved fetus has now become an integral part of her, always to remain with her. She may also have the harrowing feeling that her live body is shot through with contaminating dead matter. Where ultrasound reveals one twin having been reabsorbed, the surviving unborn twin may be unconsciously regarded as having demolished the other, eaten him/her up or greedily taken the twin's share of nourishment. This fantasy can create a prejudicial 'set' long before the surviving baby is born, labelling him/her as a 'survivor' or a 'selfish go getter', a preconceived internal image of the fetus which may persist after the birth.

30.1.4 Reactions of the partner

The male partner (or female in the case of a lesbian couple) may find miscarriage very difficult. Not receiving physical or emotional attention like the woman who has aborted, yet often suffering a similar disappointment, he is left without social acknowledgement of his plight and usually lacks opportunities among his male friends to express his grief. In addition he has not had the physical sensations that make her loss a tangible emptiness. The partner has the frustrated sense of his baby being at the mercy of his wife's body, while he, the father, is unable to ensure that she sustains the pregnancy, keeps the baby in, or even conceives again. Communication may be impaired as each partner deals alone with their complex feelings. Unconscious blame may fester in their relationship alongside unanswered questions about whose 'fault' it is, whether miscarriage was triggered by sexual intercourse or if she may be responsible for having broken some antenatal taboo or whether it occurred because of a previous abortion or is a 'blighted pregnancy' which comes from his or her 'side of the family'. Bodily disillusionment often follows miscarriage, with subsequent pregnancies being treated by both members of the couple rather gingerly and tentatively. The following pregnancy no longer can be the robust natural process of the pre-miscarriage pregnancy, and sometimes reactivates an uncompleted mourning process for the miscarried baby. Other couples may not have the courage to start another pregnancy.

It is estimated that over 6000 women or couples in the UK lose a baby through miscarriage every year according to the Health Education Council. Some of these may benefit from outpatient counselling from their obstetrician or GP. Others might wish to join or create a self-help group and women who have experienced a traumatic or repeat miscarriage may benefit from contacting a support group such as the Miscarriage Association to attain a better understanding of the problems associated with their miscarriage. Psychotherapy might be requested by women whose complex feelings preclude considering a further pregnancy until this interrupted one is resolved [4].

KEY POINTS

*Miscarriage, particularly in late pregnancy, can constitute a major life event for a woman and her family. Information about the cause of loss reduces the generalized sense of guilt and confusion and facilitates healing, so that the next pregnancy is not hampered by unresolved painful issues from this abortive one.

*'Missed abortions' involving a long wait for the dead baby to be expelled are harrowing for the bereaved mother who needs help to tide her over this period of carrying death and undergoing a fruitless birth.

*Similarly a life-threatening event, such as an ectopic pregnancy, confronts the couple with dangerous aspects of creativity, with the need to evaluate whether to take the risk of another attempt to have a baby, and indeed, the possibility that reproductive capacity has been technically impaired. During the long interim period of waiting for the all important 'verdict' on their fertility the woman, and her partner too, may need therapy to come to terms with the shock of emergency and drastic shifts in their identities.

*After a miscarriage, the interrupted psychological process of pregnancy is replaced by a new process of accommodating to loss, not only loss of the baby and all the hopes and expectations invested in it, but loss of the pregnancy and disruption of the fertile aspects of the woman and her sense of femininity.

*The social and professional 'conspiracy of silence' and discomfort about death before birth, often prevent the bereaved woman/couple from expressing grief once initial numbness has passed. Yet mourning for what is gone is necessary to make place for future creativity. Grieving the gap created by the absense of a baby never encountered is difficult, and may be helped by making the loss more tangible – through ritual, by seeing and/or naming the baby, writing fantasies about him/her, talking about the sensations of pregnancy as well as the events of the miscarriage – thus constructing memories of a precious experience rather than a 'non-event'.

*Despite yearning for a baby, unresolved self-blame and marital conflicts may lead to sexual difficulties and fear of becoming pregnant again, as do underlying guilt about having 'failed' the baby or partner and resentment about being singled out by fate or 'rejected' by the baby. *Pregnancies following miscarriage are inevitably accompanied by a loss of trust in the body's natural capacity to function unmonitored, and a high level of tension and vigilance are to be expected. Partners, too, may need help in resolving issues of frustration, blame and anxiety.

30.1.5 Ectopic pregnancy

When implantation has developed outside the uterine cavity, the woman, experiencing symptoms of nausea or breast enlargement, suspects conception yet may receive a negative pregnancy test result. In such cases, the crisis of ectopic pregnancy poses a double disillusionment – the life-threatening shock side by side with the belated discovery of pregnancy now obsolete. Once the immediate surgery and risk are over, the patient, particularly one who has had difficulty conceiving, may feel emotionally cheated of her brief pregnancy which she did not even experience as such. She may have irrational feelings of anger towards her lover who 'put the baby in the wrong place' or guilt about her own lack of provision of a roomy and safe place for the pregnancy to grow. Nightmares and fantasies about the cramped doomed baby are part of a process of coming to terms with her own strangled hopes and a pregnancy that was but was not ('the ectopic pregnancy just confirmed what I always felt – that I had bad insides. It's left me with a great void of loneliness and guilt. As if I was careless with a treasure I didn't even know I had'). Although young (40% of cases occur between 20 and 29 years), her prognosis for a future normal pregnancy is fraught with risk, and the woman may feel doomed to fail. If she was aware of the pregnancy, her reaction will be similar to that following miscarriage yet coupled with the existential shock of having been so close to a brush with Death. Her partner, too, stunned by the threat of losing his woman, may weigh up the desire to have a baby with the danger of another ectopic pregnancy. On the positive side, there is a greater chance of being accepted for IVF because the ectopic pregnancy is proof of fertility despite damage to tubes.

30.2 HIGH-RISK PREGNANCIES AND MEDICAL COMPLICATIONS

30.2.1 Living with latent emergency

Chronic anxiety often accompanies conditions requiring special medical attention, bed rest or hospitalization during pregnancy, whether for threatened abortion, coexisting medical conditions or pregnancy complicated by hypertensive syndromes, threatened premature labour or placenta praevia. Not only is the pregnant woman removed from her ordinary daily routine but must be continuously vigilant for warning signs of impending crisis. The latent emergency of a high-risk pregnancy and potential high-risk infant poses a real psychological threat as physical disequilibrium tends to create additional stress, heightening the woman's anxiety and fear [5]. She feels responsible for the two lives in her body, living a restricted and cautious life yet helplessly unable to influence her physical condition. If she has other children at home, she is acutely aware that hospitalization with this baby restricts her availability to her other children as she dwells on the effects of separation and maternal deprivation. In planning nursing management, her physical needs must be weighed against the emotional needs of the entire family necessitating careful evaluation of the possibility of maintaining home-based bed-rest with appropriate medical care and domestic help.

Women suffering from pre-existing conditions such as heart disease or one exacerbated by pregnancy such as diabetes, not only have to contend with all the complex processes of pregnancy but also with monitoring and management of a serious, possibly life-threatening disorder. The patient and her family naturally become extremely dependent on professional help for informative communication, guidance about management and decision-making. The adaptive processes in this critical situation have been found to follow the usual sequential pattern of coping mechanisms, beginning with rationalization and denial of the crisis, followed by depression, disorganization and finally acceptance [6]. While she 'rests' in bed, the woman's mind is not at rest but plays out the internal scenario in a series of fantasies related to what she imagines is happening within:

a. Hypertension may be interpreted as an internal emotional conflict with the fetus raising her blood pressure.
b. Toxaemia may be unconsciously regarded as her being poisoned by the baby or vice versa and thus playing on the fantasy tandem of good mother–bad baby or bad mother–good baby contamination.
c. Placental insufficiency may be imagined as the greedy baby outstripping the placental supply or the stingy mother withholding what the baby needs for growth.
d. Anaemia may be guiltily experienced as a result of her own iron-impoverished diet or blamed onto the demanding fetus who has depleted her iron stores.

Once again, a sense of failure and inadequacy usually accompanies these syndromes, as the mother feels she is letting down her baby and partner by being unable 'simply' to be pregnant and have a baby like everyone else. As she fearfully awaits the birth, she tries to prolong this very uncomfortable and anxious time, rationalizing that every additional day in the womb brings the fetus closer to maturity and survival, yet paradoxically, she feels that their ongoing close proximity keeps them both in danger.

30.2.2 Threat to fetal health

Where a mother is incapacitated with infections such as rubella, she has the additional guilt of having introduced an extraneous factor into the pregnancy, not only endangering her own health but possibly threatening the fetus and having a long-term deleterious effect on the baby's development. The additional worry about whether the drugs that cure the mother harm the baby, highlights their symbiotic interdependence while the threat of abortion emphasizes the nature of their separateness. Venereal infections carry the added burden of stigma and risk of punitive professional disapproval when seeking help. The woman herself guiltily feels she is transferring the fruits of her dangerous sexuality to the innocent victim of her creative sexuality. AIDS is a particular case in point where an HIV positive woman unwittingly may transmit the illness to her fetus. Less dangerous but also guilt-arousing threats are mothers who cannot control their substance intake of drugs, nicotine or alcohol yet know that their behaviour is potentially damaging the fetus. In some mothers' minds, the baby is being put to the test and exposed to the worst she can offer to see whether the baby is 'strong enough' to resist her destructiveness. Far from being complacent, each drink or fix may be experienced as a battle between the 'forces of darkness and light' with the fetus often playing the part of innocence being corrupted or Good that will survive the onslaught of Evil. A woman who makes a suicide attempt during pregnancy will continue to experience guilt and fears of having damaged her baby (especially if she overdosed), long after the depression has lifted. Attempts at self-induced abortion or distress due to physical assaults on the fetus by the father have been documented [7]. All these factors are discussed in greater detail in Chapter 33.

30.3 ACCESS TO THERAPY

Many women suffering from chronic anxiety during pregnancy would welcome the opportunity to talk about their tumultuous feelings and stress-related concerns with a trained professional therapist. The pregnant woman at risk needs someone to 'keep vigil' with her during the long wait until the 'moment of truth' when the birth will reveal whether the baby has been affected by the mother's condition. She would benefit from having help to ease her difficult 'journey' by working on psychological factors influencing the physical condition or resulting from it [8]. Following a miscarriage or ectopic pregnancy, women or couples may need therapeutic intervention, especially if fertility may have been impaired. Similarly, women suffering from infectious diseases, chronic medical conditions or addictive disturbances may need help. Such intervention can be very rewarding. Since, as noted previously, in her state of heightened awareness and greater accessibility to unconscious material, the pregnant woman is amenable to psychotherapy and is usually highly motivated to 'sort herself out' before the birth [9].

30.2.4 Multiple pregnancies

A woman expecting two or more babies is having to meet greater physiological demands on her body during pregnancy. Discomfort is greater and the risk of premature labour, lower birth weight and perinatal mortality are increased; at times, these are combatted by hospitalization and bed rest during weeks 32–36. Psychologically, the mother-to-be has the complicated task of accepting a dual or multiple pregnancy. Routine ultrasound screening, repeated following first trimester bleeding, reveals that five times as many twins are conceived as are born. Physical resorption of one twin means that a mother who has been expecting two babies, has also psychically to resorb the vanished twin and adjust to one rather than two babies.

Where diagnosis is complicated, a mother may only receive news or confirmation of multiple pregnancy as late as the sixth month and suddenly finds that the baby she has been anticipating is not unique but has 'split' into two. Prenatal bonding with two or more unknown babies is more difficult unless the mother projects quite different fantasies 'into' each of her babies, articulating and heightening perceived or imagined differences between them. Sex differences revealed by ultrasound or amniocentesis may foster gender stereotyped fantasies. If the mother herself is one of twins, she may select one of her babies to represent herself. However, lacking differentiating 'tags', the mother may continue to relate to both babies as 'the same', two 'peas' inside her 'pod'-like uterus. At times she herself feels 'left out' by the twins who provide each other with company inside her, taking the nourishment they need from her but having fun without her [10]. Like her partner, she may feel excluded from immediate contact with the babies who have such intimate close physical contact with each other. Thus, a division between generations may be set up already at this point, with the parents forming one unit and the babies another, rather than the mother-baby as a unit, or a triangle of asymmetrical relationships (including the father) such as might occur in single births.

KEY POINTS

*Pregnancies following miscarriage are accompanied by a loss of trust in the body's natural capacity to function unmonitored. Partners, too, may need help in resolving issues of 'blame' and 'guilt'.

*The medical term 'abortion' offends miscarrying women.

*High-risk pregnancies entail living in a chronic state of high tension and anxiety about a possible emergency developing. Relaxation technique and biofeedback may be useful in offering the woman more control over a prolonged uncertain situation and to stall premature labour.

*Nursing management and hospitalization plans must weigh up the physical needs of the woman against the emotional needs of her family, particularly if she has young children. Home-based bed-rest should be considered where appropriate help can be made available.

*On an emotional level, conflicts and guilt about retaining their potentially dangerous mutuality affect the mother's prenatal bonding to her baby. Fears about exacerbation of her own condition as a result of the pregnancy, and/or dread of possible miscarriage or fetal abnormality add to her already considerable endurance test. These anxieties can be helped and contained by counselling or psychotherapy.

*Conditions of psychological vulnerability, depression, excessive anxiety and frank disturbance benefit from prompt treatment during pregnancy.

*Ultrasound diagnosis of multiple pregnancies allows the couple time to adjust to the idea, and discriminatory prenatal bonding may be facilitated by naming the fetuses and identifying them as separate on the screen and in movements.

Chapter 31

Disruptions around birth: prematurity and illness, still-birth and perinatal loss

31.1 PREMATURITY AND ILLNESS

'As I see it, the trauma of birth is the break in the continuity of the infant's going on being, and when this break is significant the details of the way in which the impingements are sensed, and also of the infant's reaction to them, become in turn significant factors adverse to ego development . . . In some cases this adverse factor is so great that the individual has no chance (apart from rebirth in the course of analysis) of making natural progress in emotional development, even if subsequent external factors are extremely good.' D.W. Winnicott (Birth memories, birth trauma, and anxiety, 1949, in *Through Paediatrics to Psycho-Analysis*)

31.1.1 Preterm labour and birth

Having a baby early is frightening. Nothing happens according to expectation and nothing is ready. The couple is caught unawares and usually without much warning the woman finds that pregnancy has ended and labour begun before she has completed the emotional processes of gradual separation. Invariably, she wonders why her baby wants to leave her: is there something essential lacking, something more she might have provided? Is she unable to retain good things, or useless at providing them? Has she been careless? Is she incapable of cherishing another being and if so how can she look after the baby now it is coming out? Is there something horrible in there that the baby is escaping from? Has she herself done something to trigger the expulsion of her baby? Was it sex that started the contractions? Is the baby impatient to come out and meet her or is the fetus responding to her own impatient inability to wait until the baby is ripe?

Psychologically, she is totally unprepared for birth, unless, with the aid of artificial hormonal intervention biofeedback and/or psychotherapy, she has managed to delay the onset of labour for a few days, allowing her a little time to adjust to the idea of imminent delivery and giving the fetal lungs a chance to mature before birth. Tension permeates a preterm birth as question marks hang above the delivery table – will it survive birth? will it breathe? will it be alright? can it be normal? and only then, what sex is it?

31.1.2 Bonding

Only rarely can the baby at risk be cuddled for long before it is whisked away. The premature baby looks even less like the baby-book pictures than those born at term and parents may feel desperately guilt-ridden about their initial shock and revulsion at seeing the scrawny little 'skinned rabbit' or hairy, bony E.T.–like creature. In addition to its small size, the baby might be ill and almost transparent in appearance, is likely to be weak, 'collapsed' and unresponsive. Superimposed upon the image of their healthy fantasy baby, this one seems alien and 'wrong'. When survival is in doubt, it is not unusual for parents to protect themselves from falling in love while unconsciously preparing themselves for possible loss. The mother, in particular, might feel devastatingly inadequate to the task ahead, having to defend herself against deep feelings of anxiety, deprivation and self doubt:

a. She feels she has failed to sustain her baby within her
b. The emotional process of pregnancy has been sharply curtailed, leaving her with unfinished 'business'
c. She has abruptly lost the fantasy baby of her dreams and the robust inner baby, with whom she had a relationship, has abandoned her and has been replaced with a fragile stranger
d. As a woman, she has failed to give birth normally at full term
e. The birth may have involved emergency procedures quite unlike the ideal birth she had fondly envisaged
f. The baby she has produced is puny, jaundiced, or ill and possibly at risk
g. She may not feel maternal, cannot count on the baby living, fears she may have irreversibly damaged it physically or psychologically and does not know whether she even wishes it to survive if it is impaired.

31.1.3 The parents of an incubated baby

Bonding is further complicated when the baby and mother are separated. In some cases the ill newborn may be transferred to a high-risk perinatal centre at another hospital leaving the separated mother surrounded by new mothers and their infants, marooned empty-armed and bewildered in the maternity unit geared to breastfeeding and baby-routines. If antenatal ward and Neonatal Intensive Care Unit (NICU) are geographically separated and she has had a caeserian section or is incapacitated, it may be some time before she sees her baby again. It is recommended that where the baby is transported to another centre, even an ill baby should briefly be brought to his/her parturient mother before departure and the father encouraged to act as a link between mother and baby, by staying with and caring for the baby, and then carrying information (and polaroid photographs) to the separated mother until she is able to visit. When she does get to the special care unit, the physical and psychological barrier of the incubator as well as the off-putting paraphernalia of intravenous tubings, humming ventilators and high-tech machinery attached to her baby increase her sense of alienation. The preterm baby who is meant to be inside her safe and warm, is outside, in there, seemingly being tortured, and she has allowed it to happen. Alarms go off, monitors bleep, nurses rush around in an atmosphere of tension, instigating life-saving procedures for babies at-risk while their parents stand helplessly by, with no space of their own, no expertise, no clear role to play and, at first, little understanding of the routines involved. Parents seem not to belong in the unit. The baby seems not to belong to the parents. In the early days, mothers and fathers, too, may feel afraid even to look at their painfully scrawny baby lying forlornly in the little plastic box so encumbered with electrodes, tubes and special equipment, let alone touch him or her. Their deep-seated guilt, horror and fear may drive them away or keep them rooted to the spot, paralysed by impotence and exhaustion.

Following the birth of a premature baby, many new mothers and fathers are in a shocked state of crisis and need help in adapting to life in limbo. Unless helped to establish a caring relationship with the baby some bewildered parents will detach themselves from the neonatal care unit upon maternal discharge from hospital, telephoning for information but feeling that all they can do is wait for news in their home with her empty belly and the empty crib, avoiding embarrassed friends and relatives. However, with encouragement from the staff, these parents too can allow themselves to become involved by emotionally 'rooting' for their baby's survival and actively engaging in care which it seems, can actually contribute to his/her growth. Studies have revealed that premature infants who are touched, rocked, fondled or cuddled daily during their stay in neonatal nursery display fewer breathing problems, increase their weight gain, have fewer stools and an advance in some higher central nervous system functioning which persists for months after discharge from hospital [1]. In addition to helping with practical care, parents are especially geared to provide personal warmth, intimacy, continuity, and loving stimulation for their NICU baby who is largely deprived of meaningful human experience. Giving parents opportunities for early contact with the newborn and adequate support during this crucial period while the baby is in hospital can have a positive effect not only on attachment in the unit but on the baby's behaviour and mother–baby interaction after discharge [2,3]. However, to be competently involved in care, stunned people will have to undergo the emotional unfreezing that will enable their transformation into the intuitively responsive mother and father of a critically ill or at-risk premature baby.

31.1.4 Increasing parental involvement

The double shock of preterm parenthood and an ill baby leave new parents emotionally reeling. They may need preparation before entering the NICU for the first time and, once there, explanation about the various procedures and equipment. Opportunities must be given for parents to express their initial anxieties and to voice some of the irrational feelings of self-recrimination and trepidation about their newborn's frail condition. Studies have shown that parental caresses and gentle stroking relax the baby, assist motor organization and accelerate weight gain in low birthweight babies [4,5]. Many parents not only fear touching the infant, but fear being emotionally touched by him/her. If grief and uncertainty can be experienced and expressed rather than defensively denied and held at bay, tentative parents can begin to form loving bonds even with a baby who may not survive. Some neonatologists advocate increasing parental attachment by getting the mother (or father) to try and send tactile 'messages' to the baby and watch for feedback [6].

Defensive means of coping with the stress of relating to a severely ill preterm neonate may include blaming others, including staff and each other, to avoid excessive personal guilt or self-hatred. Rather than becoming defensive themselves or irritated, members of staff should recognize these signs of maladjustment to the crisis and offer sympathy and understanding. If the marital relationship appears deadlocked, parents may require tactful referral for professional assistance, now, while it is needed. Parent groups held in some neonatal intensive care units have been found to reduce tensions and increase parental competence [7,8]. Some parents may not seem too concerned by it all. However, over-optimistic evaluation of the baby's condition could imply denial of the facts rather than ignorance. Indeed, a fairly high level of anxiety and active requests for information have been found to predict a favourable outcome after discharge from hospital [9]. Obsessional attention to the machinery may conceal a desperate attempt to bind anxiety by equipment-control or to deflect it with busyness. Rage may displace sadness or martyrdom can conceal rage. Pre-existing marital discord exacerbated by tension may erupt in mutual accusations ('her placenta was not good enough'; 'he insisted on making love and that triggered labour') or be displaced onto the staff or acted out in mishaps or somatic symptoms. The painful strain of coping with ongoing uncertainty and long stressful hours of inactive sitting by the incubator waiting for the baby to wake, both tax individual resources and expose hidden rifts and weaknesses in the relationship. However, meaningful joint efforts could bring them closer together. One study has found that more couples divorced among parents who were allowed little contact with their premature baby than among those allowed to handle and care for their infants during the first five days of life [10]. During the critical period of a premature baby's life, some parents may be deeply affected by losses of other babies in the unit while others split-off their feelings in seemingly callous detachment or evolve magical 'statistics' wishing to believe that the death of another baby lessens the chances of the demise of their own. Similarly, envious feelings directed towards other parents whose well babies leave the unit, may engender angry suspicions that the previously idealized staff are now practising favouritism or have silently 'given-up' on their baby.

In sum, mothers and fathers of a baby in an NICU are undergoing a frightening traumatic experience and need help to adjust to this prolonged state of crisis. A study of mother's emotional responses to preterm birth finds their major concerns centre on feelings of alienation and worries over the infant's survival and long-term care [11]. Evasive answers or uncoordinated communication cause further confusion and resentment at a time when the parents are already overloaded emotionally. Daily exchanges with members of staff encouraging parental observations and reporting medical information can help the parents to come to terms with the baby's condition and prognosis. Stress-support, guidance and encouragement from health professionals can help parents develop competent skills and greater satisfaction in caring for the high-risk infant after discharge [12]. Group discussions with other parents facilitate exchange of feelings and self-help resources enabling parents to feel less isolated and singled out with their painful problem. Brief individual therapy or couple counselling may release coping resources, enabling grieving parents to talk together and become more effective in supporting each other.

31.1.5 NICU staff

Professionals working with severely ill neonates are under a great deal of pressure which has been found to lead to a 'burnout' syndrome of low morale, stress-related illnesses and absenteeism. A psychotherapist working with NICU professionals in a London teaching hospital has enumerated various stressful factors which contribute to their difficulties and the mode of coping with these. Their jobs entail crucial responsibility for the lives of very fragile babies; constant exposure to technological noise and tension; need to make quick, unsupported decisions during crises; disruptive shifts and rotations; staff shortages, low status and pay; frequent death and loss of babies; exposure to ambivalent parental feelings of anger, envy and rivalry over babycare coupled with hope and idealization, while simultaneously experiencing their own professional helplessness at being unable to save babies [13]. Furthermore, staff have to face daily moral and ethical dilemmas in deciding how best to proceed in prolonging life and when to let it ebb. They have to accept that many of their caring procedures are painful and intrusive to the tiny babies in their care; that even those who survive will ultimately be removed from their nurturing and that the endearing baby's primary attachment should be to the parents. In this highly demanding profession it has been noted that with these babies whose utero-gestation has been shortened and extero-gestation lengthened, nurses provide round the clock substitute mothering requiring constant 'over-cathexis' of their tiny charges whom they are doomed to lose [14]. Some health professionals defend themselves against recurrent experiences of attachment and loss by instituting shifts and routines that militate against forming special relationships and, like the parents, employ a range of defence mechanisms from detachment, denial and avoidance to displacement, projection, splitting and manic reparation. For some NICU workers, an omnipotent drive to save previously doomed lives and an over-idealized process of caring for damaged babies and restoring them to health may signify unconscious guilt and compensation for destructive impulses. It has been suggested that staff working under such cumulative emotionally stressful conditions need:

a. A time and place for quiet reflection within a setting 'where action sometimes takes the place of thoughts'
b. A regular non-hierarchical neutral forum for expressing their anxieties and frustrations
c. A place in which to explore their observations and encourage intuitive feelings [15].

31.1.6 The experience of a preterm baby in the NICU

The incubated neonate often bonds not with a person but with a machine. We can only imagine what it must be like to be prematurely plucked from a dark, warm watery medium governed by maternal biorhythms and familiar human sounds to a space-age bombardment of unceasing activity, intense illumination, and low frequency and impulse noise. All psychoanalytical theories of primitive emotional development stress the infant's need for a loving caregiver's external organization to filter intolerable impingements, bind unintegrated experiences and help the newborn form a sense of physical and personal continuity [16]. However, for the incubated baby, human contact often involves sleep-disruptive, painful manipulations and up to 234 handling procedures and interventions in a 24-hour period by many different busy professionals [17]. Meaningful stimulation within the incubator is minimal and limited to rhythmic vibrations of monitor and ventilator and tactile contact with tubes interrupted by sudden overstimulation of too bright lights or the deafeningly loud noises of alarms sounding and objects carelessly plonked on the incubator top. It has been argued that premature infants suffer from a poor fit between their needs and the intensive care unit environment and, indeed, that some of the current special care baby unit routines may actually contribute to the imbalance of the small ill baby [18]. A review of studies into iatrogenic effects of NICU experience cites an increased occurrence of hypoxaemia, bradycardia, apnoea and behavioural distress following handling. The higher incidence of hearing loss in very low birth weight infants has been attributed to synergistic effects of noise exposure and retinopathy of prematurity has been associated with unfiltered light and sunlight [19]. The notion that newborns feel no pain is currently being questioned and revised as evidence accumulates about fetal learning capacity and neonatal heightened perceptual sensitivity and silent crying. The long-term emotional effects of prematurity and incubation are methodically very complex to tease out. Subjectively 'prems' may feel different. ('Because I was premature, I feel terribly responsible for what happened before I was even born – as if I have to compensate my parents for arriving early and make it better . . . Mum's stainless steel logic leaves me no purchase on my life – I've got nothing good to offer myself.')

31.1.7 Improved NICU care

Changes are invariably the result of questioning set practices. The query: 'Why do we do this in that way?' often leads to startling conclusions about the obsolete, and at times, damaging nature of standard procedures. Thus, we are reminded that until Barnett showed that bacterial hospital flora constituted a greater threat to the baby's health than that of the visiting mother, parents of premature infants were held at bay behind the glass walls of the corridors [20]. Until recently, inflexible regulations about visiting also isolated some mothers and fathers from their infants in intensive care, drastically increasing parental anxieties and curtailing bonding. Some changes in visiting procedure have been instigated as a result of studies demonstrating that the sooner parents see the baby the less time they have to imagine the worst and the more rapidly they can reconcile their fantasies with the baby's true physical condition [21]. In addition to researchers proposing novel ideas based on their findings, nurses and other members of staff are in an ideal position to be innovative and have the wealth of experience to recognize potential advantages of change. Thus a nurse recently invented a mobile incubator housed in an ordinary baby-pram, giving the parents a greater sense of homely normality and saving both expense and effort. A trial of light and noise reduction between 7pm and 7am in one unit, established day and night rhythms in the babies and resulted in longer sleep, shorter feeds and greater weight gain after being discharged home [22a]. Coordination of procedures by different professionals has been found to reduce adverse handling and increase the duration of rest periods for the ill infant [22b]. In some units, premature babies have been provided with means to simulate intrauterine conditions and increase stimulation, such as sheep-skin rugs or hammocks slung inside the incubator. Water-beds have been shown to provide beneficial vestibular stimulation. In West Germany, phototherapy, feeds and ministrations take place with the baby on the mother's abdomen [23]. In some NICUs parents are being encouraged to try 'kangaroo'-type skin-to-skin incubation of the baby between the mother's breasts or under the father's shirt, providing unlimited sucking, closeness, continuity and movement.

To promote mutual bonding, it has been suggested that ideally mother and premature baby need not be separated at all, but could have the baby's incubator hinged to the maternal bed, carrying resuscitation equipment as a precaution. Furthermore, radiant heat panels above the mothers bed, which allow early skin-to-skin contact and provision of privacy, have been found to promote maternal vocalization (which is minimal in intensive care nurseries) while nurse availability ensures infant safety. Extended family visits of grandparents and siblings are welcomed and 24 hour telephone communication maintained both before and after infant discharge [24]. In some units, there is a predischarge 'nesting period' in which mothers and sometimes fathers return to spend 2–3 days rooming-in with their babies in hospital, taking complete care of the infant before taking him/her home [25].

Tube-feeding the baby with breast milk and later actual breastfeeding has been found to enable mothers to overcome some feelings of failure related to prematurity; it also reinforces their sense of being special to the baby rather than feeling ineffective compared with the efficient life-saving nurses. When staff respect the parents' intuitive capacity to soothe the baby, guidance focuses on training them to observe the ill neonate for signs of stress, to do routine tasks and work as a team with the staff, nurses are thereby freed for more specialized activities. As the baby's condition improves, staff ingenuity can focus on ways to enable parents gradually to take over further aspects of care for their baby in preparation for home-coming and full-time professionally unassisted care of their child. In conclusion, it has been proposed that because there is no universal recipe for optimal physical and psychological care of the sick and preterm baby, the principle of individualized developmental care should be implemented by observing each baby, designing an individual careplan and changing it as the baby grows [26].

KEY POINTS

*Preterm labour abruptly curtails pregnancy before completion of the emotional processes of gradual separation.
*The parturient experiences guilt about her failure to sustain her baby and to give birth normally at full term. Having abruptly lost her fantasy baby before she is ready to replace it with the real one, she may not feel maternal, and have difficulty bonding with a baby who may not survive.
*Parents of an incubated baby need help to adapt to their crisis and establish a caring relationship with the baby, through early contact and meaningful interaction.
*While professional handling of the neonate may cause distress, parents are especially geared to provide personal warmth, comfort and continuity for their NICU baby who is often deprived of stimulating human contact.
*The parental burden may be eased by: daily exchanges, stress support and guidance, group discussions with other parents and brief personal therapy or couple counselling where special help is required.
*Health professionals defend themselves against recurrent experiences of attachment and loss by instituting routines that militate against forming special relationships and, like the parents, may employ defence mechanisms ranging from detachment, denial and avoidance to displacement, projection, splitting and manic reparation.
*Staff working under such cumulative emotionally stressful conditions often benefit from a staff support group and a regular non-hierarchical neutral forum for expressing anxieties and frustrations.

31.2 PERINATAL DEATH

Although advances in obstetrical and neonatal care have increased the survival rate of ever smaller and younger babies, nevertheless, according to the Health Education Council, some 6000 babies die in the UK shortly after birth. A death in the birth chamber is an obscene contradiction, an oxymoron that we have difficulty grasping. An awaited birth becomes a death or a brief life is snuffed out with all its attendant hopes and promise.

31.2.1 The process of mourning

Health professionals are no strangers to death. However, only rarely do they follow the grief-stricken person through the whole ongoing process of mourning. When death of a loved one occurs, bereavement constitutes a painful process of gradual 'detachment' of the emotions invested in the lost person to free the mourner for new attachments [27]. This transition entails emotionally reliving memories and hopes related to the dead person and, by acknowledging that he/she is no longer alive in the external world, incorporating them in the internal world.

Research into the emotional processes of mourning have established that normal grief follows a well-defined pattern. An initial sense of unreality, disbelief and numbness gives way to intense grief, unwarranted guilt and self-blame followed by irritability and anger towards others or towards the deceased for dying. Withdrawal of interest from other relationships and development of symptoms of physical distress may follow, including symptoms imitating the terminal illness of the deceased such as breathing difficulties, palpitations or motility disturbances; and depression-related symptoms of insomnia, loss of appetite and sexual desires. The bereaved person is mentally preoccupied with idealizing the dead person, experiencing his/her presence and 'forgetting' or erasing the fact of his/her demise in dreams, fantasy and reality. Gradually these experiences give way to acceptance of the death, increased social interaction and ability to integrate the dead person into the experiential history of one's being [28].

32.2.2 Reactions to a still-birth

Clearly, the more affectionate memories of a separate person that have been created, the greater the sense of loss yet, equally, the deeper the residue of loving experiences to draw upon. However, when a baby dies before the mother has had an opportunity to establish the baby as separate from herself, the death may be experienced as loss of part of her own being, like an amputation or wasted potential in herself. This vague undefined sense of dispossession and emptiness makes grieving following still-birth difficult, and parents may need help to recapture a sense of what is being mourned. A well-meaning 'conspiracy of silence' which often accompanies still-birth increases the parents' sense of a 'non-event' [29]. Whereas the impulsive reaction of staff to a still-born baby is protectively to whisk the evidence away, seclude the parents and dampen mourning reactions, bereaved mothers and fathers have found it helpful to be given time and space in which to take in the reality of the death. Due to such feedback, the old custodial approach of defending parents from the pain of losing their newborns has given way to current understanding that since attachment begins prenatally, grief following a still-birth is inevitable.

Lewis has coined the phrase 'bringing the baby back to death' to describe the assistance required to focus mourning and avoid the experience of 'a black hole in the mind' [30]. In the case of a still-birth, physicians and midwives can help parents to create memories where few exist by enabling them to see the body, or encouraging them to touch and hold the dead baby should they so wish. Given the chance to see their child, parents may need time to decide whether to do so, and whether they would want to hold and dress the dead baby, which makes the baby real as well as providing tangible proof confirming the death. Routine photography makes this decision less irreversible for parents who have chosen not to see the baby. The chance to view the body is particularly meaningful following a still-birth when the mother has been sedated, and has no evidence of the birth of her baby or its existence. Naming the baby also facilitates mourning as it provides the baby with a continuing reality, as do keepsakes of the dead baby, such as a lock of hair, record of fetal heart monitor or name bracelet. Although hospitals dispose of dead babies (sometimes in mass graves of up to 200 bodies), many parents find the process of grieving is helped by arranging their own funeral or cremation for the baby despite the lack of a death grant for still-births. The burial signifies the reality of the birth/death experience which may remain nebulous and rootless without a ceremony and a marked grave. The funeral ritual is a form of saying goodbye to the baby they brought into the world, acknowledging parenthood and responsibility that the baby is theirs rather than the hospital's, and that it is a baby rather than a 'failure'. Symbolically, interment is a means of returning him/her to a 'womb = tomb' (in 'mother earth'), a comforting idea for mothers who feel the baby was born too soon.

31.2.2 Parental grief following perinatal death

When the baby has lived even for a short while, mourning is facilitated by having had a fleeting experience of a breathing, live baby. However ill the newborn, parents need to see their baby before s/he dies. Disconnecting the dying incubated baby from tubes and electrodes to enable parents to cradle the infant and have him/her die in their arms is often a painful yet cherished experience for parents who have never held their own baby. Such contact can help them make links between the baby experienced prenatally and the dying baby and for a brief instant reconcile an image of what is with what might have been. The glimmer of hope for a future is lopped off with the death, as evident from a poignant case of a bereaved mother opening the dead baby's mouth to see where the teeth would have been and 'walking' him in her attempt to create 'memories' of the childhood that was not to be [31]. Recognition of their grief by members of staff, in the form of a hand clasp, kind word or even single flower given to commemorate the baby whose care they have shared, adds richly to the few treasured memories of this sad time. ('It's over two years since my baby died but I can't see a white flower without getting tearful. It reminds me of that long night when I held her poor little body for the first time without the tubes and rocked her as she was dying throughout those long hours. Then the nurse came in at dawn with a single white rose. I just burst into tears and released all the pent up feelings I'd been holding in all those terrible weeks of suspense.') For a first-time parent, such memories also preserve their identity as 'mother' and 'father' when this role has been stripped from them by the death as they go home empty handed.

It is helpful for parents, particularly when the baby has died of birth complications, to have ample opportunities to talk over the details of the traumatic birth and its effect on the baby. This can be painful for the birth attendants who may be plagued by their own feelings of guilt and doubts whether another procedure might have been life-saving. Klaus and Kennell have defined as the 'Lombardi syndrome' the defensiveness that arises in units where the intensive struggle for life makes contemplating loss unacceptable [32]. To complete the process of mourning, bereaved parents need to know the cause of death and to work through their irrational feelings of self-blame and be relieved of them. They need to recount regrets, hopes and fantasies. When birth coincides with death they need to disentangle these momentous events in order to sustain a belief in future live births. The mother needs validation of her own experience by seeing her grief reflected in others, in simple gestures of sympathy and acknowledgement that there has been a tragedy and that other people, staff included, care. A father, feeling he is expected to appear calm and strong, may suppress his grief response and fail to mourn. Staff mindfulness of his loss helps him grieve.

Research has distinguished between prominent maternal and paternal grief patterns 8 weeks after the infant's death: mothers tend to suffer from sleep disturbance, depression, anorexia, weight loss, nervousness and morbid preoccupation with the baby. Father's symptoms include inability to work, denial of the death and alcoholism. Reactions of guilt/anger/hostility and social withdrawal are common to both [32] although mothers have been found to express more guilt. The couple also need to recognize each other's differing experience of the death of their baby and to keep open the channels of communication between them. If there is a disparity in the phases of their grief, one may become impatient with the other's prolonged mourning, feeling over-burdened by demands or devoid of fun in the marriage. Mutual bereavement may split the couple apart or draw them closer together, depending on a variety of current and historical factors, including communication difficulties. Siblings need help in coming to terms with the death and may be hampered in their own grief process by parental emotional unavailability, overanxiety or difficulties in dealing with the loss (see Chapter 26 on sibling loss).

31.2.4 The death of one twin

This is a particularly poignant loss in its juxtaposition of a happy event with a sad one, and survival of one baby who serves as a constant and growing reminder of the loss. Parents may unconsciously feel that the wrong twin has died or that this one has lived on at the expense of the other [33]. The process of mourning might delay bonding with the live baby and interfere with normal parenting activities, particularly when the mother is severely depressed. The surviving baby may limit her opportunities to meet with other bereaved parents, and relatives/friends tend to focus on her new baby rather than allowing her to talk about the one who is absent. The dead baby cannot be wiped out of the mother's mind by well-meaning people, and every time she answers the question: 'How many children do you have?' she is lying. She may feel disloyal towards the dead baby if she enjoys her live child yet is also full of remorse at neglecting him/her in her bereaved state. Clearly the sentient baby is in need of support in this very distressing and confusing juxtaposition of life and death in the mother which few people can handle on their own without therapy. In view of possible travelling restrictions with the baby and hospital associations with the traumatic event, therapy for the mother–baby pair might have to be conducted in the home.

31.2.5 Reactions of professionals

Hospital staff are often shocked themselves by still-birth or neonatal death and fear that talking to the bereaved parents will stir up their own emotional feelings of failure, frustration and helplessness. However, for the parents a natural part of the process of grieving is an attempt to seek explanations and make sense of the unthinkable. Accusations and blame are their defensive means of deflecting pain in the form of anger, a common phase in the mourning process. It is important for the woman's future obstetric history, as well as her current bereavement, that trust in medical personnel may be restored. Equally important is the staff's own need to understand what went wrong and to be exonerated when falsely accused. This exchange is often postponed on the grounds of delicacy and naturally must take parental feelings into consideration. However, all too often, reluctance of professionals to talk to them is misinterpreted by the parents as coldness or cowardice. A comprehensive review of the literature on perinatal loss concludes that 'bereaved parents are exceptionally vulnerable to insensitive care and callous or paternalistic staff attitudes may adversely affect the mourning process' [34].

Unresolved emotional reactions of doctors and midwives to a perinatal death or still-birth may lead them to avoid the mother during or after delivery, discharge her prematurely ('see you next year!') or to concentrate on providing physical care. Communication may be stilted by attempts to steer away from the topic which they feel would upset the bereaved mother. Thus, far from providing opportunities for the parents to express their tearful emotions, these are often curtailed by distracting avoidance or 'cheering' phrases such as: 'never mind, you'll have another baby soon' disclosing the speaker's own inability to cope with loss and lack of understanding of the process of grief. The woman does not want 'another' baby. She wants this one now. She does not see her loss as 'a blessing in disguise' which implies her baby would have been a damaged monster. She needs to express what she is feeling not to be told what she ought to feel [35].

Precisely because such tragic events are uncommon in obstetric practice (one still-birth occurs in every 80 deliveries), birth attendants require training in dealing with death. Learning how to break the news of an imminent still-birth and helping the parents through a birth that does not produce life; understanding their own resistance to the painful task of informing parents of a negative prognosis and supporting them through a perinatal death, must also be coupled with personal exploration of what death in the face of birth means to people who have chosen as their life-work a profession which helps life come into being.

31.2.6 Helping bereaved parents

In general, the pattern of grief in parents who have lost a newborn is similar to bereavement following loss of other family members, acute symptoms gradually abating within the first year after the baby's death. However, unresolved grief and disordered mourning following perinatal loss has been noted in many studies, although only four investigators have examined predictors of such disturbance. These predictors include intensity of initial grief, lack of or problematic social support, previous loss, significant life stresses and crisis during pregnancy and unsatisfactory marital relationship [36]. Unfortunately, psychological factors such as antecedent mental health, childhood relationship history and maternal personality characteristics were not examined in these research projects. Bowlby has proposed a threefold division of disordered mourning: chronic unresolved mourning; prolonged absence of grief and, euphoria (yielding within a few weeks to one of two former patterns) [37]. Such disturbances may not be consciously apprehended by members of the family but are revealed in recurrent interviews with the professional. A minimum of three contacts are recommended, the first shortly following the event to convey information about the death, which, however, may not be taken in at this stage. Research has disclosed that class, gender and ethnic discriminations affect the amount of information given to parents with working-class women and Asian mothers given minimal explanations of the cause of death [38]. A further interview will be necessary within the first week or preferably during the next 2–3 days to repeat information, register birth or death, check up on milk-suppression, talk about mourning processes and enable parents to express their puzzled, sad and angry feelings. A third meeting later on, once they have surfaced, offers a further opportunity to answer questions about the birth and illness, to convey post-mortem results and provide contraceptive advice and genetic counselling about future pregnancies. This visit provides an opportunity for the doctor to find out how the whole family is coping after the baby's birth and death. Following still-births and very early deaths, this visit may coincide with the 6-week postnatal checkup point during which a 3-month follow-up can be arranged.

Discerning interviewers may uncover persistent symptoms of pathological mourning: overactivity, psychosomatic reactions, agitated depression or prolonged hostility, insomnia, anorexia or apathy. Maternal envy of pregnant women or fear of harming or stealing a baby she might encounter, may prevent a bereaved mother from leaving her home. While these fantasies are normal in the early period, their persistence, enactment or agoraphobic isolation must be regarded as pathological. In addition to possible bereavement therapy following still-birth or perinatal death parents may also need sexual counselling. Sometimes, a bereaved mother may try and fill the gap with a 'replacement baby' before the process of mourning is completed. Experts have advised against this [39] as the new baby bears the brunt of having to live up to an impossible romanticized ideal or be forever devalued and resented for not being the baby who died. Pleasure in sex following a still-birth may be inhibited by guilt and association with the tragic birth. Both sexual withdrawal for fear of another pregnancy and further loss and a compulsion to conceive in order to replace the dead baby prevent the couple drawing closer and sharing their grief during lovemaking. If a vicious circle of defensive activity to prevent mourning has been established, professional help may be needed to remove the causes of anxiety.

In all these meetings with professionals, not only are the psychological needs of the bereaved couple acknowledged but their social identity as parents is maintained in their contact with general practitioner, health visitor, obstetrician and NICU/maternity ward staff who remember their baby. The social conspiracy of silence and avoidance around still-birth or death of a neonate, is thereby broken and a space provided for open remembrance. A medical sociologist has commented that the mother-to-be's antenatal 'social process of identity construction' is reversed following death of her baby, if hospital and society conspire to deny her loss, thereby instigating a process of 'de-construction' of her motherhood [40]. Anniversaries remain particularly painful for years, and some NICUs show solidarity with the parents by sending a card from the staff to commemorate the first anniversary of the baby's death [41].

Where emotional difficulties are observed, a psychiatrist, psychotherapist or family-therapist attached to the hospital can work therapeutically with individuals or the whole bereaved family to enable them to resume their course. In some units supportive bereavement-counselling groups or hospice programmes are provided. Where these are unavailable Relate, previously known as the Marriage Guidance Council, offers private confidential counselling and organizations such as the Twins and Multiple Births Association (TAMBA, Grimsby) have support groups for those who have lost one or both twins. Other parents may benefit from joining a self-help group of bereaved parents who have experienced a perinatal death, such as the Stillbirth and Neonatal Death Society (SAND, London, who produce a booklet entitled: 'Saying Goodbye to your Baby') or Parents Experiencing Neonatal Death (PEND in America). Parents may either attend group meetings, be 'befriended' by individual couples or offered telephone counselling to help them cope with the problem themselves.

KEY POINTS

*The process of mourning a still-birth or perinatal death is complicated by dearth of memories and an embarrassed 'conspiracy of silence'.
*Professionals can help the bereaved parents to create memories of their dead baby where none exist, enabling them to see and hold the baby, name and bury him/her and to keep their status of parenthood alive, when no-one else acknowledges it.
*The death of one twin is particularly poignant, and the surviving twin may be neglected or overprotected as a result.
*Professionals may need special training to deal with bereavement, as their help during the critical period can make the difference between healthy and disordered mourning.

Chapter 32

Postnatal complications: congenital abnormalities and critical conditions in infancy

32.1 CONGENITAL ABNORMALITIES

With improved antenatal care, screening and planning pregnancies, parents expect their chosen babies to be normal. Yet, paradoxically, advances in technology have also increased the likelihood of sustaining life and increasing life-expectancy in babies who are neurologically impaired or have a significant congenital abnormality.

32.1.1 Discovery

After a woman gives birth to a baby, it may be some time before she realizes that something is wrong. Even a severely deformed baby may be whisked away before she becomes aware of the malformation and doctors may delay the difficult task of breaking the news. However, with every passing hour of not seeing the baby, parental anxiety and suspicion grows as the fears of abnormality experienced by the woman during her pregnancy are forcefully reactivated and the minutiae of the delivery room relived. A mother who has had a complicated pregnancy knows she runs the risk of not producing a healthy baby. Specialists agree that the fantasies created in this period of delay during which parents suspect abnormality and are waiting to see the baby are often more devastating than the reality of malformation. During the initial contact, as with all babies, parents have to reconcile their anticipation of an imaginary baby to perception of the real baby. However, when the baby is visibly malformed, the initial reaction is one of shock and disappointment. A number of investigators have noted greater anxiety the closer impairment is to face and head rather than other parts of the body.

Professionals must bear in mind that what at first may appear as rejection of the baby, is at this point, an inability to accept it. Acceptance of the real malformed infant requires a greater adjustment to loss of the perfect fantasy. The wrench is almost like a process of mourning in which the ideal image has to be given up in favour of the damaged one. The greater the visibility of the defect, the greater the disruption in immediate bonding. When a baby is severely deformed, in addition to reactions of guilt and bewilderment, parents may experience shame at having produced a 'faulty' baby, and being unable to love it. Waves of humiliation wash over the mother in particular, as she encounters outside herself this imperfect baby who has been part of her and come out of her, seeming to reflect the intolerable badness within her. She feels that her own inner defectiveness is revealed in the blind, mishapen, micro or hydrocephalic baby. She has failed in being unable to produce a healthy whole one. In addition to the shock of seeing the impaired infant in conditions where the abnormality can be traced to a known viral infection, X-ray irradiation or drug taking, the mother lives with the knowledge of her share of 'responsibility' in producing the defect. Her guilt and remorse while reliving each crucial phase of the teratogenic period may be excruciatingly painful, accompanied by sleeping difficulties, nightmares, depression and even suicidal ideas.

32.1.2 Stages of adjustment to malformation

Klaus and Kennell have described a regular pattern of sequence in parental adjustment to the news of abnormality, although the duration and intensity of each stage varies according to individual reactions:

Stage 1: Shock and an urge to flee.
Stage 2: Disbelief and denial of the impact of the situation. (Stages 1 and 2 have been found to be of shorter duration with parents of a baby with visible problems rather than a hidden defect.)
Stage 3: Sadness, anger and anxiety including tearfulness, rage and hesitation about becoming attached to the baby.
Stage 4: Emotional equilibrium, achieved within weeks or months.
Stage 5: Reorganization of their lives for better or worse [1].

In addition to their own emotional strengths and psychological history, reactions of the parents and their future attachment partly depend on the nature of the malformation: the degree to which it may be potentially correctable; its visibility; whether it affects the central nervous system and/or is life threatening; whether it involves a single or multiple dysfunction; if it requires further hospitalization and, if familial, the degree to which parents have had prior experience or anticipation of the disability.

Extensive experience has led clinicians to recommend that parents see their malformed baby as soon as possible, and that professionals help parents note the baby's normal and positive features (such as strength, activity, alertness). A special nurse is assigned to the mother rather than expecting her to fall in with maternity unit routines designed for mothers of normal infants, and avoid giving tranquillizers on the assumption that these blunt responses and slow parental adaptation to the problem. It is recommended that parents have prolonged contact with their malformed baby, and fathers have extended visiting times, and possibly, even take the baby home when treatment can be postponed [2].

32.1.3 Accommodating to the reality

Despite anxieties during pregnancy about giving birth to a monster, most parents have expected a normal child. The harsh reality that together they have produced an abnormal infant is a deep narcissistic blow from which the parents may not recover. Each couple deals with the initial crisis in accordance with their marital resources and individual psychological history. The loss of the dreamed-for perfect infant must be mourned before attachment to the living defective infant can take place, a process which is hindered by the sometimes overwhelming demands of the new baby [3].

To some, the fact of bearing an abnormal child may be too difficult to bear. The baby, reflecting dissociated intolerable aspects of each may be constantly projected into the other – the woman blaming her husband for the malformation, he indicting her, or both accusing the professionals or treating the baby as aberrant and belonging to no-one. Some parents may find their solution in 'aborting' the problem and ultimately separating from each other in order to project and split-off the badness in the other or institutionalizing the baby out of their lives. Others, not needing to keep the good quite so separate from the bad, may assimilate the malformed child into the family despite the strain. Depending on the extent of the disability, the family may find ways of coming to terms with the disruption to their lives, being able to develop empathy for the infant no longer seen as a repudiated part of themselves. Given time they will develop the skills to meet the child's specific needs and adjust to the limitations of corrective surgery or painful upheaval of treatment procedures. Yet other couples may continue to live with a constant sense of what has been termed 'chronic sorrow' [4], religious or existential disillusionment, social embarrassment or guilt-ridden overprotectiveness. To these, the external experience of having a deformed child continues to represent a damaged part of each of them, visible out there for all to see, a fault that will not go away and will be prominently there, showing up the mother and/or father forever. As birth of an abnormal child may exacerbate pre-existing marital discord or reveal different coping styles, partners may require ongoing individual therapy or couple-counselling to help resolve these issues and also to assist them in dealing with questions and reactions of relatives and friends [5].

Normal siblings in the family may be displaced by the special attention focused on the problem baby. Anguished pity for the abnormal infant and awareness of parental sensitivity may mean that natural jealousy is diverted into covert forms of expression, such as acting out and sleep disturbances or regression to earlier patterns of behaviour. Older siblings may require psychotherapy in their own right, as the load of guilt at being whole and successful may impede their ability to relate to the damaged brother or sister or to achieve their own full potential [6]. (These issues have been dealt with more fully in Chapter 26). The emotional experience of future pregnancies will inevitably be influenced by the tragic outcome of this one.

32.1.4 Guidelines for professionals

Ideally, difficulties arising during labour or after the birth are conveyed immediately to the parents by the obstetrician and followed-up by the paediatrician allowing for some emotional preparation, without arousing unnecessary anxiety.

If the baby is in intensive care, separation should be minimized and the mother be brought in contact with the baby as soon as possible after the birth.

Where there are two parents, information concerning their baby should be given to them together, to enable them to support each other in a time of need and to be in a position for each to supplement facts the other may not have taken in.

Only the minimal amount of information should be given at first, to enable parents to hear it and negotiate the emotional adjustment required. However, belittling the problem, raising false hopes or patronizing the parents can undermine their trust in the doctor, and aggravate their latent anger against him/her. While resultant bitterness may be generalized to affect their relationship with other health personnel and the baby too.

There must be sufficient opportunities to clarify misunderstandings and misinformation, repeated explanations will be necessary and irrational self-recriminations and guilt will need to be dispelled.

Sympathetic straightforwardness is essential. The parent's self-esteem suffers an additional blow from exposure to staff's embarrassment and inability to deal with this 'unsuccessful' delivery and defective baby.

Professionals here serve as models (for better or for worse) who the parents may emulate in breaking the news to other children and relatives. One lesson to be learned is that the ability to assimilate information is fluid and at different times now and throughout the rest of their lives, members of the family and especially other children will require 'updating' to suit their current emotional and intellectual capacities.

32.1.5 Gradual discovery of hidden impairment

Not all abnormalities are visible at birth. In cases where disability is suspected but diagnosis complex, prolonged early contact is advocated to allow time for the suspicion to be verified and also to grant the parents time to form a positive relationship with the baby before the news of possible hidden impairment is disclosed. Suspected blindness, deafness or retardation might not be confirmed for some time. Meanwhile, attachment to the baby is occurring, with contact-seeking behaviour in the baby meeting parental delight. In time, sensitive parents begin to detect a lack in their infant's response, and indeed, may alert unsuspecting professionals to the deficit. New methods of diagnosis, such as video-visualization of sight defects [7] facilitate early detection of the problem, and where possible correction of it. When bonding is established before the detection of impairment, some parents can be sensitively attuned to their baby's needs and able to compensate for the handicap by evolving appropriate skills. Thus, parents may have intuitively developed a tactile-auditory language of communication with sight-impaired newborns, or have learned to heighten tactile-visual stimulation for deaf babies. However, parents who are particularly reliant on the modality that is impaired in their infant need special guidance and possibly therapy to facilitate a flexible approach. For instance, mothers who do not enjoy physical closeness often compensate vocally and visually with sighted or hearing babies, but find no substitution with a blind and/or deaf infant who may thereby suffer understimulation and become 'impeded' in human attachments [8]. Other parents may feel so cheated and shocked by the impact of the discovery that their normal baby is not as they thought, that they need to reorientate themselves to the baby afresh or cling to false hopes of misdiagnosis or miracle cures.

32.1.6 Emotional needs of parents and nurses of abnormal babies

Following an immediate or belated diagnosis of abnormality in their baby, what parents need most of all at this early point is the knowledge that it is safe to express all their feelings of disappointment, shame and grief without being accused of rejecting the baby or failing as parents. By offering a 'containing' function for the intense emotional upheaval experienced by the mother and father, professionals can ameliorate persecutory feelings and give them a secure place in which to recover from the emotional onslaught. They thus provide a model of 'parents' who can accept the bad with the good.

Following birth, the mother is particularly responsive to non-verbal communications and will be aware of subtle nuances of distaste or pity in the attitude of the health team towards them or their baby. Since this is the parents' first contact with others' responses to the abnormal baby, these will set the tone of later interactions. The nurse who helps the new mother to hold, feed or change her baby, will be of major importance in priming the parents' attitudes towards the defect and helping them accept it. It is therefore essential that personnel who deal with high-risk mothers and/or babies have insight into their own feelings, strengths, weaknesses and defences before they can draw out the positive resources in the parents by honest and supportive care.

Younger staff members concerned with their own reproductive capacities may find the crisis of tending a defective infant especially upsetting. Reactions of disgust or overidentification with the baby are normal, but if they remain unconscious can be disruptive to professional care of the baby and family. It has been noted that in the case of some abnormalities, repulsion is so great as to jeopardize care of the baby who may be left isolated by the personnel with only minimal provision [10]. It is most helpful for professionals to have regular access to a staff group where such feelings of personal revulsion, horror or anger with parental rejection can be candidly voiced, worked on and the underlying anxieties expressed.

Most specialists suggest that 3–4 days after the birth, a multidisciplinary health team consisting of physician, social worker and/or therapist and nurse caring for the baby (and when applicable surgeon, nutritionist, physiotherapist, etc.) should meet as a coordinated team with both the parents to explain what is known about the disability, discuss realistic plans for rehabilitation and share the prognosis, particularly when the baby is to remain in hospital after the mother's discharge. Depending on the problem, they might need genetic counselling. Parents will also benefit by being informed about the relevant self-help or support groups available, such as the Spina Bifida Society, PKU Organization or Parents of Down's Syndrome, etc.

32.1.7 Professional care

Once again, as in cases of perinatal illness and death, in negotiating this life crisis of the birth of an abnormal child, sympathetic tact, professional integrity and sensitive appreciation of timing are essential. It has been advocated that suspected brain damage and retardation should not be conveyed until there is absolute certainty, as due to the complexity of diagnosis in this area even expert neurologists and neonatologists have been found to make incorrect predictions about 50% of the time, which then 'stick' to the baby despite evidence to the contrary [9].

Confirmation of a hidden disability in a child hitherto overtly accepted as normal necessitates readjustments not only by the parents but by members of the extended family and network of social contacts. As they begin to regain their balance after emotionally reeling with the shock of diagnosis, parents need much professional support, as even simple childcare tasks appear insurmountable. Care within the hospital enables them to recuperate and regain contact with the good and normal aspects of their loved infant, while finding new strengths in themselves once defensive distractions are pared away. Given stress-support and acceptance despite their imperfect child, parents can offer similar acceptance to the baby. Professional support during the baby's infancy is related to positive bonding and increased competence in parents of high-risk and atypical babies [10]. When the baby is living at home, the family may benefit from both physiotherapeutic and psychotherapeutic treatment being brought to their home. A model for such psychosocial treatment may be adapted in modified form from a 'package' of help developed within the Medical Research Council, offered for families with a mentally ill child or adult member [11].

a. **Education**: the extended family may be given talks in the home by professionals who answer their questions as well as offering written information about the condition the child suffers from.
b. **Problem solving**: the professionals focus on the problems most worrying to the parents, by breaking these down into steps, outlining possible solutions, and discussing practicalities.
c. **Improved family communication and tension reduction**: in such an emotionally fraught situation blame, guilt, despair, helplessness and anxieties are rife. Professionals can assist by reframing the enduring sense of failure as one in which strengths are emphasized, both in the index child and other family members. Intergenerational boundaries can be firmed up with parents working as a team to help all their children develop, and the peer-group of siblings pooling their own considerable resources.
d. **Expanded family networks**: housebound focus on the needy child and/ or withdrawal through shame and overload may lead to a shrinkage of the family's social network, as embarrassed friends and relatives begin to drop contact. Professionals can help by introducing the family to others with similar problems thereby relieving their sense of isolation and guilt and providing them with an outlet for expressing negative emotions safely and for discovering and developing new coping strategies. Parents can be encouraged to form or join a self-help group and the extended family's support may be fostered through increased awareness of the problem and practical help they can offer.
e. Finally, **lowering of unrealistic expectations**: in cases where the damage is irreversible, parental expectations must be realistically framed so that the capacities that are available in the child can be maximized without undue pressure to achieve the unattainable.

Clearly, ongoing contact with the family recognizes that at each developmental phase of the index child and at crucial points in the family life-cycle, new needs will arise and old solutions will no longer suffice. Further work will need to be done to accommodate emotional changes.

32.2 CRITICAL CONDITIONS IN INFANCY

32.2.1 Failure to thrive syndrome

This syndrome involves failure of a young child to achieve a physical growth rate within the normal limits, although no organic disturbance is found and prior indications of gross neurological and physical abnormalities are absent. Indeed, both physical retardation and psychological difficulties tend to dissipate and the children resume growing once they have been transferred to a different environment, or some corrective measure has produced emotional changes in their caregivers. Among the identified characteristics of failure to thrive (FTS) babies of under 4-months old, are unusual watchfulness, lack of cuddliness, little smiling, and few vocalizations. Documented characteristics of 4–10-month-old FTS children are lack of appropriate stranger anxiety, few vocalizations and delay in pre-speech complex sound utterances, deficiency in motor-skill development and extreme passivity [12]. Feeding disturbances are common among these children who apparently ingest smaller quantities of food than normal infants of the same age, or vomit after a feed. Inadequate maternal nurturance was cited as the cause of failure to thrive in early documentation of the syndrome in institutionalized children [13]. However, the syndrome also appears in babies brought up at home and in these cases the condition has been attributed to disorders in maternal attachment. Potential causative circumstances cited are disturbing events in the mother (or primary caregiver's) own life:

a. Past events: early deprivations and possible loss of parent figures; illness or death of siblings, or own babies
b. Events during pregnancy, including protracted illness or deaths of key family figures
c. Events around the FTS child's birth, such as birth complications or disruptions, prematurity, acute illness of mother or baby, or congenital defects
d. Current life events, including marital strain, financial crisis, illness or substance abuse [14]

Split-screen videotape techniques allow detailed analysis of infant–mother interaction. These studies have revealed a deficiency in the normal lively interplay and reciprocity of mother and infant. In the failure to thrive situation, there is lack of attunement between the pair, with babies wary, inattentive or withdrawn, and mothers either overloading the baby's capacity for attention [15], ignoring their cues or responding negatively to them [16]. Such asynchrony may lie in defects in the child's ability to give or respond emotionally, or the parent's or both. Some babies, such as preterm infants, may have difficulties communicating or achieving age-appropriate skills. Some may be hard-to-comfort, easily disrupted, sensitive or vulnerable. Others may be 'hard-to-love', overly demanding or with disfiguring congenital defects [17]. However, in many cases, a baby who was developmentally normal at birth develops the syndrome with a mother whose relationship to the baby is psychologically complex or one who finds little satisfaction in nurturing her child. She may be suffering from postnatal depression or psychosis, but she may also be overwhelmed by the baby's demands, emotionally unrewarded and feeling 'starved' herself, with little to offer. Fathers have been shown to influence the origins and outcome of non-organic failure to thrive through inconsistent support, participation in maladaptive patterns of parenting, and/or conflicts with the child's mother which disrupt her emotional adjustment and interaction with the baby [18]. In some cases, ongoing weekly observation of the interaction in the home can pinpoint the nature of pathological handling and unconscious collusion between caregiver(s) and baby [19]. Interaction may become increasingly impoverished as a stalemate is reached with mother and baby reacting to the highly charged feeding situation, the child with refusal to take in or retain what the mother is offering, and she, distressed, becoming belligerent or just giving up the struggle, feeling hurt, offended, angered or rejected.

(a) Psychosocial management

In some cases, the baby is hospitalized, or attends a day centre, until growth is resumed. In others, treatment takes place in the home, with professional guidance to help the parents feed and interact with the baby. Having overcome the infant's wariness, the professional must work on establishing a new rewarding cycle of parental and infant responsiveness, a series of repeated pleasurable emotional experiences which enable the infant to develop the physical mechanisms for gaining weight [20]. Where psychotherapeutic treatment has been offered, revelations about the caregiver's psychosocial history often confirm that unresolved conflicts from the past invade the current relationship with the baby. For instance, treatment conducted in the home for a young mother's teasing relationship and 'mechanical and erratic' mothering of her FTS son revealed his identification in her mind with her resented younger sister [21]. Another found a 2-year old with longstanding FTS eating for the first time after her mother had achieved insight, through a brief therapeutic encounter, that she was subtly starving her little girl who was unconsciously seen as a product of an incestuous relationship with her abusing father [22]. These invasive 'ghosts in the nursery' which interfere with the mother's recognition of the baby as a person in his or her own right, cannot be abolished without access to the mother's deepest feelings. Each treatment must be specifically devised to suit the individual family involved [23]. Increased recognition of the paternal role in non-organic failure to thrive can encourage professionals to involve fathers in family-centred interventions. Where intractable marital conflicts are affecting the infant or mother's peace of mind, marital therapy, help in the home and/or possible separation may be indicated. In sum, a treatment formulation which offers understanding support rather than criticism, and which attends to the misery of the parents as well as the child, is more likely to enable the parents to improve their parenting skills than one which focuses on weight gain alone.

32.2.2 Sudden infant death syndrome

Parents of a seemingly thriving baby will wake up one ordinary morning to find the infant dead. About two births per thousand eventuate in unexplained sudden death. This means that more than 2000 babies die of SIDS each year in Britain and around 10 000 per annum in the United States, peaking around 2 months of age. 'Crib' or 'cot death', as it is called, is responsible for more deaths in the first year of life after the first vulnerable 10 days than any other cause. SIDS is defined as sudden death unexpected by history when the post mortem fails to demonstrate an adequate cause [24]. Thus, this term has been called a 'diagnosis of ignorance', used when no other perceptible condition can be held responsible [25]. There are numerous hypotheses about the causes of SIDS, most implicating respiratory anomalies. One theory suggests that the peaked range of timing indicates vulnerability to apnoea during the crucial changeover of maturation of the glottis [26] and many other studies cite crucial neurological and psychological developmental changes occurring at this point. Lipsett, a pioneer in research into SIDS, has shown respiratory abnormalities present at birth in future crib-death cases and suggests that innate organismic defects are activated by perinatal stress. He believes a subtle but complex aberration of learning processes prevents SIDS infants from responding defensively to respiratory occlusion [27], a learning dysfunction that can be fatal at this stage when there is a marked developmental transition from involuntary reflex to a voluntary deliberate one mediated by cortical control [28].

Other researchers have explored psychosocial factors of the baby and/or parents. One explanation focuses on the interaction of psychodynamic factors of bonding with organic failure, attributing

SIDS to a prolonged 'placental' relationship in which the infant fails to respond to danger as an autonomous being [29]. The incidence of SIDS has been found to be higher in siblings born at short intervals, in twins and premature babies [30]. It has been noted that these family constellations increase the burden on the 'regulation system' of unsupported parents [31]. A detailed study of video records and non-standardized interviews with parents of 30 SIDS cases 5 months after the death concluded that three features characterize the families of many cases: fascination with the index child as special and unique; an exclusive maternal claim that prevents the father's participation in childcare; fantasy negation of the real child as an individual [32]. Another study found overly intense involvement of mother and a wish for fusion [33]. However, a retrospective study would also elicit grief responses, one of which is idealization of the dead child. One researcher links the higher incidence in the West compared with developing countries, with separate sleeping arrangements, on the assumption that SIDS may be prevented by the baby at risk being regulated by parental breathing rhythms [34]. An interesting British experiment reports a 25% reduction of SIDS due to an interventional project providing an increase of five additional home visits by health visitors in the first six postnatal months [35].

Other research has focused on behavioural characteristics of the infants – feeding difficulties, vomiting, excessive sweating, inactivity, cyanosis, shrill cry and hyperactivity, similar characteristics in infants at-risk for SIDS [36] or even prenatal factors [37]. As noted, there are methodological problems with retrospective studies following an emotive event and bereaved parents are prone to selective memories. Prospective studies which repeat these findings are therefore more meaningful. One such study which compared 81 infants at-risk with 40 healthy controls and to a retrospective study previously conducted by the same researchers on 115 SIDS victims. The at-risk group consisted of 15 siblings of SIDS victims, 28 ALTE infants (who have experienced an apparently life-threatening event) and 38 infants with severe sleep apnoea syndrome (SAS). Over 70% of each at-risk group showed strikingly different behaviour from the controls, which agreed with the characteristics listed above. In particular, babies at-risk moved very little and analysis of their spontaneous motor activity revealed that their movements also differed qualitatively, having little variability, jerkiness and fixed body postures suggesting subtle neural dysfunction [38].

Theories abound, including such unconventional studies as mapping the layout of SIDS victims' bedrooms in relation to the distribution of high-voltage pylons [39]. Until more conclusive evidence enables the construction of an all-encompassing explanation, the high-risk group can be defined in terms of a combination of predictive risk factors, such as:

a. younger mothers
b. smaller or premature infants
c. third babies or over
d. urinary tract infection in the mother during pregnancy
e. bottle rather than breast-fed babies [40].

Also associated (as in Failure to Thrive Syndrome) are: low Apgar scores; lower socioeconomic level; crowded/substandard housing conditions; maternal anaemia and minimal care during pregnancy [41].

32.2.3 Subjective experience

According to a study of 700 SIDS bereaved families, parents found that the two most distressing aspects of the tragedy were the lack of time for emotional preparation and the lack of explanation for the disaster [42]. Having discovered the body, parents are commonly horrified by the strange appearance of the dead infant. Shocked and bewildered they try to revive the baby or desperately rush to the GP or hospital. Once death is confirmed, parents still have to face a coroner's enquiry to rule out unnatural death. This usually involves a uniformed policeman or official visiting to inspect the home and question the distraught parents. Many parents resent the swiftness with which official charge is taken of their baby's body, feeling excluded and suddenly severed from their own infant with whom they had so unquestioningly played only the night before. ('One minute I had a baby and the next thing I knew was her being whisked away – first by death and then by the doctors.')

To the distraught parents the pathologist's report seems to serve no purpose as it does not relieve their anxieties and the post mortem cannot supply the cause of death. The parents are in emotional limbo. With no explanation why the death has occurred, absolutely no preparation and no-one to blame, they flail around seeking an outlet for their intense pain and confusion. Anger may be directed at the GP who did not foresee the death, God who did not prevent it or the spouse who allowed it to happen. Rage may be turned inwards into self-accusation and misguided guilt at not having recognized subtle warning signals coupled with remorse about not having done more for and with the baby while s/he was alive. Grief-stricken parents often keep hearing their baby crying or find it unbearable to be in the room where the baby died. They may flagellate themselves with regrets about all those little frustrations inflicted on the baby. They may avoid visiting places they had enjoyed together, and every outing to the shops or post office becomes a cruel reminder of happier days, fraught with the danger of meeting an acquaintance who has not heard their tragic news.

The pointlessness of so much potential being cut short so early haunts the parents. Confidence in their parenting capacities might be shattered by this terrible experience of loss. Self-doubts prevail and unconscious accusations of neglect may hamper communications between the couple. For many young parents, this is the first bereavement they have experienced and with the disaster coming so close on the heels of the joy of having a baby, they may feel unable to cope with the terrible irony of the see-saw of life. Some couples draw closer in their mutual despair; for others, loss of what bound them together may expose underlying tensions, possibly leading to severe depression, separation and divorce or even suicide. Like other cases of perinatal deaths, partners often differ in their mode of mourning which may lead to misinterpretations of each other's feelings. Grandparents and other relatives may be so greatly affected by the loss that they are unable to offer support to the bereaved couple. The untimely unexplained death may cause neighbours and friends social embarrassment, resulting in protective silence on the subject with the couple or avoidance of the bereaved parents themselves, leaving them no safety valves for their internal pressure or outlets to talk about their dead baby. Further difficulties may result from the police visit rousing suspicions of maltreatment and some grief-stricken parents find themselves ostracized and unjustly criticized.

Siblings too are shocked and need to grieve for the baby that had become part of their lives. They too may experience remorse and guilt but have fewer capacities to distinguish justified culpability from irrational guilt. If it was the sibling who found the dead infant, in the ensuing panic the toddler may have been wrongly accused of causing or con-tributing to the baby's death, a false but devastating charge that may remain with the child in years to come. Fears that s/he may also be snatched away by death often are not picked up by parents, occupied with their own sad feelings, and the surviving child may feel aband-oned and estranged from his/her mother and father in their preoccupied emotional state. It has been suggested that an effective means of repairing the injury to parental self-esteem following a perinatal loss is to encourage their care and nurturance of the other children in the family, and help them deal with the loss [43].

32.2.4 Adaptation to life after a sudden infant death

Grieving families who have no preparation for their loss need help. A social worker may provide practical help with formalities and funeral arrangements and provision for other children. Most of all parents need to thrash out the circumstances of the death and dwell on all the minutiae of the preceding and subsequent days to make these meaningful and try to integrate this tragedy into the ongoing fabric of their lives. Close family and friends can serve as sounding boards, provided they are compassionate and non-judgemental. Organizations such as the Cot Death Society provide written information, counselling and the comfort of meeting with other parents who have survived the loss of a baby. The Foundation for the Study of Infant Deaths sees its role as providing counselling with the aim of helping the parents to 'understand their baby's death, identify their fears and misconceptions, to help them share and work through their grief until they can accept their loss and face the future with confidence again' [44].

Distraught parents need explanations from professionals in the field and may want an independent medical opinion. Grief will follow the usual pattern of mourning the unexpected death of a loved-one. However, there is something particularly poignant about the sudden loss of a healthy baby – loss of future potential, loss of parenthood (with an only child), loss of all the hopes and joys invested in the infant with whom they had planned to spend a lifetime, now lopped off overnight. The family need acknowledgement and support in their bereavement and exoneration from self-recrimination and blame.

Previously infertile parents and people who have subsequently been sterilized are in need of special counselling after SIDS, as are those suspecting a hereditary factor and mothers who have suffered a postnatal depression or psychosis with this child. Where one twin has died, anxiety will naturally be high and parents should be issued with an apnoea monitor. Sudden infant death is a 'Life Event', and as such may trigger old vulnerabilities and unresolved emotional conflicts. Prolonged grief or abnormal avoidance of mourning and delayed reactions may need specialist counselling or therapy from a psychotherapist or psychiatrist, or psychoanalysis in complex cases. In all cases, current resolution of grief does not mean that it will not surface time and again in years to come, particularly at times of stress and transitions. ('It has taken years to do so, but we have found ways of incorporating the dead baby into our everyday family life. We acknowledge her absence instead of denying her presence in our thoughts.')

KEY POINTS

*Confronted with a malformed baby, parents may be unable at first to reconcile the sad reality with their fantasy anticipation. The greater the visibility of the defect, the greater the disruption to early bonding. Disgust, guilt, fear and self-recriminations are common reactions.
*Following the initial shock and urge to flee, disbelief and denial are replaced with sadness, anger and anxiety. Once these are worked through, emotional equilibrium can be regained with increased capacity to reorganize their lives to accommodate the impaired child.

*Professionals can help by conveying information directly and immediately, to be repeated at later times with explanations; staff acceptance of the baby can help the mother care for her impaired infant, and psychosocial treatment conducted in their own home may alleviate ongoing problems, improve family communication and where necessary, expand their support networks and lower unrealistic expectations.

*Failure to thrive syndrome in young infants usually reflects a disturbance of interaction between primary caregiver and baby, due to interferences in either or both.

*Sudden infant death syndrome results in parental shock and often a crisis of confidence about caretaking capacities. Most parents need help in coming to terms with this sudden and unexplained death, which inevitably affects their relationship to other children born and as yet unborn.

Chapter 33

Postnatal psychological complications

There is a substantially increased risk of mental illness in women following childbirth. Epidemiological studies conducted originally in the United States and replicated elsewhere find an 18-fold rise in mental hospital admissions within the first month postpartum compared with the 9 months of pregnancy [1]. Puerperal women have been found to be 16 times at risk of developing psychotic illness within the first three months and have a fivefold risk of neurotic illness during the first year compared with any other period in their lives [2]. Three different syndromes of postnatal mental disorders can be distinguished.

33.1 MATERNITY BLUES

The most common form of postnatal disturbance is a mild transient disturbance termed the 'baby blues', suffered by over half the population of newly delivered western mothers [3,4] during the first week to ten days following birth. The blues are characterized (Chapter 16) by weepiness, mood swings and hypersensitivity peaking around the fifth day and lasting some hours or days. The 'day five' peak is the same in primaparae and multiparae, breast- or bottle-feeders, but women who become clinically depressed later in the puerperium rate higher on depression and lability and have a more pronounced five-day peak. The finding that the day to day mood changes is virtually the same in women delivered by caesarean section as women having a vaginal delivery rules out the possibility that timing of peak disturbance is due to homegoing, as post-caesarean hospital stay is around 10 days. Women being discharged after 48 hours rate higher on 'happiness' scales but it is unclear whether this is due to the home environment or whether they are a hand-picked group of emotionally stable women [4].

This weepy oversensitive 'state', partly related to tiredness, excitement and anti-climactic feelings following a long-anticipated birth, may be likened to the birthday-child who invariably cries at his/her awaited party. However, the additional strain and emotional upheaval of becoming mother to a newborn while adjusting to strangers and a new routine in an unfamiliar medicalized environment at a time of intense arousal, also contributes to the blues. Requiring no treatment, it is so common as to be regarded as 'normal' under our current puerperal conditions in western society, although apparently uncommon in many traditional cultures. Several recent prospective studies of postnatal psychiatric disorder have found a significant correlation between the blues and subsequent postnatal depression [6]. Nevertheless, a review of the relevant literature examined reported associations between maternity blues and psychiatric disorders. The authors conclude that psychologial, social and biochemical determinants are implicated but no firm inferences on causation can yet be drawn. Conflicting results in the literature are deemed due to variations in definition and measurement of the syndrome which these authors delineate as consisting of seven symptomatic states, tearful, tired, anxious, over-emotional, up and down in mood, low spirited, muddled in thinking [7]. A later study refuse psychiatric care status associated with blues [7b].

33.2 PUERPERAL PSYCHOSIS

This is a severe but relatively infrequent illness, affecting some 0.2% of puerperal cases. The incidence appears remarkably consistent across cultures, reported as occurring in between 1 in 500 to 1 in 1000 births in the western literature [8]. Abrupt onset of hallucinations and delusions, often heralded by insomnia, usually occurs within the first 2 weeks postpartum. The clinical picture seems to differ from other psychoses in the acuteness of onset, confusional features and preoccupation with the baby. About half the patients suffer from severe depression, morbid anxiety with delusional guilt, despair and suicidal or infanticidal impulses although these are rarely acted upon [9]. When women with the diagnosis of a major depressive disorder following childbirth are compared with non-puerperal controls, they are found to be more deluded or hallucinated, more labile and more disorientated [10]. Many become disinhibited and confused. However, with prompt treatment recovery can be complete and in some cases care of the baby, under supervision, may continue adequately throughout the illness. The remainder of cases have a manic, schizo-affective or schizophrenic picture, which is unusually common in the puerperium and characteristically begins within 6–7 days of delivery [11] with risk of puerperal relapse in manic depressive women.

There are many unanswered questions but it now appears that there are subtle differences between puerperal and other psychoses, and that some indications might be present during pregnancy. One study found that 25% of women admitted within three months of delivery had consulted for psychological symptoms during pregnancy and almost 50% had had symptoms of anxiety or depression during pregnancy [12]. Patients with an early onset of affective or cycloid psychosis (within three weeks of delivery) have been found, in a prospective study, to be more suspicious, tense, anxious, but above all, excited during late pregnancy when interviewed by midwives without psychiatric training. Although the women seemed to have fewer problems, had prepared more for the child, appeared in better health and had more positive attitudes towards the baby than their controls [13], the presence of this excitement (observed by the interviewing midwives) indicated a greatly increased risk for an early postpartum psychosis, especially of a manic type [14]. In another study, early onset within two weeks of delivery of the depressed form of bipolar puerperal psychosis has been found to be associated with less anger, less self-rated emotion and more animation than other depressed patients [15]. The cause of postpartum psychoses is unknown although about half the women also have non-puerperal episodes of psychosis and/or a family history of mental illness. However, it also occurs in women who seemed previously psychologically healthy, usually after their first pregnancy. A comparison with earlier studies suggests that, in recent years, alcohol and drug abuse disorders are very much more frequent among postpartum mental patients and hospitalized cases are more severely ill than previously, since many milder disorders are treated on an out-patient basis. Prognosis for recovery is excellent but 50% suffer relapse with subsequent babies [16].

33.2.1 Effect of psychosis on the mother's attachment

Timing of onset is an important factor in determining the quality of pre-morbid bonding. If the mother has had time to care for her infant and to establish a firm positive attachment before her illness becomes florid, there is something to build upon as the acute phase subsides. During the height of the illness, the baby is often incorporated into the mother's delusional system. Babycare can sometimes continue automatically or may be neglected or affected by obsessional rituals and morbid anxiety. The nature of interaction between mother and baby can vary from gross to inappropriate overstimulation in agitated states to depressed emotional unavailability or maudlin sentimentality, inattentive lack of response due to severe retardation or hallucinatory preoccupations. Because of the familial pattern, the woman's own mother is often unable to offer strong practical support during this crisis which may re-evoke memories of her own puerperal psychosis when her daughter was a baby. Psychoanalytical studies indicate that being mothered by a psychotic mother predisposes the daughter to difficulties in mothering her own baby, which in turn, may contribute to her own puerperal disturbance.

33.2.2 Subjective experience of postpartum psychosis

The inner experience of a woman suffering from psychosis is so strange and unlike what most of us experience that it is very difficult for carers to imagine what the sufferer is going through internally. The following is an excerpt from a novel based on the author's personal experience of puerperal psychosis:

'She had been a fetus and had knitted herself together in the bed . . . All of them standing round her bed . . . pointing to the baby and to the wall. She had thrown the medicine glass at the wall and made a livid spot on it. They took away her little baby. The top of his head was soft and sunken. Down with her chin in the silk and sunk, and flowing up around her cheeks the dying. She had warmed him in the bed . . . when she came to the door she saw a groaning skeleton . . . her face was a lion coming forth to kill . . . she screamed into her hands and tore at the woman's apron . . . How could they expect her to sleep when she was going through all of it? They didn't know. She had swung about the room from the ceiling and it was a swinging from the cross. There had been the burial. She was lying quietly in the bed and being covered over her face. She was carried quietly out and put in the casket . . . down and the dirt fell in above. Down and the worms began to tremble in and out . . . They didn't understand now. They (nurses) laughed and were hard. They filed past like moving picture actresses, with trays . . . She tore from her tender skin the rough nightgown . . . She stampeded the big door, the door that led outside. I will go out of here, why am I here? She pounded with her fists on the door. It has come, the hour has come. We are all to be free . . . she turned to the opposite wall and poured forth in bitterness and weeping . . . My beautiful, my calm head. The baby was with him hidden close in the grave cloths. The little white baby with quiet eyes that would not take her milk . . . That afternoon there was a great chair out in the hall and Yahweh was sitting in it' [17].

33.2.3 Treatment of postpartum psychosis

Psychotic mothers may be treated on psychiatric wards which nowadays usually make arrangements for joint admission of mother and baby. Alternatively, she may be hospitalized in a specialized mother–baby unit where staff have expertise in containing both maternal anxieties and their own fears about allowing the mother to care for her infant. By supporting the mother in her care for her baby they promote and restore healthy bonding. Occasionally, in cases of 'interlocking' disturbance, the entire family may require admission to a special unit for long-term treatment or in other cases the mother may remain at home, with domiciliary support service and/or day hospital treatment with nursery provision, thus minimizing the disruption in a home in which there are other children to be considered. Treatment may consist of antidepressants and neuroleptic drugs, ECT and/or individual psychotherapy or counselling or family therapy.

A survey of 305 psychiatric and district general hospitals in England and Wales between 1985 and 1986 noted 140 hospitals (74 psychiatric, 66 district general hospitals), distributed fairly widely around the country, excluding northern England and central Wales, which took conjoint mother and baby psychiatric admissions, seven of them providing day-care only. Figures show that mothers and babies currently being offered inpatient care constitute only 73% of the potential demand for 2.5–3.4 admissions per 1000 births. These findings, plus the estimated average hospital stay of 11 weeks in this study [18], tallies with those of other studies [19,20]. Once the psychosis has abated, women who feel the need for it and have a capacity for insight, might benefit from psychotherapy to try and make emotional sense of the period of illness, and to support them in its aftermath, while they adjust to life at home with a baby to care for. ('Psychotherapy is the first place in nine years that I've been asked what I feel rather than been told. The psychiatrist always asks my husband how I've been as if I'm not there. They treat my illness as his problem – something that happens every time I have a baby. As if I don't suffer when I'm ill – he's the poor one whose wife is in hospital. Then, when I'm better they assume I'll just go back to being what I was before the psychosis. But it's more like bottled up feelings that erupt when I'm so tired and excited after the birth. I'd like to get the feelings out now, while I'm O.K. and then maybe next baby I won't be so ill again, but if I try to talk about things at home my husband gets alarmed or feels criticized and just won't listen'.)

33.3 POSTNATAL DEPRESSION

The term postnatal distress often includes the very prevalent condition of 'depressed mood', accompanied by tearfulness, tiredness, anxiety and irritability which is to be distinguished from a more severe crippling postnatal neurotic depression. The former mild state might almost be described as the 'necessary depression of motherhood' – recognition of the imperfection of reality compared with fantasy and coming to terms with ambivalence. Since criteria vary in different studies, and many women are never referred for psychiatric treatment, it is difficult to establish exact incidence, however, between 6 and 28% of mothers are affected. They suffer from feelings of inadequacy, anger, self-loathing, helplessness or hopelessness. Other indicators are oversensitivity, anxiety, shame and despair, and symptoms of self-neglect, disorders of sleep, libido and appetite, and suicidal ideas. While hormonal changes are often cited as causal, the fact that all women undergo these yet only few become depressed, suggests involvement of other factors, such as a biochemical imbalance (and particularly low progesterone levels) [21] and vulnerability to the psychological stresses of mothering. Indeed, one study found six cases of puerperal psychosis among adoptive mothers [22] and it is thought that about 1 in 2000 women suffer from post-adoptive depression [23]. The milder form of distress, experienced by some 33–63% of all mothers' is clearly a response to the drastic effects of this major event which dramatically alters their life-style in the post-'honeymoon' days of mothering a tiny baby.

Were we to delineate the common denominators underlying virtually all postnatal depressions, we would be likely to find a sense of being ineffectual and a failure; feelings of profound self-depreciation; worthlessness and guilt at not living up to her own expectations; fear of judgement and criticism by others and shame at being depressed rather than elated and joyful. Other subjective experiences common to most postnatally depressed mothers are anxieties about the baby's well-being and fears of harming him/her either psychologically, or physically, or being harmed by the baby. Also, feelings of overwhelming sadness at the loss of an ideal (be it economic independence or belief in her capacity to soothe a crying infant), loss of self-confidence and a fear of not having her own internal resources replenished.

33.3.1 Differing precipitants of postnatal disorders

Women have different expectations of motherhood and are therefore affected differently by the reality of the experience. As suggested in earlier chapters, the Facilitator mother who wishes to dedicate herself to an exclusive intimate relationship with the baby feels depressed when unable to achieve blissful mothering. This may occur when conditions are less than optimal, when the baby is impaired or cries a lot and will not be comforted, when she is forced to separate from the infant (due to economic pressures, medical necessity or emotional demands from partner or other children) or when her idealized unrealistic standards of mothering cannot be achieved. In other words, a Facilitator becomes depressed when she is unable to fulfil her own expectations of perfect mothering. Her self-esteem is embedded in a blissfully reciprocal baby–mother–self matrix and is threatened by non-realization of the ideal. The more idealized her prenatal conception of mothering, the greater the likelihood of reality falling short of this ideal. By contrast, a Regulator mother who expects her baby to adapt to her routine feels depressed when, unable to maintain a clear definition of herself as a 'Person', she feels her pre-maternal identity slipping away from her. Erosion of her self-esteem and sense of adult competence comes about when her baby fails to become 'regulated' and predictable and when she feels entrapped in her new role, debarred from adult company, submerged in trivia and sucked dry by a demanding baby. These experiences of depressed mood in both Facilitators and Regulators are exacerbated by economic privation, disturbed sleep and physical exhaustion, social isolation and lack of emotional support of a partner [24].

33.3.2 Aetiology of postnatal depression

Clinical depression experienced postnatally has been attributed to a variety of aetiological factors ranging from the biochemical to the psychological. However, no single causative agent has been conclusively isolated, suggesting an interaction of several variables.

Some researchers have proposed a combination of psychological, socioeconomic and/or physical contributing factors, including the birth experience itself. Brown and Harris identified four vulnerability factors which render women liable to depression when confronted with life events which reduce self-esteem, namely: loss of mother before age 11; lack of an intimate marital relationship; lack of paid employment and three or more children under 14 [25]. A researcher following their lead proposed four vulnerability factors specific to postnatal depression: lack of employment; housing problems; segregated marital role; and little previous contact with babies. The risks were seen to be intensified by higher technological birth [26]. The same factors have been reiterated in another classic study which found poor marital relations and lack of social support to be determinants of postnatal depression [27]. Other researchers noted difficulties in the parturient's relationship to her own parents and prolonged conception period in women aged 30 plus [28]. Psychoanalytically oriented investigators have always stressed the reactivation during pregnancy and postnatally of unresolved ambivalent aspects of the woman's early relationship to her parents, overidealization of motherhood and conflicts over feminine identity [29]. Taking all these factors into account, I have suggested that these historical, cultural, socioeconomic and physical factors interact to precipitate postnatal disturbance in a woman when she is prevented from actualizing her own specific expectations about motherhood. In other words, a woman is more at risk for developing postnatal depression if she is exposed to sensitizing experiences salient to her own emotional interpretation of motherhood. Birth events will be interpreted differently by the Facilitator who feels a loss of self-esteem at having 'failed' to have the natural childbirth she craved in comparison to the Regulator who feels she has controlled her birth by sophisticated technological means. Likewise, lack of employment depresses the Regulator who feels trapped at home with her baby, but the Facilitator who is forced to take up employment rather than looking after her baby will find separation depressing. Similarly, the concept of 'over-idealization' of motherhood has a different meaning when applied to the Facilitator who believes in total selfless devotion to a perfect infant and the Regulator who interprets ideal motherhood as competent management of a predictable baby.

33.3.3 Centrality of the woman's relationship to her mother

Clinical experience reveals that a woman who has unhappy recollections of her own early childhood, or who had lost her mother before being able to establish post-pubertal feminine identification with her, is liable to feel an intense sense of deprivation and sadness postnatally as she relives her own infancy in that of her son or daughter. Research into childhood antecedents of parenting patterns reveals that compared with those from intact homes, mothers who as children had themselves experienced parental death, divorce or separation, talked to their babies, touched them and looked at them significantly less often [30]. The social reality of having no mother to fall back upon in difficult times is exacerbated when a woman lacks a good mother in her internal reality as well. A mother whose own experience of being mothered was limited or disturbed may actually envy her baby the mothering s/he receives, inhibiting her own ability to mother generously. If she carries around an internal image of a hated denigrated mother, she cannot identify with her, and mothering becomes a competitive experience of rivalry and one-up-womanship. If she has defensively glorified her internal experience of her neglectful mother, she herself will become overanxious, and a non-ideal mother by comparison. Only when a woman has been able to forgive her own mother for being less than perfect can she draw on memories of loving and helpful moments rather than mistakes, losses and sad times. Depressed women who cannot engage in a lively ambivalent relationship with the internalized mothers find it difficult to have a healthy ambivalent and real relationship with the baby. Depression is often the result of unexpressed anger turned inwards rather than out. A deprived woman who feels abandoned and unable to feel angry with her idealized dead mother may get her baby to express anger towards herself by being depressedly unresponsive to his needs or feeding herself rather than him. Similarly, she may be unable even to conceive of ordinary anger towards her own baby, but turns this against herself in accusations of being a 'bad' mother, or projects her feelings into the baby who is then felt to be angry and accusing. (I'm sad cos my baby hates me')

33.3.4 Disturbance in mother–child exchange

Systematic observation of mothers and babies have disclosed several factors which appear to be of prime importance in formation of close attachments:

a. Frequent and sustained physical contact
b. The mother's ability to soothe her baby when distressed
c. Her sensitivity to her baby's signals
d. Promptness of response to crying [31].

For her baby, a depressed mother is emotionally unavailable despite her physical presence. She is inaccessible for interaction, does not mirror the infant's behaviour and reciprocal play is likely to be sporadic, interrupted and low key. For example video micro-analysis of mother–infant interaction where the mother was clinically depressed and was anxious, intrusive and rejecting in her handling of the infant, revealed extreme withdrawal and avoidant behaviour in an apparently normal 8-week-old boy [32]. Findings of detailed studies of mother–infant interaction reveal fine sensitivity in very young infants to the emotional state of the caregiver, with indications that the baby responds discriminatingly and regulates his/her own expression in appropriate and complementary ways which the mother can interpret as particular emotions. When maternal responsiveness is not forthcoming and the mother appears blank, the infant becomes withdrawn and sad after repeated attempts to solicit and reinstate interaction. When her response is inappropriate and unexpected, detached puzzlement and confusion gradually giving way to avoidance and resignation [33]. Although on observations at home depressed mothers were found to talk and play with their 2–3–year–old children as much as the non-depressed controls, analysis of their responsivity sequences revealed that depressed mothers were more likely to ignore the child, more likely to employ control and physical rather than verbal behaviour and less likely to use questions, suggestions, explanations and distractions. This study also confirmed that depressed mothers tended to have more unhappy recollections of their early life (often describing their own mothers as indifferent, harsh or irritable) and more dissatisfaction with present circumstances, rating their marriages as marked by conflict, uncooperativeness and lack of mutual interest [34]. Long-term follow-up of this and other samples of children of depressed mothers have found conspicuously low levels of attention, concentration and many behavioural problems [35]. In some cases, offspring of depressed mothers find themselves having to mother their mothers, the burden of which fosters precocious responsibility and often brittle maturity in children who forego their childhoods in caring for the parent.

A psychoanalyst coined the term 'ghosts in the nursery' [36] for the invasion of oppressive memories from the mother's own past which become enacted once again in the current relationship with her baby.

We may say that the baby of a depressed mother is burdened not only with his own mother but with hers too! It is only when the depressed mother can begin to make conscious links with her own past that she can reclaim her experience for herself and stop inflicting it unconsciously on her baby. The transmission of these unconscious conflicts over generations can result in distortions in the infant's perception of reality when this is based on intimate contact with his depressed primary caretaker. Normally, the emotional availability of the mother provides the growth-promoting matrix for receiving the infant's emotional signalling. This signalling forms the basis of the baby's communication of his needs, intentions and satisfactions [37]. When she is preoccupied, depressed or overly anxious, she cannot respond positively to his need for affirmation. She cannot serve as a 'secure base' for exploration or provide 'social referencing' [38] by signalling her appropriate fear, reassurance or warning of danger. Pleasure in social interaction is muted and where there is constant non-reciprocal 'misattunement' [39] in affective interaction between the depressed mother and her child, the baby may have to develop maladaptive defensive means of coping.

Inner city isolated depressed mothers with poor marriages are both particularly vulnerable to depression and unable to provide respite or alternative stimulation for their children. Nuclear families tend to deteriorate when the largely absent male partner seems unaware of the extent of the mother's problem or if he has a history of violence or drinking which deters the woman from confiding in him and exacerbates her depression. Other children may prematurely have to take on responsibility for mothering the baby as well as looking after a depressed mother when an unsupported family is totally reliant on its own resources.

33.3.5 Treatment for postnatal depression

Mothers suffering from postnatal depression have been found to need practical help as well as psychological support. Health Visitors influence the course of illness by listening, counselling and effectively helping sufferers to reorganize aspects of childcare [40]. Friends and Social Service agencies may provide help with housekeeping for mothers who are severely incapacitated; others may benefit from individual befriending. When both partners are willing to have treatment, marriage guidance can work towards alleviating an unsatisfactory relationship which has been identified as a contributory cause of postnatal depression in many studies. Marital therapy has the advantage of relieving the woman's experience of unsupported parenthood and being targeted as 'the patient' while allowing her an opportunity to express some of her grievances and accumulated anger towards her partner rather than directing these against herself or taking them out on her baby ('my GP says I have postnatal depression. All I know is that I feel heartbroken, angry and cheated. I've had layers of optimism slowly peeled off me by living with a man who will not touch me, blames me for becoming pregnant and makes me feel economically so insecure that I have to be strong and cold and calculating about things I love passionately. He's fond of the baby. I'm trapped. I can't leave him, because I want my baby to have a father but I also dearly wanted a partnership. Of course I'm depressed! It doesn't come from having babies – it comes from not having a proper husband. I feel he's just feigning affection. He withdrew from me when I was pregnant, just pecked my cheek, never once stroked my belly and told no-one about the baby. Then I found out he was having an affair. Now, he never confirms me as a woman – I know I'm overweight but I've just spent nine months carrying *his* baby. I'm depressed all right!').

For the baby, such therapy promises to restore the emotional focus to its rightful place so that the frustrated mother need not use the infant as an erotic, demanding or frustrating replacement for his father. Studies indicate that increasing a healthy father's involvement in childcare also gives the baby a chance to form a close relationship with a non-disturbed parent which is a protective factor against later conduct disorders [41]. However, the father may also be disturbed in his own right. Husbands of women admitted to a mother and baby unit were also found to be implicated in their wives' postnatal disorder, with 42% of fathers diagnosed as having a depressive or anxiety disorder, associated with poor marital and social functioning [42]. Health visitor support and guidance may provide the woman with a model of good mothering and individual counselling or psychotherapy for the depressed mother does the same while also offering a means to gain insight into the sources of her problems and to achieve deep long-lasting changes in her internal world. By giving the mother space and time to herself to work through her psychological experience of motherhood and her own early deprivations and conflicts, the psychotherapist is indirectly influencing the mother's ability to give similar considerations to her own baby An ideal yet rare early treatment consists of clinical intervention in the disturbed relationship between mother and baby in the home setting [43]. Alternative possibilities are therapy within a day or residential family unit, or corrective child-therapy in conjunction with maternal counselling. Another practical and economic solution may be found in befriending schemes such as Newpin [44], therapeutic nurseries or parent-participating playgroups [45] and self-help organizations such as the Association for Post-Natal Illness, NCT and PSI.

33.4 VIOLENCE AND SEXUAL ABUSE

33.4.1 Infantile love and hatred

We all have destructive tendencies within ourselves which are activated as responses to frustration, fear or pain. Parents can help their babies learn to contain and integrate their overwhelming destructive feelings by containing these for them at first, tolerating the baby's aggression and protecting her or him from intolerable frustrations. When an infant has repeated experiences of parents as helpful, soothing non-retaliative allies against his/her own internal violence, the child is reassured that these destructive fantasies are containable and do not really kill, that the parent has survived the imagined or physical onslaught and yet continues to love the baby despite his or her hatred. The infant can then retain a sense of him/herself as good and lovable despite feeling enraged, and develops a belief in others as supportive, caring and helpful. Gradually, instead of the frustrating mother or father immediately turning into horrible witchlike creatures or powerful giants in the angry child's mind, s/he can begin to see them as well intentioned despite their seeming 'badness'. Once the growing infant can hold onto the beloved 'good' mother or father even while angry with him or her, a composite picture is built up of a parent who is both loved and hated. Violence now is curbed by the desire to please and protect this ambivalently loved parent from pain inflicted by one's own hatred. 'Depressive guilt' is aroused, at having attacked and hurt the very person one loves [46]). Some psychoanalysts see this 'synthesis of loving and destructive impulses towards one and the same' figure as a turning point in the child's development [47], hitherto relating to a 'whole' person for whom the previously 'ruthless' infant now feels concern and sorrow [48].

However, if the parent is afraid of the baby's aggression he or she may act punitively, setting rigid limits or even hitting the baby in angry response to the rage. Sometimes a father may imagine he see a glint of hatred or rejection in his baby's eyes, or disobedience in his/her actions and he finds this intolerable. The baby may chew the mother's nipple or dirty the clean nappy she has just put on, drop toys repeatedly over the side of the cot or treat her as if she didn't exist. The parent's own frustration and anger may boil over and one or both may find him/herself responding to the infant as their own angry parents responded to them. In fact, at that moment, they may each identify the 'naughty' baby with a bad baby-part of themselves that their own parents could not tolerate. By punishing the actual baby the mother or father try to force the infant to be 'good', while also hitting out at the baby inside and punishing what is unacceptable in him/herself, meanwhile paradoxically also giving expression to their own unleashed infantile violence. Thus a cycle may be set up in which the angry real baby interacts with the frustrated, hurt, hostile, put-upon baby within the parent, who was once just as weak and helpless but is now big and strong enough really to lash out and cause damage. Essentially, violence against another person is a failure to respect the integrity of that individual, who in the heat of the violent act becomes a 'thing' or a split-off part of one's self.

33.4.2 Abuse of babies

When a person has grown up with an explosive model of a parent on the rampage, and has also repeatedly had his/her own aggression curbed violently, s/he will not have had opportunities to resolve acrimonious feelings, nor help in achieving healthy internal controls, containment or channelling of aggression. Although she or he may have evolved effective adult controls in ordinary situations, being in close and unremitting contact with a vulnerable, demanding and often crying baby may cause long-suppressed fury to erupt. At times of stress and frustration with the needy real baby, this maltreated child now become adult will not only fail to respond appropriately but may find him or herself unable to control an enraged reaction from escalating into physical violence and the beloved/hated baby will be on the receiving end of the abuse. In some households, one child may be singled out as the parent projects characteristics of their own abusive mother or father into the baby, who can also come to represent hostile aspects of the partner, hated sibling or as well 'wimpish' aspects of themselves. While violent infliction of 'non-accidental injury' on a baby is clearly recognized as a form of abuse, recurrent rough handling may serve the same angry end but go unacknowledged by the parent, although still traumatic for the child. Equally, other forms of emotional or sexual abuse may injure the child's self-esteem or sense of security, such that they too grow up with a sense of parent unreliability and feel themselves to be unloved and unlovable. As adults they still feel abused, and may reinforce this feeling by recurrently engendering rejecting experiences which fulfil their expectations. And as parents they feel abused by the baby whom they now abuse in retaliation. Internal damage spans a transgenerational trajectory.

33.4.3 Research into child abuse

It is difficult to estimate the incidence, population characteristics and breakdown of child abuse, both for the obvious reasons of parental secrecy and denial and due to the variety of definitions employed by researchers and welfare bodies (the latter posing problems for interpretation of results and policy making [49]). Available statistics in the UK show that 55% of reported cases of child maltreatment involve children under four years with infants under two being most at-risk for serious physical injury [50]. The NSPCC reports that child abuse and neglect lead to the most common forms of death in children under 5, with up to 200 children dying per year as a direct result of maltreatment by their parents [51]. A distinction is made between the three forms of abuse – physical, sexual and emotional, each having an active and a passive form [52].

In a self-report survey conducted among abusive parents participating in a Parents Anonymous programme, abuse patterns towards their children took the following forms [53]:

– Physical violence   (53%)
– Physical neglect   (7%)
– Sexual abuse   (4%)
– Verbal abuse   (77%)
– Emotional abuse   (43%)
– Emotional neglect   (28%)

However, the voluntary attendance and self-selection of this group makes them atypical of the population of abusers.

Research has concentrated in trying to identify psychosocial characteristics of child-abusing parents so as to develop policies for prediction, prevention and treatment. However, the characteristics isolated, such as marital instability, early parenthood, criminality and unemployment, are too prevalent to have much predictive or diagnostic power [54] raising ethical issues of wrongly labelling a family high-risk on the basis of sociodemographic checklists [55]. Although antenatal programmes and immediate postnatal services provide an obvious focus for preventive strategies and intervention programmes (providing material and educational resources, social and emotional support, more liberal ward and medical monitoring regimens), a review of 13 studies assessing outcome concludes that there is some doubt that their less than 'dramatic' impact justifies the extra cost [56]. Another review of 11 longitudinal studies finds associations of child abuse with low birth weight, pre- and perinatal problems and congenital disorders are conflicting and inconclusive [57].

As we have seen throughout this book, parental orientations and childcare behaviour are based on parents' conscious beliefs and un-conscious internal representations of themselves and others, which they have evolved (with revisions due to later encounters) from their own babyhood and experience of being parented. Some of the research into child abuse has focused on identifying patterns in the ways abusive parents view themselves and their offspring. Abusive mothers have been found to differ in their perceptions of their children, who suffer not only from the direct effects of abuse but from the resulting distorted inter-actional behaviours [58]. Thus, abusing mothers have been found to be more inconsistent and insensitive in their responses, interfere more in the child's play and bring about overdependence and an insecure attachment pattern in their children [59].

Behaviour is based on mental representations and attributions. One English study has found that abusive mothers perceive their children as more powerul than themselves and therefore blame the child when things go wrong [60]. An American study investigating internal representational models of maltreating parents has been able to identify different patterns of relationships in different subgroups. Thus, abusing mothers were found to conceptualize social relations in terms of 'power struggles over scarce emotional and material resources' while neglecting mothers appear to conceive of relationships as empty, and everyone as helpless victims, lacking control. These representational models, based on internalized distortions learned in the course of their own childhoods' interactions with attachment figures, influenced their behaviour and relationships: abusing mothers were found to be controlling and hostile with their anxiously attached children, to have 'unstable, angry and often violent relationships' with members of their network of friends and 'to maintain superficial and manipulative relationships with professionals'. Neglecting mothers were unresponsive to their passive and helpless children, while involved in 'stable but affectionless relationships with their partners', and ignored or were withdrawn from professionals [61]. Thus, not surprisingly, not only do the distorted representational models affect the relationship with the child and his/her own internal model, but they are generalized across interpersonal exchanges, and become self-fulfilling prophecies, as rigid expectations and inappropriate aggressive, passive or defensive behaviour evoke reciprocal responses in social situations.

33.4.4 Treatment of abusive parents

There is currently a law making physical punishment of children by their parents a criminal offence. Despite media coverage and the recognition of 'child-line' over the last years, child maltreatment remains a painful problem that is difficult to acknowledge. As a result, parents contacting professionals for help find their pleas may go unheard or be misinterpreted, today, as a decade ago, when this was first stated [62]. However, as guilt and confusion intensify, abusive parents may present several times with complaints that mask their real problem. Professionals thus approached by parents need to 'listen with the third ear' to detect the cry for help and convey that such help is available. The NSPCC have established a National Advisory Centre on the Battered Child in London which provides medical, psychological and psychiatric services and as children become more aware of the problem, help may be alerted through school efforts or telephone assistance. Apart from individual or family therapy, more drastic temporary solutions may be required, such as provision of day care facilities, fostering or hospit-alizing the child or family. Parents Anonymous, a self-help crisis intervention group for abusive parents, offers these families an oppor-tunity to break out of the cycle of cross-generational abuse by enabling them to feel supported and accepted despite their abusive behaviour. Such support groups provide opportunities to gain understanding of their behaviour, and to relearn ways of relating that do not result in their rejection thus finding less punitive, more rewarding ways of meeting their own needs and those of their children. In extreme cases, last resort rehabilitation opportunities may be offered after assessment under stress conditions which enables formulation of clear management and treat-ment strategies. Thus, for instance, the Marlborough Family Service in London runs a multifamily programme attended by abusive families for several months at a time. Assessment of each family's predominant pattern of interaction takes place in the context of many different activities, geared to be shared by other families, with the aim of mutual assistance, establishing parental responsibility and maximizing the possibility for change. Among other assessments, potential for rehabilitation is estimated by the extent to which parents can resolve their own marital disputes without involving their child by strengthening their own internal boundaries and reducing the inappropriate power and centrality allocated to the child [63]. Such decisions are crucial as it has been estimated that between a third and two-thirds of abused children are reabused within a few years of rehabilitation [64]. Clearly, true therapeutic change can only be the result of modifications of parental beliefs and attributions and amelioration of their own internal worlds.

33.4.5 Wife beating

It is difficult to gauge the incidence of marital violence, but a recent study reports that 22% of 1000 women interviewed admitted they had experienced a violent assault in the home in the previous year [65]. A large-scale nationally representative survey (excluding divorced people) in the USA reported over 12% of female respondents had experienced severe violence and 28% had had some kind of physical abuse [66]. Having a baby often makes a woman more emotionally, economically and legally dependent on her male partner, and less able to separate from him if he abuses her. However, studies have revealed that much wife beating begins during pregnancy, and violent incidents occur prior to marriage or cohabitation but are ignored as warning signs. Marital violence has generated various theories. However, battered wives have been shown to have few specific personality characteristics, and although profiles feature low self-esteem and high anxiety, these may be the result of the abuse rather than preceding it.

Many researchers have asserted that early exposure to parental violence has been found to underlie both male abuse and female victims, creating an 'addiction' to violence in women who seek out these encounters, familiar from childhood. A high proportion of battered wives are reported to have been beaten as children by their fathers or witnessed their mother beaten by the father or other men, and/or were sexually assaulted before marriage. However, a recent large-scale study of 3000 at-risk for developing depression (working-class women with at least one child at home) was conducted in London. Findings of a 25% rate of reported violence militated against a theory of individual pathology. Although some women had experienced violence in childhood, the main association was between early lack of care and later marital violence in women. Early neglect was seen to lead to a susceptibility rather than a pathology and was also associated with premarital pregnancy and teenage marriage, both creating marital tensions and increasing the likelihood of these women staying in their violent relationships. Furthermore, many women reported more severe violence when they were pregnant and a tragic effect on their reproductive history was that they were found to be over twice as likely as women with no marital violence to have experienced a miscarriage or still-birth (33% vs 14%, p <0.001) [67]. In their marriages, intimidation and threat usually reinforce violence, a factor which often prevents women from reporting incidents to the police or seeking medical treatment for injuries. The balance of power in the marital relationship has been found to be usually skewed towards sex-role stereotyping with unequal decision-making, little sharing of housework or childcare and often virtual isolation of the wife because of her partner's morbid jealousy, possessiveness and dependency. Sexual relations may be used by the woman to appease the husband and prevent violence, or wives may be forced to engage in sexual activities against their will.

Treatment

Since many wife beaters begin to abuse children as well, GPs or health visitors may be alerted to the problem. Although there are clearly marital problems conjoint therapy may be counterindicated as husbands may refuse to cooperate or further violence may follow disclosures during sessions. Danger must be assessed and the woman and baby removed to safety if necessary. Emergency shelters exist in most urban areas and the National Woman's Aid Federation runs refuges offering emotional support, protection and guidance about housing, legal and welfare rights. Given their current anxieties and childhood history many women benefit from long-term therapeutic help beyond the crisis period, which needs also to increase their mastery of the environment [68]. Marital counsell-ing may follow if the relationship continues. Group therapy and ongoing self-help groups may be helpful in combatting isolation and providing psychosocial insights into their interactions.

33.4.6 Sexual abuse of babies

In recent years we have become increasingly aware of the widespread prevalence of sexual abuse of children, both intrafamilial and by paedophiles outside the family. As in cases of violence and emotional maltreatment, sexual abuse, too, must be seen as an excessive or inappropriate manifestation of unconscious sexual or aggressive impulses, which are ordinarily outgrown, sublimated or socially channelled into other activities or adult relationships. In cases where a person's infan-tile fantasies have been split off from everyday life and have remained encapsulated, frozen and inaccessible to an enriching exchange with reali-ty, they may erupt in psychosomatic symptoms or outbursts of irrational action which are enactments of these hived off fantasy configurations. Babies are often the targets for misdirected powerful emotions un-consciously intended for the deprived, demanding or abused 'child within' the abuser. As we have seen, violent attacks on a baby can even begin during pregnancy. Infants may also be victims of sexual attacks, either by direct assault or through overstimulation, pathological touching or gradual induction into eroticized non-penetrative fondling, which may or may not escalate into frank abuse. Babycare, with its emphasis on bodily functions and cleansing of genitals and bottom, can engender excited feelings in vulnerable adults. Sexual activity may occur in the context of an intense relationship between a baby and a disturbed parent who has him/herself been abused as a child, driven to mindless re-enactment or unable to control or resolve feelings now re-aroused by exposure to the infant. The father or mother is caught up in a double identification with both the victimized baby and his/her own internal-ized abusive parent, resulting in active perpetration of the trauma that he/she passively experienced as a child. This physical relationship may be rationalized as an expression of love, however, once incestuous sexuality crosses generation lines it results in emotional exploitation of the child for parental gratification.

In addition to precipitous sexual arousal, and inevitable emotional chaos, the very young child is invariably confused about body boun-daries and intactness, particular if abuse has involved penetration or insertion of objects. Confusion is greater when the infant lacks words to make sense of the overwhelming internal experience and is unable to express the medley of outrage, guilt, excitement, enjoyment, humilia-tion and deep agitation accompanying maltreatment. When sadism or pain accompany seemingly caring, affectionate or pleasurable activities, anxieties about internal damage tend to combine in the victim with acceptance of blame and a self-fulfilling unconscious need for punishment. Secrecy, denial and the other parent's disbelief or tacit compliance further complicate reality testing and formation of trusting relationships.

For the professional, suspected abuse in a preverbal child presents a particularly difficult problem, necessitating physical evidence, parental confession or meticulous observation of distorted play behaviour and interaction by a specialized child-psychotherapist [69]. In older children, oversexualized bodily behaviour and compulsive masturbation may communicate abuse, as may psychosomatic or hysterical symptoms which enact a 'passive body memory', such as encopresis, difficulty in swallowing, while simultaneously indicating psychological splitting off of the traumatic experience [70].

When sexual and physical abuse are combined and parents are the abusers, the dependent child lives with the unbearable reality that the very person to whom they turn to for love and protection is their attacker. To preserve a sustaining image of a good parent, experience must be fragmented and compartmentalized – the bad denied, as the child takes to guilt onto him/herself, tries to become 'good' and continues to believe and hope that eventually comfort and love will replace pain, intrusive intimacy and hatred. Alternatively, s/he may become aggressive, provocative or seductive, to justify the parental attack. These convoluted interactions are very complicated to resolve therapeutically. A study of 66 abused children found that over a quarter had to be separated from their parents and received into care at some point, with poor prognosis attached to persistent denial of abuse by the parents, their massive use of projection and misperception of the child, and impaired relationships throughout. Workers with such families are often themselves profoundly affected by the powerful feelings aroused by abusive parents and abused children, and may find it difficult to hold onto their own helpful insights when faced with denial, rejection, controlling behaviour and attacks on the professional's capacity to think. Professional effectivity may be increased by employment of multidisciplinary teams, inter-agency cooperation and greater awareness of conflicting roles and the tendency towards splitting and over-reaching activity induced by anxiety, and fear of uncertainty [71].

Treatment

Treatment consists of long-term individual psychotherapy for child and/or adult or may involve intensive work with the whole family as a disturbed system. It may necessitate temporary or indefinite removal of the child to a foster home or admission of the entire family to a suitable therapeutic community such as that provided by the Cassel Hospital, in London [72]. In some cases brief psychotherapy has been used effectively [73].

KEY POINTS

*Three distinct forms of postnatal mental disturbance may be distinguished: maternity 'blues', postnatal depression and puerperal psychoses. Although the first condition is transient, the second will require psychotherapeutic treatment, the latter, psychiatric assessment, and probably some hospitalization, followed, once the psychosis has abated, by psychotherapy if the woman wishes it and demonstrates a capacity for insight.
*It is suggested that the most common condition, postnatal depression, is precipitated in each mother by external or intrapsychic obstacles preventing her from actualizing her own specific expectations of motherhood.
*Misattunements in the mother–child exchange are a function of mismatch between maternal receptivity and infant capacities either due to the mother's distorted perceptions and/or depressed inability to react empathically, or to the baby's failure to signal or respond. When chronic and cumulative, such disturbances can lead to distortions in the infant's perceptions of reality, relationships and self-image.
*The psychological effects of family violence and sexual abuse of babies may result in long-term disturbances of identity and interpersonal relationships arising from the distorted family interactions, expressed in a variety of ways such as psychosomatic symptoms, precocious sexual arousal, delinquent behaviour, teenage pregnancies, baby abuse and confusion about body boundaries.
*Escalation of intrafamilial disturbance and its transmission across generations prioritizes early detection of psychological problems and prompt referral for treatment, during pregnancy or as soon as possible postnatally.

CONCLUSIONS

On this rather grim note we come to the end of the book. But perhaps it is fitting, after all, as another example of how childhood impressions and identifications live on in our internal realities to influence our perceptions of others in the external world. Unconscious fantasies fluctuate dynamically, finding subtle expression in daily life as we have seen throughout this book. Sometimes, when inner tensions and intrapsychic conflicts feel intolerable and the person cannot bear dealing with them in thought, they are converted into action; historical scenes or internal battles are reenacted with self and close intimates, including children, as victims, enemies or masters. Split off contradictory parts of the self are expelled and projected onto other people who are unconsciously allocated various roles in the internal drama. One person may represent a weak part of the self to be protected while another is imbued with a different weak bit of the self to be violently attacked; yet a third is made into an unruly or dangerous part to be controlled by force and subjugated, or another may be treated as an ever-present idealized object outside oneself to replace the inaccessible internal one. In each of us, despite all our defensive manoeuvres to keep the peace, the repressed strives to find expression, in words, deeds or psychosomatic manifestations. At times, the longing to recover lost parts of ourselves and be truly known by others emerges in convoluted ways. In the search for self-understanding, we latch onto those who seem to affirm us. As we've seen the craving to be recognized can be so great that we may even submit to the domination of a person who brutally dissolves the boundaries between us and penetrates to the core. In abusive relationships the denied hated or deprived child-self hidden within finds personification in the other whom we try to omnipotentaly control by force or magically seduce into compliance.

As in all phases of the childbearing cycles, it is at nodal points of transition and times of greater uncertainty and vulnerability when we can no longer take our world for granted, that desperate measures and earlier modes of functioning are reinstated as unresolved emotional conflicts are reactivated to be compulsively repeated. Each new transition (whether it involves discovery of infertility and its treatment; the process of adoption or the three phases of pregnancy; the dislocation of abortion, miscarriage or stillbirth; or the crises of early parenthood, adolescence or menopause) old foundations fall away and safe identities fragment as the past demands reevaluation and new adjustments are required for the present. Sometimes it takes courage to face a painful truth and hold onto it without embellishing or deflecting it. Gradually finding the emotional strength and clarity necessary to come to terms with loss and change, a person may learn to relinquish cherished hopes and amend earlier self-representations and by reintegrating old and new, move on to the next phase.

Professionals, whose contact with clients coincides with crises can help through the genuine encounter of a caring relationship. Likewise, during the transitional phases of the people in their care, they will find themselves in a position to offer healing opportunities for reformulation of earlier damaging experiences. To be effective, partnerships must be based on three elements, – mutual respect for the other's subjective experience, acknowledgement of separateness and differences, and the recognition of shared responsibility. Such interactions –including those between parent and child or client and professional – foster learning and change in both partners rather than mere repetition, facilitation or regulation. In these encounters, something authentic and reciprocally enriching can begin to unfold. A fresh meeting that has never happened before.

References and notes

CHAPTER 1: THE WISH FOR A BABY – PSYCHOSOCIAL AND CULTURAL FACTORS

[1] Winnicott, D.W. (1958) *Through Paediatrics to Psycho-Analysis*, Hogarth, London.
[2] Mead, M. (1949) *Male and Female*, Victor Gollancz, London.
[3] Goodall, J. (1979) Life and death at Gombe. *National Geographic*, **155**, 5.
[4] Wilson, E.O. (1975) *Sociobiology: The New Synthesis*, Harvard University Press, Cambridge, MA.
[5] Léutenegger, W. (1977) A functional interpretation of the sacrum of *Australopithecus africanus*. *South African Journal of Science*, **73** (quoted by Fisher, 1982).
[6] We may assume that containers and hence gathering were invented by females who were hampered in their foraging by infants in arms; sharing, too, probably originated from the mother's willingness to feed and later forage for her altricial dependent children, extending to sibling care for each other.
[7] Fisher, H.E. (1982) *The Sex Contract*, Paladin, London.
[8] Zilboorg, G. (1944) Masculine and feminine. *Psychiatry*, **7**, 257–96, republished in *Psychoanalysis and Women* (ed. J. Miller-Baker), Penguin, Harmondsworth, 1974.
[9] Ornter, S. (1974) Is female to male as Nature is to Culture?, in *Woman, Culture and Society* (eds M. Rosaldo and L. Lamphere), Stanford University Press, Stanford, CA.
[10] Rosaldo, M. (1974) Overview, in *Woman, Culture & Society* (eds M. Rosaldo and L. Lamphere), Stanford University Press, Stanford, CA.
[11] World Health Organization Statistics.
[12] Badinter, E. (1981) *The Myth of Motherhood: an Historical View of the Maternal Instinct*, Souvenir Press, London.
[13] Bowlby, J. (1971) *Attachment and Loss*, Penguin, London.
[14] Greenson, R. (1968) Dis-identifying from Mother: its special importance for the boy. *International Journal of Psycho-Analysis*, **49**, 370.
[15] Tyson, P. (1982) A developmental line of gender identity, gender role, and choice of love object. *Journal of the American Psychoanalytic Association*, **230**, 61–86.
[16] Dorner, G. (1989) Significance of hormones and neurotransmitters in pre- and early postnatal life for human ontogenesis. *International Journal of Prenatal and Perinatal Studies*, **1**, 145–50.
[17] Galenson, E. and Roiphe, H. (1982) The preoedipal relationship of father,

mother, and daughter, in *Father and Child* (eds S.H. Cath, A.R. Gurwitt and J.M. Ross), Little, Brown, Boston.

[18] Erikson, E.H. (1964) Inner and outer space: reflections on womanhood, in *The Woman in America*, (ed. R.L. Lifton), Houghton Mifflin, Boston pp. 1–26.

[19] Stoller, R.J. (1976) Primary femininity. *Journal of the American Psychoanalytic Association*, **24**, 59–78.

[20] Parke, R.D. (1979) Perspectives on father–infant interaction, in *The Handbook of Infant Development* (ed. J.D. Osofsky), Wiley, New York.

[21] Kestenberg, J.S., Marcus, H., Sossin, K.M. and Stevenson, S. (1982) The development of paternal attitudes, in *Father and Child* (eds S.H. Cath, A.R. Gurwitt and J.M. Ross), Little Brown, Boston.

[22] Fast, I. (1978) Developments in gender identity: gender differentiation in girls. *International Journal of Psycho-Analysis*, **60**, 443.

[23] Jacobson, E. (1950) Development of the wish for a child in boys. *Psychoanalytic Study of the Child*, **5**, 139.

[24] Chodorow, N. (1978) *The Reproduction of Mothering – Psychoanalysis and the Sociology of Gender*, UCLA Press, Los Angeles.

[25] Horney, K. (1926) The flight from womanhood: the masculinity complex in women as viewed by men and by women, in *Feminine Psychology*, Norton, New York, 1967.

[26] Freud, S.(1932) Femininity, in *New Introductory Lectures on Psychoanalysis*, Vol. 23, Standard Edition, Hogarth, London.

[27] Torok, M. (1981) The significance of penis envy in women, in *Female Sexuality* (ed. J. Chasseguet-Smirgel), Virago, London.

[28] Klein, M. (1945) The oedipus complex in the light of early anxieties, Chapter 21 in *Love, Guilt and Reparation*, Hogarth, London, 1984.

[29] Pines, D. (1982) The relevance of early psychic development to pregnancy and abortion. *International Journal of Psycho-Analysis*, **63**, 311–20

Further reading

Evans, M. (1982) *The Woman Question – Readings on the Subordination of Women*, Fontana, London.

French, M. (1985) *Beyond Power: on Women, Men and Morals*, Abacus, London.

Goodall van Lawick, J. (1981) *In The Shadow of Man*, Collins, London.

Greer, G. (1985) *Sex and Destiny: The Politics of Human Fertility*, Picador, London.

Halliday, T. (1980) *Sexual Strategy*, Oxford University Press, Oxford.

Kessler, E.S. (1979) *Women: An Anthropological View*, Holt Rinehart and Winston, New York.

Kestenberg, J. (1975) Development of maternal feelings in early childhood. *Psychoanalytic Study of the Child*, **30**, 257.

Mead, M. and Newton, N. (1967) Cultural patterning of perinatal behaviour, in *Childbearing: its Social and Psychological Aspects* (eds S. Richardson and A. Gutmacher), Williams and Wilkins, Baltimore

Mitchell, J. (1971) *Women's Estate*, Penguin, London.

CHAPTER 2: CONSIDERING PARENTHOOD: CULTURAL, SEXUAL AND ETHNIC VARIATIONS

[1] USA Supreme Court ruling Webster v. Reproductive Health Services, 1989

requiring fetal-viability testing in abortions at 20 weeks (for implications re future of abortion rulings see, e.g. *Newsweek*, 17 July 1989).

[2] Dowrick, S. and Grundberg, S. (1980) *Why Children?*, Women's Press, London.

[3] Pines, D. (1982) The relevance of early psychic development to pregnancy and abortion. *International Journal of Psycho-Analysis*, **63**, 311–20.

[4] Klein, E. (1984) *Gender Politics*, Harvard University Press, London.

[5] Horenstein, F. (1984) Children by donor insemination: new choice for lesbians, in *Test Tube Women* (eds Arditti, Klein and Minden), Pandora Press, London.

[6] Klein, R.D. (1984) Doing it ourselves: self-insemination, in *Test Tube Women* (eds Arditti, Klein and Minden), Pandora Press, London.

[7] Feminist Self-Insemination Group (1979) *Self Insemination*, 27 Clerkenwell Close, London, WC1.

[8] Pies, C. (1988) *Considering Parenthood*, Spinsters, San Francisco.

[9] Shaw, C. (1988) Latest estimates of ethnic minority populations. *Population Trends*, **51**, OPCS.

[10] Heshey, J. (1988) Ethic minority populations of Great Britain: their size and characteristics. Demographic and Vital Statistics division. *Office of Population Censuses & Surveys*, **54**, Winter.

[11] Werner, B. (1988) Fertility trends in the UK and in 13 other developed countries 1966–1986. *Population Trends*, **51**, Spring.

[12] Shaw, (1988) *Population Trends*, **51**.

[13] 1986 population estimates, Office of Population Census and Surveys.

[14] *Labour Force Survey*, (1986) Office of Population Census and Surveys, HMSO, London, 1988.

[15] Fuller, J.H.S. and Toon, P.D. (1988) *Medical Practice in a Multicultural Society*, Heinemann, Oxford.

[16] *Labour Force Survey* (1986) Office of Population Census and Surveys, HMSO, London, 1988.

[17] McGilvray, D.B. (1982) Sexual power and fertility in Sri Lanka: Batticaloa Tamils and Mores, in *Ethnography of Fertility and Birth* (ed. C.P. MacCormack), Academic Press, New York.

[18] Balasubrahmanyan, V. (1984) Women as targets in India's family planning policy, in *Test-Tube Women*, (eds R. Arditti, R.D. Klein and S. Minden), Pandora Press, London.

[19] Pathan mothers in Bradford, Doctoral Dissertation, University of Warwick, Coventry, UK.

[20] *Labour Force Survey* (1986) Office of Population Census and Surveys HMSO, London, 1988.

[21] This section is largely drawn from Fuller, J.H.S. and Toon, P.D. (1988). *Medical Practice in a Multicultural Society*, Heinemann, Oxford.

[22] Fuller, J.H.S. and Toon, P.D. (1988) *Medical Practice in a Multicultural Society*, Heinemann, Oxford.

[23] It is useful to distinguish between various forms of male dominance practised in different societies – ranging from male supremacy and/or patriarchal exclusion of women from all political institutions and economic decision-making to separatist cultures in which each sex retains prestige (and control) in their own spheres.

[24] Fuller, J.H.S. and Toon, P.D. (1988) *Medical Practice in a Multicultural Society*, Heinemann, Oxford.

[25] Campling, P. (1989) Race, culture and psychotherapy. *Psychiatric Bulletin of the Royal College of Psychiatrists*, **13**, 550–1.

[26] Acharya, S., Moorhouse, S., Kareem, J. and Littlewood, R. (1989) Nafsiyat: a psychotherapy centre for ethnic minorities. *Psychiatric Bulletin of the Royal College of Psychiatrics*, **13**, 358–60.

[27] Larbie, J. (1985) *Black Women and the Maternity Services*, Training in Health and Race, NEC Print, Cambridge.

[28] McGilvray, D.B. (1982) Sexual power and fertility in Sri Lanka; Batticaola Tamils and Mores, in *Ethnography of Fertility and Birth* (ed. C.P. MacCornack), Academic Press, New York.

[29] See for instance, Sangari, K. (1984) If you would be the mother a son, in *Test-Tube Women* (eds Arditti, Klein amd Minden), Pandora, London.

Further reading

Badinter, E. (1980) *The Myth of Motherhood – an Historical View of the Maternal Instinct*. Souvenir Press, London.

Chodorow, N. (1978) *The Reproduction of Mothering – Psychoanalysis and the Sociology of Gender*, University of California Press, Berkley.

Dally, A. (1982) *Inventing Motherhood – the Consequences of an Ideal*. Burnett (Hutchinsons), London.

French, M. (1986) *Beyond Power: on Women, Men and Morals*, Abacus, London.

Shapiro, J. (1989) *A Child: Your Choice*, Pandora, London.

CHAPTER 3: PROLONGED INFERTILITY: PSYCHODYNAMICS AND PSYCHOLOGICAL IMPACT OF DIAGNOSIS AND TREATMENT

[1] Wright, J., Allard, M., Lecours, A. and Sabourin, S. (1989) Psychosocial distress and infertility: a review of controlled research. *International Journal of Fertility*, **34**, 126–42.

[2] Edelmann, R.J. and Connolly, K.J. (1986) Psychological aspects of infertility. *British Journal of Medical Psychology*, **59**, 209–19.

[3] Edelmann, R.J. and Golombok, S. (1989) Stress and reproductive failure. *Journal of Reproductive and Infant Psychology*, special issue on Psychology & Infertility, **7**, 79–86.

[4] Taymor, M.L. and Bresnick, E. (1979) Emotional stress and infertility. *Infertility*, **2**, 39–47.

[5] Benedek, T., Hame, G., Robbins, F.P. and Rubinstein, B. (1953) Some emotional factors in infertility. *Psychosomatic Medicine*, **15**, 485.

[6] Langer, M. (1958) Sterility and envy. *International Journal of Psycho-Analysis*, **39**, 139–43.

[7] Deutsch, H. (1945) *The Psychology of Women*. Grune and Stratton, London.

[8] Rubinstein, B.B. (1951) Emotional factors in infertility. *Fertility and Sterility*, **2**, 80.

[9] Callan, V.J. and Hennessey, F.J. (1989) Psychological adjustment to infertility: a unique comparison of two groups of infertile women, mothers and women childless by choice. *Journal of Reproductive and Infant Psychology*, special issue on Psychology and Infertility, **7**, 105–12.

[10] Soules, M.R. (1985) The in vitro fertilization rate: let's be honest with one another. *Fertility and Sterility*, **43**, 511–13, quoted in editorial. *Journal of Reproductive and Infant Psychology*, special issue on Psychology and Infertility, **7**, 63–5.

[11] Pfeffer, N. and Woolett, A. (1983) *The Experience of Infertility*, Virago, London.

[12] Connolly, K.J., Edelmann, R.J. and Cooke, I.D. (1987) Distress and marital problems associated with infertility. *Journal of Reproductive and Infant Psychology*, **5**, 49–57.

[13] Pines, D. (1990) Emotional aspects of fertility and its remedies. *International Journal of Psycho-Analysis*, **70**.

[14] Stigger, J. (1983) *Coping with Infertility*, Augsburg, Minneapolis.

[15] Raphael-Leff, J. (1986) Infertility: diagnosis or life sentence? *British Journal of Sexual Medicine*, **13**, 28–30.

[16] Brand, H.J. (1989) The influence of sex differences on the acceptance of infertility. *Journal of Reproductive and Infant Psychology*, special issue on Psychology and Infertility, **7**, 129–32.

[17] Connolly, *et al.* (1987) Distress and marital problems associated with infertility. *Journal of Reproductive and Infant Psychology*, **5**, 49–57.

[18] Raphael-Leff, J. (1989) 'The Baby Makers', presented at International Congress on Pre- and Peri-Natal Psychology and Medicine, Jerusalem, March, 1989. *British Journal of Psychotherapy*, **7**: 1992.

[19] Raval, H., Slade, P., Buck, P. and Lieberman, B.E. (1987) The impact of infertility on emotions and on the marital and sexual relationship. *Journal of Reproductive and Infant Psychology*, **5**, 221–34.

[20] Edelmann, R.J. and Connolly K.J. (1986) Psychological aspects of infertility. *British Journal of Medical Psychology*, **59**, 209–19.

[21] Cook, R., Parsons, J., Mason, B. and Golombok, S. (1989) Emotional, marital and sexual functioning in patients embarking on IVF and AID treatment for infertility. *Journal of Reproductive and Infant Psychology*, special issue on Psychology and Infertility, **7**, 87–94.

[22] Burns, L.H. (1987) Infertility as boundary ambiguity: one theoretical perspective, *Family Process*, **26**, 359–72,

[23] Leto, S. and Frensilli, F.J. (1981) Changing parameters of donor sperm. *Fertility and Sterility*, **36**, 766–70, quoted by Page, H. (1988) The increasing demand for infertility treatment. *Health Trends*, **20**, 115–17.

[24] Berger, D.M. (1980) Impotence following the discovery of azoospermia. *Fertility and Sterility*, **34**, 154–6.

[25] Note: I am indebted to a particular patient for this concept of a 'funnel', more fully described in Raphael-Leff, J. (1989) 'The Baby Makers', paper presented at International Congress on Pre- and Peri-natal Psychology and Medicine, Jerusalem, March, 1989.

[26] Ibid.

[27] Christie, G.L. (1980) The psychological and social management of the infertile couple, chapter 11, in *The Infertile Couple* (eds. Pepperell, Hudson and Wood), Churchill Livingstone, Edinburgh.

Further reading

De Cherney, A.H., Polon, M.L., Lee, R.D. and Boyers, S.P. (1988) *Decision Making in Infertility*, Decker, Toronto.

Houghton, P. and Houghton, D. (1984) *Coping with childlessness*, Allen & Unwin, London.

Klein, R.D. (ed) (1989) *Infertility – women speak out*, Pandora, London.

Winston, R. (1986) *Infertility – A Sympathetic Approach*, Dunitz, London.

CHAPTER 4: WOMB AND WORLD: THE MOTHER-TO-BE – COMMON EXPERIENCE AND CULTURAL VARIATIONS

[1]   Shaw, E. and Darling, S. (1984) *Strategies of Being Female – Animal Patterns, Human Choices*. Harvester Press, Brighton.
[2]   Feder, L. (1980) Preconceptive ambivalence and external reality. *International Journal of Psycho-Analysis*, **61**, 161.
[3]   Note: Here as elsewhere in this book, citation marks refer to direct quotes from participants in my studies unless otherwise specified.
[4]   Raphael-Leff, J. (1980) Psychotherapy with pregnant women, in *Psychological Aspects of Pregnancy, Birthing and Bonding* (ed. B. Blum), Human Sciences Press, New York, pp. 174–205.
[5]   van Gennep, A. (1960) *The Rites of Passage*, Routledge, London, 1980.
[6]   Kestenbergh, J. (1956) On the development of maternal feelings in early childhood: observations and reflections. *Psychoanalytic Study of the Child*, **11**, 257–91.
[7]   Bibring. G., Dwyer, L., Huntington, D.D. and Valenstein, A.F. (1961) A study of the psychological processes in pregnancy and the earliest mother–child relationship. *Psychoanalytic Study of the Child*, **16**, 9.
[8]   Rapoport, R. (1963) Normal crises: Family structure and mental health. *Family Practice*, **2**, 68–80.
[9]   Deutsch, H. (1945) *The Psychology of Women*, vol. 2. Grune and Stratton, London, 1980.
[10] Benedek, T. (1970) The psychobiology of pregnancy in *Parenthood – its Psychology and Psychopathology* (eds A.J. Anthony and T. Benedek), Little, Brown, Boston.
[11] Kestenberg, J.S. (1976) Regression and reintegration in pregnancy. *Journal of the American Psychoanalytic Association*, **24**, 213, Supplement: Female Psychology.
[12] Benedek, T. (1959) Parenthood as a developmental phase. *Journal of the American Psychoanalytic Association*, **7**, 379–417.
[13] Raphael-Leff, J. (1984) Myths and modes of motherhood. *British Journal of Psychotherapy*, **1**, 6–30.
[14] Mead, M. and Newton, N. (1967) Cultural patterning of perinatal behaviour, in *Childbearing: its Social and Psychological Aspects* (eds S. Richardson and A. Gutmacher), Williams and Wilkins, Baltimore.
[15] MacCormack, C.P. (ed.) (1982) *Ethnography of Fertility*, Academic Press, New York.
[16] Jimenez, M.H. and Newton, N. (1979) Activity and work during pregnancy and the postpartum period: a cross-cultural study of 202 societies. *American Journal of Obstetrics and Gynecology*, **135**, 171–6.
[17] Kitzinger, S. (1978) *Women as Mothers*, Fontana/Collins, London.
[18] Maternity Services Liaison Scheme, Tower Hamlets, London.
[19] Multi-Ethnic Women's Health Project, City & Hackney Community Health Council, London. (For a discussion of the contribution of these projects, see Raphael-Leff, J. (1988) report on meeting of Royal Society of Medicine's Forum for Maternity and the Newborn, on 'Ethnic and cultural aspects of maternity care', *Maternal and Child Health*.)
[20] Dihour, O.E. (1989) The work of the Somali Counselling Project in the UK. *Psychiatric Bulletin*, **13**, 619–21.
[21] Larbie, J. (1985) A survey of thirty young Afro-Caribbean women's experiences and perceptions of pregnancy and childbirth, *Black Women and*

the Maternity Services, Health Education Council, Training in Health and
Race. NEC Print, Cambridge.

Further reading

Ballou, J.W. (1978) *The Psychology of Pregnancy – Reconciliation and Resolution*.
Lexington Books, Toronto.
Blum, B.L. (ed.) (1980) *Psychological Aspects of Pregnancy, Birthing and Bonding*.
Human Sciences Press, New York.
Breen, D. (1975) *The Birth of a First Child*. Tavistock, London.
Shereshefsky, P.M. and Yarrow, L.J. (1973) *Psychological Aspects of First Pregnancy
and Early Post-Natal Adaptation*. Raven Press, New York.

CHAPTER 5: MATURATIONAL PHASES

[1] Raphael-Leff, J. (1980) Psychotherapy with pregnant women, in
Psychological Aspects of Pregnancy, Birthing and Bonding (ed. B. Blum), Human
Sciences Press, New York.
[2] Raphael-Leff, J. (1982) Psychotherapeutic needs of mothers-to-be, *Journal
of Child Psychotherapy*, **8**, 3.
[3] Lester, E.P. and Notman, M.T. (1986) Pregnancy, developmental crisis and
object relations: psychoanalytic considerations, *International Journal of
Psycho-Analysis*, **67**, 357–66.
[4] Kestenberg, J. (1976) Regression and reintegration in pregnancy. *Journal
of the American Psychoanalytic Association*, **24**, 213–50 (supplement, Female
Psychology).
[5] Deutsch, H. (1944) *The Psychology of Women – a psychoanalytic interpretation*. Grune and Stratton, London.
[6] Freud, S. (1916) Parapraxes. *Introductory Lectures on Psycho-Analysis*, lectures
1–5, Hogarth Press, London.
[7] Bibring, G.L. (1959) Some considerations of the psychological processes
in pregnancy. *Psychoanalytic Study of the Child*, **16**, 9.
[8] Oakley, A. (1979) *From Here to Maternity*. Penguin, London.
[9] Breen, D. (1981) *Talking with Mothers – about Pregnancy, Childbirth and Early
Motherhood*. Jill Norman, London (reissued by Free Association Press).
[10] Ferreira, A.J. (1960) The pregnant woman's emotional attitude. *Am. J.
Orthopsychiatry* **30**, 553–61.
[11] Deutsch, H. (1944) *The Psychology of Women – a psychoanalytic interpretation*. Grune and Stratton, London.
[12] Cooper, S. (1987) The fetal alcohol syndrome. *Journal of Child Psychology
and Psychiatry*, **28**, 223–7.
[13] Condon, J.T. (1986) The spectrum of fetal abuse in pregnant women. *Journal
of Nervous and Mental Disease*, **174**, 509–16.
[14] Kestenberg, J. (1975) Development of maternal feelings in early childhood.
Psychoanalytic Study of the Child, **30**, 257.
[15] Klein, M. (1955) The psycho-analytic play technique: its history and significance, in *Envy & Gratitude and Other Works*. Hogarth, London, 1984, p. 133.
[16] Ballou, J.W. (1978) *The Psychology of Pregnancy – Reconciliation and Resolution*.
Lexington Books, Toronto.
[17] Breen, D. (1975) *The Birth of a First Child*, Tavistock, London.
[18] Raphael-Leff, J. (1985) Fears and fantasies of childbirth, *PPPANA Journal*

Official publication of Pre & Perinatal Psychology Association of North America, Spring, pp. 14–17.

[19] Areskog, B., Uddenbberg, N. and Kjessler, B. (1983) Background factors in pregnant women with and without fear of childbirth. *Journal of Psychosomatic Obstetrics and Gynaecology*, **2**, 102–8.

[20] Elliott, S. *et al.* (1984) Relationship between obstetric outcome and psychological measures in pregnancy and the postnatal year. *Journal of Reproductive and Infant Psychology* **2**, 18–32.

[21] Chalmers, B. (1983) Psychosocial factors and obstetric complications. *Psychological Medicine*, **13**, 333–9.

[22] McDonald, R.L. (1968) The role of emotional factors in obstetric complications: a review, *Psychosomatic Medicine*, **30**, 222–37.

CHAPTER 7: PSYCHOTHERAPY DURING PREGNANCY

[1] Raphael-Leff, J. (1982) Psychotherapeutic needs of mothers-to-be. *Journal of Child Psychotherapy*, **8**, 3.

[2] Robin, AA (1962) The psychological changes of normal parturition, *Psychiatric Quarterly*, **36**, 129.

[3] Kumar, R. and Robson, K. (1984) A prospective study of emotional disorders in childbearing women. *British Journal of Psychiatry*, **152**, 799–806.

[4] Jarrahi-Zadeh, A., Kane, F.J., Van de Castle, R.L., Lachenbruch, P.A. and Ewing, A. (1969) Emotional and cognitive changes in pregnancy and early puerperium. *British Journal of Psychiatry*, **115**, 797–806.

[5] Bibring, G.L., Dwyer, T.F., Huntington, D.S. and Valenstein, A.F. (1961) A study of the psychological processes in pregnancy and the earliest mother–child relationship. *Psychoanalytic Study of the Child*, **16**, 9–72.

[6] Sharpe, D. (1988) Validation of the 30 item General Health Questionnaire in early pregnancy. *Psychological Medicine*, **18**, 503.

[7] Ibid.

[8] Paykel, E.S., Emms, E.M., Fletcher, J. and Rassaby, E.S. (1980) Life events and social support in puerperal depression. *British Journal of Psychiatry*, **136**, 339–46.

[9] Oakley, A. (1980) *Woman Confined – Towards a Sociology of Childbirth*. Martin Richardson, Oxford.

[10] Bourne, S. and Lewis, E. (1984) Pregnancy after stillbirth or neonatal death: psychological risks and management. *Lancet*, **ii**, 31–3.

[11] Cartwright, A. (1989) Trends in family intentions and use of contraception among recent mothers 1967–84., Institute of Social Studies, in *Population Trends*, **55**, Spring.

[12] The question of disposal of frozen embryos (where no provision has been made in advance) has given rise to incredible legal wrangles. In a recent North American case, a divorced woman's ex-husband refused her permission to have implanted any of the seven embryos he fertilized during their marriage, on the grounds that following their separation he no longer wanted to have a baby with her. Likewise, in a widely publicized case of Australian frozen embryos whose 'parents' were killed in a crash in 1983 – authorities wrestled with the question of whether the estate should inherit the embryos, or the embryos should inherit the estate! A law was subsequently passed allowing the embryos to be implanted in another woman (*The Boston Sunday Globe*, 6 August 1989).

[13] Selective abortion has become increasingly feasible as recent technological

innovations heighten the accuracy of introduction of abortefacients into specific umbilical cords or fetal sacs. In addition to the psychological sequelae common after an abortion, not only do these conflict with an ongoing viable pregnancy, but after the birth, the live baby will continue throughout his/her life to remind the parents of their burden of guilt at having chosen to terminate one or more lives while preserving another, and at times the unconscious doubt will surface as to whether they chose to keep the 'right' baby.

[14] Pfeffer, N. and Woolet, A. (1983) *The Experience of Infertility*, Virago, London.

[15] Raphael-Leff, J. (1986) Infertility: diagnosis or life sentence? *British Journal of Sexual Medicine*, **13**, 28–30.

[16] Hormann, E. (1989) Surrogacy: high risk for mother and baby. Paper presented to 4th International Conference on Pre and Perinatal Psychology, Amherst, Mass, USA, 3 August 1989.

[17] See, for instance, Danica, E. (1988) *Don't – a woman's word*, Woman's Press, London.

[18] Herman, J. and Hirschman, L. (1977) Father–Daughter Incest. *Signs. Journal of Women in Culture and Society*, **2**, 735.

[19] Burgess, A.W. and Holmstrom, L.L. (1981) Rape: sexual disruption and recovery, in *Women and Mental Health* (eds. E. Howell and M. Bayes), Basic Books, New York.

[20] Stanko, E.A. (1985) *Intimate Intrusions: Women's Experience of Male Violence*, Routledge and Kegan Paul, London.

[21] Russel, D.E.H. and Howell, N. (1983) The prevalence of rape in the United States revisited. *Signs: Journal of Women in Culture and Society*, **8**, 688.

[22] Burgess, A.W. and Holmstrom, L.L. (1974) *Rape: Victims of Crisis*. Brady, Bowrie, Md.

[23] Brown, G.W. and Harris, T.O. (1978) *Social Origins of Depression: a Study of Psychiatric Disorder in Women*. Tavistock, London.

[24] Population Trends, Office of Population Census and Surveys, HMSO, London, Spring (1988).

[25] Population Trends, 61 Office of Population Census and Surveys, HMSO, 1989.

[26] Population Trends, Office of Population Census and Surveys, HMSO, London, Winter (1988).

[27] Paykel *et. al.* (1980) Life events and social support in puerperal depression. *British Journal of Psychiatry*, **36**, 339–46.

[28] See Cox, J.I., Paykel, E.S. and Page, M.L. (1989) *Childbirth as a Life Event*, Duphar, Dorset.

[29] Milner, G. and O'Leary, M.M. (1988) Anorexia nervosa occurring in pregnancy, *Acta Psychiatrica Scandinavica*, **77**, 491–2.

[30] Brinch, M., Isager, T. and Tolstrup, K. (1988) Anorexia nervosa and motherhood: reproduction pattern and mothering behaviour of 50 women. *Acta Psychiatrica Scandinavica*, **77**, 611–17.

[31] Beary, M.D., Lacey, J.H. and Merry, J. (1986) Alcoholism and eating disorders in women of fertile age. *British Journal of Addiction*, **81**, 769–74.

[32] Cooper, S. (1987) The fetal alcohol syndrome. *Journal of Child Psychology and Psychiatry*, **28**, 223–7.

[33] Adams-Hillard, P.J. (1985) Physical abuse in pregnancy. *Obstetrics and Gynecology*, **16**, 185–90, quoted in Condon, J.T. (1986) (see below).

[34] Condon J.T. (1986) The spectrum of fetal abuse in pregnant women. *Journal*

of Nervous and Mental Disease, **174**, 509–16.

[35] Stack, J.M. (1987) Prenatal psychotherapy and maternal transference to fetus. *Infant Mental Health Journal*, **8**, 100–9.

[36] Statement from the consultation on breastfeeding/breast milk and human immunodeficiency virus (HIV), Geneva, 23–25 June 1987, WHO/SPA/IVF/87.8

[37] AIDS in the Black Community (1989) *World AIDS*, **6**, November, p. xviii. Panos Institute and Bureau of Hygiene and Tropical Diseases, London. In the UK, an organization called *'Positively Women'* offers a range of practical and emotional support services for women who are infected, have AIDS or associated conditions, including counselling on pregnancy issues. This organization and indeed some medical ethicists feel that since up to 75% of babies born to infected mothers will be healthy, it is an invasion of privacy to forbid pregnancy, particularly when, as in all life-threatening situations, the urge to procreate may give meaning to life.

[38] For instance, Phyllis Klaus has reported success in preventing precipitous labour with psychotherapeutic techniques; POP (Paediatric/Obstetric/Psychiatric) Conference, London Hospital, 27 Sept 1989.

[39] For a personal account see Saxton, M. (1984) Born and unborn: the implication of reproductive technologies for people with disabilities, in *Test Tube Women*, (eds R. Arditti, R.D. Klein and S. Minden), Pandora Press, London.

[40a] Finger, A. (1984) Claiming all of our bodies: reproductive rights and disabilities, in *Test Tube Women* (eds R. Arditti, R.D. Klein and S. Minden), Pandora Press, London.

[40b] A recently published book deals specifically with issues faced by disabled women choosing to become pregnant. Campion, M.J. (1990) *The Baby Challenge*, Routledge, London.

[41] Brodsky, A.M. (1981) A decade of feminist influence on psychotherapy, in *Women and Mental Health* (eds. E. Howell and M. Bayes), Basic Books, New York.

[42] Ernst, S. and Goodison, L. (1981) *In Our Own Hands: a Book of Self-help Therapy*, The Woman's Press, London.

[43] Foulkes, S.H. (1953) Some similarities and differences between psycho-analytic principles and group-analytic principles, *British Journal of Medical Psychology*, **26**, 30.

[44] Saravay, S.M. (1978) Psychoanalytic theory of group development. *International Journal of Group Psychotherapy*, **28**, 481–505.

[45] Scheidlinger, S. (1974) On the concept of the 'mother group', *International Journal of Group Psychotherapy*, **24**, 417–28.

[46] Schindler, W. (1966) The role of the mother in group psychotherapy. *International Journal of Group Psychotherapy*, **16**, 198–202.

[47] Bion, W.R. (1961) *Experience in Groups*, Tavistock, London.

[48] Klaus, M.H., Kennel, J.H., Robertson, S.S. and Sosa, R. (1986) Effects of social support during parturition on maternal and infant morbidity, *British Medical Journal*, **293**, 585–7.

[49] Winnicott, D.W. (1956) Primary maternal preoccupation, in *Through Paediatrics to Psycho-Analysis*, Hogarth, London, 1982.

[50] Bassen, G.R. (1988) the impact of the analyst's pregnancy on the course of analysis. *Psychoanalytic Inquiry*, **8**, 280–98.

[51] Breen, D. (1977) Some differences between group and individual therapy in connection with the therapist's pregnancy. *International Journal of Group Psychotherapy*, **27**, 499–506.

[52] Gottlieb, S. (1989) The pregnant psychotherapist: a potent transference stimulus. *British Journal of Psychotherapy*, **5**, 287–99.

[53] Raphael-Leff, J. (1980) Psychotherapy with pregnant women, in *Psychological Aspects of Pregnancy, Birthing and Bonding* (ed. B. Blum), Human Sciences Press, New York.

[54] Peterson, G., Mehl, L. and McRae, J. (1988) Relationship of psychiatric diagnosis, defenses, anxiety and stress with birth complications, chapter 37 in *Prenatal and Perinatal Psychology and Medicine* (eds. P. Fedor-Freybrgh and V. Vogel), Parthenon Press, Lancaster.

Relevant Organizations

National Aids Helpline 0800–567–123
Body Positive 071–373–9124
London Lighthouse 071–792–1200
Frontliners 071–831–0330 extension 433
Disabilities Alliance 071–240–0806
Greater London Association for the Disabled 071–274–0107
Black Women's Centre 41 Stockwell Green, SW9 071–274–9220
Black Lesbian and Gay Centre 081–885–3543

CHAPTER 8: THE FETUS: SOCIOCULTURAL BELIEFS, MATERNAL FANTASIES AND FETAL ABILITIES

[1] Egyptian papyri such as the 'Ebers papyrus' from 1550 BC also record methods of abortion ranging from herbal remedies to insertion of foreign objects to produce irritation.

[2] Susruta; Caraka, described by Gupta, D. and Datta, B. (1989) The cultural and historic evolution of medical and psychological ideas concerning conception and embryo development, in *Prenatal and Perinatal Psychology and Medicine: Encounter with the Unborn* (ed. P. Fedor-Freybergh and M.L.V. Vogel), Parthenon Books, Lancaster. Chap. 47.

[3] Galen, *Formation of the Foetus*, see Galen of Pergamos, *On the Natural Faculties* (ed. Brock), Heinemann, London.

[4] Philo (Spec. 3:108) Refers to Jewish Law.

[5] Koran cited by Moore, K.L. (1982) *The Developing Human*, W.B. Saunders, London, pp. 8–9

[6] Malinowski, B. (1916) Baloma: the Spirit of the Dead in the Trobriand Islands. *Journal Royal Anthropological Institute*, London.

[7] Caraka, (C.S.4.5). quoted by Gupta, D. and Datta, B. (1989) *Prenatal and Perinatal Psychology and Medicine* (eds P. Fedor-Freyburgh and M.L.V. Vogel), Parthenon, Lancaster, p. 525.

[8] Meggitt, M.J. (1962) *Desert People*, Angus and Robertson, London.

[9] Hakansson, T. (1989) Cross-cultural descriptions of prenatal experience chapter 49, in *Prenatal and Perinatal Psychology and Medicine: Encounter with the Unborn* (eds P. Fedor-Freybergh and M.L.V. Vogel), Parthenon Books, Lancaster.

[10] Devish, R. (1981) Semantic patterning of fertility and gynaecological healing: some anthropological perspectives, in *Reversibility of Sterilization, Psycho(patho)logical Aspects* (eds P. Nijs and I. Brosen), Acco, Leuven.

[11] Mead, M. and Newton, N. (1967) Cultural patterning of perinatal

behaviour, in *Childbearing: its Social and Psychological Aspects* (eds S. Richardson and A. Gutmacher), Williams and Wilkins, Baltimore.

[12] Mead, M. (1949) *Male and Female*, Gollancz, New York, p. 61.

[13] Jenness, (1935) quoted by Mead, M. and Newton, N. (1967) in *Childbearing: its Social and Psychological Aspects* (eds S. Richardson and A. Gutmacher), Williams and Wilkins, Baltimore, p. 153.

[14] Blackwood, (1935), quoted in Mead and Newton, *op. cit.*

[15] Holmberg, A.R. (1950) *Nomads of the Longbow: the Siriono of Eastern Bolivia*, 10, Smithsonian Institute, Washington.

[16] Mead, M. (1935) *Sex and Temperament in Three Primitive Societies*, Mentor, New York.

[17] Zeledon, M.T., Flores, R. and Villalobos, M. (1989) Sociocultural expectations and responses to the sexual identity to the unborn and newborn in San Jose, Costa Rica. *Prenatal and Perinatal Psychology and Medicine: Encounter with the Unborn* (ed. P. Fedor-Freybergh and M.L.V. Vogel), Parthenon Books, Lancaster, Chap. 50.

[18] Raphael-Leff, J. (1989) The mother mystique: psycho-sociological factors which promote an unrealistic view of mothers, in *Prenatal and Perinatal Psychology and Medicine* (eds P. Fedor-Freybergh and M.L.V. Vogel), Parthenon, Lancaster, Chap. 53.

[19] Zeanah, C.H., Keener, M.A., Stewart, M.A. and Anders, T.F. (1985) Prenatal perception of infant personality: a preliminary investigation, *Journal of the American Academy of Child Psychiatry*, **24**, 204–10.

[20] Merbert, C.J. and Kalinowski, M.F. (1986) Parent's expectations and perceptions of infant temperament: 'pregnancy status' differences. *Infant Behaviour and Development*, **9**, 321–34.

[21] Perry, S.E. (1983) Parents' perceptions of their newborn following structured interactions. *Nursing Research*, **32**, 285–9.

[22] Vaughn, B.E., Bradley, C.F., Joffe, L.S. and Braglow, P. (1987) Maternal characteristics measured prenatally are predictive of ratings of temperamental 'difficulty' on the Carey Infant temperament Questionnaire. *Developmental Psychology*, **23**, 152–61.

[23] Bowlby, J, (1980) *Loss*. Basic Books, New York.

[24] Zeanah, C.H. and Anders, T.F. (1987) Subjectivity in parent–infant relationship: a discussion of internal working models. *Infant Mental Health Journal*, **8**, 237–49.

[25] Raphael-Leff, J. (1989) Where the wild things are. *International Journal of Prenatal and Perinatal Studies*, **1**, 79–89.

[26] Bion, W.R. (1962) *Learning from Experience*, Heinemann, London.

[27] Montague, A. (1962) *Prenatal Influences*, C.C. Thomas, Springfield, Ill.

[28] Salk, L. (1973) The role of the heartbeat in the relations between mother and infant. *Scientific American*, **220**, 24–9.

[29] W.B. Cannon, see Verny, T. (1982) *The Secret Life of the Unborn Child*, Sphere Books, London, p. 30.

[30] Van den Bergh, B.R.H. (1989) The relationship between maternal emotionality during pregnancy and the behavioural development of the fetus and neonatus, in *Prenatal and Perinatal Psychology and Medicine: Encounter with the Unborn* (ed. P. Fedor-Freyberg and M.L.V. Vogel), Parthenon Books, Lancaster, Chap. 11.

[30] Benson, P., Little, B.C., Talbert, D.G., Dewhurst, J. and Priest, R.G. (1987) Foetal heart rate and maternal anxiety. *British Journal of Medical Psychology*, **60**, 151–4.

[32] Lieberman, M. on smoking, quoted by Sontag, L.W. (1970) Prenatal determinants of postnatal behaviour, in *Fetal Growth and Development* (eds. H.A. Weisman and G.R. Kerr), McGraw Hill, New York.

[33] Sontag, L.W. (1944) War and the foetal maternal relationship. *Marriage and Family Living,* **6,** 1–5.

[34] Ferreira, A.J. (1965) Emotional factors in the prenatal environment. *Journal of Nervous and Mental Diseases,* **141,** 108.

[35] Chalmers, B. (1982) Psychological aspects of pregnancy: some thoughts for the eighties. *Social Science and Medicine,* **16,** 323–31.

[36] David, H.P., Matejcek, Z., Dytrych, Z. and Schuller, V. (eds.) (1988) *Born Unwanted: Developmental Effects of Denied Abortion,* Avicenum, Prague.

[38] Piontelli, A. (1987) Infant observation from before birth. *International Journal of Psycho-Analysis,* **68,** 453–64.

[39] De Vries, J.I.P. (1982) The emergency of fetal behaviour. Qualitative aspects. *Early Human Development,* 7, 301–22, Quoted by Piontelli, A. (1987) *International Journal of Psycho-Analysis,* **68,** 453–64.

[40] Mancia, M. (1981) On the beginning of mental life in the foetus. *International Journal of Psycho-Analysis,* **62,** 351–7.

[41] See Verny, *op. cit.*

[42] Laibow, R.E. (1989) Prenatal and perinatal experience and developmental impairment, in *Prenatal and Perinatal Psychology and Medicine: Encounter with the Unborn* (eds P. Fedor-Freybergh and M.L.V. Vogel), Parthenon Books, Lancaster, Chap. 26.

[43] Farrant, G. (1987) Cellular consciousness. *Aesthema,* 7, 28–39.

[44] Van de Carr, K.R. and Lehrer, M. (1988) Effects of a prenatal intervention program, in *Prenatal and Perinatal Psychology and Medicine* (eds P. Fedor-Freybergh and M.L.V. Vogel), Parthenon, Lancaster.

[45] Edwards, A. (1988) *'Shirley Temple American Princess',* Collins, London.

[46] Kurjak, A., Jurkovic, D. and Alfirevic, Z. (1989) Fetal therapy, the state of the art, *International Journal of Prenatal and Perinatal Studies,* **1,** 21–46.

CHAPTER 9: THE PROFESSIONAL AS MEDIATOR BETWEEN MOTHER AND FETUS: ANTENATAL CARE AND ASSESSMENT

[1] Hall, M.H. (1984) Are our accepted practices based on valid assumptions? in *Pregnancy Care for the 1980's* (eds L. Zander and G. Chamberlain), Royal Society of Medicine/Macmillan Press, London.

[2] Ibid.

[3] Macintyre, S. (1984) Consumer reaction to present-day antenatal services, in *Pregnancy Care for the 1980's* (eds. L. Zander and G. Chamberlain), Royal Society of Medicine/Macmillan Press, London.

[4] House of Commons Social Services Committee (1980) Second report, *Perinatal and Neonatal Mortality,* HMSO, London quoted in *Pregnancy and Care for the 1980s* (eds L. Zander and G. Chamberlain), Royal Society of Medicine/Macmillan, London.

[5] Graham, H. and Oakley, A. (1981) Competing ideologies of reproduction: medical and maternal perspectives on pregnancy, in *Women, Health and Reproduction* (ed. M. Roberts), Routledge & Kegan Paul, London.

[6] Macintyre, S. (1984) in *Pregnancy Care for the 1980s* (eds L. Zander and G. Chamberlain), Royal Society of Medicine/Macmillan, London.

[7] Dowling, S. (1984) The provision of community antenatal care services, in *Pregnancy Care for the 1980s* (eds L. Zander and G. Chamberlain), Royal

Society of Medicine/Macmillan, London.

[8] Taylor, R.W. (1984) Community based specialist obstetric services, in *Pregnancy Care for the 1980s* (eds L. Zander and G. Chamberlain), Royal Society of Medicine/Macmillan, London.

[9] McKee, I.H. (1984) Community antenatal care: the Sighthill community antenatal scheme, in *Pregnancy Care for the 1980s* (eds L. Zander and G. Chamberlain), Royal Society of Medicine/Macmillan, London.

[10] Cartwright, M. (1979) *The Dignity of Labour: A Study of Childbearing and Induction*, Tavistock, London.

[11] Flint, C. (1984) report to Royal Society of Medicine, Forum on Maternity and The Newborn, May 1984, Royal Society of Medicine, London.

[12] British Medical Association (1974) *You and Your Baby*, p. 7, British Medical Association, London.

[13] Devisch, R. (1981) Semantic patterning of fertility and gynaecological healing: some anthropological perspectives. in *Reversibility of Sterilization. Psycho-(patho)logical Aspects* (eds. P. Nijs and I. Brosens), Acco, Leuven, Holland.

[14] BMA booklet, (1973) *You and Your Baby*, p. 19, British Medical Association, London.

[15] Bourne, G. (1975) *Pregnancy*, Pan, London.

[16] Draper, J. *et al.* (1984) Evaluation of a Community Ante-natal clinic, quoted in Beech, *Health Rights*, 1984, (see ref. 17).

[17] Beech, B. (1984) The pregnant woman's need for information, Presented to European Symposium on Clinical Pharmacology Evaluation in Drug Control, *Health Rights*, 157 Waterloo Rd, London SE1.

[18] Squire, J. (1984) Ultrasound, an unqualified acceptance of safety. *AIMS Quarterly Journal*, Summer, 1–3.

[19] *Lancet*, (Editorial) Dec. 1989, quoted by R. Fraser in lecture on 'Evaluation of maternity care', Royal Society of Medicine, Forum on Maternity and Newborn, 6 December 1989.

[20] Zander, L. (1984) Discussion, in *Pregnancy Care for the 1980s* (eds. L. Zander and G. Chamberlain), Royal Society of Medicine/Macmillan, London, p. 44.

[21] Beech, B. in lecture on 'History of the consumer movement', Royal Society of Medicine, Forum on Maternity and Newborn, 6 December 1989.

[22] Raphael-Leff, J. (1982) Restoring the focal point of childbirth, *Hampstead and Highgate Express*, 2 April 1989.

[23] Boyd, C. and Sellers, L. (1982) *The British Way of Birth*, Pan, London.

[24] Kitzinger, S. (1979) *The Good Birth Guide*, Fontana, London.

[25] Flint, C. (1986) *Sensitive Midwifery*, Heinemann Nursing, Oxford. p. 27.

[26] Klaus, M. and Kennell, J. (1976) *Maternal Infant Bonding*, Mosby, St Louis.

[27] Reading, A.E. and Cox, D.N. (1981) The effects of ultrasound examination on maternal anxiety levels. *Journal of Behavioural Medicine*, 5, 237–47.

[28] Campbell, S. *et al.* (1982) Ultrasound scanning in pregnancy: the short-term psychological effects of early real-time scans. *Journal of Psychosomatic Obstetrics and Gynaecology*, 1, 57.

[29] Tsoi, M.M. and Hunter, M. (1987) Ultrasound scanning in pregnancy: consumers' reactions, *Journal Reproductive and Infant Psychology*, 5, 43–8.

[30] Lind (1986) Editorial. *British Medical Journal*, p. 576.

[31] Hyde, B. (1988) Routine ultrasound scanning in antenatal care. *AIMS Quarterly Journal*, Spring, pp. 5–6.

[32] Farrant, W. (1983) Prenatal screening – and agenda for better practice. *Maternity Action* – Bulletin of the Maternity Alliance May/June. (based on paper: North East Thames Regional Screening Programme for the

Detection of Fetal Abnormality: some priorities for CHC action, presented to South Camden CHC, April 1980).

[33] See, for instance, debate on ethics at the Royal Society of Medicine, Forum on Maternity and the Newborn, meeting on Prenatal Screening, 7 June 1989, reported in *Maternal and Child Health*.

[34] Endres, M. (1989) The psychological effects of antenatal diagnosis on pregnancy, in *Prenatal and Perinatal Psychology and Medicine: Encounter with the Unborn* (eds P. Fedor-Freybergh and M.L.V. Vogel), Parthenon Books, Lancaster. Chap. 33.

[35] Report from 'India Today' (31.1.88) in *British Medical Journal*, 7 May 1988.

[36] Yudkin, G. (1989) From home to hospital and back in *Hidden Loss* (eds. V. Hey *et al.*), Women's Press, London.

[37] Jakobovitz, I. *Jewish Medical Ethics*. Bloch, New York.

Further reading

Garcia, J., Kilpatrick, R. and Richards, M. (1990) *The Politics of Maternity Care – Services for Childbearing Women in Twentieth Century Britain*, Clarendon, Oxford. (Unfortunately, I was unable to draw on this important book as its publication coincided with mine going to press, JRL).

Kitzinger, S. (ed.) (1989). *The Midwife Challenge*, Pandora, London.

CHAPTER 10: THE FATHER-TO-BE: MATURATION PROCESSES

[1] In 'matrilocal' societies, the children are raised in the home of the wife's blood relatives with the husband being regarded as a privileged visitor (although he will have a dominant position in his sister's family). In patriarchal families (prevailing in feudal societies from which our own has evolved) authority is concentrated in the husband's relatives and the wife will come to share her mate's residential household or locality, and rear their children there. Rarely, annual alternations may occur between the two places of abode.

[2] *Social Trends* (1988) Central Statistical Office, HMSO, London.

[3] Diodorius Siculus (60 BC), cited by Trethowan and Conlon (1965) The Couvade Syndrome. *British Journal of Psychiatry*, **111**, 57.

[4] Reik, T. (1919) *Ritual*, International Universities Press, New York.

[5] Wainright, W.H. (1966) Fatherhood as a precipitant of mental illness. *American Journal of Psychiatry*, **123**, 40.

[6] Rosenberg Zalk, S. (1980) Psychosexual conflicts in expectant fathers, in *Psychological Aspects of Pregnancy, Birthing and Bonding* (ed. B. Blum), Human Science Press, New York.

[7] Barry, H.R. and Adler, S.P. (1980) The pregnant father, in *Psychological Aspects of Pregnancy, Birthing and Bonding* (ed. B. Blum), Human Science Press, New York.

[8] Lewis, C. (1983) One hundred fathers' perception of pregnancy and birth. *Journal of Psychosomatic Obstetrics and Gynaecology*, **2**, 166.

[9] Freeman, T. (1951) Pregnancy as a precipitant of mental illness in men. *British Journal of Medical Psychology*, **29**, 49.

[10] Trethowan, W.H. and Conlon, M.F. (1965) The Couvade Syndrome. *British Journal of Psychiatry*, **111**, 57.

[11] Greenson, R. (1968) Dis-identifying from mother. *International Journal of Psycho-Analysis*, **49**, 370–4.

[12] Mead, M. (1949) *Male and Female – a study of the sexes in a changing world* Victor Gollancz, London.

[13] Mead, M. ibid, p. 160.

[14] A South Asian view holds that semen is concentrated blood. Some Pakistanis believe that as semen is hotter/stronger than female substances, the infant's blood originates from the father, rather than the Hindu idea of 'hard' structures and bones as paternally bequeathed. See Werbner, P. (1986) The 'Virgin and the Clown', *Man*, (n.s.) **21**, 227–50.

[15] Aristotle, *On the Generation of Animals*, 729, 22.

[16] Katz Rothman, B. (1982) *In Labour – Women and Power in the Birth Place*, Junction Books, London.

[17] Rich, A. (1977) The theft of childbirth, in *Seizing our Bodies – the Politics of Women's Health*, Vintage, New York

[18] Arms, S. (1977) *Immaculate Deception*, Bantam Books, New York.

[19] Shershevsky, P.M. and Yarrow, L.M. (eds) (1973) *Psychological Aspects of a First Pregnancy and Early Postnatal Adaptation*, Raven Press, New York.

[20] Feder, L. (1980) Preconceptive ambivalence and external reality. *International Journal of Psycho-Analysis*, **61**, 161.

[21] Herzog, J.M. (1982) Patterns of expectant fatherhood: a study of the fathers of a group of premature infants, in *Father and Child: Developmental and Clinical Perspectives* (eds S.H. Cath, A.R. Gurwitt and J.M. Ross), Little, Brown, Boston.

[22] Savage, W. (1984) Sexual intercourse during pregnancy and fetal distress. *British Journal of Sexual Medicine*, **11**.

[23] Freud, S. (1933) *New Introductory Lectures*, Femininity, vol. 22, Standard Edition, Hogarth, London, 1971.

[24] Mead, M. (1957) Changing patterns of parent–child relations in urban culture. *International Journal of Psycho-Analysis*, **38**, 369–78.

[25] Gerzi, S. and Berman, E. (1981) Emotional reactions of expectant fathers to their wives' first pregnancy. *British Journal of Medical Psychology*, **54**, 259.

[26] Herzog, J.M. (1982) in *Father and Child: Developmental and Clinical Perspectives* (eds S.H. Cath, A.R. Gurwitt and J.M. Ross), Little, Brown, Boston.

[27] Ibid.

[28] Robson, K., Brant, H.A. and Kumar, R. (1981) Maternal sexuality during first pregnancy and after childbirth. *British Journal of Obstetrics and Gynaecology*, **88**, 882.

[29] Gurwitt, A.R. (1982) Aspects of prospective fatherhood, in *Father and Child: Developmental and Clinical Perspectives* (eds S.H. Cath, A.R. Gurwitt and J.M. Ross), Little, Brown, Boston.

[30] Herzog, J.M. (1982) in *Father and Child* (eds S.H. Cath, A.R. Gurwitt and J.M. Ross), Little, Brown, Boston.

[31] Freud, S. (1924) *The Dissolution of the Oedipus Complex*, Vol. 19, Standard Edition, Hogarth, London, 1971.

[32] Parsons, T. and Bales, R.F. (1955) *Family, Socialization and Interaction Process*, Free Press, New York.

[33] Gilligan, C. (1982) *In a Different Voice*, Harvard University Press, Cambridge, MA.

[34] Bem, S. (1987) Probing the promise of androgyny, in *The Psychology of Women* (ed. M. Roth Walsh), Yale University Press, New Haven, Connecticut.

[35] Ibid.

[36] Raphael-Leff, J. (1985) Facilitators and Regulators, Participators and

Renouncers – mothers' and fathers' reactions to pregnancy and parent-hood. *Journal of Psychosomatic Obstetric and Gynaecology*, **4**:

CHAPTER 11: PARTICIPATORS AND RENOUNCERS, AND EXPECTANT FATHERS AT-RISK

[1] Sawin, D.B. and Parke, P.D. (1978) The father's role in infancy: a re-evaluation, *Birth and the Family Journal*, 5: 211–13.
[2] Yogman, M.W. (1982) Observations on the father–infant relationship, in *Father and Child: Developmental and Clinical Perspectives* (eds). S.H. Cath, A.R. Gurwitt and J.M. Ross), Little, Brown, Boston.
[3] Lamb, M.E. and Lamb, J.E. (1976) The nature and importance of the father-infant relationship. *Family Coordinator*, **25** 379–85.
[4] Field, T. (1978) Interaction behaviours of primary versus secondary caretaker fathers. *American Journal of Experimental Psychology*, **14** 183–4. Although all fathers engage in more game playing and less handling of infants, this study comparing primary and secondary caretaker fathers, found that the former, like mothers, engaged in more smiling and imitative grimaces and vocalizations, a difference seemingly due to greater familiarity with their infants.
[5] Chused, J.F. (1986) Consequences of paternal nurturing. *Psychoanalytic Study of the Child*, **41**, 419–38.
[6] Raphael-Leff, J. (1991) The moon hung on a navelstring. *Journal of Pre and Perinatal Psychology*, **6**, 33–35.
[7] Wainright, W.H. (1966) Fatherhood as a precipitant of mental illness. *American Journal of Psychiatry*, **123**, 40.
[8] Rosenberg Zalk, S. (1980) Psychosexual conflicts in expectant fathers, in *Psychological Aspects of Pregnancy, Birthing and Bonding* (ed. B. Blum), Human Science Press, New York.
[9] Gerzi, S. and Berman, E. (1981) Emotional reactions of expectant fathers to their wives' first pregnancy. *British Journal of Medical Psychology*, **54**, 259.
[10] Adams-Hillard, P.J. (1985) Physical abuse in pregnancy. *Obstetrics and Gynecology*, **16**, 185–190, quoted in Condon, J.T. (1986) The spectrum of fetal abuse in pregnant women. *Journal of Nervous and Mental Disease* **174**, 509–16.

Further reading

Diamond, M.J. (1986) Becoming a father: a psychoanalytic perspective on the forgotten parent. *The Psychoanalytic Review* 73, 445–68.
Greenberg, M. (1985) *The Birth of a Father*, Continuum, New York.
Parke, R.D. (1981) *Fathering*, Fontana, London.

CHAPTER 12: LESBIAN PARTNERS

[1] Wilson, E. (1989) In a different key, in *Balancing Acts: On Being a Mother* (ed. K. Gieve), Virago, London.
[2] Ibid.
[3] Ferguson, A. (1984) Sex War: the debate between radical and libertarian feminists, in *Signs: Journal of Women in Culture and Society*, **10**, 106–12,

Forum: the feminist sexuality debates.

[4] Philipson, I. (1984) The repression of history and gender: a critical perspective on the feminist sexuality debates, in *Signs: Journal of Women in Culture and Society*, **10**, 113–18, Forum: the feminist sexuality debates.

[5] Diamond, I. and Quinby, L. (1984) American feminism in the age of the body, in *Signs: Journal of Women in Culture and Society*, **10**, 119–25. Forum: the feminist sexuality debates.

[6] Vance, C.S. and Snitow, A.B. (1984) Towards a conversation about sex in feminism: a modest proposal, in *Signs: Journal of Women in Culture and Society*, **10**, 126–35, Forum: the feminist sexuality debates.

[7] Daly, M. (1979) *Gyn/Ecology. The Metaethics of Radical Feminism*, The Women's Press, London.

[8] Rich, A. (1980) Compulsory heterosexuality and lesbian existence, in *Signs: Journal of Women in Culture and Society*, **5**, 631–60 (quote, p. 649.)

[9] Krieger, S. (1982) Lesbian identity and community: recent social science literature, in *Signs: Journal of Women in Culture and Society*, **8**, 91–108 (quote, p. 95.)

[10] Freud, S. (1889) *The Complete Letters of Sigmund Freud to Wilhelm Fliess, 1887–1904* (ed. J.M. Masson), 1 August 1889, p. 364, Belknap Press, Harvard University, London.

[11] McDougall, J. (1981) Homosexuality in women, in *Female Sexuality* (ed. J. Chasseguet-Smirgel), Virago, London, p. 172.

[12] O'Connor, N. & Ryan, J. (1993) *Wild Desires & Mistaken Identities – Lesbianism and Psychoanalysis*, Virago Press

[13] Schuker, E. (1996) Analytic understanding of lesbian patients, *Journal American Psychoanalytic Association*, 44/Supplement 585-508.

[14] Peplau, L.A. and Cochran, S.D. (1980) Sex differences in values concerning love relationships. Paper presented to annual meeting of American Psychological Association, Montreal, quoted by Krieger, S. (1982) *Signs: Journal of Women in Culture and Society*, **8**, 91–108.

[15] Krestan, J.A. and Bepko, C.S. (1980) The problems of fusion in the lesbian relationship. *Family Process*, **19**, 277–89.

[16] Dominy, M.D. (1986) Lesbian–Feminist gender conceptions: separatism in Christchurch, New Zealand. *Signs: Journal of Women in Culture and Society*, **11**, 274–83.

[17] Pies, C. (1988) *Considering Parenthood*, Spinsters/Aunt Lute, San Francisco, p. 83.

[18] Hall, M. (1981) Lesbian families: cultural and clinical issues, in *Women and Mental Health* (eds. E. Howell and M. Bayes), Basic Books, New York.

Relevant organizations

Lesbian and Gay Switchboard 071–837–7324
Lesbian Line 071–251–6911
Women's Reproductive Rights Information 071–251–6332

CHAPTER 13: ANTICIPATING PARENTHOOD IN THE WEST AND OTHER CULTURES

[1] Mead, M. and Newton, N. (1967) Cultural patterning of perinatal behaviour, in *Childbearing: its Social and Psychological Aspects* (eds S. Richardson and A. Gutmacher), Williams and Wilkins, Baltimore.

[2] MacCormack, C.P. (1982) *Ethnography of Fertility and Birth*, Academic Press, London.

[3] Mead, M. and Newton, N. (1965) Conception, pregnancy, labour and the puerperium in cultural perspective, in *First International Congress of Psychosomatic Medicine and Childbirth*, Gauthier-Villars, Paris.

[4] Jiminez, M.H. and Newton, N. (1979) Activity and work during pregnancy and postpartum period: a cross-cultural study of 202 societies. *American Journal of Obstetrics and Gynaecology*, **135**, 171.

[5] Kitzinger, S. (1978) *Women as Mothers*, William Collins, Glasgow, 1981.

[6] Adapted from Mead and Newton (1967) *Childbearing: its Social and Psychological Aspects* (eds S. Richardson and A. Gutmacher), Williams and Wilkins, Baltimore.

[7] Kitzinger (1978) *Women as Mothers*, Collins, Glasgow, p. 89.

[8] Mead and Newton (1967) *Childbearing: its Social and Psychological Aspects*.

[9] Ibid.

[10] Fraser, J.G. (1922) *The Golden Bough*, MacMillan, New York, 1953.

[11] Ford, C.S. (1945) *A Comparative Study of Human Reproduction*, Yale University Publications, New Haven.

[12] Jiminez, M.H. and Newton, N. (1979) *American Journal of Obstetrics and Gynecology*, **135**, 171.

[13] World Health Organization (1976) *Training and Supervision of Traditional Birth Attendants*, Regional Office for Africa, quoted by MacCormack (1982) *Ethnography of Fertility and Birth*.

[14] De Mause, L. (1974) *The History of Childhood*, Souvenir Press, London.

[15] Nickel, H. (1988) The role of the father in care-giving and in the development of the infant: an empirical study on the impact of prenatal courses on expectant fathers, in *Prenatal and Perinatal Psychology and Medicine: Encounters with the Unborn* (eds P. Fedor-Freybergh and V. Vogel), Parthenon Press, Lancaster.

[16] Parsons, T. and Bales, R.F. (1955) *Family, Socialization and Interaction Process* Free Press, New York.

[17] Firestone, S. (1971) *The Dialectic of Sex*, Jonathan Cape, London.

[18] Friedan, B. (1963) *The Feminine Mystique*, Norton, New York.

CHAPTER 14: READJUSTING FAMILY RELATIONSHIPS

[1] Office of Population Censuses and Surveys. Population Statistics Division. *Population Trends*, 1989, 47.

[2] Newton, J. and Newson, A. (1974) *Patterns of Infant Care*, Penguin Books, London.

[3] Rossi, A. (1968) Transition to parenthood. *Journal of Marriage and the Family*, **30**, 26–39.

[4] This conceptualization is my own elaboration of the tripartite classification of public, personal and unconscious marital bonds proposed by Dicks, H.V. (1967) *Marital Tensions*, Routledge and Kegan Paul, London.

[5] Friedan, B. (1963) *The Feminine Mystique*, Penguin Books, London.

[6] Adapted from Kenkel, (1960) *The Family in Perspective*, Appelton-Century-Crofts, New York.

[7] The concept of a 'General Systems Theory' was developed by Ludwig von Bertalanffy (1968) and applied by many family therapists to describe family functioning.

[8] Skynner, A.C.R. (1976) *One Flesh: Separate Persons*, Constable, London.

[9] Minuchin, S. (1974) *Families and Family Therapy*, Harvard University Press, Cambridge, MA.

[10] Parsons, T. and Bales, R.F. (1955) *Family, Socialization and Interactive Process*, Macmillan, New York.

[11] Bott, E. (1971) *Family and Social Networks*, Tavistock, London.

[12] Bronfenbrenner, U. and Crouter, A.C. (1983) The evolution of environmental models in developmental research, in *Handbook of Child Psychology* (ed. P.H. Mussen), John Wiley, New York, pp. 357–414.

[13] Belsky, J. (1984) The determinants of parenting: a process model. *Child Development*, **55**, 83–96.

[14] Newson, J. and Newson, A. (1974) *Patterns of Infant Care*, Penguin, London.

[15] Lewis, C. (1986) *Becoming a Father*, Open University Press, Milton Keynes.

[16] Oakley, A. (1980) *Women Confined*, Martin Robertson, Oxford.

[17] Many studies have found a change in the marital power structure following the birth, with increased economic dependency of the woman who tends to take on the bulk of babycare (whether or not she is employed) even when the couple profess egalitarian attitudes. For a review of some studies see Andersen, I.(1984) Transition to parenthood research. *Journal of Psychomatic Obstetrics and Gynaecology*, **3**, 3–16.

CHAPTER 15: RE-EVALUATION OF UNCONSCIOUS CONTRACTS AND THERAPEUTIC OPPORTUNITIES

[1] Dicks, H.V. (1963) Object relations theory and marital studies. *British Journal of Medical Psychology*, **36**, 125–9.

[2] Robin Skynner observes in his book *One Flesh: Separate Persons* (1976, Constable, London) that although couples are usually attracted by shared developmental failures, the degree to which they operate at common regressed levels may be different. While tracing marital problems to unmastered developmental levels he stresses paranoid/schizoid functioning, anal-level fixation and phallic rivalry of each other's sexual roles.

[3] Mahler, M. (1972) Rapprochement subphase of the Separation–Individuation process. *Psychoanalytic Quarterly*, **41**, 487–506.

[4] Balint, M. (1968) *The Basic Fault*, Tavistock, London.

[5] Fraiberg, S. Adelson, E. and Shapiro, V. (1975) Ghosts in the nursery: a psychoanalytic approach to the problems of impaired infant–mother relationships. *Journal of the American Academy of Child Psychiatry*, **14**, 387–421.

[6] Ferriera, A.J. (1963) Family myths and homeostasis. *Archives of General Psychiatry*, **9**, 457–63.

[7] Byng-Hall, J. (1973) Family myths used as a defence in conjoint family therapy. *British Journal of Medical Psychology*, **46**, 239–50.

[8] The way in which shared unconscious fantasy operated within a family is illustrated in a 'deadlock' broken by psychotherapeutic intervention: Clulow, C., Dearnley, B. and Balfour, F. (1986) Shared fantasy and therapeutic structure in a brief marital therapy. *British Journal of Psychotherapy*, **3**, 124–32; 133–43.

[9] Skynner (1976) *One Flesh: Separate Persons*, Constable, London.

Further reading

Ernst, S. and Goodison, L. (1981) *In Our Own Hands – a Book of Self-Help Therapy*. Women's Press, London.

Karpel, M.A. and Strauss, E.S. (1983) *Family Evaluation*. Gardner Press, London.

Pincus, L. and Dare, C. (1978) *Secrets in the Family*. Faber and Faber, London.

Minuchin, S. (1974) Families and Family Theraphy. Harvard University Press, Cambridge, MA.

Skynner, R. and Cleese, J. (1983) *Families and How to Survive Them*. Methuen, London.

CHAPTER 16: HEALTH-CARE PROFESSIONALS AS GUIDES
IN THE TRANSITION TO MOTHERHOOD

[1] MacCormack, C.P. (ed.) (1982) *Ethnography of Fertility*, Academic Press, London.

[2] WHO (1966) The midwife in maternity care. *WHO Technical Report series*, 331, WHO, Geneva.

[3] van Gennep, A. (1960) *The Rites of Passage*, Routledge and Kegan Paul, London [It has been said that all van Gennep demonstrated was that everything has a beginning, a middle and an end. Nevertheless, I feel his schema is a useful one in conceptualizing Rites of Passage. For a critique of his work see *Essays on the Ritual of Social Relations* (ed. M. Gluckman), Manchester University Press (1962)]

[4] The most important feature of the transitional 'bridge' offered by the professional clearly consists of anticipatory guidance and instruction facilitating integration of different aspects of the woman's life by utilizing pregnancy not only as preparation for childbirth but for her responsibilities as a mother. In our own western societies this aspect of emotional and practical preparation for the new demands of parenthood has been sadly neglected. The few studies evaluating programmes where continuity of care has been combined with preparatory education for parenthood, emotional and social support, have found a reduction in postnatal depression in vulnerable women. (See for instance Leverton, T.L. and Elliott, S.A. (1989) Transition to parenthood groups: a preventive intervention for postnatal depression, in *The Free Woman: Women's Health in the 1990s* (eds. E.V. Van Hall and W. Everaerd), Parthenon Press, Carnforth.

[5] Menzies, I. (1960) *The Functioning of Social Systems as a Defence against Anxiety*. Tavistock Institute Human Relations, London.

[6] Ibid.

[7] Ibid.

[8] Comaroff, J. (1977) Conflicting paradigms in pregnancy: managing ambiguity in ante-natal encounters, in *Medical Encounters* (eds A. Davis and G. Horrobin), Croom Helm, London.

[9] Flint, C. (1986) *Sensitive Midwifery*. Heinemann Nursing, Oxford, p. 219.

[10] Oakley, A. (1976) Wisewoman and medicine man: changes in the management of childbirth, in *The Rights and Wrongs of Women* (eds Mitchell and A. Oakley), Penguin Books, London, pp. 24–6.

[11] Ibid., pp. 35–8.

[12] Katz Rothman, B. (1982) *In Labour: Women and Power in the Birthplace*, Junction Books, London, p. 57.

[13] Arms, S.(1975) *Immaculate Deception*, Bantam Books.

[14] Editorial (1976) *Journal of Nurse-Midwifery*, quoted by Katz Rothman (1982) *In Labour: Women and Power in the Birthplace.*

[15] Interprofessional Task Force on Health Care of Women and Children (1976) Development of Family Centered Maternity/Newborn Care in Hospitals, quoted in W.R. Arney, *Power and the Profession of Obstetrics*, University of Chicago, 1982.

[16] Willington, S. (1985) Origins of A.I.M.S., *ARMS Quarterly Journal*, Conference Bulletin.

[17] Beech, B.A. (1985) *The role of consumer advocacy in birth care*, AIMS Publication.

[18] Kloosterman, G.J. (1972) New Horizons in Midwifery, 1972 Congress of International Confederation of Midwives, quoted by AIMS (1975) *Immaculate Deception.*

[19] Newson, K. (1982) The future of midwifery. *Midwife, Health Visitor and Community Nurse*, 18, 12.

[20] Newson, K. (1984) What sort of midwifery service do we want? in *Pregnancy Care for the 1980s* (eds L. Zander and G. Chamberlain), Royal Society of Medicine, Macmillan Press, London pp. 258–620.

[21] MacFarlane, A. and Mugford, M. (1984) *Birth Counts: Statistics of pregnancy and childbirth*. HMSO, Norwich.

[22] Ibid.

[23] See Kitzinger, S. (1984) Experiences of obstetric practices in differing countries, in *Pregnancy Care for the 1980s* (eds L. Zander and G. Chamberlain), re Queen Victoria Hospital, Melbourne; also see Mehl, L.E. (1980) Psychophysiological aspects of childbirth, in *The Psychology of Birth*, L. Feher, Souvenir, London. re Mount Zion Hospital, San Francisco and Berkely Family Health Center.

[24] Inch, S.(1987) Care in labour – a need for reassessment. Report of meeting of Forum for Maternity and the Newborn, Royal Society of Medicine, 25 February 1986, *Journal of the Royal Society of Medicine*, 80, 388–92.

[25] Dewhurst, J. (1984) Which way forward for obstetrics? in *Pregnancy Care for the 1980s* (eds L. Zander and G. Chamberlain).

[26] Taylor, G.W. (1984) What are we training our general practitioners for? in *Pregnancy Care for the 1980s* (eds L. Zander and G. Chamberlain).

[27] Chapman, V. (1984) The role of the health visitor, in *Pregnancy Care for the 1980s*. (eds L. Zander and G. Chamberlain), p. 226–31.

[28] Henschel, D. (1984) What are we expecting of our midwives? in *Pregnancy Care for the 1980s*. (eds L. Zander and G. Chamberlain), p. 176–9.

[29] Jamieson, L. (1984) A midwife's perspective, in *Pregnancy Care for the 1980s*, (eds L. Zander and G. Chamberlain), p. 223–5.

[30] Flint, C. (1986) *Sensitive Midwifery*, Heinemann Nursing, Oxford.

CHAPTER 17: ANTICIPATING CHILDBIRTH

[1] See for instance Gold and Gold (1977) and Goskin, I.M. (1977) *Spiritual Midwifery*, Book Publishing Co., Somerville, Tennessee.

[2] Bradley, R. (1965) *Husband-Coached Childbirth*, Harper and Row, New York.

[3] Dick-Read, G.(1951) *Childbirth Without Fear*, Heinemann, Oxford.

[4] Newton, N., Peeler, D. and Newton, M. (1968) Effect of disturbance on labour. *American Journal of Obstetrics and Gynecology*, 101, 1096–102.

[5] Naaktgeboren, C. (1972) Human delivery in the light of biological views of parturition, in *Psychosomatic Medicine in Obstetrics and Gynecology* (ed. N. Morris), Karler, London, 1981, pp. 206–9.

[6] Enkin, N. *et al*, (1971) An adequately controlled study of the effectiveness of PPM training, 3rd International Congress of Psychomatic Medicine in Obstetrics and Gynaecology, London, April, 1971, quoted by L.E. Mehl in Feher, L. *The Psychology of Birth*, Souvenir Press, London.

[7] Charles, A.G., Norr, K.L., Block, C.R. *et al.* (1978) Obstetric and psychological effects of psychoprophylactic preparation for childbirth. *American Journal of Obstetrics and Gynecology*, **131**: 44.

[8] Jacobson (1939) *Progressive Relaxation*, Chicago, Ill: University of Chicago Press.

[9] Kitzinger, S. (1978) *The Experience of Childbirth*, Penguin, London, p. 20.

[10] Ibid p. 25.

[11] See for instance Balaskas, J. (1989) *New Active Birth – a concise guide to natural childbirth*, Unwin, London.

[12] Beech, B.L. (1987) *Who's Having Your Baby?* Camden Press, London.

[13] Tew, M. (1978) The case against hospital deliveries, in *The Place of Birth* (eds Kitzinger, S. and Davis, J.), Oxford University Press, Oxford.

[14] Campbell, R. and Macfarlane, A. (1983) *Where to be born? –* the debate and the evidence. National Perinatal Epidemiology Unit, Oxford.

[15] Tew, M. (1980) 'Is home a safer place?', *Health and Social Services Journal*, 12 Sept. (see too, Chapter 12, this book) .

[16] Government reply to 2nd report from Social Services Commission on Perinatal and Neonatal mortality, Dec. 1980, quoted in *Choosing a Home Birth*, AIMS Publications.

[17] Beech, B.L. (1987) *Who's Having Your Baby*. Camden Press, London.

[18] Chalmers, B. (1984) A conceptualization of psycho-social obstetric research. *Journal of Psychosomatic Obstetrics and Gynecology* 3, 27–35.

[19] Oakley, A. (1984) *The Captured Womb*, Blackwell, Oxford.

[20] Klein, M. (1983) Contracting for trust in family practice obstetrics. *Canadian Family Physician*, **29**, 225–7, quoted by Inch (1988) *Journal of The Royal Society of Medicine*, **81**, 120–2.

[21] Kitzinger, S. (1986) Birth plans, presented to Forum of Maternity and the Newborn, Royal Society of Medicine, 7 October 1986, reported by Inch, S. (1988) *Journal of the Royal Society of Medicine*, **81**, 120–2.

[22] Vinall, P. (1986) Purpose of the protocol, Forum of Maternity and the Newborn, Royal Society of Medicine, 7 October 1986.

[23] Forum for maternity and the Newborn Recommendations, Royal Society of Medicine, 7 October 1986.

[24] Inch, S. (1990) Historical perspective for maternity care – a pointer for the future, Report of Forum of Maternity and the Newborn, Royal Society of Medicine, meeting 6 December 1989 in *Maternal and Child Health*, forthcoming.

CHAPTER 18: THE BIRTHPLACE AND BIRTH PROCESS

[1a] Dinnerstein, D. (1976) *The Rocking of the Cradle and the Ruling of the World*, The Women's Press, London, 1987, p. 133.

[1b] In the Developing World between 60 and 80% of deliveries are performed by traditional birth attendants (TBA). In most cultures they receive some gratuity from the family, either in money or barter. These women, who

are experienced and socially well-established within the community, have a major role to play provided they can receive recognition and support within the framework of primary health care. In recent years, training is provided as part of health development programmes in many Third World countries (A 1975 WHO survey identifies 24 countries, with survey updates since then). In cooperation with community health workers, medical assistants, and provincial and regional primary health care programme staff, the following targets of training were developed:

a. to help TBA recognize early signs of danger for mother or baby during pregnancy and birth;

b. to improve practices in delivering at home with special regard to preventing infections;

c. to teach techniques of antenatal care, and refer women 'at risk' to the care of hospital midwives;

d. to improve the condition of pregnant women and their children through improved diets;

e. to improve care of the newborn;

f. to introduce child welfare clinics.

Evaluation of the programmes have been implemented in various centres, with most impressive results of TBA training being more effective in reducing neonatal morality than tetanus toxoid vaccine given twice in pregnancy. (Rachman, S. (1982), The effect of TBA and tetanus toxoid in reduction of neonatal mortality. *Journal of Tropical Pediatrics*, 28: 163–165, quoted by Krawinkel, M.B. (1988), *Traditional Birth Attendants: a study in Sudan*, in ED. Hibbs (ED.), *Children and Families: studies in prevention and intervention*, International Universities Press: Madison, Conn.)

[2]   Mead, M. and Newton, N. (1967) Cultural patterning of perinatal behaviour, in *Childbearing: its Social and Psychological Aspects* (eds S. Richardson and A. Gutmacher, Williams and Wilkins, Baltimore.

[3]   Mead, M. (1935) *Sex and Temperament in Three Primitive Societies*. Mentor, New York.

[4]   Mead, M. and Newton, N. (1967) *Childbearing: its Social and Psychological Aspects*, Williams and Wilkins, Baltimore.

[5]   Kitzinger, S. (1978) *Women as Mothers*. Fontana/Collins, London.

[6]   Jules-Rosette (1979) in MacCormack, C.P. (ed. 1982) *Ethnography of Fertility*, Academic Press, New York.

[7]   Parvati Baker, J. (1989) The Shamanic dimensions of childbirth, presented at the 4th International conference on Pre and Perinatal Psychology, Amherst, Mass, USA, August, 1989.

[8]   Lhote, H. (1944) Les Touaregs du Hoggar, Paris: Payout, quoted by Mead, M. and Newton, N. (1967) *Childbearing: its Social and Psychological Aspects*, Williams and Wilkins, Baltimore, p. 194.

[9]   Metraux, A. (1940) Ethnology of Eastern Island, quoted by Mead, M. and Newton, N. (1967) p. 190.

[10]   Odent, M. (1984) *Birth Reborn*. Random House, New York.

[11]   Flint, C. (1986) *Sensitive Midwifery*. Nursing, Heinemann, Oxford.

[12]   Kitzinger, S. (1962) *The Experience of Childbirth*, Pelican, 1978.

[13]   Mead, M. (1949) *Male and Female*, Gollancz, New York, p. 238.

[14]   Ibid, p. 154.

[15]   Ibid.

[16]   Montague, A. (1954) *The Natural Superiority of Women*, George Allan and Unwin, London.

[17] Ibid.
[18] Mead, M. and Newton, N. (1967) *Child Bearing: Its Social and Psychological Aspects*, Williams and Wilkins, Baltimore.
[19] Levi Strauss, quoted by Kitzinger, 1978 (no reference).
[20] Parvati Baker (1989) 4th International Conference on Pre- and Perinatal Psychology.
[21] Mead, M. and Newton, N. (1967) *Child Bearing*.
[22] Naroll, F., Naroll, R. and Howard, F.H. (1961) Position of women in childbirth. *American Journal of Obstetrics and Gynecology*, **82**, 943–54.
[23] Ibid.
[24] MacCormack, C.P. (ed.) (1982) *Ethnography of Fertility*, Academic Press, New York, Chapter 4.
[25] Caldyero-Barcia, R. (1979) The influence of maternal position on time of spontaneous rupture of the membranes, progress of labour and foetal head compression. *Journal of Birth and Family*, **6**, 7.
[26] Mead and Newton (1967) *Child Bearing* pp. 210–12.
[27] Thompson, quoted by Kitzinger, S. (1978) *The Experience of Childbirth*, p. 116.
[28] Caldeyro-Barcia, 1980, in MacCormack, C.P. (1982) *Ethnography of Fertility*.
[29] Kitzinger, S. (1984) Experiences of obstetric practices in differing countries, in *Pregnancy Care for the 1980s* (eds. L. Zander and G. Chamberlain), Royal Society of Medicine/Macmillan Press, London.
[30] Odent, M. (1982) *The Listener*, 11 March.
[31] Kitzinger, S. (1978) *The Experience of Childbirth*, p. 109.
[32] Schultze (1907) quoted by Mead, M. and Newton, N. (1967) *Childbearing*, p. 217.
[33] Mead, M. and Newton, M. (1967) *Childbearing*
[34] Chamberlain, G. (1984) Modern obstetrics and patient care, in *Pregnancy Care for the 1980s* (eds L. Zander and G. Chamberlain), Royal Society of Medicine/Macmillan, London, p. 153–4.
[35] Ibid.
[36] Kloosterman, G.J. (1984) The Dutch experience of domiciliary confinements, in *Pregnancy Care for the 1980s* (eds. L. Zander and G. Chamberlain), pp. 115–25.
[37] Macfarlane, A. and Mugford, M. (1984) *Birth Counts: Statistics of Pregnancy and Childbirth*, HMSO, Norwich, p. 160.
[38] Ibid., p. 159.
[39] Beech, B. (1985) presentation to WHO Interregional Conference on Appropriate Technology for Birth, Brazil, 1985, AIMS publication.
[40] Macfarlane, A. and Mugford, M. (1984) *Birth Counts*, Chapter 12, International Comparisons.
[41] Goffman, I. (1961) *Asylums*, essays on the social situation of mental patients and other inmates, Penguin, 1970 (Anchor Books, 1961).
[42] Inch, S. (1982) *Birthrights*. Hutchinson, London.
[43] Goffman, I. (1961) *Asylums*, p. 302.
[44] Ibid. p. 87.
[45] Ibid. p. 76).
[46] Mehl, L.E. (1980) Psychophysiological aspects of childbirth, Chapter 3 in *The Psychology of Birth* (ed. L. Feher), Souvenir Press, London, p. 66.
[47] Correspondence course and apprenticeship program: Box 398, Monroe, Utah 84754.
[48] Tew, M. (1984) Understanding intranatal care through mortality statistics,

in *Pregnancy Care for the 1980s* (eds. L. Zander and G. Chamberlain) Royal Society of Medicine/Macmillan, London, pp. 93–104.

[49] Alberman, E. (1984) Statistical Comparison of Home and Hospital confinements, In (Eds L. Zander and G. Chamberlain) Pregnancy Care for the 1980's, Royal Society of Medicine/MacMillan, London.

[50] Kloosterman, G.J. (1984) in *Pregnancy Care for the 1980s* (ed. L. Zander and G. Chamberlain), Royal Society of Medicine/Macmillan, London.

[51] Kohner, N. (1984) *Pregnancy Book*, Health Education Council, London.

[52] See Beech, B. (1987) *Who's Having your Baby?* Camden Press, London.

[53] Wilmott, J. (1984) The community midwife and domiciliary confinements, in *Pregnancy Care for the 1980s* (eds. L. Zander and G. Chamberlain), Royal Society of Medicine/Macmillan, London, p. 133–7.

[54] Robinson, S., Golden, J. and Bradley, S. (1981) A preliminary report on the research project on the role and responsibilities of the midwife. *Midwives Chronicle*, commissioned by Royal College of Midwives, quoted by Wilmott, (1984) in *Pregnancy Care in the 1980s*.

[55] Zander, L. (1984) The significance of the home delivery issue, in *Pregnancy Care for the 1980s* (eds. L. Zander and G. Chamberlain), Royal Society of Medicine/Macmillan, London, pp. 126–32.

[56] Monaco and Junor (1980) *Homebirth Handbook*. Stroud, Bija Press, p. 26.

[57] Ibid, p. 24.

[58] Ibid.

CHAPTER 19: UNCOMPLICATED SPONTANEOUS LABOUR

[1] Kaufman, K. (1977) The first stage of labour, in *Maternity Nursing Today*. McGraw-Hill, New York.

[2] Raphael-Leff, J. (1985) Facilitators and Regulators; Participators and Renouncers: mothers' and fathers' orientations towards pregnancy and parenthood. *Journal of Obstetrics and Gynaecology*, **4**, 169–84.

[3] Klein, M. *et al.* (1983) A comparison of low-risk women booked for delivery in two systems of care: shared care (consultant) and integrated general practice unit. *British Journal of Obstetrics and Gynaecology*, **90**, 118.

[4] Flint, C. (1986) *Sensitive Midwifery*, Heinemann Nursing, Oxford, p. 72.

[5] Raphael-Leff, J. (1986) unpublished study.

[6] Kaufman, (1977) in *Maternity Nursing Today*.

[7] Newton, N., Peeler, D. and Newton, M. (1968) Effect of disturbance on labour. *American Journal of Obstetrics and Gynaecology*, **101**, 1096–102.

[8] Naaktgeboren, C. (1972) Human delivery in the light of biological views of parturition, in *Psychosomatic Medicine in Obstetrics and Gynecology* (ed. N. Morris), Karger, Basel, London, pp. 206–9.

[9] Haire, D.B. (1971) Cultural differences in maternity care, in *Psychosomatic Medicine in Obstetrics and Gynecology* (ed. N. Morris), Karger, Basel, p. 49.

[10] Goodlin, Stanford University, quoted by Arms, S. (1977) *Immaculate Deception*, Bantam Books, New York, p. 274.

[11] Klaus, M. *et al.* (1986) Effects of social support during parturition on maternal and infant morbidity. *British Medical Journal*, **293**, 585.

[12] Flint, C. (1986) *Sensitive Midwifery*, p. 92.

[13] Opie, I. and Tatem, M. (1989) *A Dictionary of Superstitions*. Oxford University Press, University. In many societies the umbilicus is burned or made into an amulet to prevent its falling into the hands of evil spirits or illwishers. Sarnoff, J. and Ruffins, R. (1978) *Take Warning – a book of*

superstitions, Charles Scribner's sons: New York. In hospital births, the unknown fate of the cord or placenta may therefore worry some parents.

[14] Ibid. pp. 66–7.

[15] Sleep, J. *et al.* (1984) West Berkshire perineal management trial. *British Medical Journal*, **289**, 587.

[16] Beech, B. (1986) Childbirth in hospital: the choice of the mother or the right of the child. *AIMS publication*.

[17] See *AIMS Quarterly Journal* (Spring 1987), 'Just a small cut' . . .

[18] See Flint, (1986) *Sensitive Midwifery*.

[19] Klein, M. *et al.* (1983) *British Journal of Obstetrics and Gynaecology*, **90**, 118.

[20] Flint, C. (1986), *Community Midwifery*, Heinemann Nursing, Oxford.

[21] Zander, L. (1984) The significance of the home delivery issue, in *Pregnancy care for the 1980s* (eds L. Zander and G. Chamberlain), Royal Society of Medicine/Macmillan Press, London, pp. 126–32.

[22] Shaw, E. and Darling, J. (1985) Maternalism – the fathering of a myth. *New Scientist*, 14 February, 10.

Further reading

Tew, M. (1990) *Safer childbirth? – a Critical History of Maternity Care*, Chapman and Hall, London.

Cartwright, A. (1979) *The Dignity of Labour*, Tavistock, London.

CHAPTER 20: MANAGED CHILDBIRTH

[1] Macfarlane, A. and Mugford, M. (1984) *Birth Counts: Statistics of Pregnancy and Childbirth*, HMSO, Norwich.

[2] Macfarlane, A. (1977) *The Psychology of Childbirth*, Fontana, London, p. 30.

[3] Kiwanuka, A.I. and Moore, W.M.O. (1987) The changing incidence of cesarean section in the health district of central Manchester. *British Journal of Obstetrics and Gynaecology*, **94**, 440, quoted by Philipp, E. (1988) *Caesareans: An Explanation and Preparation*, Sidgewick and Jackson, London.

[4] Flamm, B.L. *et al.* (1988) Vaginal birth after caesarean section: results of a multicenter study. *American Journal of Ortho Psychiatry*, **158**, 1079–84.

[5] Chalmers, B. (1982) Psychological aspects of pregnancy: some thoughts for the eighties. *Social Science and Medicine*, **16**, 323.

[6] Macdonald, R.L. (1968) The role of emotional factors in obstetric complications: a review. *Psychosomatic Medicine*, **30**, 222.

[7] Ferreira, A. (1965) Emotional factors in prenatal environment: a review. *Journal of Nervous and Mental Disorders* **141**, 108. [However, a distinction must be made between a general state of anxiety and feelings of anxiety about childbirth; the latter has not always been found to be associated with difficult labour. See for instance Thompson, M. and Hanley, J. (1988) Factors predisposing to difficult labour in primiparae, *American Journal of Obstetrics and Gynecology*, **158**, 1074–8.

[8] Chalmers, B. (1983) Psychosocial factors and obstetric complications. *Psychological Medicine*, **13**, 333.

[9] Twining, T.C. (1983), Some inter-relationships between personality variables, obstetric outcome and perinatal mood. *Journal of Reproductive and Infant Psychology*, **1**, 11–17.,

[10] Elliott, S.A., Anderson, M. Brough, D.I., Watson, J.P. and Rugg, A.J.

(1984) Relationship between obstetric outcome and psychological measures in pregnancy and the postnatal year. *Journal of Reproductive and Infant Psychology*, **2**, 18–32. Also see Eliott, S.A., Rugg, A.J., Watson, J.P. and Brough, D.I. (1983) Mood change during pregnancy and after the birth of a child. *British Journal of Clinical Psychology*, **22**, 295–308.

[11] Mehl, L. and Peterson, G. (1981) Existential prenatal risk screening, in *Pregnancy, Birth and Parenting: Coping with Medical Issues* (ed. P. Ahmed), Elsevier-North Holland, New York.

[12] Peterson, G., Mehl, L. and McRae, J. (1988) Relationship of psychiatric diagnosis, defenses, anxiety and stress with birth complications, in *Prenatal and Perinatal Psychology and Medicine* (eds P. Fedor-Freybergh and M.L. Vogel), Parthenon Press, Lancaster, Chap. 37.

[13] Standley, K., Soule, B. and Copans, S.A. (1979) Dimensions of prenatal anxiety and their influence on pregnancy outcome. *American Journal of Obstetrics and Gynecology*, **135**, 22–6. [The reader will appreciate that a psychodynamic approach which assumes continuous operation of unconscious historically determined emotions as well as concurrent conscious responses to pregnancy and childbirth, takes for granted the inevitably complex interaction of ambivalent feelings influencing the course of labour, birth and the relationship between mother and her newborn infant.]

[14] Elliott *et al.* (1984),

[15] Raphael-Leff, J. (1985) Facilitators and Regulators; Participators and Renouncers: mothers' and fathers' orientations towards pregnancy and parenthood. *Journal of Psychosomatic Obstetrics and Gynaecology*, **4**, 169–84.

[16] Trowell, J. (1983) Emergency caesarean section: a research study of the mother/child relationship of a group of women admitted expecting a normal vaginal delivery. *Child Abuse and Neglect*, **7**, 387.

[17] Richards, M.P.M. and Bernal, J.F. (1972) An observational study of mother–infant interaction, in *Ethological Studies of Child Behaviour* (ed. N. Blurton-Jones), Cambridge University Press, Cambridge. This study, like many others following it, demonstrated that newborn babies whose mothers had received pethidine during labour were less cuddly and responsive and necessitated more maternal stimulation during feeding, thereby affecting the early mother–infant interaction.)

[18] See Macfarlane and Mugford (1984) *Birth Counts*.

[19] Klaus, M. and Kennell, J. (1989) The effects of continual social support during birth on maternal and infant morbidity, in *Prenatal and Perinatal Psychology and Medicine*, (eds P. Fedor-Freybergh and M.L. Vogel), Parthenon Press, Lancaster, Chap. 43.

[20] Jacoby, A. (1987) Women's preferences for and satisfaction with current procedure in childbirth – findings from a national study, *Midwifery*, **3**, 117–24.

[21] St James-Roberts, I. (1987) Linking pre- and peri-natal adversities with child development. *Child: Care, Health and Development*, **13**, 207–25.

[22] Chamberlain, D. (1986) Reliability of birth memories: evidence from mother and child pairs in hypnosis. *Journal of the American Academy of Medical Hypnoanalysts*, **1**, 88.

[23] Laibow, R. (1988) Prenatal and perinatal psychology and medicine (eds P. Fiedor-Fieybagh and M.L. Vogel). Parthenon Press, Lancaster.

[24] Grof, S. (1985) *Beyond the Brain, Death and Transcendence in Psychotherapy*, State University of New York Press, Albany, NY.

[25] English Butterfield, J. (1985) *Different Doorway: Adventures of a Caesarean Born*, Point Reyes Station, CA: Earth Heart.

[26a] Flint, C. (1986) *Sensitive Midwifery*, Heinemann Nursing, Oxford, p. 117.

[26b] Raphael-Leff, J. (1985) Facilitators and Regulators: Participators and Renouncers: mothers and fathers orientating towards pregnancy and parenthood. *J. Psycho. Obstet. Gynaecol.* **4**, 169–84.

[27] See for instance Trowell, J. (1983) *Child Abuse and Neglect*, 7, 387.

[28] Flint, (1986) *Sensitive Midwifery*, p. 120.

[29] Flamm *et al.* (1988).

[30] Philipp, E. (1988) *Caesareans: an Explanation and Preparation*. Sidgwick and Jackson, London.

[31] Mitchell, K. and Nason, M. (1981) *Cesarean Birth: a Couples' Guide for Decision and Preparation*. Harbor, San Francisco.

[32] Pitt, B. (1968) 'Atypical' depression following childbirth. *British Journal of Psychiatry*, **114**, 1325–35.

[33] Dalton, K. (1971) Prospective study into puerperal depression. *British Journal of Psychiatry*, **118**, 689–92.

[34] Jacobsen, L., Kaij, L. and Nilssen, A. (1965) Postnatal mental disorders in an unselected sample: frequency and predisposing factors, *British Medical Journal*, **1**, 1640–3 (quoted by Elliott *et al.* 1984).

[35] Trowell (1983) *Child Abuse and Neglect*, 7, 387.

[36] Helfer, R.E. (1975) The relationship between lack of bonding and child abuse and neglect, in Klaus, M. *et al*, *Maternal Attachment and Mothering Disorders*, sponsored by Johnson and Johnson, 1974.

[37] Meyer, L.D. (1979) *The Cesarean (R)evolution: a handbook for parents and Childbirth Educators*, Chas. Franklin Press, Edmond, WA.

[38] Richards, M. (1978) *New Scientist*, 847.

[39] Carway, E. and Brackbill, Y. (1970) Delivery medication and infant outcome: an empirical study, in *Effects of Obstetrical Medication on the Foetus and Infant* (eds. W. Bowes *et al.*), Monograph of Society for Research in Child Development, **35**. [However a more recent review of many studies have found conflicting evidence about long-term effects: see for instance Kraemer, H.C. *et al.* (19850) Obstetric drugs and infant behaviour: a reevaluation, *Journal of Pediatric Psychology*, **10**, 345–54.

[40] Sameroff, A.J. (ed.) (1978) Organization and stability of newborn behaviour: a commentary on the Brazelton Neonatal Behavioural Assessment Scale. *Monographs of the Society for Research in Child Development*, **43**, 5–6.

[41] Salk, L. *et al.* (1985) Relationship of maternal and perinatal conditions to eventual adolescent suicide. *Lancet*, **i**, 624.

[42] Oakley, A. (1980) *Women Confined: Towards a Sociology of Childbirth*, Martin Robertson, Oxford.

CHAPTER 21: THE NEWBORN: PARENTAL RESPONSES AND NEONATAL SENSORY AND COGNITIVE ABILITIES

[1] Robson, K. and Kumar, R. (1980) Delayed onset of maternal affection after childbirth. *British Journal of Psychiatry*, **136**, 347.

[2] Robson, K.S. and Moss, H.A. (1970) Patterns and determinants of maternal attachment. *Journal of Pediatrics*, **77**, 976–85.

[3] Macfarlane, A. (1977) *The Psychology of Childbirth*, Fontana, Glasgow, pp. 51–4.

[4] Klaus, M. and Kennell, J. (1970) Human maternal behaviour at first contact with her young. *Pediatrics*, **46**, 187–92.

[5] Wolff, P.H. (1963) Observations on the development of smiling, in *Determinants of Infant Behaviour* (ed. B.M. Foss), Methuen, London.

[6] Klaus, M. and Kennell, J. (1976) *Maternal–Infant Bonding*, C.V. Mosby, St Louis, MO.

[7] Kennell, J. and Klaus, M.(1984) Mother–Infant Bonding: Weighing the Evidence. *Developmental Review*, **4**, 275–82.

[8] Benedek, T. (1959) Parenthood as a developmental phase: a contribution to the libido theory. *Journal of the American Psychoanalytic Association*, **7**, 389.

[9] Rosenblatt, J. *et al.* (1962) Progress in the study of maternal behaviour in the rat: hormonal, nonhormonal, sensory and developmental aspects. *Advances in the Study of Behaviour*, **10**, 226.

[10] See Klaus, M. and Kennell, J. (1983) *Bonding – the Beginnings of Parent–Infant Attachment*. Mosby, St Louis, MO, pp. 457–50.

[11] Bowlby, J. (1977) The making and breaking of affectional bonds: I. aetiology and psychopathology in the light of attachment theory. *British Journal of Psychiatry*, **130**, 201.

[12] Macfarlane, A. (1977) *The Psychology of Childbirth*, Fontana, Glasgow.

[13] Condon, W.S. and Sander, L.W. (1974) Neonate movement is synchronized with adult speech: interactional participation and language acquisition. *Science*, **183**, 99.

[14] Stern, D. (1985) *The Interpersonal World of the Infant*. Basic Books, New York.

[15] Richards, M. (1980) *Infancy*, Mutimedia, Holland.

[16] Klaus, M. and Kennell, J. (1983) Parent to infant bonding: setting the record straight. *Journal of Pediatrics*, 10, 575–6. [In my view, some confusion about the effects of early contact on bonding appears to have arisen due to lack of conceptual distinction between cases of parental choice determining the degree of contact with the newborn compared with the psychological impact on bonding of being denied wished-for access to the baby].

[17] Balint, M. (1948) Individual differences of behaviour in early infancy and an objective method for recording them. *Journal of Genetic Psychology*, **73**, 57–79; 81–117.

[18] Korner, A.F. (1971) Individual differences at birth: implications for early experience and later development. *American Journal of Orthopsychiatry*, **41**, 608–19.

[19] Lipsett, L. (1979) The newborn as informant, in *Infants at Risk – assessment of cognitive functioning* (eds R.B. Kearsley and I.E. Sigel), Lawrence Erlbaum, Hillsdale, NJ.

[20] Brazelton, T.B. (1973) The effects of prenatal drugs on the behaviour of the neonate. *American Journal of Psychiatry*, **126**, 1261–6.

[21] Rutter, M. (1974) Dimensions of parenthood: some myths and some suggestions, in DHSS Report, *The Family in Society: Dimensions of Parenthood*, HMSO, London.

[22] St James-Roberts, I. and Wolke, D. (1988) Convergences and discrepancies among mothers' and professionals' assessments of difficult neonatal behaviour, *Journal Child Psychology and Psychiatry*, **29**, 21–42.

[23] Zeanah, C.H. and Anders, T.F. (1987) Subjectivity in parent–infant relationships: a discussion of internal working models. *Infant Mental Health Journal*, **8**, 237–49.

[24] St James-Roberts, I. and Wolke, D. (1989) Do obstetric factors affect mother's perception of her new-born's behaviour? *British Journal of*

Developmental Psychology, 7, 141–58.

[25] Winnicott, D.W. (1956) Primary maternal preoccupation, in *Through Paediatrics to Psycho-Analysis*. Hogarth Press, London, p. 302.

[26] Raphael-Leff, J. (1986) Facilitators and Regulators: conscious and unconscious processes in pregnancy and early motherhood. *British Journal of Medical Psychology*, 59, 43.

[27] Shaw, E. and Darling, J. (1984) *Strategies of Being Female: Animal Patterns, Human Choices*, Harvester Press, Brighton.

[28] Greenberg, M. & Morris, N. (1974) Engrossment: the newborn's impact upon the father. *American Journal of Orthopsychiatry*, 44, 520.

[29] Parke, R.D. (1979) Perspectives on father–infant interaction, in *The Handbook of Infant Development* (ed. J. Osofsky), Wiley, New York, quoted in Klaus & Kennell, *Bonding* (1983).

[30a] Rodholm, M. (1981) Effects of father–infant post-partum contact on their interaction 3 months after birth. *Early Human Development*, 5, 79, quoted in Klaus and Kennell (1983).

[30b] Field, T. and Widmayer, S. (1980) Developmental follow-up of infants delivered by caesarean section and general anaesthesia. *Infant Behaviour and Development*, 3, 253–64.

[31] Greenberg, M. and Morris, N. (1974) *American Journal of Orthopsychiatry*, 44, 520.

[32] Rodholm (1981) *Early Human Development*, 5, 79.

[33] Lang, Raven cited by Klaus, M. and Kennell, S. (1983) *Bonding*, p. 21.

[34] Stern, D. (1985) *The Interpersonal World of the Infant.*

[35] Caplan, G. (1973) *The First Twelve Months of Life*. Grosset and Dunlap, New York.

[36] Chamberlain, D. (1983) The cognitive newborn: a scientific update. *British Journal of Psychotherapy*, 42, 30–71.

[37] Macfarlane, A. (1975) Olfaction in the development of social preferences in the human neonate, in *Parent–Infant Interaction* (ed. M. Hofer), Elsevier, Amsterdam.

[38] DeCasper, A.J. and Fifer, W.P. (1980) Of human bonding: newborns prefer their mothers' voices. *Science*, 208, 1174.

[39] Wolff, P.H. (1959) Observations on newborn infants, *Psychosomatic Medicine*, 21, 110–18.

[40] Brazleton, T.B. (1981) *On Becoming a Family*.

[41] Brackbill, Y. (1987) Obstetrical medications and infant behaviour, in *Handbook of Infant Development*, (ed. J.D. Osofsky), Wiley, New York.

[42] Field, T.M., Woodson, R., Greenberg, R. and Cohen, D. (1982) Discrimination and imitation of facial expression by neonates. *Science*, 218, 179–81.

[43] Emde, R.N. (1988) Development terminable and interminable. *International Journal of Psycho-Analysis*, 69, 283–96.

[44] Murray, L. and Trevarthen, C.B. (1986) The infant's role in mother–infant communication. *Journal of Child Language*, 13, 1.

[45] Bruner, J.S. (1977) Early social interaction and language acquisition, in *Studies in Mother–Infant Interaction* (ed. H.R. Schaffer), Academic Press, London.

[46] Bower, T.G.R. (1974) *Developments in Infancy*. Freeman, San Francisco.

[47] Stern, (1985) *The Interpersonal World of the Infant*.

[48] Murray, L. (1989) Winnicott and the developmental psychology of infancy. *British Journal of Psychotherapy*, 5, 333–48.

[49] Truby, H.M. (1975) Prenatal and neonatal speech, prespeech and an infantile speech lexicon, in *Child Language*, special issue of *Word*, 27, quoted

by Chamberlain (1983) *British Journal of Psychotherapy*, **4**, 30–71.

[50] Wasz-Hockert *et al.* (1968) quoted in Chamberlain (1983) *British Journal of Psychotherapy*, p. 18.

[51] Meltzoff, A.N. and Moore, M.K. (1977) Imitation of facial and manual gestures by human neonates. *Science*, **198**, 75.

[52] Carpenter, G. (1974) Mother's face and the newborn. *New Scientist*, 21 March.

[53] Sherrod, L.R. (1981) Issues in cognitive-perceptual development: the special case of social stimuli, in *Infant Social Cognition* (eds M.E. Lamb and L.R. Sherrod), Erlbaum, Hillsdale, NJ.

[54] Klaus, M. and Kennell, J. (1983) *Bonding*, New American Library, Mosby, St Louis.

[55] Winnicott, D.W. (1971) *Playing and Reality*, Penguin, London, 1980.

[56] Bion, W.R. (1967) *Second Thoughts*. Maresfield reprints, London.

CHAPTER 22: EARLY DAYS: GETTING ACQUAINTED

[1] Winnicott, D.W. (1952) Anxiety associated with insecurity, in *Through Paediatrics to Psycho-Analysis*, Hogarth, London, Chap. 8, 1982.

[2] Ainsworth, M.D.S., Bell, S.M. and Stayton, D.J. (1974) Infant–mother attachment and social development: socialization as a product of reciprocal responsiveness to signals, in *The Integration of a Child into a Social World* (ed. M.P.M. Richards), Cox and Wyman, London.

[3] Herzog, J.M. (1982) Patterns of expectant fatherhood: a study of the fathers of a group of premature infants, in *Father and Child – Developmental and Clinical Perspectives* (eds. S.H. Cath, A.R. Gurwitt and J. Munder Ross), Little, Brown, Boston, Chap. 19.

[4] Field, T. and Widmayer, S. (1980) Developmental follow-up of infants delivered by caesarian section and general anesthesia, *Infant Behaviour and Development*, **3**, 253–64.

[5] Winnicott, D.W. (1965) *The Family and Individual Development*, Tavistock, London.

[6] Benedek, T. (1970) Motherhood and nurturing, in *Parenthood – Its Psychology and Psychopathology* (eds. E.J. Anthony and T. Benedek), Little, Brown, Boston, Chap. 6.

[7] Opie, I. and Tatem, M. (eds) (1989) *A Dictionary of Superstitions*, Oxford University Press, Oxford.

[8] Freud, S. (1913) *Totem and Taboo*, S.E. vol. XIII, Hogarth, London.

[9] Opie and Tatem (1989) *Dictionary of Superstitions*.

[10] Frazer, J.G. (1953) *The Golden Bough*. MacMillan, New York.

[11] Hamilton, A. (1970) Nature and nurture: childrearing in north-central Arnheim Land, unpublished MA thesis, University of Sydney (quoted by Trevarthen 1979, in *Human Ethology: Claims and Limits of a New Discipline*).

[12] Carek, D.J. and Capelli, A.J. (1981) Mothers' reactions to their newborn infants. *American Academy of Child Psychiatry*, **20**, 16–31.

[13] Raphael-Leff, J. (1990) The moon hung by a navelstring. in press.

[14] Galenson, E. and Roiphe, H. (1982) The preoedipal relationship of a father, mother and daughter, in *Father and Child* (eds S.H. Cath, A.R. Gurwitt and J. Munder Ross), Chapter 9.

[15] Yogman, M.W. (1982) Observations on the father–infant relationship, in *Father and Child*, (eds Cath, Gurwitt and Munder Ross), Chap. 6.

[16] Burlingham, D. (1973) The preoedipal infant–father relationship.

Psychoanalytic Study of the Child, **28**, 23–48.

[17]   Lamb, M.E. and Frodi, A.M. (1982) Varying degrees of paternal involvement in infant care, in *Parenting and Child Development* (ed. M.E. Lamb), Erlbaum, Hillsdale, NJ.

[18]   Dorner, (1989) Significance of hormones and neurotransmitters in pre- and early postnatal life for human ontogenesis. *International Journal of Prenatal and Perinatal Studies*, **1**, 145–50.

[19]   Trevarthen, C. (1979) Instincts for human understanding and for cultural cooperation: their development in infancy, in *Human Ethology: Claims and Limits of a New Discipline* (eds von Cranach *et al*), Maison des Sciences de l'Homme/Cambridge University Press, Cambridge, p. 551.

[20]   See Erikson, E. (1964) Inner and outer space: reflections on womanhood, in *The Woman in America* (ed. R. Lifton), Houghton Mifflin, Boston.

[21]   Kestenberg, J. (1968) Outside and inside, male and female. *Journal of the American Psychoanalytic Association*, **16**, 457–520.

[22]   Stoller, R.J. (1968) *Sex and Gender*. Hogarth Press, London.

[23]   Trager, J. (1989) Forget those headlines about circumcision. *Medical Tribune (USA)*, **30**, 16.

[24]   Winberg, J. *et al.* (1989) *Lancet*, 18 March.

[25]   Freud, S. (1910) *Leonardo da Vinci and a Memory of his Childhood*, footnote p. 95, added 1919. Standard Edition. vol. XI. Hogarth, London.

[26]   Service at a Circumcision, *Authorized Daily Prayer Book* of the United Congregations of the British Empire, p. 305. Eyre and Spottiswoode, London, 1935.

[27]   Fuller, J.H.S. and Toon, P.D. (1988) *Medical Practice in a Multicultural Society*, Heinemann, Oxford.

[28]   St James-Roberts, I. and Wolke, D. (1988) Convergences and discrepancies, among mothers' and professionals' assessments of difficult neonatal behaviour. *Journal of Child Psychology and Psychiatry*, **29**, 21–42.

[29]   Rubin, R. (1961) Puerperal change, *Nursing Outlook*, **9**, 753–5.

[30]   Pitt, B. (1982) Puerperal depression. *Psychiatric Problems in Women*, Smith Kline and French publications, Hertfordshire, Vol. 1.1.

Further reading

Miller, L., Rustin, M., Rustin, M. and Shuttleworth, J. (1989) *Closely Observed Infants*. Duckworth, London.

Winnicott, D.W. (1988) *Human Nature*, Free Association Books, London.

Daws, D. (1989) *Through the Night*, Duckworth Books, London.

CHAPTER 23: POSTPARTUM PROFESSIONAL CARE

[1]   Alder, E. and Bancroft, J. (1988) The relationship between breast feeding persistence, sexuality and mood in postpartum women. *Psychological Medicine*, **18**, 389–96.

[2]   Pines, D. (1986) A woman's unconscious use of her body, a psychoanalytic perspective, Carol Dilling memorial lecture, New York (unpublished).

[3]   Welldon, E.V. (1988) *Mother, Madonna, Whore – the Idealization and Denigration of Motherhood*, Free Association Books, London, p. 120.

[4]   Newson, J. and Newson, A. (1969) *Patterns of Infant Care*. Penguin Books, London.

[5]   Price, J. (1987) *Motherhood – What it Does to Your Mind*. Pandora, London.

[6]   Wright, P. (1988) Learning experiences in feeding behaviour during

infancy. *Journal of Psychosomatic Research*, **32**, 613–19.

[7] Simsarian, F.P. and McLennon, P.S. (1942) Feeding behaviour of an infant during the first 12 weeks of life on a self-demand schedule. *Journal of Pediatrics*, **20**, 93, quoted by Inch, S. (1987).

[8] Hall, B. (1975) Changing composition of milk and early development of an appetite control, *Lancet*, i, 779–81.

[9] Alberts, E., Kalverboer, A.F. and Hopkins, B. (1983) Mother–infant dialogue in the first days of life: an observational study during breast-feeding. *Journal of Child Psychology and Psychiatry*, **24**, 145–61.

[10] Copies of the code are available from The Baby Milk Action Coalition, 34 Binco Grove, Cambridge CB1 4TS.

[11] Garforth, S. (1987) Policy and practice in midwifery study, reported by Inch, S. *Journal of the Royal Society of Medicine*, **80**, 53–8.

[12] Ibid.

[13] Inch, S. (1987) Difficulties with breastfeeding: midwives in disarray? report on meeting of RSM Forum of Maternity and the Newborn, 2 December 1985, *Journal of the Royal Society of Medicine*, **80**, 53–8.

[14] Winnicott, D.W. (1969) Breastfeeding as a communication. *Maternal and Child Care*, **5**, 147–50.

[15] Goffman, I. (1961) *Asylums*, Penguin Books, London.

[16] Beech, B. (1987) *Who's having your baby?* Camden Press, London.

[17] Currer, C. (1983) Pathan mothers in Bradford, report to DHSS. Warwick University (unpublished).

[18] Ibid.

[19] Gideon, H. (1962) A baby is born in the Punjab. *American Anthropologist*, **64**, 1220–34.

[20] See Graves, R. and Patai, R. (1965) *Hebrew Myths*, Cassel, London.

[21] Grundulis, H., Scott, P.H. Belton, N.R. and Wharton, B.A. (1986) Combined deficiencies of iron and vitamin D in Asian toddlers. *Archives of Disease in Childhood*, **61**, 843–8.

[22] Fenton, T.R., Bhat, R., Davies, A. and West, R. (1989) Maternal insecurity and failure to thrive in Asian children. *Archives of Disease in Childhood*, **64**, 369–72.

[23] Currer, C. (1983) Pathan mothers in Bradford.

[24] Barnett, S. (1989) Working with interpreters, in *Working with Bilingual Language Disability* (ed. D. Duncan), Chapman & Hall, London, Chap. 7.

Further reading

Stern, D.N. (1985) *The Interpersonal World of the Infant*. Basic Books, New York.

Garcia, J., Kilpatrick, R. and Richards, M. (eds) (1990) *The Politics of Maternity Care – Services for Childbearing Women in Twentieth Century Britain*, Clarendon, London.

Jacoby, A. (1987) Women's preferences for and satisfaction with current procedures in childbirth – findings from a national study. *Midwifery*, **3**, 117–24.

Oppong, C. (ed) (1985) *Female and Male in West Africa*, George Allen and Unwin, London.

Daws, D. (1985) Two papers on working in a baby clinic: I Standing next to the weighing scales. *Journal of Child Psychotherapy*, **11**, 77–85. II Sleep problems in babies and young children. *Journal of Child Psychotherapy*, **11**, 87–96.

CHAPTER 24: FIRST SIX WEEKS: DIFFERING PATTERNS OF
MATERNAL AND PATERNAL ADJUSTMENT

[1] For a description of this very complicated process, called 'projective identification', see for instance: Bion, W.R. (1959) Attacks on linking. *International Journal of Psycho-Analysis*, **40**, 308–15 (republished in Bion, W.R.
(1967) *Second Thoughts*, Heinemann, London, pp. 93–109.) Also Ogden,
T.H. (1979) On projective identification. *International Journal of Psycho-
Analysis*, **60**, 357–73.

[2a] Raphael-Leff, J. (1989) Where the wild things are. *International Journal of
Prenatal and Perinatal Studies*, **1**, 79–89.

[2b] Main, M. (1989) Parental careism to infant-initiated contact is correlated
with the parents' own rejection during childhood: the effects of experience
on signals of security with respect to attachment. In *Touch* (eds Blazelton,
T.B. and Barnard, V.) International Universities Press, New York.

[3] Brody, S. (1970) A mother is being beaten: an instinctual derivative and
infant care, in *Parenthood – its Psychology and Psychopathology* (eds E.J.
Anthony and T. Benedek), Little, Brown, Boston, p. 30.

[4] Brazelton, T.B. (1981) *On Becoming a Family*, Delacorte Press, New York.

[5] Ainsworth, M.D.S., Bell, S.M. and Stayton, D.J. (1974) Infant–mother
attachment and social development: socialization as a product of reciprocal
responsiveness to signals, in *The Integration of a Child into a Social World*
(ed. M.P.M. Richards), Cox and Wyman Cambridge University Press,
London.

[6] Daws, D. (1989) *Through the night*, Duckworth, London.

[7] Paykel, E.S., Emms, E.M., Fletcher, J. and Tassaby, E.S. (1980) Life events
and social support in puerperal depression. *British Journal of Psychiatry*,
136, 339–47.

[8] Oakley, A. (1980) *Women Confined: Towards a Sociology of Childbirth*, Martin
Robertson, Oxford:

[9] Breen, D. (1975) *Birth of the First Child*. Tavistock, London.

[10] Raphael-Leff, J. (1985) Facilitators and Regulators: Vulnerability to Postnatal
Disturbance. *Journal of Psychosomatic Obstetrics and Gynaecology*, **4**, 151–68.

[11] Ibid.

[12a] Freud, S. (1939) *Moses and Monotheism*. S.E. **23**, Hogarth, London.

[12b] Samuels, A. (1988) A relation called father. *British Journal of Psychotherapy*,
4, 416–26.

[13] Rosaldo, M.Z. (1974) Women, culture and society: a theoretical overview,
in *Woman, Culture and Society* (eds M.Z. Rosaldo and L. Lamphere),
Stanford University Press, Stanford.

[14] Abelin, E.L. (1975) Some further observations and comments on the earliest
role of the father. *International Journal of Psycho-Analysis*, **56**, 293–302.

[15] Lacan, J. (1966) *Ecrits*, Tavistock, London.

[16] Lewis, C. (1989) Fathers and postnatal disturbance: what can we learn from
studies of the transition to parenthood. *Marce Society Bulletin*, Spring.

[17] Zaslow, M., Pedersen, F., Suwalsky, J., Rabinovich, B. and Cain, R. (1986)
Fathering during the infancy period: implications of the mother's employment role. *Infant Mental Health Journal*, **7**, 225.

[18] Hwang, P. (1988) Swedish Fathers and Childbearing, lecture, Marce
Society Conference on Mental Illness in the Puerperium, Keele University.

[19] Cath, S.H. (1986) Fathering from infancy to old age: a selective overview
of recent psychoanalytic contributions. *The Psychoanalytic Review*, **73**, 469–79.

[20] Biller, H.B. (1974) *Paternal Deprivation*, Lexington Books, Massachusetts.

[21] Atkins, R.N. (1982) Discovering daddy: the mother's role, in *Father and Child – Developmental and Clinical Perspectives* (eds S.H. Cath, A.R. Gurnitt and J. Munder Ross), Little, Brown, Boston, Chap. 8.

[22] Belsky, J. and Voling, B. (1987) Mothering, fathering and marital interaction in the family triad during infancy, in *Men's Transition to Parenthood* (eds P. Bermnan and F. Pedersen), Lawrence Erlbaum, New Jersey.

[23] Ferketich, S.L. and Mercer, R.T. (1989) Men's health status during pregnancy and early fatherhood. *Research, Nursing, Health*, **12**, 137–48.

[24] Biller (1974) *Paternal Deprivation*.

[25] Yogman, M.W. (1982) Observations on the father–infant relationship, in *Father and Child: Developmental and Clinical Perspectives* (eds S.H. Cath, A.R. Gurwitt and J.M. Ross), Little, Brown, Boston.

[26] Parke, R. and Sawin, D.B. (1980) The family in early infancy, in *Father–Infant Relationship* (ed. F.A. Pederson), New York, pp. 65–91.

[27] Macoby, E. and Jacklin, C. (1974) *The Psychology of Sex Differences*, Stanford University Press, Los Angeles.

[28] Pederson, F.A., Anderson, B. and Kain, R., (1980) Parent–infant and husband–wife interactions observed at 5 months, in *Father–Infant Relationship* (ed. F.A. Pederson), Praeger, New York.

[29] Gunsberg, L. (1982) Selected critical review of psychological investigations of the early father–infant relationship, chapter 4 in *Father and Child* (eds S.H. Cath *et al*). Little, Brown, Boston.

[30] Lamb, M.E. (ed.) (1976) *The Role of the Father in Child Development*, Wiley, New York.

[31] Abelin, E. (1980) Triangulation, in *Rapprochement* (eds R. Lacks, S. Bach and E.J. Burland), Aaronson, New York, pp. 151–69.

[32] Ross, J.M. (1982) In search of fathering: a review, chapter 2 in *Father and Child* (eds S.H. Cath *et al*.)

[33] Chassueguet-Smirgel *et al.* (1981) *Female Sexuality – New Psychoanalytic Views*, Virago, London.

[34] Tyson, P. (1982) A developmental line of gender identity, gender role and choice of love object. *Journal of the American Psychoanalytic Association*, **30**, 61–86.

[35] Brazelton, T.B. *et al.* (1970) The infant as a focus for family reciprocity, in *The Child and its Family* (eds M. Lewis and L.A. Rosenblum), Plenum, New York, pp. 62–80.

[36] Burgner, M. (1985) The oedipal experience: effects on development of an absent father. *International Journal of Psycho-Analysis*, **66**, 311–20.

[37] Layland, R.W. (1981) In search of a loving father. *International Journal of Psycho-Analysis*, **62**, 215–24, p. 216.

[38] Chused, J.F. (1986) Consequences of paternal nurturing. *Psychoanalytic Study of the Child*, **41**, 419–38.

[39] Pruett, K.D. (1983) Infants of primary nurturing fathers, *Psychoanalytic Study of the Child*, **38**, 257–77.

[40] Yogman, M.W. (1984) The father's role with preterm and fullterm infants, in *Frontiers of Infant Psychiatry*, Vol. II, (eds J.D. Call, E. Galenson and R.L. Tyson), Basic Books, New York.

[41] Field, T. (1978) Interaction behaviours of primary vs. secondary caretaker fathers. *Developmental Psychology*, **14**, 183–4.

[42] Raphael-Leff, J. (1983) Facilitators and Regulators: two approaches to mothering. *British Journal of Medical Psychology*, **56**, 379–90.

CHAPTER 25: FIRST SIX WEEKS: RELATIONSHIP OF THE PARENTS

[1]   Rossi, A. (1968) Transition to parenthood. *Journal of Marriage and the Family*, **30**, 26–39.
[2]   Andersen, I. (1984) Transition to parenthood research, review article. *Journal of Psychosomatic Obstetrics and Gynaecology*, **3**, 3–16.
[3]   Shereshefsky, P.M. and Yarrow, L.M. (eds) (1973) *Psychological Aspects of a First Pregnancy and Early Postnatal Adaptation*, New York.
[4]   Scott-Hayes, G. (1983) Marital adaptation during pregnancy and after childbirth. *Journal of Reproductive and Infant Psychology*, **1**, 18–28.
[5]   Meyerowitz, J.H. and Feldman, H. (1966) Transition to parenthood, *Psychiatric Research Report*, **20**, 78, quoted by Andersen (1984).
[6]   Oakley, A. (1980) *Women Confined: Towards a Sociology of Childbirth*, Robertson, Oxford.
[7]   Entwistle, D.R. and Doering, S.G. (1980) *The First Birth*, John Hopkins University Press, Baltimore, MD.
[8]   Lewis, C. (1986) *Becoming a Father*, Open University Press, Milton Keynes.
[9]   Russel, C.S. (1974) Transition to parenthood: problems and gratifications. *Journal of Marriage and the Family*, **36**, 294–350.
[10] Sollie, D.L. and Miller, B.C. (1980) The transition to parenthood is a critical time for building family strengths, in *Family Strengths, Positive Models for Family Life* (eds N. Stinennet *et al.*), University of Nebraska Press, Omaha, NE, quoted by Andersen (1984).
[11] Skynner, A.C.R. (1976) *One Flesh, Separate Persons: Principles of Family and Marital Psychotherapy*, Constable, London.
[12] Benedek, T. (1959) Parenthood as a developmental phase: a contribution to the libido theory. *Journal of the American Psychoanalytic Association*, **7**, 389.
[13] Brody, S. (1970) A mother is being beaten: an instinctual derivative and infant care, in *Parenthood – its Psychology and Psychopathology* (eds E.J. Anthony and T. Benedek), Little, Brown, Boston.
[14] Skynner (1970) *One Flesh, Separate Persons*.
[15] Johnson, A.M. (1953) Factors in the etiology of fixations and symptom choice. *Psychoanalytic Quarterly*, **22**, 475–96, quoted by Benedek (1959).
[16] Daniels, P. and Weingarten, K. (1982) *Sooner or Later – the Timing of Parenthood in Adult Lives*. W.W. Norton, London.
[17] Ibid.
[18] Alder, E. and Bancroft, J. (1988) The relationship between breast feeding persistence, sexuality and mood in postpartum women. *Psychological Medicine*, **18**, 389–96.
[19] Sleep, J. *et al.* (1984) West Berkshire perineal management trial. *British Medical Journal*, **289**, 587.
[20] Flint, C. (1986) *Sensitive Midwifery*, Heinemann Nursing, Oxford.

Further reading

Chalmers, B. (1984) *Early Parenthood – Heaven or Hell*, Juta, Cape Town.
Gieve, K. (ed.) (1989) *Balancing Acts – On Being a Mother*, Virago, London.
Greenberg, M. (1985) *The Birth of a Father*, Continuum, New York.
Price, J. (1988) *Motherhood – What it Does to Your Mind*, Pandora, London.

Relevant organizations

The Parent Network, 44–46 Caversham Road, London NW5 2DS (parents discussion groups about family relationships).

La Leche League, 27 Old Gloucester Street, London WC1. (Breastfeeding promotion)

Association for Breastfeeding Mothers, 10 Hersell Road, London SE23 1EN (nationwide 24 hour advice line).

National Childbirth Trust, Alexandra House, Oldham Terrace, Acton, London W3 (breastfeeding counsellors and postnatal groups).

CHAPTER 26: SIBLINGS

[1] Solnit, A.J. (1983) The sibling experience. *Psychoanalytic Study of the Child,* **38**, 281–4.
[2] Henchie, quoted by Trause M.A. and Irvin, N.A. (1983) Care of the sibling in *Bonding* (eds M.H. Klaus and J.H. Kennell), New American Library, St Louis, pp. 76–92.
[3] Sostek and Read, quoted by Trause and Irvin (1983) in *Bonding.*
[4] Henchie, quoted in Trause and Irvin (1983) in *Bonding.*
[5] Trause M.A. and Irvin, N.A. (1983) Care of the Sibling, in *Bonding.*
[6] American College of Obstetrics and Gynecology (1979) Survey of sibling participation in hospital births, quoted by Trause and Irvin (1983) in *Bonding.*
[7] Mehl, L. (1980) Psychophysiological aspects of childbirth, in *The Psychology of Birth* (ed. L. Feher), Souvenir Press, London.
[8] See Neubauer, P.B. (1983) The importance of the sibling experience. *Psychoanalytic Study of the Child,* **38**, 325–36.
[9] Fraiberg, S. (1959) *The Magic Years,* Scribner's, New York, p. 280f, quoted by Colona, A.B. and Newman, L.M. (1983) Psychoanalytic literature on siblings, *Psychoanalytic Study of the Child,* **38**, 285–309.
[10] Freud, A. and Dann, S. (1951) An experiment in group upbringing. *Psychoanalytic Study of the Child ,* **6**, 127–68.
[11] Provence, S. and Solnit, A.J. (1983) Development-promoting aspects of the sibling experience. *Psychoanalytic Study of the Child,* **38**, 337–51.
[12] Freud, S. (1921) *Group psychology and the analysis of the ego.* S.E. **18**, 67–143.
[13] Kris, M. and Ritvo, S. (1983) Parents and siblings: their mutual influence, *Psychoanalytic Study of the Child,* **38**, 311–24.
[14] Abarbanel, J. (1983) The revival of the sibling experience during the mother's second pregnancy. *Psychoanalytic Study of the Child,* **38**, 353–79.
[15] Kris and Ritvo (1983) Parents and siblings.
[16] Ibid.
[17] Trause, M.A. and Irvin, N.A. (1983) Care of the sibling, in *Bonding.*
[18] Kennedy, H. (1985) Growing up with a handicapped sibling. *Psychoanalytic Study of the Child,* **40**, 255–74.
[19] Miller, L., Rustin, M.M. and Shuttleworth, J. (1989) Kathy and Suzanne: Twin Sisters, in *Closely Observed Infants,* Duckworth, London.
[20] Stern, D.N. (1971) A micro-analysis of mother–infant interaction: behaviours regulating social contact between a mother and her three and a half month old twins. *Journal of the American Academy of Child Psychiatry,* **10**, 501–17.
[21] Piontelli, A. (1989) A study on twins before and after birth, *International Review of Psycho-Analysis,* **16**, 413–26.

[22] Klaus, M. and Kennell, J. (1983) *Bonding*, New American Library, Mosby, St Louis.

[23] Rutter, M. (1981) *Maternal Deprivation Reassessed*, Penguin, London.

[24] Raphael-Leff, J. (1990) If Oedipus was an Egyptian. *International Review of Psycho-Analysis*, **20**, 309–35.

[25] Bender, H. (1990) On the outside looking in: sibling perceptions, dreams and anxieties about premature infants, in *Prenatal and Perinatal Psychology and Medicine*, Vol. 2 (ed. F. Freybegh) Proceedings of International Conference 'Encounter with the Newborn', Jerusalem, April, 1988, Parthenon Press, Cairnforth.

[26] Lewis, H.A. (1980) A stillbirth or other perinatal death, in *Psychological Process of Pregnancy, Birthing and Bonding* (ed. B. Blum), New York, Human Sciences Press.

[27] Bowlby, J. (1980) *Attachment and Loss*, vol. III. *Loss*. Basic Books, New York.

[28] Nagera, H. (1970) Childrens' reactions to the death of important objects. *Psychoanalytic Study of the Child*, **25**, 360–400.

[29] Leon, I.G. (1986) Intrapsychic and family dynamics in perinatal sibling loss. *Infant Mental Health Journal*, **7**, 200–13.

[30] Sekaer, C. and Katz, S. (1986) On the concept of mourning in childhood. *Psychoanalytic Study of the Child*, **41**, 287–314.

Relevant organizations

TAMBA (The Twins and Multiple Birth Association), 292 Valley Road, Lillington, Leamington Spa CV32 7UE (offers support when one twin dies).

Twins and Multiple Births, 54 Windmill Drive, Croxley Green, Rickmansworth, Herts WD3 3FE.

CHAPTER 27: ADOLESCENT PARENTS

[1] Erlich, H.S. (1986) Denial in adolescence: some paradoxical aspects, *Psychoanalytic Study of the Child*, **41**, 315–36.

[2] Pines, D. (1988) Adolescent pregnancy and motherhood: a psychoanalytic perspective. *Psychoanalytic Inquiry*, **8**, 234–51.

[3a] Simms, M. and Smith, C. (1982) Teenage mothers and abortion. *British Journal of Sexual Medicine*, **9**, 45–7.

[3b] Hibbs, E.D. and Sansbury, D.L. (1988) The impact of the finality of family and peer relations on adolescent pregnancy. In *Children and Families: studies in prevention and intervention*. (ed E.D. Hibbs) International Universities Press, Madison, Conn.

[4] Simms, M. and Smith, C. (1984) Teenage mothers: some views on health visitors. *Health Visitor*, **57**, 269–70.

[5] Anastasiow, N.J. (1987) Programs developed in response to teen pregnancies. *Infant Mental Health Journal*, **8**, 65.

[6] Crockenberg, S.B. (1986) Professional support for adolescent mothers: who gives it, how adolescent mothers evaluate it, what they would prefer. *Infant Mental Health Journal*, **7**, 49.

[7] Dunst, C.J., Vance, S.D. and Cooper, C.S. (1986) A social systems perspective of adolescent pregnancy: determinants of parent and parent–child behaviour. *Infant Mental Health Journal*, **7**, 34–48.

[8] Osofsky, J.D. and Eberhart-Wright, A. (1988) Affective exchanges between

high risk mothers and infants. *International Journal of Psycho-Analysis,* **69**, 221–32.

[9]　Fraiberg, S. (1987) The adolescent mother and her infant, in *Selected Writings of Selma Fraiberg,* Ohio University Press.

[10]　Blos, P. (1983) The contribution of psychoanalysis to the psychotherapy of adolescents. *Psychoanalytic Study of the Child,* **38**, 577–600, p. 19.

[11]　Ibid.

[12]　Simms, M. and Smith, C. (1982) Young fathers: attitudes to marriage and family life. *The Father Figure,* Tavistock, London.

Further reading

Esman, A.H. (1975) *The Psychology of Adolescence,* International Universities Press, New York.

Kennedy, R., Heymans, A. and Tischler, L. (1987) *The Family as In-Patient – Families and Adolescents at the Cassel Hospital.* Free Associations Books, London.

Lamb, M. *et al.* (1986) Characteristics of married and unmarried adolescent mothers and their partners, *Journal of Youth and Adolescence,* **15**, 487–96.

Laufer, M. and Laufer, M.E. (eds) (1989) *Developmental Breakdown and Psychoanalytic Treatment in Adolescence – Clinical Studies,* Yale University Press, London and New Haven.

Nathanson, M. *et al.* (1986) Family functioning and the adolescent mother. *Adolescence,* **21**, 827–42.

Relevant organizations

Gingerbread, 25 Wellington Street, London WC2E 7BN (nationwide self-help groups for single parents).

MAMA (Meet A Mother Association) 5 Westbury Gardens, Luton, Beds. (countrywide local groups).

Home Start, 140 New Walk, Leicester, LE1 7JL (Countrywide scheme offering practical help in the home and friendship for families with young children).

CHAPTER 28: ADOPTION

[1]　See for instance 'Single, pregnant and thinking about adoption', a pamphlet distributed by BAAF (British Agencies for Adoption and Fostering) which offers information about the various options and stresses: 'If after considering all the possibilities, you decide on adoption, you should not feel that you are abandoning your baby. Although it is a difficult decision to make, it is a responsible and caring one'.

[2]　BAAF (1987) *Explaining Adoption.* London.

[3]　Lindsay, J. and Monserrat, C. (1990) *Adoption Awareness.* Morning Glory Press, California.

[4]　Reich, D. (1990) Working with mothers who lost a child through adoption. *Post-adoption Centre,* discussion papers, no. 5.

[5]　Post-adoption Centre (1990) Groups for women who have parted with a child for adoption, discussion papers, no. 2.

[6]　Ibid.

[7]　Reich, D. (1990) Preparing people to adopt babies and young children, *Post-adoption Centre,* discussion papers, no. 1.

[8]　Sabatello, U., Natali, P. and Giannotti, A. (1989) Pre-adoptive diagnosis:

the meaning of a crisis. *British Journal of Psychotherapy,* **6**, 160–9.

[9] Hormann, E. (1989) The bonding process in a planned adoption. *International Journal of Prenatal and Perinatal Studies,* **1**, 75–8.

[10] Blum, H.P. (1983) Adoptive parents: generative conflict and generational continuity. *Psychoanalytic Study of the Child,* **38**, 141–63.

[11] Brinich, P.M. (1980) Some potential effects of adoption. *Psychoanalytic Study of the Child,* **35**, 107–33.

[12] Blum (1983) Adoptive parents.

[13] Brinich (1980) Some potential effects of adoption.

[14] Ibid.

[15] Nickman, S.L. (1985) Losses in adoption, *Psychoanalytic Study of the Child,* **40**, 365–98.

[16] Brodzinsky, D.M. *et al.* (1985) Children's knowledge of adoption, in *Thinking about the Family* (eds R. Ashmore and D.M. Brodzinsky), Earlbaum, Hillsdale, NJ.

[17] Nickman (1985) Losses in adoption.

[18] Brinich (1980) Some potential affects of adoption.

[19] Reich (1990) *Post-adoption Centre,* discussion paper, no. 1, p. 6.

[20] Nickman (1985) Losses in adoption.

[21] Burnell, A. (1990) Explaining adoption to children who have been adopted: how do we find the right words?', *Post-adoption Centre,* discussion papers, no. 3.

[22] Ibid., p. 12.

[23] Fitsell, A. (1990) Adoption issues for Lesbian women. *Post-adoption Centre,* discussion papers, no. 4.

Further reading

NORCAP *Shared Experiences.*

Arms, S. (1990) *Adoption: A handful of hope,* Celestial Arts, Berkeley.

Lifton, B.J. (1988) *Lost and Found: the adoption experience,* Harper and Row, New York.

Inglis, K. (1984) *Living Mistakes,* Allen and Unwin, London.

Saunders, P. and Sitterly, N. *Search Aftermath and Adjustments – Adoptees' Search,* USA.

Toynbee, P. (1985) *Lost Children,* Hutchinson, London.

Silverman, P.R. (1982) *Helping Women Cope with Grief,* Sage Human Services Guide, California.

Relevant organizations

BAAF: British Agencies for Adoption and Fostering, 11 Southwark Street, London SE1 1RQ. 071-407-8800

Life, 118/120 Warwick Street, Leamington Spa CV32 4QY.

NORCAP: National Organization for the Counselling of Adoptees and Parents, 3 New High Street, Headington, Oxford, OX3 5AJ.

Post-adoption Centre, Interchange Building, 15 Wilkin Street, London NW5 3NG.

CHAPTER 29: INTERRUPTED PREGNANCIES: ABORTIONS

[1] Deutsch, H. (1945) *Psychology of Women,* Vol. IIT, Routledge, London.

[2] Office of Population Censuses and Surveys. Population Statistics Division. *Population Trends,* 1989, 47.

[3] Ibid.
[4] See for instance Centre for Disease Control: Abortion Surveillance: US Department of Health, Education and Welfare, Public Health Service.
[5] Pines, D. (1988) Adolescent pregnancy and motherhood: a psychoanalytical perspective. *Psychoanalytic Inquiry*, **8**, 234–51.
[6] Brazzle and Acock (1988) Influence of attitudes, significant others and aspirations on how adolescents intend to resolve a premarital pregnancy, *Journal of Marriage and the Family*, **50**, 413–25.
[7] Simms, M. and Smith, C. (1982) Teenage mothers and abortion. *British Journal of Sexual Medicine*, **9**, 45–7.
[8] Hatcher, S. (1973) The adolescent experience of pregnancy and abortion: a developmental analysis, quoted by Francke (1978) *The Ambivalence of Abortion*, Penguin, London.
[9] Leschot, N.J., Verjaal, M. and Treffers, P.E. (1982) Therapeutic abortion on genetic indications – a detailed follow-up study of 20 patients. *Journal of Psychosomatic Obstetrics and Gynaecology*, **1**, 47–57.
[10] Francke, L.B. (1978) *The Ambivalence of Abortion*, Penguin, London.
[11] Berry, S. (1977) Abortion, in *Maternity Nursing Today*, McGraw–Hill, New York.
[12] Recent development of an abortion-inducing self-administered pill evokes new political and ethical issues about medical control, woman's responsibility for her reproductive body and the legal status of a fetus.
[13] Francke (1978) *The Ambivalence of Abortion*.
[14] Boston Women's Collective (1979) *Our Bodies, Ourselves*, Penguin, London.
[15] Greer, H.S., Lal, S., Lewis, S.C., Belsey, E.M. and Beard, R.W. (1976) Psychological consequences of therapeutic abortion. *British Journal of Psychiatry*, **128**, 74–9.
[16] Although some GPs are trained to offer sex-therapy, a non-orgasmic post abortion sufferer may prefer to attend a group specifically run for women with her problem (The Women's Therapy Centre, 6 Manor Gardens, London N7) or to be referred as a couple to a sex-therapy clinic. For others, the presenting sexual difficulties are merely a secondary symptom of unresolved emotional issues which require personal psychotherapy.

Further reading

Biro, F.M. *et al.* (1986) Acute and long term consequences of adolescents who choose abortions. *Pediatric Annals*, **15**, 667–73.
Gilligan, C. (1982) *In a Different Voice*, Harvard University Press, Cambridge, MA. (A study of the distinctive approach to women to moral dilemmas of conflicting responsibilities when considering abortion.)
Katz Rothman, B. (1989) *The Tentative Pregnancy – Prenatal Diagnosis and the Future of Motherhood*, Pandora, London.

Relevant organizations

SAFTA (Support after Termination for Foetal Abnormality) 29/30 Soho Square, London W1V 6JB. (Personal befriending and telephone support for couples after termination for abnormality offered by fellow sufferers.)
Sickle Cell Society, Green Lodge, Barretts Green Road, London NW10 7AP.
WHRRIC: Women's Health and Reproductive Rights Information Centre, 52–4 Featherstone Street, London EC1. (Provides a range of broadsheets on

different aspects of women's experience including abortion and miscarriage.)
Confidential counselling on unwanted pregnancy is offered by many *pregnancy advisory services* such as National Marriage Guidance Council; Pregnancy Advisory Service; Marie Stopes and Brook Advisory Centres (headquarters all in London).

CHAPTER 30: PREBIRTH LOSS AND PREGNANCY COMPLICATIONS

[1]	Lovell, A. (1983) Some questions of identity: late miscarriage, stillbirth and perinatal loss. *Social Science Medicine*, **17**, 755–61, no. 11.
[2]	Hey, V., Itzin, C., Saunders, L. and Speakman, M.A. (eds) (1989) *Hidden Loss: Miscarriage and Ectopic Pregnancy*, The Women's Press, London.
[3]	Ridley, R. (1988) Its not like losing a real baby is it? in *AIMS Quarterly Journal*, Summer, p. 9.
[4]	Couple, individual or group psychotherapy may be offered to work through the unresolved grief reactions, to improve impaired relationships between the spouse and or mother and other children due to the effect of the miscarriage. See for instance: Stirtzinger, R. and Robinson, G.E. (1989) The psychologic effects of spontaneous abortion, *Canadian Medical Association Journal*, **140**, 799–801.
[5]	O'Neil Lowe, (1977) High-risk complications of pregnancy, in *Maternity Nursing Today*, McGraw Hill, New York.
[6]	For signs of normal and pathological grief see for instance: Hall, R.C., Beresford, T.P. and Quinones, J.E. (1987) Grief following spontaneous abortion. *Psychiatry Clinics North America*, **10**, 405–20.
[7]	Condon, J.T. (1986) The spectrum of fetal abuse in pregnant women, *Journal of Nervous and Mental Disease*, **174**, 509–16.
[8]	Pregnancy following on previous miscarriages due to a known medical condition, or high-risk pregnancies in which the process of adaptation and bonding is delayed, may benefit from additional attention. See for instance Rogers, M.P. (1989) Psychologic aspects of pregnancy in patients with rheumatic diseases. *Rheumatic Diseases Clinics North America*, **15**, 361–74.
[9]	Psychological conditions during pregnancy often foreshadow postnatal complications and as such will be dealt with in Chapter 33. However, even quite brief psychotherapeutic intervention during pregnancy can do much to alleviate the difficulty, and reduce the possibility of puerperal illness. See for instance: Chiesa, M.C. (1985) Brief focal psychotherapy with a pregnant woman presenting with nightmares of killing her baby: a case study. *British Journal of Psychotherapy*, **2**, 42–9.
[10]	For a description of prenatal relating between twins observed on ultrasound see: Piontelli, A. (1989) A study on twins before and after birth. *International Review of Psycho-Analysis*, **16**, 413–26.

Further reading

Borg, S. and Lasker, J. (1983) *When Pregnancy Fails*, Routledge and Kegan Paul, London.
Friedman, R. and Gradstein, B. (1982) *Surviving Pregnancy Loss*, Little, Brown, Boston.
Oakley, A., McPherson, A. and Roberts, H. (1990) *Miscarriage*. Penguin, London.

Relevant organizations

The Miscarriage Association (P.O. Box 24, Ossett, West Yorkshire WF5 9XG). (Publishes a newsletter and runs post-miscarriage self-help support groups nationwide.)

Stitch Network, 15 Matcham Road, London E11 3LE (publications and contacts for women with incompetent cervix)

British Diabetic Association, 10 Queen Anne Street, London W1M 0BD.

Association to Combat Huntington's Chorea, Borough House, 34A Station Road, Hinckley, Leicestershire LE10 1AP.

Disabled Parents Contact Register, c/o National Childbirth Trust, Alexandra House, Oldham Terrace, Acton, London W3.

CHAPTER 31: DISRUPTIONS AROUND BIRTH: PREMATURITY AND ILLNESS, STILL-BIRTH AND PERINATAL LOSS

[1] Klaus, M. and Kennell, J. (1983) *Bonding*, New American Library, Mosby, St Louis.

[2] Whiten, A. (1977) Assessing the effects of perinatal events on the success of the mother–infant relationship, in *Studies in Mother-Infant Interaction* (ed. H.R. Schaffer), Academic Press, London.

[3] Seashore, M.J. *et al.* (1973) The effects of denial of early mother–infant interaction on maternal self-confidence. *Journal of Personality and Social Psychology*, **26**, 369–78.

[4] Rice, R.D. (1977) Neurophysiological development in premature infants following stimulation. *Developmental Psychology*, **13**, 69–76.

[5] Adamson-Macedo, E.N. (1985) Effects of tactile stimulation on very low birthweight infants – a two year follow-up study. *Current Psychological Research and Reviews*, **6**, 305–8.

[6] Klaus and Kennell (1983) *Bonding*.

[7] De Leeuw, R. (1982) Neonatal intensive care – impact on families, *Journal of Psychosomatic Obstetrics and Gynaecology*, **1**, 120–3.

[8] Minde, K. *et al.* (1980) Self-help groups in a premature nursery – a controlled evaluation. *Journal of Pediatrics*, **96**, 933–40.

[9] Mason, cited by Klaus and Kennell, (1983) *Bonding*.

[10] Seashore *et al.* (1973) The effects of denial.

[11] Pederson, R.D. *et al.* (1987) Maternal emotional responses to preterm birth. *American Journal of Orthopsychiatry*, **57**, 15–21.

[12] Crnic, K.A., Greenberg, M.T. and Slough, N.M. (1986) Early stress and social support influences on mothers' and high-risk infants' functioning in late infancy. *Infant Mental Health Journal*, **7**, 19–33.

[13] Bender, H. (1988) Psychological aspects of prematurity and of neonatal intensive care: a working report, in *Prenatal and Perinatal Psychology and Medicine* (eds F. Freybegh and V. Vogel), Parthenon Press, Carnforth, Lancs.

[14] Freud, W.E. (1988) Prenatal attachment, the perinatal continuum and the psychological side of neonatal intensive care in *Prenatal and Perinatal Psychology and Medicine* (eds F. Freybergh and V. Vogel), Parthenon Press, Carnforth, pp. 226–7.

[15] Bender (1988) Psychological aspects of prematurity.

[16] See for instance, Winnicott, D.W. (1945) Primitive emotional development,

in *Through Paediatrics to Psycho-Analysis*, Hogarth, London 1982.

[17] Murdoch, D.R. and Darlow, B.A. (1984) Handling during neonatal intensive care. *Archives of Disease in Childhood*, **59**, 957–61, quoted by Wolke (1987) Environmental and developmental neonatology.

[18] Wolke, D. (1987) Environmental and developmental neonatology. *Journal of Reproductive and Infant Psychology*, **5**, 17–42.

[19] For a review of these see Wolke (1987).

[20] Freud, W.E. (1988) Prenatal attachment.

[21] Klaus and Kennel (1983) *Bonding*.

[22a] Mann, N.P. *et al.* (1986) Effect of night and day on preterm infants in a newborn nursery: randomised trial. *British Medical Journal*, **293**, 1265–7, cited in Wolke (1987).

[22b] Koriver, A.F. (1988) Early intervention with pre-term infants in *Children and Families: studies in prevention and intervention* (ed E.D. Hibbs), International Universities Press, Madison, Conn.

[23] Freud, W.E. (1988) Prenatal attachment.

[24] Klaus and Kennel (1983) *Bonding*.

[25] Macfarlane, A. (1977) *The Psychology of Birth*, Fontana, London.

[26] Wolke (1987) Environmental and developmental neonatology.

[27] Freud, S. (1917) *Mourning and Melancholia*, S.E. 14, Hogarth, London, 1971.

[28] Parkes, C.M. (1972) *Bereavement: Studies of Grief in Adult Life*. International Universities Press, New York.

[29] Bourne, S. (1968) The psychological effect of stillbirths on women and their doctors. *Journal Royal College of General Practitioners*, **16**, 103–12.

[30] Lewis, E. (1976) Management of stillbirth, coping with an unreality. *Lancet*, **ii**, 620.

[31] Ibid.

[32] Tudelope, D.I. *et al* (1986) Neonatal death: grieving families. *Medical Journal of Australia*, **144**, 290–2, quoted by Zeanah (1989).

[33] Whelan, M. (1985) *Infant observations, unpublished archives*. British Institute of Psychoanalysts.

[34] Zeanah, C.H. (1989) Adaptation following perinatal loss: a critical review. *Journal American Academy of Child and Adolescent Psychiatry*, **28**, 467–80.

[35] Chalmers, B. (1984) *Early Parenthood: Heaven or Hell*. Juta, Cape Town.

[36] Zeanah (1989) Adaptation following perinatal loss.

[37] Bowlby, J. (1980) *Attachment and Loss*, vol. III, Basic Books, New York.

[38] Lovell, A. (1983) Some questions of identity: Late miscarriage, stillbirth and perinatal loss. *Social Science Medicine*, **17**, 755–61.

[39] Davis, D.L., Stewart, M. and Harmon, R.J. (1989) Postponing pregnancy after perinatal death: perspectives on doctor advice. *Journal American Academy of Child and Adolescent Psychiatry*, **28**, 481–7.

[40] Lovell (1983) Some questions of identity.

[41] Bender (1988) Psychological aspects of prematurity.

Further reading

Berkowitz, G.S. and Kasl, S.V. (1983) The role of psychological factors in spontaneous preterm delivery. *Journal of Psychosomatic Research*, **27**, 283–90.

Omer, H. and Everly, G.S. (1988) Psychological factors in preterm labour: critical review and theoretical synthesis. *American Journal of Psychiatry*, **145**, 1507–13.

Redshaw, M., Rivers, M. and Rosenblatt, D. (1985) *Born Too Soon*. Oxford University Press, Oxford.

Relevant organizations

Association for Spina Bifida and Hydrocephalus, 22 Upper Woburn Place, London WC1H 0EP.

Bliss link, 44/45 Museum Street, London WC1. (Support groups for parents of babies in special care).

Caesarean Support Network, 11 Duke Street, Astley, Lancaster M29 7BG.

Nippers, 49 Allison Road, Acton, London W3 (Support groups for parents of premature babies and those in special care).

Scottish Premature Babies Support Group, 5 Boghead Road, Lenzie, Glasgow.

SANDS (Stillbirth and Neonatal Death Society), 28 Portland Place, London, W1.

Compassionate Friends, 5 Lower Clifton Hill, Clifton, Bristol BS8 1BT. (for bereaved parents)

CRUSE (Bereavement Care), 126 Skeen Road, Richmond, Surrey, TW9 1VE.

Voluntary Council for Handicapped Children, National Children's Bureau, 8 Wakeley Street, London EC1V 7QE. (For information about rights and organizations dealing with disability).

AIMS, Association for Improvement of Maternity Services, 40 Kingswood, Queens Park, London NW6.

CHAPTER 32: POSTNATAL COMPLICATIONS: CONGENITAL ABNORMALITIES AND CRITICAL CONDITIONS IN INFANCY

[1] Klaus, M. and Kennell, J. (1983) *Bonding*, New American Library, Mosby, St Louis.

[2] Ibid.

[3] Solnit, A.J. and Stark, M.H. (1961) Mourning and the birth of a defective child. *Psychoanalytic Study of the Child*, **16**, 523–37.

[4] Olshansky, quoted by Klaus and Kennell (1983) *Bonding*.

[5] Fleishman, A.R. and Sands, F.D. (1980) The birth of an abnormal child, in *Psychological Aspects of Pregnancy, Birthing and Bonding* (ed. B. Blum), Human Sciences Press, New York.

[6] Kennedy, H. (1985) Growing up with a handicapped sibling. *Psychoanalytic Study of the Child*, **40**, 255–74.

[7] Atkinson, J. and Braddick, O. (1989) Cambridge University Visual Development Unit Study of 3000 babies, reported in *Observer*, 12 November 1989.

[8] Fraiberg, S. (1987) The development of attachments in babies blind from birth. *Selected Writings of Selma Fraiberg*, Ohio University Press.

[9] McCarty and Scipien (1977) Interuterine growth deviations, in *Maternity Nursing Today*, McGraw–Hill, New York.

[10] Crnic, K.A., Greenberg, M.T. and Slough, N.M. (1986) Early stress and social support influences on mothers' and high-risk infants' functioning in late infancy. *Infant Mental Health Journal*, **7**, 19–33.

[11] Leff, J.P., Kuipers, L., Berkowitz, R., Eberlein-Freis, R. and Sturgeon, D. (1982) A controlled trial of intervention in the families of schizophrenic patients. *British Journal of Psychiatry*, **141**, 121–34.

[12] Lipsitt, L.P. (1979) Critical conditions in infancy: a psychological perspective. *American Psychology*, **34**, 973–80.

[13] Spitz, R.A. (1945) Hospitalism. *The Psychoanalytic Study of the Child*, Vol. I. International Universities Press, New York.

[14] Barbero, G. (1975) Failure to thrive, in *Maternal Attachment and Mothering*

Disorders, Johnson and Johnson, New Brunswick, NJ.

[15]   Brazelton, T.B. (1975) Mother–infant reciprocity, in *Maternal Attachment and Mothering Disorders* (eds M.H. Klaus, T. Leger and M.A. Trause), Johnson and Johnson, New Brunswick, NJ.

[16]   Pollitt, E., Eichler, A.W. and Chan, C.K. (1975) Psychosocial development and behaviour of mothers of failure to thrive children. *American Journal of Orthopsychiatry,* **45**, 525–37.

[17]   Loewald, E.L. (1985) Psychotherapy with parents and child in failure-to-thrive. *Psychoanalytic Study of the Child,* 40, 345–63.

[18]   Drotar, D. and Strum, L. (1987) Paternal influences in non-organic failure to thrive: implications for psychosocial management. *Infant Mental Health Journal,* **8**, 37.

[19]   See for instance Crick, P. and Cantle, A. (1989) Finding the infant in the Infant Observation. *British Psycho-Analytical Society Bulletin,* September 1989.

[20]   Brazelton (1975) Mother–infant reciprocity.

[21]   Fraiberg, S. (1975) Billy: psychological intervention for a failure-to-thrive infant, in *Maternal Attachment and Mothering Disorders* (eds M.H. Klaus, T. Leger and M.A. Trause), Johnson and Johnson, New Brunswick, NJ.

[22]   Mayer, E.L. (1986) A note on oedipal guilt and a failure-to-thrive child. *International Review of Psycho-Analysis,* **13**, 487–9.

[23]   Aquarone, S. (1989) Early interventions in disturbed mother–infant relationships. *Infant Mental Health Journal,* **9**, 340.

[24]   von Lupke, H. (1989) Towards an integrative approach on sudden infant death syndrome SIDS. *International Journal of Prenatal and Perinatal Studies,* **1**, 275–7.

[25]   Lipsitt (1979) Critical conditions in infancy.

[26]   MacKenna, J.J. (1987) An anthropological perspective on the sudden infant death syndrome (SIDS): the role of breathing cues and speech breathing adaptations. *Medical Anthropology,* **10**, 1–103.

[27]   Lipsitt (1979) Critical conditions in infancy.

[28]   Lipsitt, L.P. (1978) Perinatal indicators and early psycho-physiological precursors of crib death, in *Early Developmental Hazards: Predictors and Precautions* (ed. F.D. Horowitz), Westview Press, New York, pp. 11–29.

[29]   von Lupke, H. (1989) The problem of SIDS is more than the problem of SIDS. *International Journal of Prenatal and Perinatal Studies,* **1**, 278–86.

[30]   Valdes-Dapena, M. (1980) Sudden infant death syndrome: a review of the medical literature 1974–1979. *Pediatrics,* **66**, 597–614.

[31]   von Lupke (1989) The problem of SIDS.

[32]   Stork, J. (1989) The phenomenon of 'cot death' from a psychological point of view. *International Journal of Prenatal and Perinatal Studies,* **1**, 287–94.

[33]   Ibid.

[34]   MacKenna (1987) An anthropological perspective on SIDS.

[35]   Carpenter, R.G. *et al* (1988) Prevention of unexpected infant death. A review of risk-related intervention in six centres. *Annals of New York Academy of Science,* **533**, 96–103.

[36]   Einspieler, C. (1990) Behavioural characteristics of SIDS victims and infants at risk for SIDS, in *Prenatal and Perinatal Psychology and Medicine,* Vol. 2, proceedings of International Conference 'Encounter with the Newborn', Jerusalem, April, 1988 (ed. F. Freybergh), Parthenon Press, Carnforth, Lancs.

[37]   von Lupke, H. (1990) The mutual absence as a problem in SIDS – pre and

postnatal aspects, presented to International Conference 'Encounter with the Newborn', Jerusalem, April, 1988.

[38] Einspieler (1990) Behavioural characteristics of SIDS victims.

[39] Coghill, R. (1989) Electromagnetic fields and sudden unexpected death in infancy: a discussion paper presented to Royal Society of Medicine Forum on Maternity and the Newborn, February, 1989.

[40] Carpenter, and Emery, (1974) Identification and follow up of infants at risk of sudden death in infancy. *Nature*, **250**, 729.

[41] Lipsitt (1979) Critical conditions in infancy.

[42] Limerick (1976) Counselling needs after a cot death, *Marriage Guidance*, July/August, p. 118.

[43] Furman, E. (1978) The death of a newborn: care of the parents. *Birth and Family Journal*, **5**, 214–18.

[44] Limerick (1976) Counselling needs after a cot death.

Further reading

Balarajan, R. and Botting, B. (1989) Perinatal mortality in England and Wales: variations by mother's country of birth (1982–85). *Health Trends*, **21**, 79–83.

Farel, A.M., Bailey, D.B. and O'Donnell, K.J. (1987) A new approach for training infant intervention specialists. *Infant Mental Health Journal*, **8**, 76.

Relevant organizations

Cleft Lip and Palate Association, 1 Eastwood Gardens, Kenton, Newcastle-upon-Tyne.

Down's Syndrome Association, 4 Oxford Street, London W1N 9FL.

MENCAP, Royal Society for Mentally Handicapped Children and Adults, 123 Golden Lane, London EC1Y 0RT.

Muscular Dystrophy Group of Great Britain, Nattrass House, 35 Macauley Road, London SW4 0PQ.

National Association for Deaf-Blind and Rubella Handicapped, 311 Gray's Inn Road, London WC1X 8PT,

Sickle Cell Society, c/o Brent Community Health Council, 16 High Street, Harlesden, London NW10 4LX.

Spastics Society, 12 Park Crescent, London W1N 4EQ.

Thalassemia Society, 107 Nightingale Lane, London N8.

Foundation for the Study of Infant Deaths, 4 Grosvenor Place, London SW1X 7HD.

CHAPTER 33: POSTNATAL PSYCHOLOGICAL COMPLICATIONS

[1] Brockington, I.F. (1985) Mental disorder occurring in mothers of young children: a summary of the Marce Society presentation to a meeting with the Chief Scientist and representative of the Department of Health of England and Wales, 20 Feb. 1985, *Marce Society Bulletin*, Autumn, 20–38.

[2] Price, J. (1988) *Motherhood: What it Does to Your Mind*. Pandora Press, London.

[3] A review of the anthropological literature on childbirth provides little evidence for postnatal depression, suggesting that the ubiquitous blues may represent a western culture bound syndrome resulting in lowered

self-esteem in the absence of family rituals and structuring of postpartum events, dearth of social recognition of a mother's role transition and lack of protection and instrumental support. See for instance: Stern, G. and Kruckman, L. (1983) Multi-disciplinary perspectives on post-partum depression: an anthropological critique. *Social Science and Medicine*, **17**, 1027–41.

[4] With reference to East Africa Cox, J.L. (1988) Childbirth as a life event: sociocultural aspects of postnatal depression. *Acta Psychiatrica Scandanavia*, supplement, **344**, 75–83.

[5] Kendell *et al.* (1984) Day-to-day mood changes after childbirth. *British Journal of Psychiatry* , **145**, 620–5.

[6] Hapgood, C.C., Elkind, G.S. and Wright, J.J. (1988) Maternity blues: phenomena and their relationship to alter postpartum depression. *Australia, New Zealand Psychiatry*, **22**, 229–306.

[7] Kennerly, H. and Gath, D. (1986) Maternity blues reassessed. *Psychiatric Development*, **4**, 1–17.

[7b] Kennely, H. *et al.*, (1989) *Br. J. Psych*, **155**, 367–73.

[8] Brockington, I.F., Margison, F.R., Scofield, E. and Knight, R.J. (1988) The clinical picture of the depressed form of puerperal psychosis. *Journal of Affective Disorders*, **15**, 29–37.

[9] Pitt, B. (1968) 'Atypical' depression following childbirth. *British Journal of Psychiatry*, **114**, 1325–35.

[10] Dean, C. and Kendell, R.E. (1981) The symptomatology of puerperal illnesses. *British Journal of Psychiatry*, **139**, 128–33.

[11] Harding, J.J. (1989) Postpartum psychiatric disorders: a review. *Comprehensive Psychiatry*, **30**, 109–12.

[12] Dean and Kendall (1981) The symptomatology of puerperal illnesses.

[13] McNeil, T.F. (1988) A prospective study of postpartum psychoses in a high-risk group. 3. Relationship to mental health characteristics during pregnancy. *Acta Psychiatrica Scandinavica*, **77**, 604–10.

[14] McNeil, T.F. (1989) Women with non-organic psychosis, *Acta. Psychiat. Scand*. **78**, 603–9.

[15] Brockington, I.F., Margison, F.R., Scofield, E. and Knight, R.J. (1988). The clinical picture of the depressed form of puerperal psychosis. *Journal of Affective Disorders*, **15**, 29–37.

[16] Bagedahl-Strindlund, M. (1986) Parapartum mental illness: timing of illness onset and its relation to symptoms and sociodemographic characteristics. *Acta Psychiatrica Scandinavica*, **74**, 490–6.

[17] Coleman, E.H. (1930) *The Shutter of Snow*, Virago, London, 1981, pp. 3–9. The material from *The Shutter of Snow* by Emily Holmes Coleman is reproduced by permission of Virago Press, © The Estate of Emily Holmes Coleman 1974.

[18] Aston, A. and Thomas, L. (1987) Mother and baby psychiatric facilities in England and Wales, 1985–6. *Marce Society Bulletin*, Summer, 2–12.

[19] Kumar, R. (1986) Admitting mentally ill mothers with their babies into psychiatric hospitals. *Bulletin of the Royal College of Psychiatrists*, **10**, 169–72.

[20] Shawcross, C.R. and McCrae, Y. (1986) Mother and baby facilities in England. *Bulletin of the Royal College of Psychiatrists*, **10**, 50–1.

[21] Dalton, K. (1989) Successful prophylactic progesterone for idiopathic postnatal depression. *International Journal of Prenatal and Perinatal Studies*, **1**, 323–8.

[22] Tetlow, C. (1955) Psychosis of childbearing. *Journal of Mental Science*, **101**, 629–39.

[23] Welburn, V. (1980) *Postnatal Depression*, Manchester University Press, Manchester.

[24] Raphael-Leff, J. (1985) Facilitators and Regulators: vulnerability to postnatal disturbance. *Journal of Psychosomatic Obstetrics and Gynaecology*, 4, 151–68.

[25] Brown, G. and Harris, T. (1978) *The Social Origins of Depression*, Tavistock, London.

[26] Oakley, A. (1980)*Women Confined: Towards a Sociology of Childbirth*. Martin Robertson, Oxford.

[27] Paykel, E.S., Emms, E.M., Fletcher, J. and Tassaby, E.S. (1980) Life events and social support in puerperal depression. *British Journal of Psychiatry*, 136, 339–47.

[28] Kumar, R. and Robson, K.M. (1984) A prospective study of emotional disorders in childbearing women. *British Journal of Psychiatry*, 144, 35–47.

[29] See, for instance, Lomas, P. (1960) Dread of envy as a factor in the aetiology of puerperal breakdown. *British Journal of Medical Psychology*, 33, 105.

[30] Wolkind, S. (1985) The first five years: pre-school children and their families in the inner city, in *Recent Research in Developmental Pathology* (ed. J.E. Stevenson), *Journal of Child Psychology and Psychiatry*, supplement 4.

[31] Ainsworth, M.D.S., Bell, S.M. and Stayton, D.J. (1974) Infant–mother attachment and social development: socialization as a product of reciprocal responsiveness to signals, in *The Integration of a Child into a Social World* (ed. M.P.M. Richards), Cox and Wyman, Cambridge University Press, London.

[32] Murray, L. (1988) Effects of postnatal depression on infant development: direct studies of early mother–infant interactions, in *Motherhood and Mental Illness*, vol. II (eds I. Kumar and I. Brockington), John Wright, London.

[33] Murray, L. and Trevarthen, C. (1985) Emotional regulation of interactions between 2 month olds and their mothers, in *Social Perception in Infants* (eds T.M. Field and N.A. Fox), Ablex, New Jersey.

[34] Pound, A., Puckering, C., Cox, T. and Mills, M. (1988) The impact of maternal depression on young children. *British Journal of Psychotherapy*, 4, 240–52.

[35] Caplan, H.L., Coghill, S.R., Alexandra, H. *et al.* (1989) Maternal depression and the emotional development of the child. *British Journal of Psychiatry*, 154, 818–22.

[36] Fraiberg, S., Adelson, E. and Shapiro, V. (1975) Ghosts in the nursery: a psychoanalytic approach to the problems of impaired infant–mother relationships. *Journal of the American Academy of Child Psychiatry*, 14, 387–421.

[37] Emde, R.N. and Easterbrooks, M.A. (1989) Assessing emotional availability in early development, in *Early Identification of Children at Risk: an International Perspective* (eds R. Emde and J. Sullivan), Plenum, New York.

[38] Bowlby, J. (1980) *Attachment and Loss*, vol. III. *Loss*. Basic Books, New York.

[39] Stern, D. (1985) *The Interpersonal World of the Infant*, New York: Basic Books.

[40] In a treatment programme developed in Edinburgh, health visitors received a manual and three sessions of instruction on postnatal depression and non-directive counselling. In a controlled study they were found to reduce depressive illness in 69% of vulnerable mothers visited for eight successive weeks (compared with 38% recovery in the control group). See Holden, J.M., Sagovsky, R. and Cox, J.L. (1989) Counselling in a general practice setting: controlled study of health visitors' intervention in treatment of postnatal depression. *British Medical Journal*, 298, 223–6.

[41] Rutter, M. (1966) *Children of Sick Parents*, Oxford University Press, Oxford.

[42] Harvey, I. and McGrath, G. (1988) Psychiatric morbidity in spouses of

women admitted to a mother and baby unit. *British Journal of Psychiatry*, **152**, 506–10.

[43] Fraiberg, S. (1980) *Selected Writings of Selma Fraiberg*, Ohio University Press.

[44] Pound, A. and Mills, M. (1990) An evaluation of NEWPIN: home visiting and befriending scheme in South London. *British Journal of Psychotherapy*, in press.

[45] Because they are self-staffed, parent-run playgroups are very cheap to operate after the initial outlay for equipment, toys and materials (often obtainable secondhand). In addition to minimizing separation and parents providing each other with role models and practical support, the advantage of a parent participating playgroup [such as PACT (Parents and Children Together) which I founded in the Hampstead Community Centre in 1978] is flexibility, offering a facility which consumers can attend as seldom or frequently as they like, become as involved in the running of the group as they wish and either stay to participate and/or chat or leave their child in the custody of another familiar adult. For a general overview and action research study of regular day-care for under fives see Menzies, Lyth, I. (1989) *The Dynamics of the Social*, Chapter 9, Free Association Books.

[46] Klein, M. (1937) Love, guilt and reparation, in *Love, Hate and Reparation*, Hogarth, London, 1967. (Reprinted in 1981 in *Love, Guilt and Reparation and other works 1921–1945*, Hogarth.)

[47] Although we can only speculate as to the emotional dynamics and fantasies of a preverbal baby, most clinicians who observe babies directly agree on the occurrence of specific adaptive phases of development, including a 'quantum leap' soon after six months when the baby appears not only to have a sense of his/her own self and feelings but recognizes that other people do, and that they relate to each other and interact emotionally. Psychoanalytical theoreticians focus on different aspects of this momentous change: Mahler defines it as 'hatching' (Mahler, M.S., Pine, F. and Bergman, A. (1975) *The Psychological Birth of the Human Infant*, Hutchinson, London); Stern refers to it as 'intersubjective relatedness' (Stern, D.N. (1973) *The Interpersonal World of the Infant*, Basic Books, New York); Klein calls this the 'depressive position' (Klein (1937) *Love, Hate and Reparation*); Winnicott would describe it as 'the age of concern' (Winnicott (1945) Primitive emotional development).

[48] Winnicott, D.W. (1945), Primitive emotional development, chapter 12, in *Through Paediatrics to Psycho-Analysis*, Hogarth, London, 1982.

[49] Hallet, C. (1988) Research in child abuse: some observations on the knowledge base. *Journal of Reproductive and Infant Psychology*, special issue on Early Child Maltreatment, **6**, 119–24.

[50] Creighton, S.J. (1987) Quantitative assessment of child abuse, in *Child Abuse: An Educational Perspective* (ed. P. Maher), Blackwell, Oxford.

[51] NSPCC (National Society for Prevention of Cruelty to Children) (1985), Child abuse deaths. *Information Briefing no. 5*.

[52] Browne, K.D. (1988) The naturalistic context of family violence and child abuse, in *Human Aggression: Naturalistic approaches* (eds J. Archer and K. Browne), Routledge, London quoted in editorial K. Brown, early child maltreatment: an interdisciplinary approach, *Journal of Reproductive and Infant Psychology*, **6**, 115.

[53] Wheat, P. (1979) *Hope for the Children*, A personal history of Parents Anonymous, Winston Press, Minneapolis.

[54] Hallet (1988) Research in child abuse.

[55] Leventhal, J.M. (1988) Can child maltreatment be predicted during the perinatal period: evidence from longitudinal cohort studies. *Journal of Reproductive and Infant Psychology*, **6**, 139–82.

[56] Gough, D. and Taylor, J. (1988) Child abuse prevention: studies of ante-natal and post-natal services, *Journal of Reproductive and Infant Psychology*, **6**, 217–28.

[57] Starr, R.H. (1988) Pre- and perinatal risk and physical abuse, *Journal of Reproductive and Infant Psychology*, **6**, 125–38.

[58] Browne, K.D. and Saqi, S. (1988) Mother–infant interaction and attachment in physically abusing families, *Journal of Reproductive and Infant Psychology*, **6**, 163–82.

[59] Ibid.

[60] Stratton, P. and Swaffer, R. (1988) Maternal causal beliefs for abused and handicapped children. *Journal of Reproductive and Infant Psychology*, **6**, 201–16.

[61] Crittenden, P.M. (1988) Distorted patterns of relationship in maltreating families: the role of internal representational models, *Journal of Reproductive and Infant Psychology*, **6**, 183–200.

[62] Boston Women's Health Collective (1978) *Ourselves and Our Children*, Penguin, London.

[63] Asen, K., George, E., Piper, R. and Stevens, A. (1989) *Child Abuse and Neglect*, **13**, 45–57.

[64] Rivara, F.P. (1985) Physical abuse in children under two: a study of therapeutic outcome. *Child Abuse and Neglect*, **9**, 81–7.

[65] Jones, T., McClean, B. and Young, J. (1986) *The Islington Crime Survey*, Gower, Aldershot, quoted by Andrews and Brown (1988) Marital violence in the community.

[66] Straus, M., Gelles, R. and Steinmetz, S. (1980) *Behind Closed Doors: Violence in the American Family*. Anchor, New York.

[67] Andrews, B. and Brown, G. (1988) Marital violence in the community: a biographical approach. *British Journal of Psychiatry*, **153**, 305–12.

[68] Star *et al.* (1981) Psychosocial aspects of wife battering, in *Women and Mental Health* (eds Howell and Bayes), Basic Books, New York.

[69] Sinason, V. (1988) Dolls and bears: from symbolic equation to symbol. The significance of different play material for sexually abused children and others. *British Journal of Psychotherapy*, **4**, 349–63.

[70] Vizard, E. (1988) Child sexual abuse – the child's experience. *British Journal of Psychotherapy*, **5**, 77–91.

[71] Trowell, J. (1986) Physical abuse of children. *Psychoanalytic Psychotherapy*, **2**, 63–73.

[72] Kennedy, R., Heymans, A. and Tischler, L. (1986) *The Family as In-Patient: Families and Adolescents at the Cassel Hospital*. Free Association Books, London.

[73] Counsellors at Shanti, a women's counselling service in Brixton have found that rewarding group or individual therapeutic work can be done with mothers who themselves suffered sexual or physical abuse in childhood, in brief-psychotherapy consisting of a contract for 16 sessions. An independent evaluation study has not yet born results but in an unpublished paper entitled 'Family rupture and strategies for survival', M. Mills and C. Topolski have conveyed their clinical findings. On the issue of how to distinguish 'true' reports of sexual abuse from 'fantasy' (an issue which has preoccupied therapists since Freud), they note the therapists' awareness of a struggle to tell; the use of non-adult language in the telling; clarity of

description once the screen memory has been dropped and the woman's sense of herself as having only a sexual value (paper present to Applied Section of the British Institute of Psychoanalysis, 27.6.90).

[74] Bass, E. and Davis, L. (1988) *The Courage to Heal*, a guide for women survivors of child sexual abuse, Harper and Row, New York.

Further reading

Bentovim, A., Elton, E., Hildebrand, J. *et al.* (eds) (1988) *The Treatment of Sexual Abuse in the Family*, John Wright, Bristol.

Edwards, S. (1989) *Policing Domestic Violence*, Sage, London.

Horley, S. (1988) *Love and Pain*, Survival Handbook, London.

Leff, J. and Isaacs, A. (1990) Psychiatric Examination in Clinical Practice, Blackwells, London.

Osborne, K. (1982) Sexual violence, chapter 3 in *Development of the Study of Criminal Behaviour* (ed. P. Feldman) Wiley, London.

Welburn, V. (1980) *Postnatal Depression*, Manchester University Press, Manchester.

Relevant organizations

Association for Postnatal Illness, 7 Gowan Avenue, London SW6.

Cry-sis, BM Box Crysis, London, WC1N 3XX. 071–404–5011.

Marcé Society. An international society for the understanding, prevention and treatment of mental illness related to childbearing. Secretary, Dr Adler, Queen Margaret College, Clerwood Terrace, Edinburgh, EH12 8TS. Tel. 031–317–3000.

OPUS, 106 Godstone Road, Whyteleafe, Croydon CR3 0EB. (Support groups and day centres for families under stress.) 081–645–0469.

Parents Anonymous, 6–9 Manor Gardens, London N7 6LA (nightline – 01–669–8900: for parents who fear they could hurt their babies)

Childline 0800–1111 A 24 hour confidential counselling for victims, abusers and professionals.

Incest Crisis Line 081–422–5100

PSI: Postpartum Support International, 927 North Kellogg Ave, Santa Barbara, CA 93111, USA.

Sex Abuse Crisis Line 081–985–0044 (Thur 7–10pm) For boys and young men.

London Women's Aid 52–54 Featherstone Street, EC1. 071–251–6537.

Help to leave violent men, refuges and legal advice.

Appendix A

INTERACTION OF PSYCHOLOGICAL AND SOCIAL FACTORS INFLUENCING BREAST FEEDING

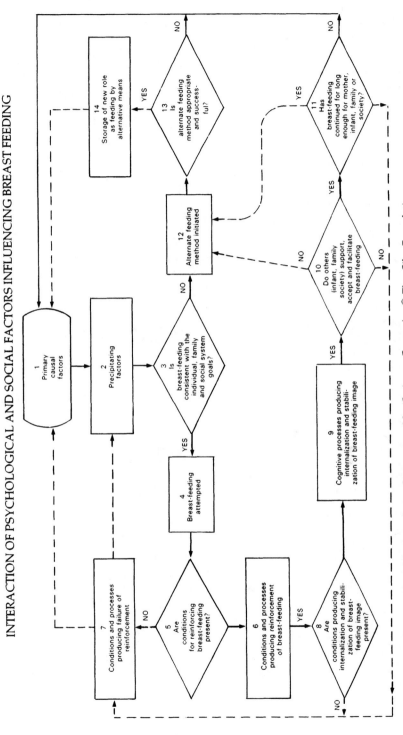

Reproduced by permission of Ciba Foundation Symposium No 45; Arnon Bentovin. © The Ciba Foundation.

Some Useful Organisations 2005*

Association for Postnatal Illness
Helpline: 0207 386 0868
www.apni.org

Marce Scoiety for prevention and treatment of mental illness related to childbearing www.marcesociety.com

Cry-sis
Helpline & local support for those caring for a crying or sleepless newborn
tel: 0207 404 5011
www.cry-sis.

Contact a Family
For families of special need children
Freephone: 0808 808 3555
www.cafamily.org.uk

Fathers Network – to celebrate and support fathers of children with developmental needs
www.fathersnetwork.org

TAMBA –twins & multiple births
www.tamba.org
Twinline tel: 0800 138 0509
Support & information

La Leche League international
www.lalecheleague.org

Association for breastfeeding mothers
www.abm.me.uk

Fathers Direct
tel: 020 7920 9491
www.fathersdirect.com

Fathers – helping you become a better dad www.fathers.com

SANDS –Stillbirth & Neonatal Death Society www.uk-sands.org

Cruse Bereavement Care
National helpline (national rate):
0870 167 1677
www.crusebereavmentcare.org.uk

PIP – Parent Infant Project
Anna Freud Centre
21 Maresfield Gardens,
London NW3 5SD
0207-794-2313
www.annafreud.org

School of Infant Mental Health
www.infantmentalhealth.com

Tavistock Clinic
Under-5's & Infant Mental Health
120 Belsize Lane, London NW3 5BA
020 7435 7111 www.tavi-port.org

The Association of Child Psychotherapists
120 West Heath Road
London NW3 7TU
tel: 020 8458 1609
email: acp@dial.pipex.com

The Scottish Child Psychotherapy Trust
13 Park Terrace
Glasgow G3 6BY
tel: 0141 353 3399
fax: 0141 332 3999

Childcare Link
Information about child care
Freephone: 0800 096 0296
www.childcarelink.gov.uk

Childline UK tel: 08001111
Childline Ireland ISPCC
Tel: 1800 666 666
see: www.childlike.org

*More organizations appear at the end of the references to each chapter.
Contact details change over time and not all of these have been updated..
Check websites for your local resources.

Author Index

Locations are shown as page number and reference number, e.g. 394 [14]. Where one page of the Reference List contains similarly-numbered items from different chapters, the chapter number is also included e.g. 517 [(Ch. 15)8]. Page number and [FR] indicates that the item will be found under Further Reading, e.g. 538[FR]. Page numbers up to 497 are to references in the body of the text, and from 498 onwards to items in the Reference List.

Subject Index

References are to page numbers. References of the form 507[37] are to page number and note number on that page.

Appendix B - 2004
Facilitators & Regulators
Questionnaire (FRQ)*

Question 1: *Do you have a daily routine (for youngest child)? YES/NO (please specify)*
[leave 6 free linesl *When did it begin?*
Scoring:
0 Extreme Facilitator NO routine; nothing at all specified.
I Moderate Facilitator says YES but nothing specific itemized or says NO and very few general activities enumerated (such as play, lunch, nap)
2 Reciprocator group some set sequences
3 Moderate Regulator detailed times/activities; some flexibility
4 Extreme Regulator inflexible specification of times/activities
Note: Where routine was begun at 1 year plus, deduct 1 from score
Question 2:
2a. *In general, which do you believe (about breast or bottle) during the first three months: Tick one.*
0___*Babies should be fed whenever and for as long as they want*
1___*Babies should be allowed unrestricted sucking including night feeds but the idea of 'mealtimes' should be introduced*
2___*Babies should be fed when they are clearly hungry*
3___*Babies should be fed adjustable quantities at specified times but not at night*
4___.*Babies should be fed a set amount by schedule (3—4 hourly with no 'snacking' in between)*
2b. *Ideally, at what age do you think weaning should occur?*
Note: in a culture-bound activity such as this, solid feeds and weaning times must be adjusted to suit local feeding recommendations and changing habits. (b) is scored if it falls in the extremes — +1 for very early or —1 for very Fate weaning.
Question 3: *When do you believe the baby starts communicating with you? [How?]*
Scoring:
O Extreme Facilitator: during pregnancy/before birth
I Moderate Facilitator: at birth
2 Reciprocator group: within the first 2 weeks
3 Moderate Regulator: next 6 weeks
4 Extreme Regulator: after 2 months
[*Note:* focus on baby's intentional efforts at communication]
Question 4: *Which best describes your feelings during the first weeks:*
0___*my baby seemed still part of me*
1___*my baby seemed an outgoing sociable person*
2___*my baby seemed separate but not yet sociable*
Question 5: *How would you describe your interaction with your baby:*
0___*I adapt myself to my baby*
1___*We negotiate between us*
2___*The baby adapts to the household routine*

Total Scores:
Extreme Facilitator: 0—2 Moderate Facilitator: 3—5
Reciprocator group: 6—10
Moderate Regulator: 11—13 Extreme Regulator: 14—16
Conflicted group: People whose moderate scores are composed of a combination of high and low scores on questions 1, 2, 3 constitute a separate group

The questionnaire has been modified to assess beliefs rather than activities. It can therefore be used earlier than 6 months (and in the form of expectations during pregnancy). This version is applicable to first babies only.

[Only italicised words (no scoring notes/numbers) should appear on questionnaire].

Readers wishing to use the questionnaire please contact the author: Joan Raphael-Leff 1 South Hill Park Gardens, London NW3 2TD.   Raphael@leff.co.uk

Appendix C - 2004

PPQ –Placental Paradigm Questionnaire

PPQ: JOAN RAPHAEL-LEFF, 2004
NOTE: Scores should be removed before the questionnaire is administered.

Most women experience very strong emotions and reactions during pregnancy that can sometimes feel difficult to cope with. But each woman has her own personal experience and we would like to know about yours. There are no right or wrong answers, so just respond as honestly and as quickly as you can. All of your answers are confidential.

This section is about your feelings towards yourself during this pregnancy.

1. **I feel more of a woman now that I'm pregnant.**
    - 0   Yes, much more
    - 1   Yes, somewhat
    - 2   Not very much
    - 3   No, I don't ever feel this

2. **I worry that the baby inside me knows everything about me, including bad things**
    - 0   No, not at all
    - 1   Hardly ever
    - 2   Yes, sometimes
    - 3   Yes, very often

3. **My body will 'know' how to give birth naturally without medical help**
    - 0   Strongly agree
    - 1   Agree
    - 2   Disagree
    - 3   Definitely disagree

4. **I doubt I have enough goodness inside me for both of us**
    - D3   Often
    - D2   Sometimes
    - D1   Hardly ever
    - D0   Never

5. **I have day-dreams about the baby**
    - 3   Never.
    - 2   Hardly ever
    - 1   Yes, sometimes
    - 0   Yes, very often

6. **I worry that my bad thoughts during pregnancy may affect my**
   baby

       A0   No, not at all
       A1   Hardly ever
       A2   Yes, sometimes
       A3   Yes, very much

7. **I feel in touch with my emotions**

       0   More than before I became pregnant
       1   As much as before
       2   Less than before
       3   Not at all

8. **Pregnancy is the peak of my female experience.**

       0   I definitely agree
       1   I quite agree
       2   I disagree
       3   Definitely not

9. **Strange thoughts pop into my mind about harming the baby**

       3   Quite often
       2   Some of the time
       1   Rarely
       0   Never

10. **Pregnancy makes me feel special**

        0   I definitely agree
        1   Agree
        2   Disagree
        3   Definitely disagree

This section is about your feelings towards the baby that you are carrying

11. **I feel I have a lovely baby inside me.**

        0   Yes, most of the time
        1   Yes, some of the time
        2   Not very much
        3   No, never

12. **I believe newborn babies need a routine**

        3   Strongly agree
        2   Agree
        1   Disagree
        0   Definitely disagree

13. **I experience the baby inside me as being hard to satisfy.**

        0   No, not at all
        1   Hardly ever
        2   Yes, sometimes
        3   Yes, very much

14. In some ways I feel my baby tries to communicate with me
   0   I definitely agree
   1   Agree
   2   Disagree
   3   Definitely disagree

15. The baby seems like an intruder or parasite
   0   No, not at all
   1   Occasionally
   2   Quite a lot
   3   Very much so

16. I feel as though the baby might damage me inside.
   3   Yes, most of the time
   2   Yes, some of the time
   1   Not very often
   0   No, never

17. I experience the baby inside me as friendly.
   0   Yes, most of the time
   1   Yes, some of the time
   2   Not very much
   3   No, never

This section concerns your more general feelings about this pregnancy.

18. I find myself talking to the baby
   3   No, not at all
   2   Hardly ever
   1   Yes, sometimes
   0   Yes, very often

19. I experience panic attacks
   A3   Quite often
   A2   Sometimes
   A1   Hardly ever
   A0   Never

20. I feel as though there is a battle going on inside me between what I need for myself and what the baby wants from me.
   3   Yes, most of the time
   2   Yes, some of the time
   1   Not very much
   0   No, never

21. This pregnancy is perfect.
   0   I strongly agree
   1   Agree
   2   Disagree
   3   I definitely disagree

22. Both the baby and I are enjoying pregnancy.

    0   Strongly agree
    1   Agree
    2   Disagree
    3   Definitely disagree

23. I feel uneasy about sharing my body with the baby.

    3   Much of the time
    2   Some of the time
    1   Not very often
    0   I never feel this

24. I go about my life just as if I am not pregnant

    3   Yes, most of the time
    2   Yes, some of the time
    1   Not very often
    0   No, never

25. Over the past months, I have felt very unhappy without knowing why

    D0   No, not at all
    D1   Hardly ever
    D2   Yes, sometimes
    D3   Yes, most of the time

26. I worry I will lose control during the labour

    3   Yes, very often
    2   Yes, quite a lot
    1   Only sometimes
    0   No, never

27. During this pregnancy I have had thoughts of harming myself

    D0   No, never
    D1   Hardly ever
    D2   Occasionally
    D3   Yes, very often

28. I have felt anxious and don't know why

    A3   Much of the time.
    A2   Some of the time.
    A1   Not very often.
    A0   Never

*PPQ: JOAN RAPHAEL-LEFF, 2004**
ITEMS & SCORES:

This questionnaire is a screening device for specific antenatal emotional disturbance, based on representation of the self, baby and pregnancy. It detects depression and anxiety (high D and A scores respectively) and in addition, delineates the predominant defences – idealization, persecution, obsession and detachment.

It may also be used to determine Orientation:

Emotional state:	items:
Depression	4; 25; 27
Anxiety	6; 19; 28

Defences:	items:	
Idealisation	8; 10; 11; 21	(low scores)
Persecution	15; 16; 20; 23	(high scores)
Obsession	2; 9; 26	(high scores)
Detachment	5; 7; 18; 24	(high scores)

ORIENTATIONS: Different approaches to parenting, discernable during pregnancy are predictive of postnatal interactive styles - with Facilitators adapting to the baby; Regulators expecting the baby to adapt and Reciprocators negotiating each incident on its own merits. Precipitants and the nature of postnatal disturbance differ according to orientation. Discrepancies between expectations and reality of labour affect both Facilitators and Regulators (according to their own wish for a 'natural' or a 'civilised' birth respectively); in addition, Facilitators respond with depression to disappointments in their own anticipated perfect mothering. Reciprocators tend to be resilient, but those who are vulnerable, antenatal depression predicts postnatal disturbance (see Sharp & Bramwell below).

Facilitator	1; 3; 14 + idealisation (above)
Reciprocator	17; 22 (and all intermediate scores)
Regulator	12; 13 [14] + persecution (above)
Conflicted	moderate scores composed of both extremes

NOTE:
Depression and Anxiety may be experienced by both Facilitators and Regulators, but these will differ respectively in quality from self-castigation when linked to idealization or forms of persecutory anxiety such as contamination anxiety.

A previous version [PPP] composed of 20 items from my earlier questionnaires and work was standardised by Linda Charles (2000) as part of her (unpublished) PhD project

RELEVANT REFERENCES:
Raphael-Leff J (1985) Facilitators and Regulators, Participators and Renouncers:
    mothers' and fathers' orientations towards pregnancy and parenthood. *Journal of Psychosomatic Obstetrics and Gynaecology*, 4:169-184.
_____ (1985)Facilitators and Regulators: vulnerability to postnatal disturbance *Journal of Psychosomatic Obstetrics and Gynaecology*, 4:151-168
_____ (1986) Facilitators and Regulators: conscious and unconscious processes in pregnancy and early motherhood. *British Journal of Medical Psychology*, 59:43-55.
_____ (1987) Facilitators and Regulators: vulnerability to postnatal disturbance, in *The Year Book of Psychiatry & Applied Mental Health*, eds. Freedman et al., Chicago:Year Book Medical Publishers
_____ (1997) Procreative Process, Placental Pardigm and perinatal psychotherapy, *Journal American Psychoanalyic Association,* Female Psychology supplement 44:373-399
_____ (2001)'Primary Maternal Persecution', Chapter 3 in *Forensic Psychotherapy* and Psychopathology Winnicottian Perspectives (ed.) Brett Kahr, London: Karnac Books.

Pregnancy and Early Motherhood

The following questions ask about women's experience of pregnancy and early motherhood. They ask you for your thoughts and feelings about the birth of your baby and what you expect it to be like. They also ask about your expectations of your future baby and early motherhood. Please just **say how you generally feel now**. There are no right or wrong answers.

Instructions

For each of the following questions we would like to know the way you generally feel.

Please make a clear tick (✓) in one of the boxes to tell us how much your feelings are nearer to the words on the left, or to the words on the right. Please try to decide either way – only use the middle box if your feelings are no nearer to one end than the other.

Question 1.   If you try to imagine your labour...

(a) Does it seem...

MOSTLY
EXCITING   [__]...[__]...[__]...[__]...[__]...[__]...[__]   MOSTLY
EXHAUSTING

(b) Would you prefer it to be....

CONTROLLED
BY THE
MIDWIFE OR
DOCTOR   [__]...[__]...[__]...[__]...[__]...[__]...[__]   CONTROLLED
BY YOU

(c) Would you prefer to spend time...

MOSTLY LYING
DOWN   [__]...[__]...[__]...[__]...[__]...[__]...[__]   MOSTLY
WALKING
ABOUT

(d) Would you prefer to spend time...

MOSTLY BEING
MONITORED   [__]...[__]...[__]...[__]...[__]...[__]...[__]   MOSTLY NOT
BEING
MONITORED

(e) Would you rather...

MOSTLY BE
LEFT WITH A   [__]...[__]...[__]...[__]...[__]...[__]...[__]   MOSTLY HAVE
MIDWIVES OR

PARTNER, MUM   DOCTORS WITH
OR FRIEND   YOU

(f) Do you imagine you will…

BEHAVE LIKE   [__]…[__]…[__]…[__]…[__]…[__]…[__]   SHOW ANOTHER
YOUR USUAL   SIDE OF
SELF   YOURSELF

(g) I think of my labour as…

MOSTLY BEING   [__]…[__]…[__]…[__]…[__]…[__]…[__]   MOSTLY BEING
STARTED BY   STARTED BY MY
MY BABY   OWN BODY

Question 2. What are your feelings about the birth…?

(a) I feel…
MY BODY   [__]…[__]…[__]…[__]…[__]…[__]…[__]   MY BODY
WILL   NEEDS TO BE
KNOW   TRAINED TO
WHAT TO   KNOW WHAT
DO   TO DO

(b) Mostly I am...

DREADING   [__]…[__]…[__]…[__]…[__]…[__]…[__]   LOOKING
IT   FORWARD
TO IT

(c) I would prefer the birth to be…

HELPED A   [__]…[__]…[__]…[__]…[__]…[__]…[__]   AS 'NATURAL'
LOT BY   AS POSSIBLE
MEDICAL
EQUIPMENT

(d) I feel that birth is mainly…

A   [__]…[__]…[__]…[__]…[__]…[__]…[__]   A SPECIAL
PERSONAL   HOSPITAL
EVENT   EVENT
BETWEEN
MOTHER
AND BABY

(e) Giving birth will mostly be…

FULL OF   [__]…[__]…[__]…[__]…[__]…[__]…[__]   FULL OF
PAIN   PLEASURE

(f) Do you mostly imagine yourself…

GIVING   [_]...[_]...[_]...[_]...[_]...[_]...[_]   BEING
BIRTH TO   DELIVERED
THE BABY   BY THE
YOURSELF   MIDWIFE

Question 3. What do you imagine the baby will be like at first?

(a) ...
FITTING EASILY   [_]...[_]...[_]...[_]...[_]...[_]...[_]   TAKING OVER
INTO YOUR LIFE   EVERYTHING
                                                             YOU DO

(b) ...
A STRANGER   [_]...[_]...[_]...[_]...[_]...[_]...[_]   SOMEONE THAT
AT FIRST   YOU KNOW
                                                               ALREADY

(c) ...
MOSTLY   [_]...[_]...[_]...[_]...[_]...[_]...[_]   MOSTLY NEEDY
DEMANDING   AND HELPLESS

(d) ...
ABLE TO TELL   [_]...[_]...[_]...[_]...[_]...[_]...[_]   UNABLE TO
WHO YOU ARE   TELL YOU
FROM EARLY   APART FROM
ON   OTHER PEOPLE
                                                               EARLY ON

Question 3 *(continued)* What do you imagine the baby will be like at first?

(e) ...
BORN BEING   [_]...[_]...[_]...[_]...[_]...[_]...[_]   BORN NEEDING
ABLE   HELP TO LEARN
TO   HOW TO COM -
COMMUNICATE   MUNICATE
WITH YOU

(f) ...
BORN   [_]...[_]...[_]...[_]...[_]...[_]...[_]   AS THE
KNOWING   MOTHER YOU
WHAT IS BEST   KNOW WHAT'S
FOR HIM/HER   BEST

Question 4. How do you intend to feed your baby?

(a) To begin with, do you intend to...

FEED YOUR   [_]...[_]...[_]...[_]...[_]...[_]...[_]   FEED YOUR
BABY   BABY
ON DEMAND   AT SET TIMES

(b) After several months, do you intend to...

FEED YOUR   [_]...[_]...[_]...[_]...[_]...[_]...[_]   FEED YOUR
BABY   BABY
ON DEMAND   AT SET TIMES

(c) Do you intend to...

MOSTLY   [_]...[_]...[_]...[_]...[_]...[_]...[_]   MOSTLY BOTTLE
BREAST   FEED
FEED

Question 5. How do you imagine <u>yourself</u> in the first few weeks?

(a)...

     [_]...[_]...[_]...[_]...[_]...[_]...[_]   MOSTLY THE
MOSTLY   SAME PERSON
A MOTHER   AS USUAL

(b) ...

MOSTLY   [_]...[_]...[_]...[_]...[_]...[_]...[_]   MOSTLY
TRYING TO   ADAPTING TO
GET THE BABY   THE BABY
TO ADAPT TO
A ROUTINE

(c) ...

MOSTLY   [_]...[_]...[_]...[_]...[_]...[_]...[_]   MOSTLY
FEELING   FEELING
FULFILLED   TRAPPED

(d) ...

VERY MUCH   [_]...[_]...[_]...[_]...[_]...[_]...[_]   MOSTLY
CHANGED BY   UNCHANGED
BECOMING A
MOTHER

(e) ...

MOSTLY   [_]...[_]...[_]...[_]...[_]...[_]...[_]   MOSTLY
WAITING FOR   ENJOYING THE
THINGS TO   NEW WAY OF
GET BACK TO   LIFE
NORMAL

The Antenatal Maternal Orientation Measure (AMOM; Sharp & Bramwell, 2004). was developed from the third trimester version of the Facilitator Regulator Questionnaire (FRQIII, Raphael-Leff, 1985). It assesses women's expectations across five domains: (1) labour - 7 items, (2) childbirth - 6 items, (3) the newborn baby - 6 items, and (4) feeding method and style – 3 items and (5) self as a new mother - 5 items. For scoring guidelines and any other queries please contact Dr Helen Sharp, Department of Clinical Psychology, University of Liverpool, The Whelan Building, Quadrangle, Brownlow Hill, Liverpool, UK, L69 3GB. Tel: + 44 (0)151-794-5529. Fax: +44 (0)151-794-5537. Email:hmsharp@Liverpool.ac.uk.

Reference

Sharp, H.M. and Bramwell, R (2004). An empirical evaluation of a psychoanalytic theory of mothering orientation: implications for the antenatal prediction of postnatal depression. *Journal of Reproductive and Infant Psychology*, **22**(2), 71-89.